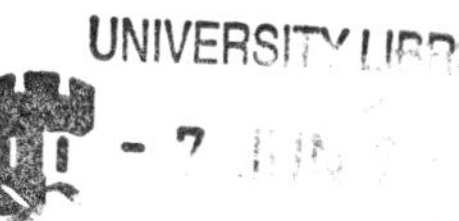

CONTENTS

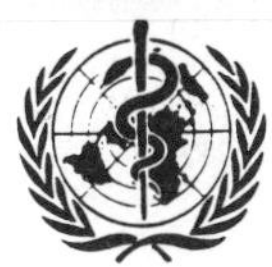

WORLD HEALTH ORGANIZATION

INTERNATIONAL AGENCY FOR RESEARCH ON CANCER

IARC MONOGRAPHS

ON THE

EVALUATION OF CARCINOGENIC RISKS TO HUMANS

Alcohol Drinking

VOLUME 44

This publication represents the views and expert opinions of an IARC Working Group on the Evaluation of Carcinogenic Risks to Humans, which met in Lyon,

13-20 October 1987

IARC MONOGRAPHS

In 1969, the International Agency for Research on Cancer (IARC) initiated a programme on the evaluation of the carcinogenic risk of chemicals to humans involving the production of critically evaluated monographs on individual chemicals. In 1980, the programme was expanded to include the evaluation of the carcinogenic risk associated with exposures to complex mixtures.

The objective of the programme is to elaborate and publish in the form of monographs critical reviews of data on carcinogenicity for chemicals and complex mixtures to which humans are known to be exposed, and on specific occupational exposures, to evaluate these data in terms of human risk with the help of international working groups of experts in chemical carcinogenesis and related fields, and to indicate where additional research efforts are needed.

This project was supported by PHS Grant No. 6 UO1 CA33193-06 awarded by the US National Cancer Institute, Department of Health and Human Services.

ISBN 92 832 1244 4

ISSN 0250-9555

Distributed for the International Agency for Research on Cancer
by the Secretariat of the World Health Organization

PRINTED IN THE UK

NOTE TO THE READER

The term 'carcinogenic risk' in the *IARC Monographs* series is taken to mean the probability that exposure to an agent will lead to cancer in humans.

Inclusion of an agent in the *Monographs* does not imply that it is a carcinogen, only that the published data have been examined. Equally, the fact that an agent has not yet been evaluated in a monograph does not mean that it is not carcinogenic.

The evaluations of carcinogenic risk are made by international working groups of independent scientists and are qualitative in nature. No recommendation is given for regulation or legislation.

Anyone who is aware of published data that may alter the evaluation of the carcinogenic risk of an agent to humans is encouraged to make this information available to the Unit of Carcinogen Identification and Evaluation, International Agency for Research on Cancer, 150 cours Albert Thomas, 69372 Lyon Cedex 08, France, in order that the agent may be considered for re-evaluation by a future Working Group.

Although every effort is made to prepare the monographs as accurately as possible, mistakes may occur. Readers are requested to communicate any errors to the Unit of Carcinogen Identification and Evaluation, so that corrections can be reported in future volumes.

IARC WORKING GROUP ON THE EVALUATION OF CARCINOGENIC RISKS TO HUMANS: ALCOHOL DRINKING

Lyon, 13-20 October 1987

Members[1]

F. Berrino, National Institute for the Study and Treatment of Tumours, via Venezian 1, Milan, Italy

M. Grant, Division of Mental Health, World Health Organization, 1211 Geneva 27, Switzerland

L. Griciute, Oncological Institute of the Lithuanian SSR, 341 Dzerhinsky Shosse, 232021 Vilnius, Lithuanian SSR, USSR

B. Holmberg, Department of Toxicology, National Institute of Occupational Health, 17184 Solna, Sweden

A.J. McMichael, Community Medicine Department, University of Adelaide, Adelaide SA 5000, Australia (*Vice-chairman*)

O. Møller-Jensen, Danish Cancer Registry, 66 Landskronagade, 2100 Copenhagen Ø, Denmark (*Chairman*)

L. Nykänen, Alko Ltd, The Finnish State Alcohol Company Research Laboratories, PO Box 350, 00101 Helsinki 10, Finland

G. Obe, Free University of Berlin, Division of Biology (FB23), Institute of General Genetics (WEI), Arnimallee 5-7, 1000 Berlin (West) 33, Federal Republic of Germany

J.K. Reddy, Northwestern University, The Medical School, Ward Memorial Building, 303 East Chicago Avenue, Chicago, IL 60611, USA

R. Room, Alcohol Research Group, 1816 Scenic Avenue, Berkeley, CA 94709, USA

M. Salaspuro, Research Unit of Alcohol Diseases, University Central Hospital of Helsinki, Tukholmankatu 8C, 00290 Helsinki, Finland

[1]Unable to attend: C.S. Lieber, Alcohol Research and Treatment Center, Section of Liver Disease and Nutrition, 130 West Kingsbridge Road, Bronx, NY 10468, USA; S. Takayama, National Cancer Centre Research Institute, 5-1-1 Sukkiji-5-chome, Tokyo 104, Japan

H. Sancho-Garnier, Department of Medical Statistics, Gustave Roussy Institute, rue Camille Desmoulins, 94805 Villejuif Cedex, France

B.A. Schwetz, Systemic Toxicology Branch, Division of Toxicology Research and Testing, National Institute of Environmental Health Sciences, PO Box 12233, Research Triangle Park, NC 27709, USA

F.M. Sullivan, Department of Pharmacology, United Medical and Dental School of Guy's and St Thomas' Hospitals, London SE1 9RT, UK

R.G. Thurman, Department of Pharmacology, University of North Carolina, 1106 Faculty Laboratory Office, Building 231H, Chapel Hill, NC 27514, USA

D. Trichopoulos, Department of Hygiene and Epidemiology, University of Athens, School of Medicine, Athens 11527, Greece

M.D. Waters, Genetic Toxicology Division (MD-68), US Environmental Protection Agency, Health Effects Research Laboratory, PO Box 12233, Research Triangle Park, NC 27711, USA

W. Willett, Harvard School of Public Health, Channing Laboratory, 180 Longwood Avenue, Boston, MA 02113, USA

R.A. Woutersen, TNO-CIVO Toxicology and Nutrition Institute, PO Box 360, 3700 AJ Zeist, The Netherlands

Observers

Representative of the National Cancer Institute

J. Rice, NCI-Frederick Cancer Research Facility, Building 538, Frederick, MD 21701, USA

Representative of the Commission of the European Communities

E. Krug, Commission of the European Communities, Health and Safety Directorate, Bâtiment Jean Monnet, 2920 Luxembourg, Grand Duchy of Luxembourg

Representatives of the Chemical Manufacturers' Association

C.H. Tamburro, Department of Community Health, Liver Research Center, Suite 119A, Health Science Center, University of Louisville, Louisville, KY 40292, USA

W.J. Waddell, Pharmacology/Toxicology Department, Health Science Center, University of Louisville, Louisville, KY 40292, USA

Representative of the International Federation of Wines and Spirits

B. Le Bourhis, International Federation of Wines and Spirits, 103 Boulevard Haussmann, 75008 Paris, France

Representative of the International Life Sciences Institute

C.I. Chappel, CanTox Inc., 1196 Botany Hill, Oakville, Ontario L6J 6J5, Canada

Representative of the International Programme on Chemical Safety

E. Smith, Division of Environmental Health, World Health Organization, 1211 Geneva 27, Switzerland

Representative of Systembolaget and the International Council on Alcohol and Addictions

G. Romanus, Systembolaget, 10397 Stockholm, Sweden

Secretariat

A. Aitio, Unit of Carcinogen Identification and Evaluation (*Officer-in-charge*)
H. Bartsch, Unit of Environmental Carcinogenesis and Host Factors
J.R.P. Cabral, Unit of Mechanisms of Carcinogenesis
E. Cardis, Unit of Biostatistics Research and Informatics
J. Estève, Unit of Biostatistics Research and Informatics
M. Friesen, Unit of Environmental Carcinogenesis and Host Factors
M.-J. Ghess, Unit of Carcinogen Identification and Evaluation
E. Heseltine, Lajarthe, Montignac, France
J. Kaldor, Unit of Biostatistics Research and Informatics
T. Kauppinen, Unit of Carcinogen Identification and Evaluation
D. Mietton, Unit of Carcinogen Identification and Evaluation
R. Montesano, Unit of Mechanisms of Carcinogenesis
I. O'Neill, Unit of Environmental Carcinogenesis and Host Factors
C. Partensky, Unit of Carcinogen Identification and Evaluation
I. Peterschmitt, Unit of Carcinogen Identification and Evaluation, Geneva, Switzerland
E. Riboli, Unit of Analytical Epidemiology
D. Shuker, Unit of Environmental Carcinogenesis and Host Factors
L. Shuker, Unit of Carcinogen Identification and Evaluation (*Co-secretary*)
L. Tomatis, Director
V. Turusov, Office of the Director
A. Tuyns, Lyon, France
H. Vainio, Institute of Occupational Health, Helsinki, Finland
J.D. Wilbourn, Unit of Carcinogen Identification and Evaluation (*Co-secretary*)
H. Yamasaki, Unit of Mechanisms of Carcinogenesis

Secretarial assistance

J. Cazeaux
M. Lézère
S. Reynaud

The *Monographs* represent the first step in carcinogenic risk assessment, which involves examination of all relevant information in order to assess the strength of the available evidence that, under certain conditions of exposure, an agent could alter the incidence of cancer in humans. The second step is quantitative risk estimation, which is not usually attempted in the *Monographs*. Detailed, quantitative evaluations of epidemiological data may be made in the *Monographs*, but without extrapolation beyond the range of the data available. Quantitative extrapolation from experimental data to the human situation is not undertaken.

These monographs may assist national and international authorities in making risk assessments and in formulating decisions concerning any necessary preventive measures. **No recommendation is given for regulation or legislation, since such decisions are made by individual governments and/or other international agencies**. The *IARC Monographs* are recognized as an authoritative source of information on the carcinogenicity of chemicals and complex exposures. A users' survey, made in 1984, indicated that the *Monographs* are consulted by various agencies in 45 countries. Each volume is printed in 4000 copies for distribution to governments, regulatory bodies and interested scientists. The *Monographs* are also available *via* the Distribution and Sales Service of the World Health Organization.

3. SELECTION OF TOPICS FOR MONOGRAPHS

Topics are selected on the basis of two main criteria: (a) that they concern agents for which there is evidence of human exposure, and (b) there is some evidence or suspicion of carcinogenicity. The term agent is used to include individual chemical compounds, groups of chemical compounds, physical agents (such as radiation), biological factors (such as viruses) and mixtures of agents such as occur in occupational exposures and as a result of personal and cultural habits (like smoking and dietary practices). Chemical analogues and compounds with biological or physical characteristics similar to those of suspected carcinogens may also be considered, even in the absence of data on carcinogenicity.

The scientific literature is surveyed for published data relevant to an assessment of carcinogenicity; the IARC surveys of chemicals being tested for carcinogenicity(8) and directories of on-going research in cancer epidemiology(9) often indicate those agents that may be scheduled for future meetings. An ad-hoc working group convened by IARC in 1984 gave recommendations as to which chemicals and exposures to complex mixtures should be evaluated in the *IARC Monographs* series(10).

As significant new data on subjects on which monographs have already been prepared become available, re-evaluations are made at subsequent meetings, and revised monographs are published.

4. DATA FOR MONOGRAPHS

The *Monographs* do not necessarily cite all of the literature on a particular agent. Only those data considered by the Working Group to be relevant to making an evaluation are included.

IARC MONOGRAPHS PROGRAMME ON THE EVALUATION OF CARCINOGENIC RISKS TO HUMANS[1]

PREAMBLE

1. BACKGROUND

In 1969, the International Agency for Research on Cancer (IARC) initiated a programme to evaluate the carcinogenic risk of chemicals to humans and to produce monographs on individual chemicals. The *Monographs* programme has since been expanded to include consideration of exposures to complex mixtures of chemicals (which occur, for example, in some occupations and as a result of human habits) and of exposures to other agents, such as radiation and viruses. With Supplement 6(1), the title of the series was modified from *IARC Monographs on the Evaluation of the Carcinogenic Risk of Chemicals to Humans* to *IARC Monographs on the Evaluation of Carcinogenic Risks to Humans*, in order to reflect the widened scope of the programme.

The criteria established in 1971 to evaluate carcinogenic risk to humans were adopted by the working groups whose deliberations resulted in the first 16 volumes of the *IARC Monographs* series. Those criteria were subsequently re-evaluated by working groups which met in 1977(2), 1978(3), 1979(4), 1982(5) and 1983(6). The present preamble was prepared by two working groups which met in September 1986 and January 1987, prior to the preparation of Supplement 7 to the *Monographs*(7).

2. OBJECTIVE AND SCOPE

The objective of the programme is to prepare, with the help of international working groups of experts, and to publish in the form of monographs, critical reviews and evaluations of evidence on the carcinogenicity of a wide range of agents to which humans are or may be exposed. The *Monographs* may also indicate where additional research efforts are needed.

[1]This project is supported by PHS Grant No. 6 UO1 CA33193-06 awarded by the US National Cancer Institute, Department of Health and Human Services, and with a subcontract to Tracor Jitco, Inc. and Technical Resources, Inc. Since 1986, this programme has also been supported by the Commission of the European Communities.

ERRATUM

IARC Monographs, Volume 44, Alcohol Drinking

Due to errors in the printing of this volume, the following copy of the Preamble should be read in place of that in Volume 44.

IARC MONOGRAPHS PROGRAMME ON THE EVALUATION OF CARCINOGENIC RISKS TO HUMANS[1]

PREAMBLE

1. BACKGROUND

In 1969, the International Agency for Research on Cancer (IARC) initiated a programme to evaluate the carcinogenic risk of chemicals to humans and to produce monographs on individual chemicals. The *Monographs* programme has since been expanded to include consideration of exposures to complex mixtures of chemicals (which occur, for example, in some occupations and as a result of human habits) and of exposures to other agents, such as radiation and viruses. With Supplement 6(1), the title of the series was modified from *IARC Monographs on the Evaluation of the Carcinogenic Risk of Chemicals to Humans* to *IARC Monographs on the Evaluation of Carcinogenic Risks to Humans*, in order to reflect the widened scope of the programme.

The criteria established in 1971 to evaluate carcinogenic risk to humans were adopted by the working groups whose deliberations resulted in the first 16 volumes of the *IARC Monographs* series. Those criteria were subsequently re-evaluated by working groups which met in 1977(2), 1978(3), 1979(4), 1982(5) and 1983(6). The present preamble was prepared by two working groups which met in September 1986 and January 1987, prior to the preparation of Supplement 7 to the *Monographs*(7).

2. OBJECTIVE AND SCOPE

The objective of the programme is to prepare, with the help of international working groups of experts, and to publish in the form of monographs, critical reviews and evaluations of evidence on the carcinogenicity of a wide range of agents to which humans are or may be exposed. The *Monographs* may also indicate where additional research efforts are needed.

[1]This project is supported by PHS Grant No. 6 UO1 CA33193-06 awarded by the US National Cancer Institute, Department of Health and Human Services, and with a subcontract to Tracor Jitco, Inc. and Technical Resources, Inc. Since 1986, this programme has also been supported by the Commission of the European Communities.

The *Monographs* represent the first step in carcinogenic risk assessment, which involves examination of all relevant information in order to assess the strength of the available evidence that, under certain conditions of exposure, an agent could alter the incidence of cancer in humans. The second step is quantitative risk estimation, which is not usually attempted in the *Monographs*. Detailed, quantitative evaluations of epidemiological data may be made in the *Monographs*, but without extrapolation beyond the range of the data available. Quantitative extrapolation from experimental data to the human situation is not undertaken.

These monographs may assist national and international authorities in making risk assessments and in formulating decisions concerning any necessary preventive measures. **No recommendation is given for regulation or legislation, since such decisions are made by individual governments and/or other international agencies.** The *IARC Monographs* are recognized as an authoritative source of information on the carcinogenicity of chemicals and complex exposures. A users' survey, made in 1984, indicated that the *Monographs* are consulted by various agencies in 45 countries. Each volume is printed in 4000 copies for distribution to governments, regulatory bodies and interested scientists. The *Monographs* are also available *via* the Distribution and Sales Service of the World Health Organization.

3. SELECTION OF TOPICS FOR MONOGRAPHS

Topics are selected on the basis of two main criteria: (a) that they concern agents for which there is evidence of human exposure, and (b) there is some evidence or suspicion of carcinogenicity. The term agent is used to include individual chemical compounds, groups of chemical compounds, physical agents (such as radiation), biological factors (such as viruses) and mixtures of agents such as occur in occupational exposures and as a result of personal and cultural habits (like smoking and dietary practices). Chemical analogues and compounds with biological or physical characteristics similar to those of suspected carcinogens may also be considered, even in the absence of data on carcinogenicity.

The scientific literature is surveyed for published data relevant to an assessment of carcinogenicity; the IARC surveys of chemicals being tested for carcinogenicity(8) and directories of on-going research in cancer epidemiology(9) often indicate those agents that may be scheduled for future meetings. An ad-hoc working group convened by IARC in 1984 gave recommendations as to which chemicals and exposures to complex mixtures should be evaluated in the *IARC Monographs* series(10).

As significant new data on subjects on which monographs have already been prepared become available, re-evaluations are made at subsequent meetings, and revised monographs are published.

4. DATA FOR MONOGRAPHS

The *Monographs* do not necessarily cite all of the literature on a particular agent. Only those data considered by the Working Group to be relevant to making an evaluation are included.

With regard to biological and epidemiological data, only reports that have been published or accepted for publication in the openly available scientific literature are reviewed by the working groups. In certain instances, government agency reports that have undergone peer review and are widely available are considered. Exceptions may be made on an ad-hoc basis to include unpublished reports that are in their final form and publicly available, if their inclusion is considered pertinent to making a final evaluation (see pp. 27 *et seq.*). In the sections on chemical and physical properties and on production, use, occurrence and analysis, unpublished sources of information may be used.

5. THE WORKING GROUP

Reviews and evaluations are formulated by a working group of experts. The tasks of this group are five-fold: (i) to ascertain that all appropriate data have been collected; (ii) to select the data relevant for the evaluation on the basis of scientific merit; (iii) to prepare accurate summaries of the data to enable the reader to follow the reasoning of the Working Group; (iv) to evaluate the results of experimental and epidemiological studies; and (v) to make an overall evaluation of the carcinogenicity of the agent to humans.

Working Group participants who contributed to the consideration and evaluation of the agents within a particular volume are listed, with their addresses, at the beginning of each publication. Each participant who is a member of a working group serves as an individual scientist and not as a representative of any organization, government or industry. In addition, representatives from national and international agencies and industrial associations are invited as observers.

6. WORKING PROCEDURES

Approximately one year in advance of a meeting of a working group, the agents to be evaluated are announced and participants are selected by IARC staff in consultation with other experts. Subsequently, relevant biological and epidemiological data are collected by IARC from recognized sources of information on carcinogenesis, including data storage and retrieval systems such as CANCERLINE, MEDLINE and TOXLINE. Bibliographical sources for data on genetic and related effects and on teratogenicity are the Environmental Mutagen Information Center and the Environmental Teratology Information Center, both located at the Oak Ridge National Laboratory, USA.

The major collection of data and the preparation of first drafts of the sections on chemical and physical properties, on production and use, on occurrence, and on analysis are carried out under a separate contract funded by the US National Cancer Institute. Efforts are made to supplement this information with data from other national and international sources. Representatives from industrial associations may assist in the preparation of sections on production and use.

Production and trade data are obtained from governmental and trade publications and, in some cases, by direct contact with industries. Separate production data on some agents may not be available because their publication could disclose confidential information.

Information on uses is usually obtained from published sources but is often complemented by direct contact with manufacturers.

Six months before the meeting, reference material is sent to experts, or is used by IARC staff, to prepare sections for the first drafts of monographs. The complete first drafts are compiled by IARC staff and sent, prior to the meeting, to all participants of the Working Group for review.

The Working Group meets in Lyon for seven to eight days to discuss and finalize the texts of the monographs and to formulate the evaluations. After the meeting, the master copy of each monograph is verified by consulting the original literature, edited and prepared for publication. The aim is to publish monographs within nine months of the Working Group meeting.

7. EXPOSURE DATA

Sections that indicate the extent of past and present human exposure, the sources of exposure, the persons most likely to be exposed and the factors that contribute to exposure to the agent under study are included at the beginning of each monograph.

Most monographs on individual chemicals or complex mixtures include sections on chemical and physical data, and production, use, occurrence and analysis. In other monographs, for example on physical agents, biological factors, occupational exposures and cultural habits, other sections may be included, such as: historical perspectives, description of an industry or habit, exposures in the work place or chemistry of the complex mixture.

The Chemical Abstracts Services Registry Number, the latest Chemical Abstracts Primary Name and the IUPAC Systematic Name are recorded. Other synonyms and trade names are given, but the list is not necessarily comprehensive. Some of the trade names may be those of mixtures in which the agent being evaluated is only one of the ingredients.

Information on chemical and physical properties and, in particular, data relevant to identification, occurrence and biological activity are included. A separate description of technical products gives relevant specifications and includes available information on composition and impurities.

The dates of first synthesis and of first commercial production of an agent are provided; for agents which do not occur naturally, this information may allow a reasonable estimate to be made of the date before which no human exposure to the agent could have occurred. The dates of first reported occurrence of an exposure are also provided. In addition, methods of synthesis used in past and present commercial production and different methods of production which may give rise to different impurities are described.

Data on production, foreign trade and uses are obtained for representative regions, which usually include Europe, Japan and the USA. It should not, however, be inferred that those areas or nations are necessarily the sole or major sources or users of the agent being evaluated.

Some identified uses may not be current or major applications, and the coverage is not necessarily comprehensive. In the case of drugs, mention of their therapeutic uses does not necessarily represent current practice nor does it imply judgement as to their clinical efficacy.

Information on the occurrence of an agent in the environment is obtained from data derived from the monitoring and surveillance of levels in occupational environments, air, water, soil, foods and animal and human tissues. When available, data on the generation, persistence and bioaccumulation of the agent are also included.

Statements concerning regulations and guidelines (e.g., pesticide registrations, maximal levels permitted in foods, occupational exposure limits) are included for some countries as indications of potential exposures, but they may not reflect the most recent situation, since such limits are continuously reviewed and modified. The absence of information on regulatory status for a country should not be taken to imply that that country does not have regulations with regard to the agent.

The purpose of the section on analysis is to give the reader an overview of current methods cited in the literature, with emphasis on those widely used for regulatory purposes. No critical evaluation or recommendation of any of the methods is meant or implied. Methods for monitoring human exposure are also given, when available. The IARC publishes a series of volumes, *Environmental Carcinogens: Selected Methods of Analysis*(11), that describe validated methods for analysing a wide variety of agents.

8. BIOLOGICAL DATA RELEVANT TO THE EVALUATION OF CARCINOGENICITY TO HUMANS

The term 'carcinogen' is used in these monographs to denote an agent that is capable of increasing the incidence of malignant neoplasms; the induction of benign neoplasms may in some circumstances (see p. 21) contribute to the judgement that an agent is carcinogenic. The terms 'neoplasm' and 'tumour' are used interchangeably.

Some epidemiological and experimental studies indicate that different agents may act at different stages in the carcinogenic process, probably by fundamentally different mechanisms. In the present state of knowledge, the aim of the *Monographs* is to evaluate evidence of carcinogenicity at any stage in the carcinogenic process independently of the underlying mechanism involved. There is as yet insufficient information to implement a classification of agents according to their mechanism of action(6).

Definitive evidence of carcinogenicity in humans is provided by epidemiological studies. Evidence relevant to human carcinogenicity may also be provided by experimental studies of carcinogenicity in animals and by other biological data, particularly those relating to humans.

The available studies are summarized by the working groups, with particular regard to the qualitative aspects discussed below. In general, numerical findings are indicated as they appear in the original report; units are converted when necessary for easier comparison. The Working Group may conduct additional analyses of the published data and use them in

their assessment of the evidence and may include them in their summary of a study; the results of such supplementary analyses are given in square brackets. Any comments are also made in square brackets; however, these are kept to a minimum, being restricted to those instances in which it is felt that an important aspect of a study, directly impinging on its interpretation, should be brought to the attention of the reader.

9. EVIDENCE FOR CARCINOGENICITY IN EXPERIMENTAL ANIMALS

For several agents (e.g., 4-aminobiphenyl, bis(chloromethyl)ether, diethylstilboestrol, melphalan, 8-methoxypsoralen (methoxsalen) plus UVR, mustard gas and vinyl chloride), evidence of carcinogenicity in experimental animals preceded evidence obtained from epidemiological studies or case reports. Information compiled from the first 41 volumes of the *IARC Monographs*(12) shows that, of the 44 agents for which there is *sufficient* or *limited evidence* of carcinogenicity to humans (see pp. 27-28), all 37 that have been tested adequately experimentally produce cancer in at least one animal species. Although this association cannot establish that all agents that cause cancer in experimental animals also cause cancer in humans, nevertheless, **in the absence of adequate data on humans, it is biologically plausible and prudent to regard agents for which there is *sufficient evidence* (see p. 28) of carcinogenicity in experimental animals as if they presented a carcinogenic risk to humans.**

The monographs are not intended to summarize all published studies. Those that are inadequate (e.g., too short a duration, too few animals, poor survival; see below) or are judged irrelevant to the evaluation are generally omitted. They may be mentioned briefly, particularly when the information is considered to be a useful supplement to that of other reports or when they provide the only data available. Their inclusion does not, however, imply acceptance of the adequacy of the experimental design or of the analysis and interpretation of their results. Guidelines for adequate long-term carcinogenicity experiments have been outlined (e.g., ref. 13).

The nature and extent of impurities or contaminants present in the agent being evaluated are given when available. Mention is made of all routes of exposure by which the agent has been adequately studied and of all species in which relevant experiments have been performed. Animal strain, sex, numbers per group, age at start of treatment and survival are reported.

Experiments in which the agent was administered in conjunction with known carcinogens or factors that modify carcinogenic effects are also reported. Experiments on the carcinogenicity of known metabolites and derivatives may be included.

(*a*) *Qualitative aspects*

The overall assessment of the carcinogenicity of an agent involves several considerations of qualitative importance, including (i) the experimental conditions under which the test was performed, including route and schedule of exposure, species, strain, sex, age, duration of follow-up; (ii) the consistency with which the agent has been shown to be carcinogenic, e.g., in how many species and at which target organs(s); (iii) the spectrum of neoplastic

response, from benign tumours to malignant neoplasms; and (iv) the possible role of modifying factors.

Considerations of importance to the Working Group in the interpretation and evaluation of a particular study include: (i) how clearly the agent was defined; (ii) whether the dose was adequately monitored, particularly in inhalation experiments; (iii) whether the doses used were appropriate and whether the survival of treated animals was similar to that of controls; (iv) whether there were adequate numbers of animals per group; (v) whether animals of both sexes were used; (vi) whether animals were allocated randomly to groups; (vii) whether the duration of observation was adequate; and (viii) whether the data were adequately reported. If available, recent data on the incidence of specific tumours in historical controls, as well as in concurrent controls, should be taken into account in the evaluation of tumour response.

When benign tumours occur together with and originate from the same cell type in an organ or tissue as malignant tumours in a particular study and appear to represent a stage in the progression to malignancy, it may be valid to combine them in assessing tumour incidence. The occurrence of lesions presumed to be preneoplastic may in certain instances aid in assessing the biological plausibility of any neoplastic response observed.

Among the many agents that have been studied extensively, there are few instances in which the only neoplasms induced were benign. Benign tumours in experimental animals frequently represent a stage in the evolution of a malignant neoplasm, but they may be 'endpoints' that do not readily undergo transition to malignancy. However, if an agent is found to induce only benign neoplasms, it should be suspected of being a carcinogen and it requires further investigation.

(*b*) *Quantitative aspects*

The probability that tumours will occur may depend on the species and strain, the dose of the carcinogen and the route and period of exposure. Evidence of an increased incidence of neoplasms with increased exposure strengthens the inference of a causal association between exposure to the agent and the development of neoplasms.

The form of the dose-response relationship can vary widely, depending on the particular agent under study and the target organ. Since many chemicals require metabolic activation before being converted into their reactive intermediates, both metabolic and pharmacokinetic aspects are important in determining the dose-response pattern. Saturation of steps such as absorption, activation, inactivation and elimination of the carcinogen may produce nonlinearity in the dose-response relationship, as could saturation of processes such as DNA repair(14,15).

(*c*) *Statistical analysis of long-term experiments in animals*

Factors considered by the Working Group include the adequacy of the information given for each treatment group: (i) the number of animals on study and the number examined histologically, (ii) the number of animals with a given tumour type and (iii) length of survival. The statistical methods used should be clearly stated and should be the generally accepted techniques refined for this purpose(15,16). When there is no difference in survival

between control and treatment groups, the Working Group usually compares the proportions of animals developing each tumour type in each of the groups. Otherwise, consideration is given as to whether or not appropriate adjustments have been made for differences in survival. These adjustments can include: comparisons of the proportions of tumour-bearing animals among the 'effective number' of animals alive at the time the first tumour is discovered, in the case where most differences in survival occur before tumours appear; life-table methods, when tumours are visible or when they may be considered 'fatal' because mortality rapidly follows tumour development; and the Mantel-Haenszel test or logistic regression, when occult tumours do not affect the animals' risk of dying but are 'incidental' findings at autopsy.

In practice, classifying tumours as fatal or incidental may be difficult. Several survival-adjusted methods have been developed that do not require this distinction(15), although they have not been fully evaluated.

10. OTHER RELEVANT DATA IN EXPERIMENTAL SYSTEMS AND HUMANS

(*a*) *Structure-activity considerations*

This section describes structure-activity correlations that are relevant to an evaluation of the carcinogenicity of an agent.

(*b*) *Absorption, distribution, excretion and metabolism*

Concise information is given on absorption, distribution (including placental transfer) and excretion. Kinetic factors that may affect the dose-reponse relationship, such as saturation of uptake, protein binding, metabolic activation, detoxification and DNA-repair processes, are mentioned. Studies that indicate the metabolic fate of the agent in experimental animals and humans are summarized briefly, and comparisons of data from animals and humans are made when possible. Comparative information on the relationship between exposure and the dose that reaches the target site may be of particular importance for extrapolation between species.

(*c*) *Toxicity*

Data are given on acute and chronic toxic effects (other than cancer), such as organ toxicity, immunotoxicity, endocrine effects and preneoplastic lesions. Effects on reproduction, teratogenicity, feto- and embryotoxicity are also summarized briefly.

(*d*) *Genetic and related effects*

Tests of genetic and related effects may indicate possible carcinogenic activity. They can also be used in detecting active metabolites of known carcinogens in human or animal body fluids, in detecting active components in complex mixtures and in the elucidation of possible mechanisms of carcinogenesis.

The available data are interpreted critically by phylogenetic group according to the endpoints detected, which may include DNA damage, gene mutation, sister chromatid exchange, micronuclei, chromosomal aberrations, aneuploidy and cell transformation. The

concentrations (doses) employed are given and mention is made of whether an exogenous metabolic system was required. When appropriate, these data may be represented by bar graphs (activity profiles), with corresponding summary tables and listings of test systems, data and references. Detailed information on the preparation of these profiles is given in an appendix to those volumes in which they are used.

Positive results in tests using prokaryotes, lower eukaryotes, plants, insects and cultured mammalian cells suggest that genetic and related effects (and therefore possibly carcinogenic effects) could occur in mammals. Results from such tests may also give information about the types of genetic effects produced by an agent and about the involvement of metabolic activation. Some endpoints described are clearly genetic in nature (e.g., gene mutations and chromosomal aberrations), others are to a greater or lesser degree associated with genetic effects (e.g., unscheduled DNA synthesis). In-vitro tests for tumour-promoting activity and for cell transformation may detect changes that are not necessarily the result of genetic alterations but that may have specific relevance to the process of carcinogenesis. A critical appraisal of these tests has been published(13).

Genetic or other activity detected in the systems mentioned above is not always manifest in whole mammals. Positive indications of genetic effects in experimental mammals and in humans are regarded as being of greater relevance than those in other organisms. The demonstration that an agent can induce gene and chromosomal mutations in whole mammals indicates that it may have the potential for carcinogenic activity, although this activity may not be detectably expressed in any or all species tested. The relative potency of agents in tests for mutagenicity and related effects is not a reliable indicator of carcinogenic potency. Negative results in tests for mutagenicity in selected tissues from animals treated *in vivo* provide less weight, partly because they do not exclude the possibility of an effect in tissues other than those examined. Moreover, negative results in short-term tests with genetic endpoints cannot be considered to provide evidence to rule out carcinogenicity of agents that act through other mechanisms. Factors may arise in many tests that could give misleading results; these have been discussed in detail elsewhere(13).

The adequacy of epidemiological studies of reproductive outcomes and genetic and related effects in humans is evaluated by the same criteria as are applied to epidemiological studies of cancer.

11. EVIDENCE FOR CARCINOGENICITY IN HUMANS

(*a*) *Types of studies considered*

Three types of epidemiological studies of cancer contribute data to the assessment of carcinogenicity in humans — cohort studies, case-control studies and correlation studies. Rarely, results from randomized trials may be available. Case reports of cancer in humans exposed to particular agents are also reviewed.

Cohort and case-control studies relate individual exposure to the agent under study to the occurrence of cancer in individuals, and provide an estimate of relative risk (ratio of incidence in those exposed to incidence in those not exposed) as the main measure of association.

In correlation studies, the units of investigation are usually whole populations (e.g., in particular geographical areas or at particular times), and cancer incidence is related to a summary measure of the exposure of the population to the agent under study. Because individual exposure is not documented, however, a causal relationship is less easy to infer from correlation studies than from cohort and case-control studies.

Case reports generally arise from a suspicion, based on clinical experience, that the concurrence of two events — that is, exposure to a particular agent and occurrence of a cancer — has happened rather more frequently than would be expected by chance. Case reports usually lack complete ascertainment of cases in any population, definition or enumeration of the population at risk and estimation of the expected number of cases in the absence of exposure.

The uncertainties surrounding interpretation of case reports and correlation studies make them inadequate, except in rare instances, to form the sole basis for inferring a causal relationship. When taken together with case-control and cohort studies, however, relevant case reports or correlation studies may add materially to the judgement that a causal relationship is present.

Epidemiological studies of benign neoplasms and presumed preneoplastic lesions are also reviewed by working groups. They may, in some instances, strengthen inferences drawn from studies of cancer itself.

(*b*) *Quality of studies considered*

It is necessary to take into account the possible roles of bias, confounding and chance in the interpretation of epidemiological studies. By 'bias' is meant the operation of factors in study design or execution that lead erroneously to a stronger or weaker association between an agent and disease than in fact exists. By 'confounding' is meant a situation in which the relationship between an agent and a disease is made to appear stronger or to appear weaker than it truly is as a result of an association between the agent and another agent that is associated with either an increase or decrease in the incidence of the disease. In evaluating the extent to which these factors have been minimized in an individual study, working groups consider a number of aspects of design and analysis as described in the report of the study. Most of these considerations apply equally to case-control, cohort and correlation studies. Lack of clarity of any of these aspects in the reporting of a study can decrease its credibility and its consequent weighting in the final evaluation of the exposure.

Firstly, the study population, disease (or diseases) and exposure should have been well defined by the authors. Cases in the study population should have been identified in a way that was independent of the exposure of interest, and exposure should have been assessed in a way that was not related to disease status.

Secondly, the authors should have taken account in the study design and analysis of other variables that can influence the risk of disease and may have been related to the exposure of interest. Potential confounding by such variables should have been dealt with either in the design of the study, such as by matching, or in the analysis, by statistical adjustment. In cohort studies, comparisons with local rates of disease may be more

appropriate than those with national rates. Internal comparisons of disease frequency among individuals at different levels of exposure should also have been made in the study.

Thirdly, the authors should have reported the basic data on which the conclusions are founded, even if sophisticated statistical analyses were employed. At the very least, they should have given the numbers of exposed and unexposed cases and controls in a case-control study and the numbers of cases observed and expected in a cohort study. Further tabulations by time since exposure began and other temporal factors are also important. In a cohort study, data on all cancer sites and all causes of death should have been given, to avoid the possibility of reporting bias. In a case-control study, the effects of investigated factors other than the agent of interest should have been reported.

Finally, the statistical methods used to obtain estimates of relative risk, absolute cancer rates, confidence intervals and significance tests, and to adjust for confounding should have been clearly stated by the authors. The methods used should preferably have been the generally accepted techniques that have been refined since the mid-1970s. These methods have been reviewed for case-control studies(17) and for cohort studies(18).

(*c*) *Quantitative considerations*

Detailed analyses of both relative and absolute risks in relation to age at first exposure and to temporal variables, such as time since first exposure, duration of exposure and time since exposure ceased, are reviewed and summarized when available. The analysis of temporal relationships can provide a useful guide in formulating models of carcinogenesis. In particular, such analyses may suggest whether a carcinogen acts early or late in the process of carcinogenesis(6), although such speculative inferences cannot be used to draw firm conclusions concerning the mechanism of action of the agent and hence the shape (linear or otherwise) of the dose-response relationship below the range of observation.

(*d*) *Criteria for causality*

After the quality of individual epidemiological studies has been summarized and assessed, a judgement is made concerning the strength of evidence that the agent in question is carcinogenic for humans. In making their judgement, the Working Group considers several criteria for causality. A strong association (i.e., a large relative risk) is more likely to indicate causality than a weak association, although it is recognized that relative risks of small magnitude do not imply lack of causality and may be important if the disease is common. Associations that are replicated in several studies of the same design or using different epidemiological approaches or under different circumstances of exposure are more likely to represent a causal relationship than isolated observations from single studies. If there are inconsistent results among investigations, possible reasons are sought (such as differences in amount of exposure), and results of studies judged to be of high quality are given more weight than those from studies judged to be methodologically less sound. When suspicion of carcinogenicity arises largely from a single study, these data are not combined with those from later studies in any subsequent reassessment of the strength of the evidence.

If the risk of the disease in question increases with the amount of exposure, this is considered to be a strong indication of causality, although absence of a graded response is

not necessarily evidence against a causal relationship. Demonstration of a decline in risk after cessation of or reduction in exposure in individuals or in whole populations also supports a causal interpretation of the findings.

Although the same carcinogenic agent may act upon more than one target, the specificity of an association (i.e., an increased occurrence of cancer at one anatomical site or of one morphological type) adds plausibility to a causal relationship, particularly when excess cancer occurrence is limited to one morphological type within the same organ.

Although rarely available, results from randomized trials showing different rates among exposed and unexposed individuals provide particularly strong evidence for causality.

When several epidemiological studies show little or no indication of an association between an agent and cancer, the judgement may be made that, in the aggregate, they show evidence of lack of carcinogenicity. Such a judgement requires first of all that the studies giving rise to it meet, to a sufficient degree, the standards of design and analysis described above. Specifically, the possibility that bias, confounding or misclassification of exposure or outcome could explain the observed results should be considered and excluded with reasonable certainty. In addition, all studies that are judged to be methodologically sound should be consistent with a relative risk of unity for any observed level of exposure to the agent and, when considered together, should provide a pooled estimate of relative risk which is at or near unity and has a narrow confidence interval, due to sufficient population size. Moreover, no individual study nor the pooled results of all the studies should show any consistent tendency for relative risk of cancer to increase with increasing amount of exposure to the agent. It is important to note that evidence of lack of carcinogenicity obtained in this way from several epidemiological studies can apply only to the type(s) of cancer studied and to dose levels of the agent and intervals between first exposure to it and observation of disease that are the same as or less than those observed in all the studies. Experience with human cancer indicates that, for some agents, the period from first exposure to the development of clinical cancer is seldom less than 20 years; latent periods substantially shorter than 30 years cannot provide evidence for lack of carcinogenicity.

12. SUMMARY OF DATA REPORTED

In this section, the relevant experimental and epidemiological data are summarized. Only reports, other than in abstract form, that meet the criteria outlined on pp. 16-17 are considered for evaluating carcinogenicity. Inadequate studies are generally not summarized: such studies are usually identified by a square-bracketed comment in the text.

(*a*) *Exposures*

Human exposure is summarized on the basis of elements such as production, use, occurrence in the environment and determinations in human tissues and body fluids. Quantitative data are given when available.

(*b*) *Experimental carcinogenicity data*

Data relevant to the evaluation of the carcinogenicity of the agent in animals are summarized. For each animal species and route of administration, it is stated whether an

increased incidence of neoplasms was observed, and the tumour sites are indicated. If the agent produced tumours after prenatal exposure or in single-dose experiments, this is also indicated. Dose-response and other quantitative data may be given when available. Negative findings are also summarized.

(*c*) *Human carcinogenicity data*

Results of epidemiological studies that are considered to be pertinent to an assessment of human carcinogenicity are summarized. When relevant, case reports and correlation studies are also considered.

(*d*) *Other relevant data*

Structure-activity correlations are mentioned when relevant.

Toxicological information and data on kinetics and metabolism in experimental animals are given when considered relevant. The results of tests for genetic and related effects are summarized for whole mammals, cultured mammalian cells and nonmammalian systems.

Data on other biological effects in humans of particular relevance are summarized. These may include kinetic and metabolic considerations and evidence of DNA binding, persistence of DNA lesions or genetic damage in humans exposed to the agent.

When available, comparisons of such data for humans and for animals, and particularly animals that have developed cancer, are described.

13. EVALUATION

Evaluations of the strength of the evidence for carcinogenicity arising from human and experimental animal data are made, using standard terms.

It is recognized that the criteria for these evaluations, described below, cannot encompass all of the factors that may be relevant to an evaluation of the carcinogenicity of an agent. In considering all of the relevant data, the Working Group may assign the agent to a higher or lower category than a strict interpretation of these criteria would indicate.

(*a*) *Degrees of evidence for carcinogenicity in humans and in experimental animals and supporting evidence*

It should be noted that these categories refer only to the strength of the evidence that these agents are carcinogenic and not to the extent of their carcinogenic activity (potency) nor to the mechanism involved. The classification of some agents may change as new information becomes available.

(i) *Human carcinogenicity data*

The evidence relevant to carcinogenicity from studies in humans is classified into one of the following categories:

Sufficient evidence of carcinogenicity: The Working Group considers that a causal relationship has been established between exposure to the agent and human cancer. That is, a positive relationship has been observed between exposure to the agent and cancer in

studies in which chance, bias and confounding could be ruled out with reasonable confidence.

Limited evidence of carcinogenicity: A positive association has been observed between exposure to the agent and cancer for which a causal interpretation is considered by the Working Group to be credible, but chance, bias or confounding could not be ruled out with reasonable confidence.

Inadequate evidence of carcinogenicity: The available studies are of insufficient quality, consistency or statistical power to permit a conclusion regarding the presence or absence of a causal association.

Evidence suggesting lack of carcinogenicity: There are several adequate studies covering the full range of doses to which human beings are known to be exposed, which are mutually consistent in not showing a positive association between exposure to the agent and any studied cancer at any observed level of exposure. A conclusion of 'evidence suggesting lack of carcinogenicity' is inevitably limited to the cancer sites, circumstances and doses of exposure and length of observation covered by the available studies. In addition, the possibility of a very small risk at the levels of exposure studied can never be excluded.

In some instances, the above categories may be used to classify the degree of evidence for the carcinogenicity of the agent for specific organs or tissues.

(ii) *Experimental carcinogenicity data*

The evidence relevant to carcinogenicity in experimental animals is classified into one of the following categories:

Sufficient evidence of carcinogenicity: The Working Group considers that a causal relationship has been established between the agent and an increased incidence of malignant neoplasms or of an appropriate combination of benign and malignant neoplasms (as described on p. 21) in (a) two or more species of animals or (b) in two or more independent studies in one species carried out at different times or in different laboratories or under different protocols.

Exceptionally, a single study in one species might be considered to provide sufficient evidence of carcinogenicity when malignant neoplasms occur to an unusual degree with regard to incidence, site, type of tumour or age at onset.

In the absence of adequate data on humans, it is biologically plausible and prudent to regard agents for which there is *sufficient evidence* of carcinogenicity in experimental animals as if they presented a carcinogenic risk to humans.

Limited evidence of carcinogenicity: The data suggest a carcinogenic effect but are limited for making a definitive evaluation because, e.g., (a) the evidence of carcinogenicity is restricted to a single experiment; or (b) there are unresolved questions regarding the adequacy of the design, conduct or interpretation of the study; or (c) the agent increases the incidence only of benign neoplasms or lesions of uncertain neoplastic potential, or of certain neoplasms which may occur spontaneously in high incidences in certain strains.

Inadequate evidence of carcinogenicity: The studies cannot be interpreted as showing either the presence or absence of a carcinogenic effect because of major qualitative or quantitative limitations.

Evidence suggesting lack of carcinogenicity: Adequate studies involving at least two species are available which show that, within the limits of the tests used, the agent is not carcinogenic. A conclusion of evidence suggesting lack of carcinogenicity is inevitably limited to the species, tumour sites and doses of exposure studied.

(iii) *Supporting evidence of carcinogenicity*

The other relevant data judged to be of sufficient importance as to affect the making of the overall evaluation are indicated.

(*b*) *Overall evaluation*

Finally, the total body of evidence is taken into account; the agent is described according to the wording of one of the following categories, and the designated group is given. The categorization of an agent is a matter of scientific judgement, reflecting the strength of the evidence derived from studies in humans and in experimental animals and from other relevant data.

Group 1 — The agent is carcinogenic to humans.

This category is used only when there is *sufficient evidence* of carcinogenicity in humans.

Group 2

This category includes agents for which, at one extreme, the degree of evidence of carcinogenicity in humans is almost sufficient, as well as agents for which, at the other extreme, there are no human data but for which there is experimental evidence of carcinogenicity. Agents are assigned to either 2A (probably carcinogenic) or 2B (possibly carcinogenic) on the basis of epidemiological, experimental and other relevant data.

Group 2A — The agent is probably carcinogenic to humans.

This category is used when there is *limited evidence* of carcinogenicity in humans and *sufficient evidence* of carcinogenicity in experimental animals. Exceptionally, an agent may be classified into this category solely on the basis of *limited evidence* of carcinogenicity in humans or of *sufficient evidence* of carcinogenicity in experimental animals strengthened by supporting evidence from other relevant data.

Group 2B — The agent is possibly carcinogenic to humans.

This category is generally used for agents for which there is *limited evidence* in humans in the absence of *sufficient evidence* in experimental animals. It may also be used when there is *inadequate evidence* of carcinogenicity in humans or when human data are nonexistent but there is *sufficient evidence* of carcinogenicity in experimental animals. In some instances, an agent for which there is *inadequate evidence* or no data in humans but *limited evidence* of carcinogenicity in experimental animals together with supporting evidence from other relevant data may be placed in this group.

Group 3 — The agent is not classifiable as to its carcinogenicity to humans.

Agents are placed in this category when they do not fall into any other group.

Group 4 — The agent is probably not carcinogenic to humans.

This category is used for agents for which there is *evidence suggesting lack of carcinogenicity* in humans together with *evidence suggesting lack of carcinogenicity* in experimental animals. In some circumstances, agents for which there is *inadequate evidence* of or no data on carcinogenicity in humans but *evidence suggesting lack of carcinogenicity* in experimental animals, consistently and strongly supported by a broad range of other relevant data, may be classified in this group.

References

1. IARC (1987) *IARC Monographs on the Evaluation of Carcinogenic Risks to Humans*, Supplement 6, *Genetic and Related Effects: An Updating of Selected* IARC Monographs *from Volumes 1 to 42*, Lyon
2. IARC (1977) *IARC Monographs Programme on the Evaluation of the Carcinogenic Risk of Chemicals to Humans. Preamble* (*IARC intern. tech. Rep. No. 77/002*), Lyon
3. IARC (1978) *Chemicals with* Sufficient Evidence *of Carcinogenicity in Experimental Animals* — IARC Monographs *Volumes 1-17* (*IARC intern. tech. Rep. No. 78/003*), Lyon
4. IARC (1979) *Criteria to Select Chemicals for* IARC Monographs (*IARC intern. tech. Rep. No. 79/003*), Lyon
5. IARC (1982) *IARC Monographs on the Evaluation of the Carcinogenic Risk of Chemicals to Humans*, Supplement 4, *Chemicals, Industrial Processes and Industries Associated with Cancer in Humans (IARC Monographs, Volumes 1 to 29)*, Lyon
6. IARC (1983) *Approaches to Classifying Chemical Carcinogens According to Mechanism of Action* (*IARC intern. tech. Rep. No. 83/001*), Lyon
7. IARC (1987) *IARC Monographs on the Evaluation of Carcinogenic Risks to Humans*, Supplement 7, *Overall Evaluations of Carcinogenicity: An Updating of* IARC Monographs *Volumes 1 to 42*, Lyon
8. IARC (1973-1986) *Information Bulletin on the Survey of Chemicals Being Tested for Carcinogenicity*, Numbers 1-12, Lyon

   Number 1 (1973) 52 pages
   Number 2 (1973) 77 pages
   Number 3 (1974) 67 pages
   Number 4 (1974) 97 pages
   Number 5 (1975) 88 pages
   Number 6 (1976) 360 pages

Number 7 (1978) 460 pages
Number 8 (1979) 604 pages
Number 9 (1981) 294 pages
Number 10 (1983) 326 pages
Number 11 (1984) 370 pages
Number 12 (1986) 385 pages

9. Muir, C. & Wagner, G., eds (1977-87) *Directory of On-going Studies in Cancer Epidemiology 1977-87* (*IARC Scientific Publications*), Lyon, International Agency for Research on Cancer

10. IARC (1984) *Chemicals and Exposures to Complex Mixtures Recommended for Evaluation in* IARC Monographs *and Chemicals and Complex Mixtures Recommended for Long-term Carcinogenicity Testing* (*IARC intern. tech. Rep. No. 84/002*), Lyon

11. *Environmental Carcinogens. Selected Methods of Analysis:*

Vol. 1. *Analysis of Volatile Nitrosamines in Food* (*IARC Scientific Publications No. 18*). Edited by R. Preussmann, M. Castegnaro, E.A. Walker & A.E. Wasserman (1978)

Vol. 2. *Methods for the Measurement of Vinyl Chloride in Poly(vinyl chloride), Air, Water and Foodstuffs* (*IARC Scientific Publications No. 22*). Edited by D.C.M. Squirrell & W. Thain (1978)

Vol. 3. *Analysis of Polycyclic Aromatic Hydrocarbons in Environmental Samples* (*IARC Scientific Publications No. 29*). Edited by M. Castegnaro, P. Bogovski, H. Kunte & E.A. Walker (1979)

Vol. 4. *Some Aromatic Amines and Azo Dyes in the General and Industrial Environment* (*IARC Scientific Publications No. 40*). Edited by L. Fishbein, M. Castegnaro, I.K. O'Neill & H. Bartsch (1981)

Vol. 5. *Some Mycotoxins* (*IARC Scientific Publications No. 44*). Edited by L. Stoloff, M. Castegnaro, P. Scott, I.K. O'Neill & H. Bartsch (1983)

Vol. 6. N-*Nitroso Compounds* (*IARC Scientific Publications No. 45*). Edited by R. Preussmann, I.K. O'Neill, G. Eisenbrand, B. Spiegelhalder & H. Bartsch (1983)

Vol. 7. *Some Volatile Halogenated Hydrocarbons* (*IARC Scientific Publications No. 68*). Edited by L. Fishbein & I.K. O'Neill (1985)

Vol. 8. *Some Metals: As, Be, Cd, Cr, Ni, Pb, Se, Zn* (*IARC Scientific Publications No. 71*). Edited by I.K. O'Neill, P. Schuller & L. Fishbein (1986)

Vol. 9. *Passive Smoking* (*IARC Scientific Publications No. 81*). Edited by I.K. O'Neill, K.D. Brunnemann, B. Dodet & D. Hoffmann (1987)

12. Wilbourn, J., Haroun, L., Heseltine, E., Kaldor, J., Partensky, C. & Vainio, H. (1986) Response of experimental animals to human carcinogens: an analysis based upon the IARC Monographs Programme. *Carcinogenesis*, *7*, 1853-1863

13. Montesano, R., Bartsch, H., Vainio, H., Wilbourn, J. & Yamasaki, H., eds (1986) *Long-term and Short-term Assays for Carcinogenesis — A Critical Appraisal* (*IARC Scientific Publications No. 83*), Lyon, International Agency for Research on Cancer

14. Hoel, D.G., Kaplan, N.L. & Anderson, M.W. (1983) Implication of nonlinear kinetics on risk estimation in carcinogenesis. *Science*, *219*, 1032-1037

15. Gart, J.J., Krewski, D., Lee, P.N., Tarone, R.E. & Wahrendorf, J. (1986) *Statistical Methods in Cancer Research*, Vol. 3, *The Design and Analysis of Long-term Animal Experiments* (*IARC Scientific Publications No. 79*), Lyon, International Agency for Research on Cancer

16. Peto, R., Pike, M.C., Day, N.E., Gray, R.G., Lee, P.N., Parish, S., Peto, J., Richards, S. & Wahrendorf, J. (1980) *Guidelines for simple, sensitive significance tests for carcinogenic effects in long-term animal experiments.* In: *IARC Monographs on the Evaluation of the Carcinogenic Risk of Chemicals to Humans*, Supplement 2, *Long-term and Short-term Screening Assays for Carcinogens: A Critical Appraisal*, Lyon, pp. 311-426

17. Breslow, N.E. & Day, N.E. (1980) *Statistical Methods in Cancer Research*, Vol. 1, *The Analysis of Case-control Studies* (*IARC Scientific Publications No. 32*), Lyon, International Agency for Research on Cancer

18. Breslow, N.E. & Day, N.E. (1987) *Statistical Methods in Cancer Research*, Vol. 2, *The Design and Analysis of Cohort Studies* (*IARC Scientific Publications No. 82*), Lyon, International Agency for Research on Cancer

PREAMBLE

With regard to biological and epidemiological data, only reports that have been published or accepted for publication in the openly available scientific literature are reviewed by the working groups. In certain instances, government agency reports that have undergone peer review and are widely available are considered. Exceptions may be made on an ad-hoc basis to include unpublished reports that are in their final form and publicly available, if their inclusion is considered pertinent to making a final evaluation (see pp. 27 *et seq.*). In the sections on chemical and physical properties and on production, use, occurrence and analysis, unpublished sources of information may be used.

5. THE WORKING GROUP

Reviews and evaluations are formulated by a working group of experts. The tasks of this group are five-fold: (i) to ascertain that all appropriate data have been collected; (ii) to select the data relevant for the evaluation on the basis of scientific merit; (iii) to prepare accurate summaries of the data to enable the reader to follow the reasoning of the Working Group; (iv) to evaluate the results of experimental and epidemiological studies; and (v) to make an overall evaluation of the carcinogenicity of the agent to humans.

Working Group participants who contributed to the consideration and evaluation of the agents within a particular volume are listed, with their addresses, at the beginning of each publication. Each participant who is a member of a working group serves as an individual scientist and not as a representative of any organization, government or industry. In addition, representatives from national and international agencies and industrial associations are invited as observers.

6. WORKING PROCEDURES

Approximately one year in advance of a meeting of a working group, the agents to be evaluated are announced and participants are selected by IARC staff in consultation with other experts. Subsequently, relevant biological and epidemiological data are collected by IARC from recognized sources of information on carcinogenesis, including data storage and retrieval systems such as CANCERLINE, MEDLINE and TOXLINE. Bibliographical sources for data on genetic and related effects and on teratogenicity are the Environmental Mutagen Information Center and the Environmental Teratology Information Center, both located at the Oak Ridge National Laboratory, USA.

The major collection of data and the preparation of first drafts of the sections on chemical and physical properties, on production and use, on occurrence, and on analysis are carried out under a separate contract funded by the US National Cancer Institute. Efforts are made to supplement this information with data from other national and international sources. Representatives from industrial associations may assist in the preparation of sections on production and use.

Production and trade data are obtained from governmental and trade publications and, in some cases, by direct contact with industries. Separate production data on some agents may not be available because their publication could disclose confidential information.

Information on uses is usually obtained from published sources but is often complemented by direct contact with manufacturers.

Six months before the meeting, reference material is sent to experts, or is used by IARC staff, to prepare sections for the first drafts of monographs. The complete first drafts are compiled by IARC staff and sent, prior to the meeting, to all participants of the Working Group for review.

The Working Group meets in Lyon for seven to eight days to discuss and finalize the texts of the monographs and to formulate the evaluations. After the meeting, the master copy of each monograph is verified by consulting the original literature, edited and prepared for publication. The aim is to publish monographs within nine months of the Working Group meeting.

7. EXPOSURE DATA

Sections that indicate the extent of past and present human exposure, the sources of exposure, the persons most likely to be exposed and the factors that contribute to exposure to the agent under study are included at the beginning of each monograph.

Most monographs on individual chemicals or complex mixtures include sections on chemical and physical data, and production, use, occurrence and analysis. In other monographs, for example on physical agents, biological factors, occupational exposures and cultural habits, other sections may be included, such as: historical perspectives, description of an industry or habit, exposures in the work place or chemistry of the complex mixture.

The Chemical Abstracts Services Registry Number, the latest Chemical Abstracts Primary Name and the IUPAC Systematic Name are recorded. Other synonyms and trade names are given, but the list is not necessarily comprehensive. Some of the trade names may be those of mixtures in which the agent being evaluated is only one of the ingredients.

Information on chemical and physical properties and, in particular, data relevant to identification, occurrence and biological activity are included. A separate description of technical products gives relevant specifications and includes available information on composition and impurities.

The dates of first synthesis and of first commercial production of an agent are provided; for agents which do not occur naturally, this information may allow a reasonable estimate to be made of the date before which no human exposure to the agent could have occurred. The dates of first reported occurrence of an exposure are also provided. In addition, methods of synthesis used in past and present commercial production and different methods of production which may give rise to different impurities are described.

Data on production, foreign trade and uses are obtained for representative regions, which usually include Europe, Japan and the USA. It should not, however, be inferred that those areas or nations are necessarily the sole or major sources or users of the agent being evaluated.

Some identified uses may not be current or major applications, and the coverage is not necessarily comprehensive. In the case of drugs, mention of their therapeutic uses does not necessarily represent current practice nor does it imply judgement as to their clinical efficacy.

Information on the occurrence of an agent in the environment is obtained from data derived from the monitoring and surveillance of levels in occupational environments, air, water, soil, foods and animal and human tissues. When available, data on the generation, persistence and bioaccumulation of the agent are also included.

Statements concerning regulations and guidelines (e.g., pesticide registrations, maximal levels permitted in foods, occupational exposure limits) are included for some countries as indications of potential exposures, but they may not reflect the most recent situation, since such limits are continuously reviewed and modified. The absence of information on regulatory status for a country should not be taken to imply that that country does not have regulations with regard to the agent.

The purpose of the section on analysis is to give the reader an overview of current methods cited in the literature, with emphasis on those widely used for regulatory purposes. No critical evaluation or recommendation of any of the methods is meant or implied. Methods for monitoring human exposure are also given, when available. The IARC publishes a series of volumes, *Environmental Carcinogens: Selected Methods of Analysis*(11), that describe validated methods for analysing a wide variety of agents.

8. BIOLOGICAL DATA RELEVANT TO THE EVALUATION OF CARCINOGENICITY TO HUMANS

The term 'carcinogen' is used in these monographs to denote an agent that is capable of increasing the incidence of malignant neoplasms; the induction of benign neoplasms may in some circumstances (see p. 21) contribute to the judgement that an agent is carcinogenic. The terms 'neoplasm' and 'tumour' are used interchangeably.

Some epidemiological and experimental studies indicate that different agents may act at different stages in the carcinogenic process, probably by fundamentally different mechanisms. In the present state of knowledge, the aim of the *Monographs* is to evaluate evidence of carcinogenicity at any stage in the carcinogenic process independently of the underlying mechanism involved. There is as yet insufficient information to implement a classification of agents according to their mechanism of action(6).

Definitive evidence of carcinogenicity in humans is provided by epidemiological studies. Evidence relevant to human carcinogenicity may also be provided by experimental studies of carcinogenicity in animals and by other biological data, particularly those relating to humans.

The available studies are summarized by the working groups, with particular regard to the qualitative aspects discussed below. In general, numerical findings are indicated as they appear in the original report; units are converted when necessary for easier comparison. The Working Group may conduct additional analyses of the published data and use them in their assessment of the evidence and may include them in their summary of a study; the results of such supplementary analyses are given in square brackets. Any comments are also made in square brackets; however, these are kept to a minimum, being restricted to those instances in which it is felt that an important aspect of a study, directly impinging on its interpretation, should be brought to the attention of the reader.

9. EVIDENCE FOR CARCINOGENICITY IN EXPERIMENTAL ANIMALS

For several agents (e.g., 4-aminobiphenyl, bis(chloromethyl)ether, diethylstilboestrol, melphalan, 8-methoxypsoralen (methoxsalen) plus UVR, mustard gas and vinyl chloride), evidence of carcinogenicity in experimental animals preceded evidence obtained from epidemiological studies or case reports. Information compiled from the first 41 volumes of the *IARC Monographs*(12) shows that, of the 44 agents for which there is *sufficient* or *limited evidence* of carcinogenicity to humans (see pp. 27-28), all 37 that have been tested adequately experimentally produce cancer in at least one animal species. Although this association cannot establish that all agents that cause cancer in experimental animals also cause cancer in humans, nevertheless, **in the absence of adequate data on humans, it is biologically plausible and prudent to regard agents for which there is *sufficient evidence* (see p. 28) of carcinogenicity in experimental animals as if they presented a carcinogenic risk to humans.**

The monographs are not intended to summarize all published studies. Those that are inadequate (e.g., too short a duration, too few animals, poor survival; see below) or are judged irrelevant to the evaluation are generally omitted. They may be mentioned briefly, particularly when the information is considered to be a useful supplement to that of other reports or when they provide the only data available. Their inclusion does not, however, imply acceptance of the adequacy of the experimental design or of the analysis and interpretation of their results. Guidelines for adequate long-term carcinogenicity experiments have been outlined (e.g., ref. 13).

The nature and extent of impurities or contaminants present in the agent being evaluated are given when available. Mention is made of all routes of exposure by which the agent has been adequately studied and of all species in which relevant experiments have been performed. Animal strain, sex, numbers per group, age at start of treatment and survival are reported.

Experiments in which the agent was administered in conjunction with known carcinogens or factors that modify carcinogenic effects are also reported. Experiments on the carcinogenicity of known metabolites and derivatives may be included.

(*a*) *Qualitative aspects*

The overall assessment of the carcinogenicity of an agent involves several considerations of qualitative importance, including (i) the experimental conditions under which the test was performed, including route and schedule of exposure, species, strain, sex, age, duration of follow-up; (ii) the consistency with which the agent has been shown to be carcinogenic, e.g., in how many species and at which target organs(s); (iii) the spectrum of neoplastic response, from benign tumours to malignant neoplasms; and (iv) the possible role of modifying factors.

Considerations of importance to the Working Group in the interpretation and evaluation of a particular study include: (i) how clearly the agent was defined; (ii) whether the dose was adequately monitored, particularly in inhalation experiments; (iii) whether the doses used were appropriate and whether the survival of treated animals was similar to that of controls; (iv) whether there were adequate numbers of animals per group; (v) whether animals of both sexes were used; (vi) whether animals were allocated randomly to groups; (vii) whether the duration of observation was adequate; and (viii) whether the data were adequately reported. If available, recent data on the incidence of specific tumours in historical controls, as well as in concurrent controls, should be taken into account in the evaluation of tumour response.

When benign tumours occur together with and originate from the same cell type in an organ or tissue as malignant tumours in a particular study and appear to represent a stage in the progression to malignancy, it may be valid to combine them in assessing tumour incidence. The occurrence of lesions presumed to be preneoplastic may in certain instances aid in assessing the biological plausibility of any neoplastic response observed.

Among the many agents that have been studied extensively, there are few instances in which the only neoplasms induced were benign. Benign tumours in experimental animals frequently represent a stage in the evolution of a malignant neoplasm, but they may be 'endpoints' that do not readily undergo transition to malignancy. However, if an agent is found to induce only benign neoplasms, it should be suspected of being a carcinogen and it requires further investigation.

(*b*) *Quantitative aspects*

The probability that tumours will occur may depend on the species and strain, the dose of the carcinogen and the route and period of exposure. Evidence of an increased incidence of neoplasms with increased exposure strengthens the inference of a causal association between exposure to the agent and the development of neoplasms.

The form of the dose-response relationship can vary widely, depending on the particular agent under study and the target organ. Since many chemicals require metabolic activation before being converted into their reactive intermediates, both metabolic and pharmacokinetic aspects are important in determining the dose-response pattern. Saturation of steps such as absorption, activation, inactivation and elimination of the carcinogen may produce nonlinearity in the dose-response relationship, as could saturation of processes such as DNA repair(14,15).

(*c*) *Statistical analysis of long-term experiments in animals*

Factors considered by the Working Group include the adequacy of the information given for each treatment group: (i) the number of animals on study and the number examined histologically, (ii) the number of animals with a given tumour type and (iii) length of survival. The statistical methods used should be clearly stated and should be the generally accepted techniques refined for this purpose(15,16). When there is no difference in survival between control and treatment groups, the Working Group usually compares the proportions of animals developing each tumour type in each of the groups. Otherwise, consideration is given as to whether or not appropriate adjustments have been made for differences in survival. These adjustments can include: comparisons of the proportions of tumour-bearing animals among the 'effective number' of animals alive at the time the first tumour is discovered, in the case where most differences in survival occur before tumours appear; life-table methods, when tumours are visible or when they may be considered 'fatal' because mortality rapidly follows tumour development; and the Mantel-Haenszel test or logistic regression, when occult tumours do not affect the animals' risk of dying but are 'incidental' findings at autopsy.

In practice, classifying tumours as fatal or incidental may be difficult. Several survival-adjusted methods have been developed that do not require this distinction(15), although they have not been fully evaluated.

10. OTHER RELEVANT DATA IN EXPERIMENTAL SYSTEMS AND HUMANS

(*a*) *Structure-activity considerations*

This section describes structure-activity correlations that are relevant to an evaluation of the carcinogenicity of an agent.

(*b*) *Absorption, distribution, excretion and metabolism*

Concise information is given on absorption, distribution (including placental transfer) and excretion. Kinetic factors that may affect the dose-reponse relationship, such as saturation of uptake, protein binding, metabolic activation, detoxification and DNA-repair processes, are mentioned. Studies that indicate the metabolic fate of the agent in experimental animals and humans are summarized briefly, and comparisons of data from animals and humans are made when possible. Comparative information on the relationship between exposure and the dose that reaches the target site may be of particular importance for extrapolation between species.

(*c*) *Toxicity*

Data are given on acute and chronic toxic effects (other than cancer), such as organ toxicity, immunotoxicity, endocrine effects and preneoplastic lesions. Effects on reproduction, teratogenicity, feto- and embryotoxicity are also summarized briefly.

(*d*) *Genetic and related effects*

Tests of genetic and related effects may indicate possible carcinogenic activity. They can also be used in detecting active metabolites of known carcinogens in human or animal body fluids, in detecting active components in complex mixtures and in the elucidation of possible mechanisms of carcinogenesis.

The available data are interpreted critically by phylogenetic group according to the endpoints detected, which may include DNA damage, gene mutation, sister chromatid exchange, micronuclei, chromosomal aberrations, aneuploidy and cell transformation. The concentrations (doses) employed are given and mention is made of whether an exogenous metabolic system was required. When appropriate, these data may be represented by bar graphs (activity profiles), with corresponding summary tables and listings of test systems, data and references. Detailed information on the preparation of these profiles is given in an appendix to those volumes in which they are used.

Positive results in tests using prokaryotes, lower eukaryotes, plants, insects and cultured mammalian cells suggest that genetic and related effects (and therefore possibly carcinogenic effects) could occur in mammals. Results from such tests may also give information about the types of genetic effects produced by an agent and about the involvement of metabolic activation. Some endpoints described are clearly genetic in nature (e.g., gene mutations and chromosomal aberrations), others are to a greater or lesser degree associated with genetic effects (e.g., unscheduled DNA synthesis). In-vitro tests for tumour-promoting activity and for cell transformation may detect changes that are not necessarily the result of genetic alterations but that may have specific relevance to the process of carcinogenesis. A critical appraisal of these tests has been published(13).

Genetic or other activity detected in the systems mentioned above is not always manifest in whole mammals. Positive indications of genetic effects in experimental mammals and in humans are regarded as being of greater relevance than those in other organisms. The demonstration that an agent can induce gene and chromosomal mutations in whole mammals indicates that it may have the potential for carcinogenic activity, although this activity may not be detectably expressed in any or all species tested. The relative potency of agents in tests for mutagenicity and related effects is not a reliable indicator of carcinogenic potency. Negative results in tests for mutagenicity in selected tissues from animals treated *in vivo* provide less weight, partly because they do not exclude the possibility of an effect in tissues other than those examined. Moreover, negative results in short-term tests with genetic endpoints cannot be considered to provide evidence to rule out carcinogenicity of agents that act through other mechanisms. Factors may arise in many tests that could give misleading results; these have been discussed in detail elsewhere(13).

The adequacy of epidemiological studies of reproductive outcomes and genetic and related effects in humans is evaluated by the same criteria as are applied to epidemiological studies of cancer.

11. EVIDENCE FOR CARCINOGENICITY IN HUMANS

(*a*) *Types of studies considered*

Three types of epidemiological studies of cancer contribute data to the assessment of carcinogenicity in humans — cohort studies, case-control studies and correlation studies. Rarely, results from randomized trials may be available. Case reports of cancer in humans exposed to particular agents are also reviewed.

Cohort and case-control studies relate individual exposure to the agent under study to the occurrence of cancer in individuals, and provide an estimate of relative risk (ratio of incidence in those exposed to incidence in those not exposed) as the main measure of association.

In correlation studies, the units of investigation are usually whole populations (e.g., in particular geographical areas or at particular times), and cancer incidence is related to a summary measure of the exposure of the population to the agent under study. Because individual exposure is not documented, however, a causal relationship is less easy to infer from correlation studies than from cohort and case-control studies.

Case reports generally arise from a suspicion, based on clinical experience, that the concurrence of two events — that is, exposure to a particular agent and occurrence of a cancer — has happened rather more frequently than would be expected by chance. Case reports usually lack complete ascertainment of cases in any population, definition or enumeration of the population at risk and estimation of the expected number of cases in the absence of exposure.

The uncertainties surrounding interpretation of case reports and correlation studies make them inadequate, except in rare instances, to form the sole basis for inferring a causal relationship. When taken together with case-control and cohort studies, however, relevant case reports or correlation studies may add materially to the judgement that a causal relationship is present.

Epidemiological studies of benign neoplasms and presumed preneoplastic lesions are also reviewed by working groups. They may, in some instances, strengthen inferences drawn from studies of cancer itself.

(*b*) *Quality of studies considered*

It is necessary to take into account the possible roles of bias, confounding and chance in the interpretation of epidemiological studies. By 'bias' is meant the operation of factors in study design or execution that lead erroneously to a stronger or weaker association between an agent and disease than in fact exists. By 'confounding' is meant a situation in which the relationship between an agent and a disease is made to appear stronger or to appear weaker than it truly is as a result of an association between the agent and another agent that is associated with either an increase or decrease in the incidence of the disease. In evaluating the extent to which these factors have been minimized in an individual study, working groups consider a number of aspects of design and analysis as described in the report of the study. Most of these considerations apply equally to case-control, cohort and correlation studies. Lack of clarity of any of these aspects in the reporting of a study can decrease its credibility and its consequent weighting in the final evaluation of the exposure.

Firstly, the study population, disease (or diseases) and exposure should have been well defined by the authors. Cases in the study population should have been identified in a way that was independent of the exposure of interest, and exposure should have been assessed in a way that was not related to disease status.

Secondly, the authors should have taken account in the study design and analysis of other variables that can influence the risk of disease and may have been related to the exposure of interest. Potential confounding by such variables should have been dealt with either in the design of the study, such as by matching, or in the analysis, by statistical adjustment. In cohort studies, comparisons with local rates of disease may be more appropriate than those with national rates. Internal comparisons of disease frequency among individuals at different levels of exposure should also have been made in the study.

Thirdly, the authors should have reported the basic data on which the conclusions are founded, even if sophisticated statistical analyses were employed. At the very least, they should have given the numbers of exposed and unexposed cases and controls in a case-control study and the numbers of cases observed and expected in a cohort study. Further tabulations by time since exposure began and other temporal factors are also important. In a cohort study, data on all cancer sites and all causes of death should have been given, to avoid the possibility of reporting bias. In a case-control study, the effects of investigated factors other than the agent of interest should have been reported.

Finally, the statistical methods used to obtain estimates of relative risk, absolute cancer rates, confidence intervals and significance tests, and to adjust for confounding should have been clearly stated by the authors. The methods used should preferably have been the generally accepted techniques that have been refined since the mid-1970s. These methods have been reviewed for case-control studies(17) and for cohort studies(18).

(*c*) *Quantitative considerations*

Detailed analyses of both relative and absolute risks in relation to age at first exposure and to temporal variables, such as time since first exposure, duration of exposure and time since exposure ceased, are reviewed and summarized when available. The analysis of temporal relationships can provide a useful guide in formulating models of carcinogenesis. In particular, such analyses may suggest whether a carcinogen acts early or late in the process of carcinogenesis(6), although such speculative inferences cannot be used to draw firm conclusions concerning the mechanism of action of the agent and hence the shape (linear or otherwise) of the dose-response relationship below the range of observation.

(*d*) *Criteria for causality*

After the quality of individual epidemiological studies has been summarized and assessed, a judgement is made concerning the strength of evidence that the agent in question is carcinogenic for humans. In making their judgement, the Working Group considers several criteria for causality. A strong association (i.e., a large relative risk) is more likely to indicate causality than a weak association, although it is recognized that relative risks of small magnitude do not imply lack of causality and may be important if the disease is common. Associations that are replicated in several studies of the same design or using different epidemiological approaches or under different circumstances of exposure are more likely to represent a causal relationship than isolated observations from single studies. If there are inconsistent results among investigations, possible reasons are sought (such as differences in amount of exposure), and results of studies judged to be of high quality are given more weight than those from studies judged to be methodologically less sound. When suspicion of carcinogenicity arises largely from a single study, these data are not combined with those from later studies in any subsequent reassessment of the strength of the evidence.

If the risk of the disease in question increases with the amount of exposure, this is considered to be a strong indication of causality, although absence of a graded response is not necessarily evidence against a causal relationship. Demonstration of a decline in risk after cessation of or reduction in exposure in individuals or in whole populations also supports a causal interpretation of the findings.

Although the same carcinogenic agent may act upon more than one target, the specificity of an association (i.e., an increased occurrence of cancer at one anatomical site or of one morphological type) adds plausibility to a causal relationship, particularly when excess cancer occurrence is limited to one morphological type within the same organ.

Although rarely available, results from randomized trials showing different rates among exposed and unexposed individuals provide particularly strong evidence for causality.

When several epidemiological studies show little or no indication of an association between an agent and cancer, the judgement may be made that, in the aggregate, they show evidence of lack of carcinogenicity. Such a judgement requires first of all that the studies giving rise to it meet, to a sufficient degree, the standards of design and analysis described above. Specifically, the possibility that bias, confounding or misclassification of exposure or outcome could explain the observed results should be considered and excluded with reasonable certainty. In addition, all studies that are judged to be methodologically sound should be consistent with a relative risk of unity for any observed level of exposure to the agent and, when considered together, should provide a pooled estimate of relative risk which is at or near unity and has a narrow confidence interval, due to sufficient population size. Moreover, no individual study nor the pooled results of all the studies should show any consistent tendency for relative risk of cancer to increase with increasing amount of exposure to the agent. It is important to note that evidence of lack of carcinogenicity obtained in this way from several epidemiological studies can apply only to the type(s) of cancer studied and to dose levels of the agent and intervals between first exposure to it and observation of disease that are the same as or less than those observed in all the studies. Experience with human cancer indicates that, for some agents, the period from first exposure to the development of clinical cancer is seldom less than 20 years; latent periods substantially shorter than 30 years cannot provide evidence for lack of carcinogenicity.

12. SUMMARY OF DATA REPORTED

In this section, the relevant experimental and epidemiological data are summarized. Only reports, other than in abstract form, that meet the criteria outlined on pp. 16-17 are considered for evaluating carcinogenicity. Inadequate studies are generally not summarized: such studies are usually identified by a square-bracketed comment in the text.

(*a*) *Exposures*

Human exposure is summarized on the basis of elements such as production, use, occurrence in the environment and determinations in human tissues and body fluids. Quantitative data are given when available.

(*b*) *Experimental carcinogenicity data*

Data relevant to the evaluation of the carcinogenicity of the agent in animals are summarized. For each animal species and route of administration, it is stated whether an increased incidence of neoplasms was observed, and the tumour sites are indicated. If the agent produced tumours after prenatal exposure or in single-dose experiments, this is also indicated. Dose-response and other quantitative data may be given when available. Negative findings are also summarized.

(*c*) *Human carcinogenicity data*

Results of epidemiological studies that are considered to be pertinent to an assessment of human carcinogenicity are summarized. When relevant, case reports and correlation studies are also considered.

(*d*) *Other relevant data*

Structure-activity correlations are mentioned when relevant.

Toxicological information and data on kinetics and metabolism in experimental animals are given when considered relevant. The results of tests for genetic and related effects are summarized for whole mammals, cultured mammalian cells and nonmammalian systems.

Data on other biological effects in humans of particular relevance are summarized. These may include kinetic and metabolic considerations and evidence of DNA binding, persistence of DNA lesions or genetic damage in humans exposed to the agent.

When available, comparisons of such data for humans and for animals, and particularly animals that have developed cancer, are described.

13. EVALUATION

Evaluations of the strength of the evidence for carcinogenicity arising from human and experimental animal data are made, using standard terms.

It is recognized that the criteria for these evaluations, described below, cannot encompass all of the factors that may be relevant to an evaluation of the carcinogenicity of an agent. In considering all of the relevant data, the Working Group may assign the agent to a higher or lower category than a strict interpretation of these criteria would indicate.

(*a*) *Degrees of evidence for carcinogenicity in humans and in experimental animals and supporting evidence*

It should be noted that these categories refer only to the strength of the evidence that these agents are carcinogenic and not to the extent of their carcinogenic activity (potency) nor to the mechanism involved. The classification of some agents may change as new information becomes available.

(i) *Human carcinogenicity data*

The evidence relevant to carcinogenicity from studies in humans is classified into one of the following categories:

Sufficient evidence of carcinogenicity: The Working Group considers that a causal relationship has been established between exposure to the agent and human cancer. That is, a positive relationship has been observed between exposure to the agent and cancer in studies in which chance, bias and confounding could be ruled out with reasonable confidence.

Limited evidence of carcinogenicity: A positive association has been observed between exposure to the agent and cancer for which a causal interpretation is considered by the Working Group to be credible, but chance, bias or confounding could not be ruled out with reasonable confidence.

Inadequate evidence of carcinogenicity: The available studies are of insufficient quality, consistency or statistical power to permit a conclusion regarding the presence or absence of a causal association.

Evidence suggesting lack of carcinogenicity: There are several adequate studies covering the full range of doses to which human beings are known to be exposed, which are mutually consistent in not showing a positive association between exposure to the agent and any studied cancer at any observed level of exposure. A conclusion of 'evidence suggesting lack of carcinogenicity' is inevitably limited to the cancer sites, circumstances and doses of exposure and length of observation covered by the available studies. In addition, the possibility of a very small risk at the levels of exposure studied can never be excluded.

In some instances, the above categories may be used to classify the degree of evidence for the carcinogenicity of the agent for specific organs or tissues.

(ii) *Experimental carcinogenicity data*

The evidence relevant to carcinogenicity in experimental animals is classified into one of the following categories:

Sufficient evidence of carcinogenicity: The Working Group considers that a causal relationship has been established between the agent and an increased incidence of malignant neoplasms or of an appropriate combination of benign and malignant neoplasms (as described on p. 21) in (a) two or more species of animals or (b) in two or more independent studies in one species carried out at different times or in different laboratories or under different protocols.

Exceptionally, a single study in one species might be considered to provide sufficient evidence of carcinogenicity when malignant neoplasms occur to an unusual degree with regard to incidence, site, type of tumour or age at onset.

In the absence of adequate data on humans, it is biologically plausible and prudent to regard agents for which there is *sufficient evidence* of carcinogenicity in experimental animals as if they presented a carcinogenic risk to humans.

Limited evidence of carcinogenicity: The data suggest a carcinogenic effect but are limited for making a definitive evaluation because, e.g., (a) the evidence of carcinogenicity is restricted to a single experiment; or (b) there are unresolved questions regarding the adequacy of the design, conduct or interpretation of the study; or (c) the agent increases the incidence only of benign neoplasms or lesions of uncertain neoplastic potential, or of certain neoplasms which may occur spontaneously in high incidences in certain strains.

Inadequate evidence of carcinogenicity: The studies cannot be interpreted as showing either the presence or absence of a carcinogenic effect because of major qualitative or quantitative limitations.

Evidence suggesting lack of carcinogenicity: Adequate studies involving at least two species are available which show that, within the limits of the tests used, the agent is not carcinogenic. A conclusion of evidence suggesting lack of carcinogenicity is inevitably limited to the species, tumour sites and doses of exposure studied.

(iii) *Supporting evidence of carcinogenicity*

The other relevant data judged to be of sufficient importance as to affect the making of the overall evaluation are indicated.

(*b*) *Overall evaluation*

Finally, the total body of evidence is taken into account; the agent is described according to the wording of one of the following categories, and the designated group is given. The categorization of an agent is a matter of scientific judgement, reflecting the strength of the evidence derived from studies in humans and in experimental animals and from other relevant data.

Group 1 — The agent is carcinogenic to humans.

This category is used only when there is *sufficient evidence* of carcinogenicity in humans.

Group 2

This category includes agents for which, at one extreme, the degree of evidence of carcinogenicity in humans is almost sufficient, as well as agents for which, at the other extreme, there are no human data but for which there is experimental evidence of carcinogenicity. Agents are assigned to either 2A (probably carcinogenic) or 2B (possibly carcinogenic) on the basis of epidemiological, experimental and other relevant data.

Group 2A — The agent is probably carcinogenic to humans.

This category is used when there is *limited evidence* of carcinogenicity in humans and *sufficient evidence* of carcinogenicity in experimental animals. Exceptionally, an agent may be classified into this category solely on the basis of *limited evidence* of carcinogenicity in humans or of *sufficient evidence* of carcinogenicity in experimental animals strengthened by supporting evidence from other relevant data.

Group 2B — The agent is possibly carcinogenic to humans.

This category is generally used for agents for which there is *limited evidence* in humans in the absence of *sufficient evidence* in experimental animals. It may also be used when there is *inadequate evidence* of carcinogenicity in humans or when human data are nonexistent but there is *sufficient evidence* of carcinogenicity in experimental animals. In some instances, an agent for which there is *inadequate evidence* or no data in humans but *limited evidence* of carcinogenicity in experimental animals together with supporting evidence from other relevant data may be placed in this group.

Group 3 — The agent is not classifiable as to its carcinogenicity to humans.

Agents are placed in this category when they do not fall into any other group.

Group 4 — The agent is probably not carcinogenic to humans.

This category is used for agents for which there is *evidence suggesting lack of carcinogenicity* in humans together with *evidence suggesting lack of carcinogenicity* in experimental animals. In some circumstances, agents for which there is *inadequate evidence* of or no data on carcinogenicity in humans but *evidence suggesting lack of carcinogenicity* in experimental animals, consistently and strongly supported by a broad range of other relevant data, may be classified in this group.

References

1. IARC (1987) *IARC Monographs on the Evaluation of Carcinogenic Risks to Humans*, Supplement 6, *Genetic and Related Effects: An Updating of Selected* IARC Monographs *from Volumes 1 to 42*, Lyon
2. IARC (1977) *IARC Monographs Programme on the Evaluation of the Carcinogenic Risk of Chemicals to Humans. Preamble* (*IARC intern. tech. Rep. No. 77/002*), Lyon
3. IARC (1978) *Chemicals with* Sufficient Evidence *of Carcinogenicity in Experimental Animals* — IARC Monographs *Volumes 1-17* (*IARC intern. tech. Rep. No. 78/003*), Lyon
4. IARC (1979) *Criteria to Select Chemicals for* IARC Monographs (*IARC intern. tech. Rep. No. 79/003*), Lyon
5. IARC (1982) *IARC Monographs on the Evaluation of the Carcinogenic Risk of Chemicals to Humans*, Supplement 4, *Chemicals, Industrial Processes and Industries Associated with Cancer in Humans (IARC Monographs, Volumes 1 to 29)*, Lyon
6. IARC (1983) *Approaches to Classifying Chemical Carcinogens According to Mechanism of Action* (*IARC intern. tech. Rep. No. 83/001*), Lyon
7. IARC (1987) *IARC Monographs on the Evaluation of Carcinogenic Risks to Humans*, Supplement 7, *Overall Evaluations of Carcinogenicity: An Updating of* IARC Monographs *Volumes 1 to 42*, Lyon
8. IARC (1973-1986) *Information Bulletin on the Survey of Chemicals Being Tested for Carcinogenicity*, Numbers 1-12, Lyon

    Number 1 (1973) 52 pages
    Number 2 (1973) 77 pages
    Number 3 (1974) 67 pages
    Number 4 (1974) 97 pages
    Number 5 (1975) 88 pages
    Number 6 (1976) 360 pages

Number 7 (1978) 460 pages
Number 8 (1979) 604 pages
Number 9 (1981) 294 pages
Number 10 (1983) 326 pages
Number 11 (1984) 370 pages
Number 12 (1986) 385 pages

9. Muir, C. & Wagner, G., eds (1977-87) *Directory of On-going Studies in Cancer Epidemiology 1977-87* (*IARC Scientific Publications*), Lyon, International Agency for Research on Cancer

10. IARC (1984) *Chemicals and Exposures to Complex Mixtures Recommended for Evaluation in* IARC Monographs *and Chemicals and Complex Mixtures Recommended for Long-term Carcinogenicity Testing* (*IARC intern. tech. Rep. No. 84/002*), Lyon

11. *Environmental Carcinogens. Selected Methods of Analysis:*

Vol. 1. *Analysis of Volatile Nitrosamines in Food* (*IARC Scientific Publications No. 18*). Edited by R. Preussmann, M. Castegnaro, E.A. Walker & A.E. Wasserman (1978)

Vol. 2. *Methods for the Measurement of Vinyl Chloride in Poly(vinyl chloride), Air, Water and Foodstuffs* (*IARC Scientific Publications No. 22*). Edited by D.C.M. Squirrell & W. Thain (1978)

Vol. 3. *Analysis of Polycyclic Aromatic Hydrocarbons in Environmental Samples* (*IARC Scientific Publications No. 29*). Edited by M. Castegnaro, P. Bogovski, H. Kunte & E.A. Walker (1979)

Vol. 4. *Some Aromatic Amines and Azo Dyes in the General and Industrial Environment* (*IARC Scientific Publications No. 40*). Edited by L. Fishbein, M. Castegnaro, I.K. O'Neill & H. Bartsch (1981)

Vol. 5. *Some Mycotoxins* (*IARC Scientific Publications No. 44*). Edited by L. Stoloff, M. Castegnaro, P. Scott, I.K. O'Neill & H. Bartsch (1983)

Vol. 6. N-*Nitroso Compounds* (*IARC Scientific Publications No. 45*). Edited by R. Preussmann, I.K. O'Neill, G. Eisenbrand, B. Spiegelhalder & H. Bartsch (1983)

Vol. 7. *Some Volatile Halogenated Hydrocarbons* (*IARC Scientific Publications No. 68*). Edited by L. Fishbein & I.K. O'Neill (1985)

Vol. 8. *Some Metals: As, Be, Cd, Cr, Ni, Pb, Se, Zn* (*IARC Scientific Publications No. 71*). Edited by I.K. O'Neill, P. Schuller & L. Fishbein (1986)

Vol. 9. *Passive Smoking* (*IARC Scientific Publications No. 81*). Edited by I.K. O'Neill, K.D. Brunnemann, B. Dodet & D. Hoffmann (1987)

12. Wilbourn, J., Haroun, L., Heseltine, E., Kaldor, J., Partensky, C. & Vainio, H. (1986) Response of experimental animals to human carcinogens: an analysis based upon the IARC Monographs Programme. *Carcinogenesis*, *7*, 1853-1863

13. Montesano, R., Bartsch, H., Vainio, H., Wilbourn, J. & Yamasaki, H., eds (1986) *Long-term and Short-term Assays for Carcinogenesis — A Critical Appraisal* (*IARC Scientific Publications No. 83*), Lyon, International Agency for Research on Cancer

14. Hoel, D.G., Kaplan, N.L. & Anderson, M.W. (1983) Implication of nonlinear kinetics on risk estimation in carcinogenesis. *Science*, *219*, 1032-1037

15. Gart, J.J., Krewski, D., Lee, P.N., Tarone, R.E. & Wahrendorf, J. (1986) *Statistical Methods in Cancer Research*, Vol. 3, *The Design and Analysis of Long-term Animal Experiments* (*IARC Scientific Publications No. 79*), Lyon, International Agency for Research on Cancer

16. Peto, R., Pike, M.C., Day, N.E., Gray, R.G., Lee, P.N., Parish, S., Peto, J., Richards, S. & Wahrendorf, J. (1980) *Guidelines for simple, sensitive significance tests for carcinogenic effects in long-term animal experiments.* In: *IARC Monographs on the Evaluation of the Carcinogenic Risk of Chemicals to Humans*, Supplement 2, *Long-term and Short-term Screening Assays for Carcinogens: A Critical Appraisal*, Lyon, pp. 311-426

17. Breslow, N.E. & Day, N.E. (1980) *Statistical Methods in Cancer Research*, Vol. 1, *The Analysis of Case-control Studies* (*IARC Scientific Publications No. 32*), Lyon, International Agency for Research on Cancer

18. Breslow, N.E. & Day, N.E. (1987) *Statistical Methods in Cancer Research*, Vol. 2, *The Design and Analysis of Cohort Studies* (*IARC Scientific Publications No. 82*), Lyon, International Agency for Research on Cancer

ALCOHOL DRINKING

1. GENERAL INTRODUCTION: ALCOHOL DRINKING AND THE PUBLIC HEALTH

The terms 'alcohol' and 'alcoholic beverages' tend to be used interchangeably to designate the product consumed, and the same practice has been followed in this monograph. A distinction is made, however, between alcohol or alcoholic beverages and the substance ethanol. This monograph includes only data relevant to the consumption of alcoholic beverages by humans: occupational exposures to ethanol and exposures other than by drinking were not considered by the Working Group.

Most human societies have made and used alcoholic beverages. The major exceptions, prior to contact with European cultures, were the Pacific Islanders and the indigenous populations of most of North America (Marshall, 1979). The distillation of alcoholic beverages has a long tradition on the Eurasian continent, beginning in the Far East and moving to Europe *via* Arabia about a millenium ago (Anon., 1966; Lord, 1979). Traditional alcoholic beverages are fermentation products of a wide variety of organic materials, including grain (beer, *shochu*), fruit (wine, cider), sap (palm wine, pulque) and honey (mead); even wood has been used occasionally (Treml, 1982). Since distillation was traditionally associated with pharmacy, many substances other than ethanol have often been included intentionally in distilled drinks. Thus, traditional alcoholic beverages and commercially produced beverages contain many constituents other than ethanol and water (see p. 71).

Alcoholic beverages have a wide variety of functions for humans. They quench thirst, in some parts of the world more hygienically than local water supplies; they are nutritional and, in some situations, can lead to excess caloric intake or an unbalanced diet (Balboni, 1963). It has been estimated that alcohol may provide as much as one-quarter of the caloric intake of male agricultural workers in wine production areas (Lolli *et al.*, 1958). Alcohol has also been used medicinally in many cultures and is present as a solvent in pharmaceutical preparations. It is used in many cultures as a psychoactive substance (Marshall, 1979).

Alcoholic beverages have diverse symbolic functions: alcohol is used in many religious observances; it is often associated with feasting and celebration; having or sharing a drink may be a ritual of solidarity or friendship, of sealing an agreement, of marking a rite of passage or of indicating that normal social constraints are suspended. In different cultures, various powers are attributed to drinking, and diverse behaviours are associated with drunkenness (MacAndrew & Edgerton, 1969; Marshall, 1979). In some societies, intoxication leads to and, to some extent, is used to explain disruptive or violent behaviour.

Abstaining from drinking has also often had a sociocultural meaning. For Muslims, abstention is both a religious duty and a mark of differentiation from those of other faiths.

In ancient China, abstention was expected of those holding government offices (Cherrington, 1924). In nineteenth century Britain, serious persons who wanted to better the lot of their children signed a pledge of abstinence (Harrison, 1971).

In cultures where alcohol is valued, access to it has often been the prerogative of those of higher status. This may reflect a scarcity value, an ideology that intoxication is appropriate only for those of higher status, or fear that intoxication may produce insurrection. It is notable that the access of groups of persons who have been considered to be of socially subordinate status, such as women and children, has frequently been limited (Knupfer & Room, 1964). However, abstinence among women has decreased dramatically in many countries, and, in a number of countries, young people have also increased their drinking (World Health Organization, 1980).

In traditional societies, the availability of alcoholic beverages depended mainly on agricultural abundance and climate. In a tropical climate, production of alcoholic beverages may be a simple task, whereas in preindustrial times, in regions such as Iceland, alcoholic beverages were all imported (Room, 1983). Alcohol has long been an item of trade: the abundance of amphoras from the classical world testifies to the long-standing importance of wine in Mediterranean trade patterns (Johnson, 1985). The spread of distilled beverages in the seventeenth and eighteenth centuries partly reflects their function as a form of agricultural surplus that did not spoil and was relatively transportable (Rorabaugh, 1979).

In traditional societies with no cash economy and poor transportation connections, fermented beverages were, and still are, consumed relatively quickly after their production, before spoiling. Such production is frequently seasonal — for example, at harvest time or on festive occasions — and is often associated with a culturally sanctioned drinking pattern or intermittent extreme intoxication, where all the alcoholic beverage produced for the occasion is rapidly consumed. In such circumstances, variations in agricultural supply can limit drinking (Anon., 1966).

Such traditional societies have gradually disappeared over the last few centuries as more peoples are incorporated into a global market economy (Wolf, 1982). Groups moving from a traditional into an urban cash economy often preserve their drinking patterns initially, but engage in them more frequently (Caetano *et al.*, 1983). In general, the advent of industrially produced alcoholic beverages with an indefinite shelf-life, improvements in transportation and participation in a cash economy have erased constraints on availability of alcohol. Under these circumstances, constraints on consumption depend on state controls on availability and price and, for example, on religious and social limitations.

With time, home-made and locally produced alcoholic beverages tend to be replaced by industrially produced alcohol (World Health Organization, 1980). In the USA and the UK, industrially brewed beer replaced cider in the nineteenth century (Anon., 1966). Today, the process continues in countries such as Zambia and Mexico, as lager-style beer replaces opaque beer and pulque. The attractiveness of industrially produced alcoholic beverages is enhanced by the cosmopolitan, high-status connotations given to them by advertisers (Moser, 1985; Rosovsky, 1986). Governments also have a fiscal interest in the industrialization of production, since it facilitates the collection of revenues based on drinking. Although the epidemiological evidence reviewed in this monograph is based primarily on commercially produced alcoholic beverages, it should be kept in mind that much of the world's alcohol consumption is of noncommercially produced alcoholic beverages (Walsh & Grant, 1985).

Even in Europe, the current level of availability of alcoholic beverages is a relatively recent historical phenomenon. In the seventeenth and eighteenth centuries, spirits shifted from a pharmaceutical status to an item of everyday consumption, as industrial production methods flooded the market. Technological innovations transformed beer production, starting in the latter part of the nineteenth century, from a craft producing beverages for local and immediate consumption to an integrated industry producing a beverage that could be transported worldwide and stored almost indefinitely (Anon., 1966). Improvements in agricultural methods and the development of disease-resistant vines have allowed greatly increased wine production and consumption. Thus, wine consumption in France quadrupled in the last decades of the nineteenth century (Johnson, 1985).

Effects of drinking

Alcohol consumption is associated with many health problems, which can be divided into three main types: chronic physical problems, casualty and disability problems, and mental problems.

Physical health problems include, notably, cirrhosis of the liver (discussed on pp. 146-147), cancers at various sites (discussed in section 5, p. 153), effects on the developing embryo and fetus (discussed on pp. 148-151), and other diseases affecting the gastrointestinal, cardiovascular, respiratory, nervous and reproductive systems (World Health Organization, 1980). The relationship between alcohol intake and the occurrence of cardiovascular disease appears to be J-shaped, with the risk for abstainers being slightly higher than that in moderate drinkers (i.e., those consuming fewer than two or three drinks per day) and substantially lower than that for heavy drinkers (Marmot, 1984). The reduced incidence of coronary heart disease may explain the lower total mortality among moderate drinkers which has often been found in relation to alcohol intake. Possible confounding effects of socioeconomic variables cannot be excluded in the light of their correlation with past alcohol consumption, and data with regard to women are limited (Marmot, 1984; Friedman & Kimball, 1986).

Alcohol is causally implicated in many types of casualty, including road-traffic deaths, drownings, burns, falls, suicides and acute poisoning. Mental problems associated with drinking include a wide range of neurological consequences of prolonged heavy consumption, depression and other mental disorders. A prominent adverse consequence of drinking is the alcohol dependence syndrome (World Health Organization, 1980), a term which encompasses both physical and psychological aspects of addiction to alcohol (Edwards *et al.*, 1977; Walsh & Grant, 1985). The pharmacological basis of alcohol dependence has been reviewed (Edwards *et al.*, 1977).

Although, at an individual level, alcohol consumption can be associated with domestic violence and neglect, and criminal behaviour, and, at a collective level, can result in loss of production due to absenteeism and reduced efficiency (World Health Organization, 1980), the drinking of alcoholic beverages is a source of pleasure and of solace to many people and facilitates human contacts in many societies.

In studying potential causal relations between alcohol consumption and health or social problems, it is important to consider and investigate the aspect of alcohol consumption that may be involved — total volume of ethanol consumption, frequency of bouts of drunkenness or length of time spent with the amount of blood-alcohol above a given level. Questions of exposure measurement in epidemiological studies are discussed in detail in section 5.1 (p. 153).

Responding to alcohol-related problems

Efforts by society to reduce the toll of alcohol-related problems are cited in the earliest written records of mankind. Societies and ethnic groups in which there are now few alcohol-related problems reacted in different ways: for example, during several Chinese dynasties severe controls were enacted on drinking, while Israelite prophets preached against drunkenness and its consequences. The prohibitions on drinking in the Koran were proclaimed in response to a situation in Middle Eastern societies during the sixth century.

Until the late nineteenth century, governmental actions to reduce alcohol-related problems rarely took account of public health issues (Walsh & Grant, 1985); authorities were more concerned with social disorder, destitution, vagrancy and vices, which were seen as being due to drinking. The role of drinking casualties did not become a matter of policy concern until the age of railways and automobiles, and the involvement of drinking in such specific disorders as cirrhosis and delirium tremens was clarified only in the nineteenth century. Although small groups of physicians actively pressed for temperance policies in a number of countries, the consequences of drinking usually played a small part in policy decisions during this period (Bruun, 1985). As a reaction to prohibitionist claims, there was a tendency in the medical literature of the 1940s and 1950s in some countries to discount any chronic biological consequences of drinking; in the 1940s, a review of findings on the biological effects of drinking disclaimed any connection between drinking and cancer, and even questioned a direct relationship with cirrhosis (Haggard & Jellinek, 1942).

Since the Second World War, public health considerations have taken priority in actions to combat alcohol-related problems. Responding to the high prevalence of alcohol-related medical problems among their patients, French doctors led the way to some extent, with the concept of the 'alcoholization' of society (Jellinek, 1954). In other countries in the 1950s, actions to reduce the role of alcohol-related traffic casualties had been instituted (Moore & Gerstein, 1981; Mäkelä *et al.*, 1981). Otherwise, the responsibility of public health officials in the management of alcohol-related problems was limited to the provision of treatment for relatively marginalized populations of 'alcoholics', without regard to the general population of 'normal drinkers' (Room, 1984). Arguments for instituting preventive activities orientated towards the long-term biological consequences of drinking are a relatively new phenomenon in many countries, although they have become widespread in recent years (see, for example, Bruun *et al.*, 1975; World Health Organization, 1980).

Increased interest in the chronic biological effects of drinking also reflects objective conditions: in most industrialized societies, alcohol consumption levels, after having reached a low in the 1930s, rose steeply in the period after the Second World War, resulting in substantial increases in mortality from cirrhosis and in other indicators of biological effects (Mäkelä *et al.*, 1981). In many countries, alcohol consumption levels have now stabilized, but at much higher levels than earlier in the century. In the meantime, the number of known chronic biological effects of alcohol has grown considerably, although dose-response curves are not well established. In particular, the importance of the pattern of drinking, as distinct from the overall volume of drinking, is not well understood for many conditions.

Societies have adopted a number of strategies to diminish alcohol-related problems (Moore & Gerstein, 1981). Some measures aim at reducing the consequences without necessarily affecting drinking patterns themselves; others aim at structuring drinking and associated behaviour in order to minimize harmful effects; and a third type aims at reducing the level of consumption, particularly heavy drinking (Bruun *et al.*, 1975). While the first two types of measure are important elements of an overall plan to tackle social and casualty problems, the third type is the most important with regard to chronic biological consequences.

In most societies, there is some form of control to restrict the availability of alcohol. The state may monopolize the sale or production of alcohol, or may license others to sell or produce on condition that they comply with licence requirements. Commonly, some limits are placed on the hours and conditions of sale. Investigation of the effectiveness of such actions suggests that it is limited unless the restrictions are very stringent. Price control, normally through excise taxes, has been used for a long time but is often motivated more by fiscal interest than by concern for the public health. Recently, there has been renewed interest in, and evidence of the effectiveness of, taxes as a constraint on consumption levels (Grant, 1985). Other controls that have proved effective include rationing the supply available to any one individual and setting minimum age levels below which drinking is not permitted. Control measures are most likely to be effective in the long term when popular support is substantial. Major reductions in the consumption level in a society tend to occur either in situations of social crisis, such as war, or in response to large-scale popular movements and shifts in consciousness concerning drinking (Moser, 1985).

Education and public persuasion campaigns have been a popular strategy for prevention in all societies concerned about the level of alcohol-related problems. Such campaigns are unlikely to be strongly effective if they are pursued in isolation from other strategies (World Health Organization, 1980; Moser, 1985).As with cigarette smoking, education and persuasion efforts are likely to be potentiated in periods of shift in popular sentiments concerning drinking. In the period after the Second World War, many industrial societies built up extensive alcoholism treatment systems, partly with the aim of reducing the rate of alcohol-related problems in the population (Mäkelä *et al.*, 1981). While such treatment is crucial, studies have shown that there is a substantial relapse rate after any type of treatment, suggesting that the provision of treatment and early case finding is only moderately effective in preventing future alcohol problems (Miller & Hester, 1986). It is in this context and because of growing popular opinion to reduce alcohol consumption in many countries that broader approaches to alcohol problems have come to the fore (World Health Organization, 1980; Walsh & Grant, 1985).

2. WORLDWIDE PRODUCTION AND USE OF ALCOHOLIC BEVERAGES

2.1 Worldwide production

(*a*) *Kinds of alcoholic beverages*

The Standard International Trade Classification (SITC; United Nations, 1961) defines the following classes of alcoholic beverages, which corresponds to the Brussels Tariff Nomenclature (BTN) of the Customs Cooperation Council:

SITC				BTN
112	Alcoholic beverages			
	112.1	Wine of fresh grapes (including grape must)		
		112.1(1)	Grape must, in fermentation or with fermentation arrested, otherwise than by the addition of alcohol	22.04
		112.1(2)	Wine of fresh grapes; grape must with fermentation arrested by the addition of alcohol	22.05
		112.1(3)	Vermouths and other wines of fresh grapes flavoured with aromatic extracts	22.06
	112.2	Cider and fermented beverages (not elsewhere specified)		22.07
	112.3	Beer (including ale, stout, porter)		22.03
	112.4	Distilled alcoholic beverages		22.09

Most of the available data refer to three groups of alcoholic beverages: beer, wine and distilled spirits. These classes are based on raw materials and production methods, not on ethanol content, but the classes are not clear-cut. Fortified wines, for example, are classified as wines, even though spirits are added during their production; while wine blended with distilled beverages to make a cocktail belongs to the category 'distilled spirits', as do aperitifs, unless they are made of wine from fresh grapes. In the tables in this section, other kinds of fermented beverages, such as cider, fruit wines, rice wine, saké, palm wine, cactus wine and pulque, are sometimes included in statistics for other groups; for instance, fruit wines are counted as wines. The quantities of these other beverages are small in a global perspective, although they are important at a national level.

In addition to commercial production, various types of home-produced alcoholic beverages are common in many countries, particularly in developing countries. It is hard to estimate the quantities of such beverages that are consumed, and very little documentation exists on their chemical composition and possible toxicity.

Table 1 summarizes the average ethanol content and content per glass of some alcoholic beverages. It is worth noting that the amount of ethanol consumed in a standard measure of most drinks is approximately the same for beer, wine and spirits. The ethanol content of beverages can be measured either by weight or by volume. In this section of the monograph, ethanol content is given by volume; the conversion factor is 1 ml = 789 mg.

Table 1. Approximate ethanol content of various alcoholic beverages per drink[a]

Beverage	Ethanol content (%)		Average standard glass		Ethanol per drink	
	Vol.	Weight	USA (fl oz (ml))	Europe (ml)	ml	g
Beer	5	4	12 (350)	250	12–17.5	10–14
Wine	12	10	4 (120)	100	12–14.5	10–12
Spirits	40	32	1.5 (45)	35	14–18	11–14.2

[a]Adapted from Hoofdproduktschap voor Akkerbouwprodukten (1984); Anon. (1985a)

(b) *Production methods*

The production of beer, wine and spirits can be outlined as follows:

beer is brewed by fermenting malted barley, and occasionally other cereals, to which hops are added;

wine is made by fermenting grape juice (white wine) or crushed grapes (red wine and rosé). In fortified wines, such as sherry and port, distilled spirits are added;

distilled spirits are made from different sources of starch or sugar: cereals, molasses (from sugar beets), grapes, potatoes, cherries, plums or other fruits; when the sugar has fermented, the liquid is distilled.

(i) *Beer* (from Jackson, 1982)

In the basic recipe for brewing beer, barley is turned into malt, the malt is cooked in hot water, hops are added as a flavouring and preserving agent, and yeast is introduced to induce fermentation. Modern industrial processes have, in some cases, replaced traditional brewing practices, resulting in substantial variations in composition.

Without malting, the barley grain cannot be fermented; its starches have to be broken down into their component sugars, maltose and dextrin, and it is principally maltose that is later converted to ethanol and carbon dioxide through fermentation. Controlled germination is induced by steeping the barley in water. Traditionally, the grain is spread on a floor during the malting period, which may last for a week or ten days. Germination is then arrested by drying, or by roasting if a dark beer is to be produced. When other grains such as rice and corn are used, the carbohydrates are made soluble by precooking.

The malt and other grains are mixed with hot water to form a mash, which is heated for up to 6 h. A clarified liquid, known as the wort, is extracted and fed into a brewing kettle, where it is heated to boiling point and boiled for 1-2.5 h. Hops are then added. After brewing, the spent hops are removed, and the wort is cooled before being transferred to the fermentation vessel, where the yeast is added.

Fermentation is basically of two types — bottom fermentation (producing lager-type beers) and top fermentation (producing ales and stouts or dark beers) — distinguished by the location of the yeast in the fermentation vessel. Bottom fermentation takes place at low temperatures. Primary fermentation (one or two weeks) is carried out at approximately 5-10°C; secondary fermentation ('maturing', 'ageing', 'ripening', 'conditioning', 'lagering') takes place at an even lower temperature (≤2°C) for four weeks or more. When the beer reaches condition it is usually filtered. Top fermentation takes place at higher temperatures; primary fermentation, at 15-20°C, lasts for about a week, and maturation at the brewery lasts for only a few days. Traditional English ale, one of the most typical top-fermented beers, is not filtered, so that secondary fermentation continues while the beer is in the barrel.

Beer may or may not be pasteurized; pasteurization stabilizes the beer, but also affects the taste. Bottled beer is more likely to be pasteurized to enable longer storage, and is also more likely to contain preservatives. Draught beer is more commonly sold unpasteurized, but this varies in different parts of the world.

The ethanol content of beer is often measured by weight. Beer may vary in ethanol content from 2.25% by volume to over 10%. German beers usually contain about 5% alcohol, as do US beers; English ales usually contain 2.5-5.5% by volume (mild ale, 2.5-3.5%; bitter ale, 3-5.5%). Recent developments in different countries include stronger beers, also called 'malt liquors', containing up to 10% ethanol, and weaker beers, so-called 'low-alcohol' beers. In western Australia, for instance, a beer with only 0.9% ethanol has taken 15% of the beer market (Smith, 1987). In many countries, taxation and sales regulations are related to ethanol content — stronger beers are more heavily taxed and sold only in special outlets.

(ii) *Wine* (from Johnson, 1985)

Wine is made basically by fermentation of grapes, during which their sugar content, or part of it, is converted into ethanol and carbon dioxide by yeast. Traditionally, the natural yeasts on the grape skins are used, but in modern industrial wine-making yeast may be added.

White wine is made by fermenting only the grape juice obtained by pressing grapes. To make red wine, the grapes are crushed, and fermentation takes place before the juice is separated from the residue. Rosé wine is made by fermentation beginning when the grapes are crushed; however, the juice is run into a separate vat after a short time. Red wine gets its colour from the skin of the grapes, and its chemical composition is altered due to the presence of tannins in the skin. The sweetness of the wine depends on the sweetness of the grapes and on the length of fermentation; in the production of sweet wines, fermentation must be stopped before all of the sugar is converted into ethanol. Fermentation can be stopped by adding sulphites or by filtering off the yeast; it can also be stopped by adding alcohol (generally brandy) to raise the level up to or exceeding 15%, as for fortified wines, such as sherry and port (Lord, 1979).

Fermentation usually takes about two weeks at 24°C for red wine and four to six weeks at 15.5°C for white wines. This is followed by a second fermentation, the malolactic fermentation, during which bacteria work on the malic acid to convert it to lactic acid, which is less sharp to the taste. The second fermentation may take place in barrels, during which the wine extracts different substances from the wood. In the case of sparkling wines, the second fermentation takes place in bottles and may continue for several months; the carbon dioxide content determines the extent to which the wine will be sparkling. Maturation continues during storage, which may last for several years. Red wines of high quality are often stored for a long time; white wines are generally consumed within a few years, with the exception of wines such as sweet French Sauternes and Italian Tokay wines.

The ethanol content of wine usually varies from 8 to 15% by volume. Recently, light wines with an ethanol content of 4.5% were introduced onto markets such as the USA, primarily as 'low-calorie' wines. In so-called nonalcoholic wines, the ethanol content has been reduced to 0.5% (Hiaring, 1986).

Although grapes are by far the most common raw material for wine, it can also be made from other fruits and from berries, particularly in countries where grapes are not grown. Cider, which is fermented from apples or pears, is a common alcoholic beverage in many countries, although its consumption has declined in industrialized areas.

(iii) *Spirits* (from Lord, 1979)

Spirits are made by distilling a liquid, or wash, that contains ethanol produced by fermentation of a base ingredient that contains sugar or starch. The purpose of distillation is to increase the ethanol content and to eliminate fractions of the base liquid that are not wanted in the final product. The process of distilling involves heating the liquid so that ethanol and other volatile substances evaporate, passing the vapours through a cooling system, and collecting the liquid which then contains less water and other unwanted substances. The liquid may be redistilled, or rectified, several times to increase its purity: this process leads ultimately to a colourless neutral spirit, which can then be flavoured. In many cases, some of the original flavouring components of the base liquid are retained. The traditional distilling process is carried out in a 'pot-still', and is still used in the production of cognac, malt whisky, most Irish whiskeys and some of the flavouring used in liqueurs. For many other spirits, distillation is performed in a 'continuous still', consisting of two or three columns; the heat of the product at the end of the process is used to warm the cold liquid that enters the system. The pot-still allows greater retention of the original flavouring elements in the base liquid, while continuous distillation is more efficient. After distillation, water is often added to achieve the desired strength of the beverage.

Spirits are made from many raw materials; these may contain sugar, such as sugar cane, molasses, grapes and other fruits, or starch which is converted into sugar by malting, such as grains and potatoes. Wood is also used as a raw material. Brandies are made from a fruit mash or from wine; cognac and other varieties are made from grapes, but numerous other types are made from other fruits, such as apples, pears, pineapples, plums and strawberries. Malted grains are the base of all types of whisky. Scotch malt whisky is made almost entirely from barley, but in other whiskies grains such as maize, oats, rye and wheat are used. Gins and vodkas are produced from grain or potatoes; both are distilled to a fairly high ethanol content, sometimes filtered through charcoal to attain purity, and then, in the case of gin, flavoured. Sugar cane and molasses are used to produce rum; and the Mexican spirit, tequila, is distilled from a mash made from cactus.

Flavouring is an important part of spirits. The large variety of substances used in flavouring can be grouped into three main categories: herbs and spices, seeds and plants, and fruits. The flavours can be obtained from the raw ingredients by pressure, by extraction or by distillation from an alcoholic solution. One or more ingredients may be soaked in alcohol, which is sometimes warmed to hasten the process. Another method is to mix the ingredient with alcohol and then distil the mixture; the condensed vapour then contains a high proportion of both ethanol and the flavouring components of the added ingredient, provided these components are volatile. Many flavouring ingredients may be used in a single beverage. The recipes are often closely guarded secrets, but it is well known that ingredients such as angelica, aniseed, blackcurrant, camomile, caraway, cinnamon, cloves, coffee, juniper, lavender, lemon, orange and rose petals are used, as are many other fruits and berries. Aperitifs and appetizers are among the richly flavoured spirits, as are liqueurs. A list of flavour compounds is given in Appendix 1.

The ethanol content of spirits varies. Generally speaking, whisky, vodka, schnapps, rum, liqueurs and brandies contain around 40% ethanol by volume, but may be stronger. Aperitifs usually have an ethanol content of around 20%. There are three different ways of indicating the ethanol content. In this monograph, the simple percentage by volume is used, which is also called the French or Gay-Lussac system. American proof is equal to twice the percentage of ethanol by volume; thus, spirits that contain 50% ethanol are 100 proof. The British proof system is slightly more complicated, 100 proof containing 57% ethanol by volume and pure (100% ethanol) alcohol being 175 proof.

(iv) *Mixed drinks*

Beer, wine and spirits may be consumed without adding any other liquid. In some countries, however, beer and wine are consumed as mixtures with other beverages, and, in the case of wine, mixed with water. Mixtures of spirits and soft drinks are sold; spirits may be drunk with ice or water, or mixed with other beverages in various dilutions.

(c) *Production volumes*

The available figures on production of and trade in alcoholic beverages have been reviewed by Walsh and Grant (1985), and the following discussion relies mainly upon that report.

The production of alcoholic beverages has increased substantially in most parts of the world since the Second World War, and world production of alcohol showed an 83% increase between the early 1960s and 1983 (Kortteinen, 1986). Overall commercial production of alcoholic beverages between 1965 and 1980 increased by 50%, measured in terms of 100% ethanol content. On a per head basis, the increase during the same period was 15% (Table 2).

(i) *Beer*

World commercial production of beer more than doubled between 1960 and 1980; and, in terms of weight, over half of the world's alcohol is now produced in the form of beer (Kortteinen, 1986). As shown in Table 3, Europe, the USA and Canada accounted for almost 80% of the total production in 1960; although these areas increased their production very rapidly, their share of world production had fallen to 70% by 1980, because of the even more rapid increase in production in other regions. It should be noted that information on the production of beer by traditional, small-scale methods is not included in these figures, although it may be considerable in certain parts of the world, notably in West and Central Africa. World production per head rose by 50% during the period 1960-80, with Europe, North America, Australia and New Zealand remaining the areas with the highest production per head. As shown in Table 4, seven of the ten largest producers in 1960 were still among the ten largest producers in 1981; Japan, Mexico, Brazil and Nigeria were among the 25 largest producers in that year.

(ii) *Wine*

Wine production has increased since the Second World War, except in North Africa, where there was a reduction following the emigration of a large part of the French population. In terms of weight, about one-fifth of all alcoholic beverages now produced are as wine (Kortteinen, 1986). Since 1950, wine production has increased by about 80%, and, since 1965, by a little over 20%. Since, in general, this growth has parallelled the population growth since the War, current world production per head is about the same as in the 1950s. Wine-growing has always been concentrated in Europe and in areas of European settlement (Table 5). Table 6 shows the production in the largest producing countries: ten countries accounted for 84.4% of world production in 1965 and for 80.5% in 1980.During the 1980s, production in the 'new' wine countries has continued to increase, while the surplus in traditional European wine-producing countries has led to attempts to limit the volume of production and emphasize prestigious varieties.

(iii) *Spirits*

Table 7 presents available data on the production of spirits in 1965 and 1980. These figures are less complete than those for production of beer and wine, especially in Latin America. Three-quarters of the amount recorded in 1965, and slightly more in 1980, was produced in Europe, the USSR, the USA and Canada; a fall in production over the period was seen in Latin America, but increases were notable in the USA, Canada, Japan, Europe

Table 2. Total commercial production of alcoholic beverages (beer, wine and spirits)[a]

Region or country	1965								1980							
	Beer		Wine		Spirits		Total		Beer		Wine		Spirits		Total	
	Volume[b]	Per head[c]	Volume	Per head	Volume	Per head	Volume	Per head	Volume	Per head	Volume	Per head	Volume	Per head	Volume	Per head
Africa	0.35	0.1	2.5	0.8	0.2	0.1	3.1	1.0	1.9	0.4	1.2	0.3	0.2	0.1	3.3	0.7
Asia, excluding Japan	0.3	0.0	0.1	0.0	0.7	0.0	1.1	0.1	1.1	0.0	0.2	0.0	3.0	0.1	4.3	0.2
Japan	0.9	0.9	0.0	0.0	1.2	1.2	2.1	2.1	2.0	1.7	0.0	0.0	2.6	2.2	4.6	4.0
Australia and New Zealand	0.7	5.0	0.1	0.7	0.1	0.7	0.9	6.4	1.0	5.6	0.5	2.8	0.4	2.2	1.9	10.6
Oceania, excluding Australia and New Zealand	0.0	0.0	0.0	0.0	0.0	0.0	0.0	0.0	0.1	2.0	0.0	0.0	0.0	0.0	0.1	2.0
North America	5.4	2.7	1.0	0.5	3.2	1.5	9.6	4.7	11.0	4.5	2.2	0.9	6.5	2.7	19.7	8.1
Latin America and Caribbean	1.1	0.4	2.75	1.1	2.3	0.9	6.1	2.4	3.3	0.9	3.5	1.0	2.0	0.5	6.8	2.4
Europe, excluding the USSR	10.9	2.4	22.8	5.1	5.1	1.1	38.8	8.7	16.2	3.3	26.3	5.4	10.2	2.1	52.7	10.9
USSR	1.4	0.6	1.5	0.6	7.4	3.2	10.3	4.4	2.7	1.0	3.5	1.3	8.8	3.3	15.0	5.6
World	22.4	0.7	30.9	0.9	20.5	0.6	73.8	2.2	39.3	0.9	37.5	0.8	33.3	0.8	110.1	2.5

[a] From Walsh & Grant (1985); based on an assumed ethanol content of: beer, 4.4%; wine, 11.0%; spirits, 40%. Totals may not equal the sum of the individual entries since these have been rounded off.

[b] Million hectolitres of ethanol

[c] Litres of ethanol

Table 3. Commercial beer production[a]

Region or country	1960		1970		1980	
	Total[b]	Per head[c]	Total	Per head	Total	Per head
Africa	5.0	1.8	16.6	4.7	43.6	9.3
Asia, excluding Japan	3.2	0.2	10.0	0.5	25.1	1.0
Japan	9.3	9.9	30.0	28.8	45.5	38.7
Australia and New Zealand	13.0	102.4	18.9	122.7	23.2	130.3
Oceania, excluding Australia and New Zealand	0.0	0.0	0.1	2.5	1.6	32.0
North America	122.2	61.4	173.8	77.2	249.4	101.4
Latin America and Caribbean	25.3	11.8	50.2	17.7	73.9	20.1
Europe, excluding the USSR	197.5	46.4	304.7	71.7	368.8	76.2
USSR	25.0	11.7	41.9	19.6	61.3	23.0
World	400.5	13.4	646.2	17.6	892.4	20.2

[a]From Walsh & Grant (1985)
[b]Million hectolitres
[c]Litres

Table 4. Commercial beer production by major producing countries (total production in million hectolitres)[a]

Country	1960	Country	1981
USA	110.8	USA	227.3
Germany, Federal Republic of	53.7	Germany, Federal Republic of	93.7
United Kingdom	43.4	USSR	62.9
USSR	25.0	United Kingdom	61.7
France	16.7	Japan	46.4
Czechoslovakia	14.1	Mexico	29.3
German Democratic Republic	13.4	Brazil	24.3
Canada	11.4	German Democratic Republic	24.1
Australia	10.5	Czechoslovakia	23.9
Belgium	10.1	Canada	22.7
Japan	9.3	France	21.7
Mexico	8.5	Spain	20.9
Poland	6.7	Australia	19.8
Colombia	6.1	Netherlands	16.6
Brazil	5.7	Belgium	13.8
Austria	5.1	Yugoslavia	12.2
Ireland	4.1	Venezuela	12.0
Denmark	4.0	Colombia	12.0
Netherlands	3.6	Romania	11.5
Hungary	3.6	Poland	10.5
Spain	3.4	South Africa	10.4
Switzerland	3.3	Italy	9.0
Italy	2.5	Denmark	8.1
Venezuela	2.4	Nigeria	8.0
Sweden	2.4	Austria	8.0

[a]From Walsh & Grant (1985)

Table 5. Commercial wine production[a]

Region or country	1948–52		1965		1980	
	Total[b]	Per head[c]	Total	Per head	Total	Per head
Africa	17.1	7.8	23.0	7.4	10.9	2.3
Asia	0.5	0.0	1.3	0.1	2.6	0.1
Australia and New Zealand	1.5	15.0	1.8	12.9	4.6	25.8
Oceania, excluding Australia and New Zealand	0.0	0.0	0.0	0.0	0.0	0.0
North America	9.2	5.5	9.2	4.3	19.7	8.0
Latin America	16.5	10.0	25.0	10.0	32.7	8.9
Europe, excluding the USSR	141.3	36.0	207.4	46.6	238.7	49.3
USSR	0.3	0.2	13.4	5.8	32.2	12.1
World	186.4	7.5	281.1	8.4	341.6	7.7

[a]From Walsh & Grant (1985)
[b]Million hectolitres
[c]Litres

Table 6. Commercial wine production by major producing countries (in million hectolitres)[a]

Country	1965	Country	1980
France	68.4	Italy	75.0
Italy	68.2	France	69.1
Spain	26.5	Spain	42.6
Argentina	18.3	USSR	32.2
Portugal	14.7	Argentina	23.3
Algeria	14.0	USA	18.0
USSR	13.4	Portugal	9.4
USA	8.5	Romania	7.6
Romania	5.2	Germany, Federal Republic of	7.1
Yugoslavia	5.2	Yugoslavia	6.9
Germany, Federal Republic of	4.6	South Africa	6.3
Greece	4.1	Chile	5.7
Chile	3.6	Australia	4.7
South Africa	3.6	Greece	4.4
Morocco	3.5	Bulgaria	4.0
Bulgaria	3.4	Austria	3.1
Hungary	2.2	Poland	3.0
Brazil	1.9	Brazil	2.7
Tunisia	1.8	Algeria	2.6
Australia	1.8	Hungary	2.4
Poland	1.6	Czechoslovakia	1.4
Austria	1.4	Morocco	1.0
Switzerland	1.0	Canada	1.0
Uruguay	0.9	Switzerland	0.8
Canada	0.8	Turkey	0.7
Czechoslovakia	0.7	Tunisia	0.7
Turkey	0.5	Mexico	0.7
Cyprus	0.3	Cyprus	0.6
Peru	0.1	Uruguay	0.5
		New Zealand	0.5

[a]From Walsh & Grant (1985)

Table 7. Commercial production of spirits[a]

Region or country	1965		1980	
	Total[b]	Per head[c]	Total	Per head
Africa	0.4	0.1	0.4	0.1
Asia, excluding Japan	1.8	0.1	7.4	0.3
Japan	2.9	2.9	6.4	5.5
Australia and New Zealand	0.2	1.3	0.1	0.4
Oceania, excluding Australia and New Zealand	0.0	0.0	0.0	0.0
North America	8.1	3.8	16.6	6.7
Latin America and Caribbean	5.7	2.3	4.9	1.3
Europe, excluding the USSR	12.7	2.9	25.5	5.3
USSR	18.5	7.9	22.0	8.2
World	50.3	1.5	83.3	1.9

[a] From Walsh & Grant (1985)
[b] Million hectolitres
[c] Litres

and the USSR. World production of spirits increased by 65% between 1965 and 1980 and production per head by slightly over 25%. The principal producing countries are listed in Table 8. The five largest producers (the USSR, the USA, the UK, France and the Federal Republic of Germany) accounted for over 71% of total production in 1965, but by 1980 this figure had fallen to 54%. Production of spirits rose rapidly between 1965 and 1980 in many countries, notably in the Republic of Korea, Cuba, Mexico and the Philippines. Production by home distilling is not included in the figures, but, in some countries where beverage taxes, and thus retail prices, are high, illegal distilling can be widespread.

Table 8. Commercial production of spirits by major producing countries (in million hectolitres)[a]

Country	1965	1980[b]	Country	1965	1980[b]
USSR	18.5	22.0	Mexico	0.6	1.5
USA	7.7	14.9	Philippines	0.5	1.1
United Kingdom	3.6	4.9	Canada	0.4	1.7
France	3.4	2.8	Bulgaria	0.4	0.5
Germany, Federal Republic of	3.3	3.9	Czechoslovakia	0.4	1.3
			Sweden	0.4	0.5
Japan	2.9	6.4	Colombia	0.3	NA
Spain	2.0	3.1	Hungary	0.2	1.1
Poland	2.0	5.3	Finland	0.2	0.6
Brazil	2.0	NA	Austria	0.2	0.4
Argentina	1.6	NA	Algeria	0.2	NA
Republic of Korea	0.9	5.1	Cuba	0.2	0.4
German Democratic Republic	0.8	2.1	Jamaica	0.2	0.2
			Estimated world total	51.2	89.5

[a] From Walsh & Grant (1985)
[b] 1980 or nearest year with available data; NA, not available

2.2 International trade

International trade in alcoholic beverages has increased in volume and in value over the years, although only a small part of production is traded, accounting for about one-half of 1% of total world trade in the market economy countries during the period 1976-80 (Walsh & Grant, 1985). In general, it is the higher priced products that are traded internationally, mostly between a few industrialized countries. Exports to developing countries consist predominantly of beer.

(a) Beer

Beer is a relatively low-value, bulky commodity and would not therefore be expected to figure prominently in long-distance international trade; technical problems of storage and conservation also render transport of beer over long distances difficult. This situation is changing with improvements in technology (pasteurization and shipping in containers), although it is estimated that only about 2.4% of world production of beer entered into international trade in 1981, compared to 1.6% in 1960 (Walsh & Grant, 1985). Table 9 shows the relative distribution of international trade in beer between market economy countries. Imports to developing market economy countries fell during the 1970s, as production of beer under licence from a parent European or North American company in these countries increased (Walsh & Grant, 1985). The effect of this development on the economy of developing countries is still unclear, but reductions in imports of beer may be offset, at least partly, by increases in imports of raw materials (Kortteinen, 1986). The gross flow of trade in beer exaggerates its net impact on consumption, since several importing countries are also significant exporters.

Table 9. Percentage distribution of international trade in beer by value[a]

Imports			Exports		
Country	1971	1980	Country	1971	1980
USA	14.9	40.8	Netherlands	17.0	30.8
France	10.5	12.0	Germany, Federal Republic of	19.4	17.8
United Kingdom	21.6	7.9	Belgium and Luxembourg	7.0	8.9
Italy	3.4	6.1[b]	Denmark	19.0	8.8
Developing market economy countries	24.8	19.7[b]	United Kingdom	6.6	4.7
			Ireland	10.5	4.0
Other countries	24.8	13.5	Other countries	20.5	25.0

[a] From Walsh & Grant (1985)
[b] 1978

(b) Wine

The trade in wine is dominated by a few industrialized countries. Table 10 shows the percentage distibution of trade in wine between market economy countries; France alone accounted for almost half the total exports of wine, and its share increased slightly between 1973 and 1980. The proportion of the total production of wine that entered into international trade increased from 5.2% in 1965 to 12.4% in 1980, and this, in combination with the increase in travelling, has contributed to the spread of wine drinking to countries outside viticultural regions. Table 11 illustrates the importance of wine exports to four main trading countries. As with beer, however, some of the leading exporters also import wine, in particular France and the Federal Republic of Germany.

Table 10. Percentage distribution of international trade in wine by value in the market economy countries[a]

Imports			Exports		
Country	1973	1980	Country	1973	1980
USA	16.1	18.6	France	43.0	44.7
Germany, Federal Republic of	19.3	18.2	Italy	16.6	21.1
United Kingdom	13.7	14.7	Spain	10.1	9.8
Belgium and Luxembourg	6.5	8.6	Germany, Federal Republic of	5.1	8.9
France	10.8	7.8	Portugal	7.0	6.2
Switzerland	7.0	6.7	Algeria	8.5	–
Netherlands	4.1	6.4	All other market economy countries	3.5	3.1
Canada	9.7	9.3			
Denmark	1.6	2.2			
Italy	3.4	2.1			
All other market economy countries	14.0	11.6			

[a]From Walsh & Grant (1985)

(c) Spirits

As with beer and wine, only the more expensive spirits tend to enter into international trade. Most spirits are exported from the UK, France and Canada (Table 12), where the volumes in 1980 were 5.6, 3.1 and 1.6 million hl, respectively. Imports to the USA in 1979 amounted to 7.7 million hl. The rapid growth in exports ceased during the late 1970s and early 1980s, possibly as a result of economic recession, shortage of foreign exchange and increased consumption of cheaper domestic substitutes. The drop in exports of Scotch whisky to Latin America (especially to Venezuela) and to Nigeria is particularly notable. The importance of the USA as an importer of spirits is clear but has declined, and a wider range of countries now import significant quantities of spirits (Walsh & Grant, 1985).

Table 11. Exports of wine by four main trading countries[a]

Country	1965		1973		1980	
	Volume (million hl)	% of domestic production	Volume (million hl)	% of domestic production	Volume (million hl)	% of domestic production
France	4.1	6.0	9.0	10.8	11.8	17.0
Italy	2.4	3.5	9.5	12.3	14.7	19.6
Spain	2.2	8.3	3.8	9.5	6.1	14.3
Portugal	2.5	17.0	2.0	18.0	1.4	21.2

[a]From Walsh & Grant (1985)

Table 12. Percentage distribution of international trade in spirits by value in the market economy countries[a]

Imports[b]			Exports[c]		
Country	1970	1979	Country	1970	1980
USA	54.8	31.6	United Kingdom	50.0	49.6
Germany, Federal Republic of	5.8	8.3	France	19.2	25.7
United Kingdom	4.9	7.3	Canada	17.5	6.8
Japan	1.4	7.0	Ireland	0.2	2.3
France	3.9	4.1	USA	2.4	1.8
Italy	2.5	3.7	Netherlands	1.4	1.7
Belgium and Luxembourg	1.8	3.3	Spain	0.7	1.3
Canada	3.1	2.7	Mexico	0.2	1.0
Other market economy countries	21.8	32.0	Other market economy countries	8.4	9.8

[a]From Walsh & Grant (1985)
[b]Total value (in US $): 1970, 900 million; 1979, 3500 million
[c]Total value (in US $): 1970, 900 million; 1980, 3900 million

2.3 Trends in consumption

By the middle of the nineteenth century, intake of alcoholic beverages was high in most countries in Europe and North America, but, at the turn of the century, there was a decline in consumption which continued until the period between the two world wars. This downward trend was particularly strong with respect to distilled beverages, and especially pronounced in the spirit-drinking countries of northern and eastern Europe compared to countries with a high daily intake of wine. Such patterns ('long waves') of consumption of alcoholic beverages are notable in two respects: firstly, they are surprisingly common across countries, despite differences in general economic development and in drinking habits. Secondly, none of the factors commonly proposed to explain these consumption habits — such as buying power, amount of leisure time, social misery or industrialization and urbanization — presents patterns of variation over time similar to the variations in consumption of alcoholic beverages (Mäkelä *et al.*, 1981). A partial explanation of lower consumption in the first decades of the twentieth century in many industrialized countries may be the influence of the reform movements, including the international temperance movement, in preceding decades.

In contrast, the last few decades have been a period of increasing consumption in developed countries, with some countries approaching the peak levels of the nineteenth century. The largest growth rates have been recorded in countries with originally relatively low levels of average consumption; a few viticultural countries with very high initial levels of consumption showed no increase. In different countries, patterns of drinking tended to be aligned with type of beverage, but changes in economic structure and living conditions, large-scale migration, increased economic independence and relative isolation from wider social networks of individuals and families during the postwar period in industrialized countries led to weakening of local and subcultural traditions and to a more international pattern of consumption. The increase in consumption of alcoholic beverages slowed down or levelled off in many countries in the 1970s, and some decreases were recorded. This phenomenon has been explained partially by economic difficulties experienced in most industrialized countries and by changes in living conditions and life styles (Mäkelä *et al.*, 1981).

In the developing countries, the variation in trends over the last 30 years has undoubtedly been greater. Most of the available information points toward increases in consumption, except in areas such as Muslim countries (Moser, 1985). In many developing countries local alcohol industries, which provide a base for other industries (glass, packaging, etc.), have been encouraged, as they serve as a source of state revenue and obviate the use of foreign exchange for imported beverages. Once developed, these industries tend to create their own demand, so that the overall rates of consumption rise. In most cases, new factories produce European-style beverages — beer or spirits; and in parts of the developing world, European-style beverages are gradually replacing traditional beverages, although at present both types are consumed. Improvements in transportation and distribution also tend to have a direct, dramatic effect on the trade and consumption of alcoholic beverages (Marshall, 1982; Rootman & Moser, 1984).

(*a*) *Total consumption per head*

There are wide variations in the rates of consumption of alcoholic beverages between countries and regions. Total consumption of alcohol per head is often calculated as the difference between the quantities produced and imported and the quantities exported and in stock, or on the basis of sales statistics collected for taxation purposes. Neither calculation includes noncommercial production of alcoholic beverages or tax-free importation by individual travellers between countries. A report from the Addiction Research Foundation (1985) in Toronto, Canada, covering 164 countries, gives estimated consumption of 100% alcohol per head for the period 1970-77 (Table 13); two-thirds of the countries experienced an increase in consumption per head, and 10% a doubling of consumption per head, but only 2% showed a decrease of 50% or more. For the period before 1970 and after 1977, data are available for a smaller number of industrialized countries only (Table 13). Table 14 summarizes the changes over the period 1970-77 in different regions of the world; increases can be seen for most regions and for each type of beverage. Sales of spirits, wine and beer per head in some countries in 1985 are shown in Table 15.

In alcohol-producing areas, consumption is dominated by the type of beverage that is produced, which usually accounts for most of the increase in consumption, although other beverages also contribute significantly. In countries where wine is drunk, for instance, there has been a marked increase in consumption of beer and spirits; whereas, in countries where beer was the preferred drink, consumption of wine and spirits has become more general (Walsh & Grant, 1985; Horgan *et al.*, 1986). Overall, there has been no very marked shift in the relative standing of the categories of alcoholic beverages. In both 1960 and 1981, commercially produced beer, wine and spirits contributed approximately equal amounts to world ethanol consumption. The share of beer in the total has risen slightly, however, while that of wine has declined (Walsh & Grant, 1985).

Table 16 shows the growth in consumption of alcoholic beverages for selected countries in which total consumption increased very rapidly over the period 1960-81. With the sole exception of spirits in Austria, consumption of *all* beverages increased in these countries over that period. The rate of increase in the Republic of Korea, the Netherlands and Japan was exceptionally high, and other countries in Africa, Latin America and Asia are already in the initial stages of what may become a similar trend, although the increase may at present be confined to a single beverage (typically beer).

(*b*) *Beer consumption*

Table 17 shows the consumption of beer per head in 1960 and 1981 in the 25 largest consumer countries. The figures are not directly comparable because of differences in population structure: in countries in which a large proportion of the population is under 15 years of age, the average consumption of the drinking population is greater than that shown

Table 13. International statistics: consumption of commercial alcohol (as ethanol) per head for 1960, 1970, 1977 and 1985

Country or area	Ethanol (litres per head)[a]			
	1960[b]	1970[c]	1977[c]	1985[d]
Africa				
Algeria	2.0	0.3	–	–
Angola	–	2.7	2.2	–
Benin	–	0.6	1.2	–
Botswana	–	3.7	2.5	–
Burkina Faso	–	2.3	2.4	–
Burundi	–	13.7	13.8	–
Cameroon	–	6.7	7.0	–
Cape Verde	–	1.0	1.7	–
Central African Republic[e]	–	2.0	–	–
Chad	–	0.5	0.4	–
Comoros	–	0.1	0.1	–
Congo	–	1.4	2.6	–
Côte d'Ivoire	–	1.3	2.0	–
Egypt	–	0.1	0.1	–
Ethiopia	–	0.8	–	–
Gabon	–	3.9	9.6	–
Gambia	0.2	2.0	1.3	–
Ghana	–	1.0	–	–
Guinea	–	0.1	0.1	–
Guinea-Bissau	–	2.9	2.2	–
Kenya	–	1.7	–	–
Liberia	–	0.6	–	–
Libyan Arab Jamahiriya	–	0.01	–	–
Losotho	–	1.7	1.5	–
Madagascar	–	0.7	0.9	–
Malawi	–	2.3	3.0	–
Mali	–	1.0	1.0	–
Mauritania	–	0.1	0.1	–
Mauritius	–	1.4	–	–
Morocco	0.6	0.4	–	–
Mozambique	–	0.8	0.5	–
Niger	–	0.1	0.1	–
Nigeria	–	3.8	3.7	–
Réunion	–	4.0	5.4	–
Rwanda	–	5.4	5.1	–
Sao Tome and Principe	–	5.8	3.6	–
Senegal	–	0.3	0.4	–
Sierra Leone	–	0.2	0.2	–
Somalia	–	0.02	0.01	–
South Africa	1.8	4.3	5.2	4.3
Sudan	–	1.2	–	–
Swaziland	–	3.5	4.0	–
Togo	–	1.4	2.2	–
Tunisia	–	0.8	0.5	–
Uganda	–	12.6	11.7	–
United Republic of Tanzania	–	4.6	4.0	–
Zaire	–	2.7	2.9	–
Zambia	–	3.5	3.1	–
Zimbabwe	–	0.8	0.8	–

Table 13. (contd)

Country or area	Ethanol (litres per head)[a]			
	1960[b]	1970[c]	1977[c]	1985[d]
America, North				
Antigua and Barbuda	-	5.1	3.3	-
Bahamas	-	11.0	9.7	-
Barbados	-	8.0	16.2	-
Belize	-	4.6	2.8	-
Bermuda	-	6.4	6.3	-
Canada	4.8	6.5	8.5	8.0
Costa Rica	-	1.4	2.4	-
Cuba	-	1.5	-	-
Dominica	-	3.7	2.9	-
Dominican Republic	-	2.0	2.1	-
El Salvador	-	0.7	1.8	-
Grenada	-	2.3	2.4	-
Guadeloupe	-	6.5	9.0	-
Guatemala	-	1.4	1.9	-
Haiti	-	4.0	3.9	-
Honduras	-	1.3	1.4	-
Jamaica	-	2.1	2.6	-
Martinique	-	9.5	10.1	-
Mexico	-	2.1	2.4	-
Netherlands Antilles	-	4.4	7.0	-
Nicaragua	-	3.0	2.7	-
Panama	-	2.9	2.8	-
Puerto Rico	-	-	-	-
Saint Christopher and Nevis	-	3.3	2.1	-
Saint Lucia	-	4.7	3.8	-
Saint Vincent and the Grenadines	-	1.4	1.3	-
Trinidad and Tobago	-	2.9	5.2	-
USA	5.2	6.8	8.1	8.0
America, South				
Argentina	9.7	13.1	14.0	8.7
Bolivia	1.6	1.8	2.0	-
Brazil	0.7	2.2	2.4	-
Chile	7.0	6.5	7.1	-
Colombia	2.2	2.2	2.5	-
Ecuador	-	0.9	-	-
French Guinea	-	12.1	10.3	-
Guyana	-	3.5	4.9	-
Paraguay	-	2.1	2.8	-
Peru	-	2.4	2.5	-
Suriname	-	4.3	3.7	-
Uruguay	-	5.6	-	-
Venezuela	-	3.7	4.1	-

Table 13. (contd)

Country or area	Ethanol (litres per head)[a]			
	1960[b]	1970[c]	1977[c]	1985[d]
Asia				
Afghanistan	–	–	–	–
Bangladesh	–	–	–	–
Bhutan	–	2.7	2.7	–
Brunei Darussalam	0.4	0.9	–	–
Burma	–	0.1	–	–
China	–	0.1	–	–
Cyprus	3.3[f]	3.3	3.8	5.6
Democratic Kampuchea	–	0.6	–	–
Democratic People's Republic of Korea	–	2.9	3.4	–
Democratic Yemen	–	0.6	0.3	–
Hong Kong	–	1.8	2.2	–
India	–	–	0.01	–
Indonesia	–	0.02	–	–
Iran (Islamic Republic of)	–	0.2	–	–
Iraq	–	0.2	0.4	–
Israel	2.3[f]	2.8	2.9	–
Japan	–	4.9	–	5.7
Jordan	–	0.1	–	–
Lao People's Democratic Republic	–	0.4	0.3	–
Lebanon	–	1.9	–	–
Macao	–	2.1	2.8	–
Malaysia	–	6.6	6.3	–
Mongolia	–	1.1	2.0	–
Nepal	–	–	–	
Pakistan	–	–	–	–
Philippines	–	3.0	–	–
Republic of Korea	–	3.6	7.0	–
Saudi Arabia	–	–	0.02	–
Singapore	–	1.4	1.7	–
Sri Lanka	–	0.3	–	–
Syrian Arab Republic	–	0.2	–	–
Thailand	–	0.4	0.6	–
Turkey	0.3[f]	0.5	–	1.0
Viet Nam	–	0.3	–	–
Yemen	–	–	–	–
Europe				
Albania	–	0.6	0.6	–
Austria	8.7	11.9	11.5	9.9
Belgium	6.4	8.9	10.1	10.5
Bulgaria	3.8	7.2	–	8.7
Czechoslovakia	5.5	9.1	9.9	9.1
Denmark	4.2	6.3	8.8	9.9
Faröe Islands	–	2.5	3.8	–
Finland	1.8	4.5	6.9	6.5
France	17.3	19.6	17.3	13.3
German Democratic Republic	4.6	6.3	9.1	10.3
Germany, Federal Republic of	6.9	11.2	12.2	10.8

Table 13. (contd)

Country or area	Ethanol (litres per head)[a]			
	1960[b]	1970[c]	1977[c]	1985[d]
Greece	–	5.9	6.3	–
Hungary	6.2	10.1	13.6	11.5
Iceland	1.7	2.7	3.2	4.0
Ireland[g]	3.4	4.2	5.8	6.2
Italy	12.2	14.5	12.4	11.6
Luxembourg	8.3	10.2	14.4	13.0
Malta	–	2.3	3.3	–
Netherlands	2.5	5.7	8.9	8.5
Norway	2.6	3.6	4.5	4.1
Poland	3.8	5.1	8.2	7.0
Portugal	10.4	9.9	14.0	13.1
Romania	4.1	6.3	–	–
Spain	10.3[f]	11.3	12.8	11.8
Sweden	3.7	5.6	6.0	5.0
Switzerland	9.8	10.5	10.6	11.2
United Kingdom	5.1	5.2	6.8	7.1
Yugoslavia	4.7	7.6	6.9	7.7
Oceania				
Australia	6.5	8.2	9.8	9.4
Fiji	–	1.3	2.0	–
French Polynesia	–	9.1	9.0	–
New Caledonia	–	8.6	5.9	–
New Hebrides	–	1.9	1.6	–
New Zealand	6.5	6.7	8.4	9.2
Papua New Guinea	–	0.5	0.7	–
Samoa	–	0.5	1.0	–
Solomon Islands	–	0.3	0.3	–
Tonga	–	0.3	0.7	–
USSR	3.7	5.1	5.2	8.4

[a]Figures were converted into ethanol on the basis of the following average values for ethanol by volume: beer, 5%; fermented beverages, 12%; wine, 12%; vermouths and similar beverages, 18%; distilled beverages, 40%; –, no country- or beverage-specific data available.
[b]From Finnish Foundation for Alcohol Studies (1977)
[c]From Addiction Research Foundation (1985)
[d]From Systembolaget (1986)
[e]Population figures for 1970 are estimates based on the 1968 'recensement instantané' of 1968.
[f]1963
[g]Figures for 1970 are for the 12 months ending 31 March of that year; figures for 1977 correspond to the 12-month period ending 31 December of that year.

Table 14. Percentage change in consumption of commercial alcoholic beverages (as ethanol) per head by type of beverage in six WHO regions, 1970-77[a]

Beverage	Africa	Americas	Eastern Mediter-ranean	Europe	South-east Asia	Western Pacific
Wine	-16.7	6.9	0.0	-4.2	0.0	200.0
Beer	9.1	17.1	8.3	15.6	100.0	20.7
Spirits	11.1	8.8	71.4	4.3	20.0	-24.3
All alcoholic beverages	7.3	11.3	12.5	3.0	25.0	-4.4

[a]From Moser (1985)

Table 15. Sales of alcoholic beverages in litres per head, 1985[a]

Country	Spirits[b]	Wine	Beer
France	5.8	80	40
Portugal	2.0	87	38
Luxembourg	6.3	57	120
Spain	7.5	48	61
Italy	3.0	85	22
Hungary	13.5	25	92
Switzerland	5.5	50	69
Germany, Federal Republic of	5.9	26	146
Belgium	5.3	23	121
German Democratic Republic	12.0	10	142
Austria	3.8	34	112
Denmark	4.0	21	119
Australia	3.3	21	116
New Zealand	4.3	14	115
Czechoslovakia	8.4	16	131
Argentina	2.5	60	10
Bulgaria	7.5	22	60
Netherlands	5.6	15	84
USSR	14.0	13	24
USA	6.8	9	90
Canada[c]	6.6	10	83
Yugoslavia	5.0	26	50
United Kingdom	4.3	10	109
Poland	11.5	8	30
Finland	7.5	4	59
Ireland	4.4	4	100
Japan	6.0	1	38
Cyprus	5.3	12	42
Sweden	5.1	12	35
South Africa	2.8	10	40
Norway	3.5	5	45
Iceland	5.6	7	17
Turkey	1.6	1	4

[a]From Systembolaget (1986)
[b]Values converted from 50% ethanol to litres of beverage with an ethanol content of 40% (a common strength of distilled beverages) by the Working Group
[c]1984

Table 16. Growth in commercial alcoholic beverage consumption (in litres of ethanol per head) in countries in which it has increased rapidly[a]

Country	1960				1981				Increase 1960–81 (%)
	Beer	Wine	Spirits	Total	Beer	Wine	Spirits	Total	
Republic of Korea	0.1	–	0.7	0.8	1.5	–	5.4	6.9	762
Netherlands	1.0	0.2	1.1	2.3	3.9	1.4	2.6	7.9	243
Japan	1.1	1.3[b]	1.2	3.6	4.3	2.2[b]	3.2	9.7	169
Finland	1.1	0.1	1.3	2.5	2.5	0.5	2.8	5.8	132
German Democratic Republic	3.1	0.3	0.6	4.0	5.7	1.8	1.5	9.0	125
Canada	3.4	0.4	1.4	6.2	6.2	1.1	4.8	12.1	95
Germany, Federal Republic of	2.5	0.2	1.5	4.2	3.8	1.0	3.3	8.1	93
Mexico	1.0	–	0.5	1.5	1.8	–	0.9	2.7	80
Hungary	1.6	3.2	1.4	7.2	3.9	3.5	4.8	12.2	69
Poland	1.0	0.4	2.4	3.8	1.3	0.8	4.3	6.4	68
Denmark	4.2	1.1	1.9	7.2	6.5	2.2	2.9	11.9	61
Austria	3.2	2.3	2.4	7.9	4.6	3.8	1.5	9.9	25

[a] From Walsh & Grant (1985)
[b] Including saké

Table 17. Consumption of commercially produced beer per head (in litres)[a]

Country	1960	Country	1981
Luxembourg	116.4	Germany, Federal Republic of	147.0
Belgium	112.0	German Democratic Republic	141.4
Australia	101.9	Czechoslovakia	140.1
Czechoslovakia	100.1	Gabon	135.0
New Zealand	100.0	Australia	134.4
Germany, Federal Republic of	95.7	Denmark	131.0
United Kingdom	85.1	Belgium	124.0
German Democratic Republic	79.5	Luxembourg	118.6
Austria	71.9	New Zealand	117.7
Denmark	71.4	Ireland	116.4
Ireland	67.3	United Kingdom	111.5
Switzerland	62.9	Austria	104.8
Canada	60.0	USA	93.3
USA	57.9	Netherlands	89.6
Colombia	43.4	Hungary	88.0
Hungary	36.8	Canada	86.4
Venezuela	36.0	Venezuela	79.9
France	35.3	Switzerland	71.0
Sweden	31.1	Bulgaria	60.9
Chile	30.0	Finland	57.1
Cuba	25.1	Spain	55.2
Finland	25.0	Romania	45.0
Norway	24.5	Colombia	45.0
Netherlands	23.8	Norway	44.8
Mexico	22.9	France	44.0

[a] From Walsh & Grant (1985)

by the figures per head. Table 18 gives the average consumption of beer per person 15 years or older, from which it can be seen that some countries with a young population, such as Venezuela, Colombia, Mexico and Panama, are ranked higher. In 1960, high levels of beer consumption were recorded mainly in Europe, North America, Australia and New Zealand, and in a few Latin American countries; in 1981, while consumption had increased in all those countries where it was already high in 1960, a wider range of Latin American countries were among high-consumer countries, as were Gabon and South Africa (Walsh & Grant, 1985).

Consumption of commercially produced beer increased in many countries over the period 1960-81 (Table 19). Although in many instances consumption per head in 1981 was

Table 18. Consumption of commercially produced beer per person aged 15 and over (in litres)[a]

Country	1960	Country	1981
New Zealand	149.2	Australia	184.1
Belgium	147.4	Germany, Federal Republic of	183.7
Australia	145.6	Czechoslovakia	181.9
Luxembourg	145.5	Gabon	180.0
Czechoslovakia	137.1	German Democratic Republic	179.0
Germany, Federal Republic of	122.7	Ireland	168.7
United Kingdom	109.1	Denmark	167.9
German Democratic Republic	101.9	New Zealand	165.8
Ireland	96.1	Belgium	159.0
Denmark	95.2	Luxembourg	148.2
Switzerland	93.9	United Kingdom	142.9
Austria	92.1	Venezuela	140.2
Canada	89.6	Austria	136.1
USA	83.9	USA	122.8
Colombia	72.3	Netherlands	117.9
Venezuela	65.5	Canada	115.2
Chile	50.0	Hungary	111.4
France	47.1	Switzerland	89.9
Cuba	41.8	Colombia	81.8
Mexico	41.6	Bulgaria	78.1
Sweden	39.9	Spain	76.7
Finland	35.7	Mexico	74.1
Poland	35.1	Finland	73.2
Netherlands	34.0	Panama	64.0
Norway	33.1	Romania	60.0
		South Africa	59.7
		Norway	58.2
		Sweden	57.2
		France	57.1
		Japan	51.8
		Peru	51.2
		Portugal	50.8

[a]From Walsh & Grant (1985)

Table 19. Consumption[a] of commercially produced beer (in litres per head) in countries or areas in which there has been a marked increase over the period 1960–81[b]

Country or area	1960	1973	1981
Africa			
Cameroon	5.0	22.0	33.1
Congo	4.3	18.5	42.7
Côte d'Ivoire[c]	3.3[d]	12.4	20.0
Gabon	12.0[d]	35.6	135.0
Kenya	4.8	10.0	16.7
Namibia	12.6	22.9	47.1
South Africa[c]	4.2	14.3	34.6
America, Central and Caribbean			
Costa Rica[c]	6.8	10.8	21.7
Dominican Republic	3.1	12.7	17.0
Jamaica	9.2	29.1	27.0
Mexico[c]	22.9	32.0	40.0
Nicaragua	2.8	13.3	16.4
Panama	14.3	22.5	47.4
Trinidad and Tobago	11.0	23.5	28.3
America, South			
Bolivia	4.6	8.3	24.6
Brazil	9.3[d]	14.0	19.8
Ecuador	9.2	12.5	35.7
Paraguay	2.8	8.3	23.9
Peru	14.6	23.3	29.2
Suriname	7.3	22.3	32.8
Venezuela	36.0	40.8	86.0
Asia			
Cyprus[c]	8.2	20.5	34.7
Hong Kong[c]	3.8	16.1	23.0
Japan[c]	9.8	34.9	39.4
Republic of Korea	0.7	2.6	14.5
Philippines[c]	3.3	8.5	14.9
Europe[c]			
Bulgaria	13.0	43.6	60.9
Finland	25.0	54.5	57.1
Greece	5.5	13.3	34.6
Hungary	36.8	61.6	88.0
Italy	5.1	15.7	17.9
Netherlands	23.8	73.5	89.6
Portugal	3.0	26.0	36.6
Romania	8.8	27.0	45.0
Spain	11.0	42.6	55.2
USSR	11.9	20.4	23.4
Yugoslavia	6.7	37.2	79.9[e]

[a]Based on production data, unless otherwise specified
[b]From Walsh & Grant (1985)
[c]Based on consumption data
[d]1965
[e]1980

still relatively modest, the rate of increase in these countries was such that, if it were sustained for another decade, the level of beer consumption per head would be higher than that recorded in Norway and the Netherlands in 1960. There is currently no evidence of a levelling off in this rate. The appearance of so many developing countries in Africa, Latin America, the Caribbean and Asia on this table is an indication of recent trends in beer consumption (Walsh & Grant, 1985).

(*c*) *Wine consumption*

Wine-producing areas, such as France and Italy, tend also to be areas of highest wine consumption (Table 20). Countries in which rapid changes (growth or decline) in wine consumption have been seen are listed in Table 21: important increases occurred during the 1960s in several northern European countries, in North America and in Australia. In general, this reflects a diversification of drinking patterns, as the new beverage (wine) is added to the already fairly large amounts of beer and spirits consumed. The decline in wine consumption in France, Italy and Portugal, where consumption was previously very high, is an important trend. In Italy, the decline has been offset by increased beer consumption, while in France and Portugal total alcohol consumption has declined (Walsh & Grant, 1985).

Increased wine production in the USA, Spain and Australia in recent years, in conjunction with the marked fall in consumption in the heaviest wine-drinking countries, has given rise to a growing surplus of production over consumption. The potential for increased consumption outside the areas of Mediterranean culture is illustrated by the rapid growth of wine drinking in Scandinavia during the last three decades. People in this region formerly consumed almost exclusively beer and spirits, but during the 1960s their levels of wine consumption rose rapidly without a corresponding fall in drinking of other alcoholic beverages. The growing popularity of wine was thus an important factor in the increase in total consumption of alcoholic beverages (Walsh & Grant, 1985).

(*d*) *Consumption of spirits*

In many of the countries that are the world's largest producers of spirits, there is a high consumption per person. In Table 22, countries are ranked according to consumption of spirits per head in 1960 and 1981; countries in which there was a substantial increase in consumption of spirits during that period are listed in Table 23.

There is a tendency to an 'internationalization' of drinking habits following the increased ease of communication. An example is the increase in wine consumption in many countries where traditionally beer and spirits have dominated; the new drinking habits are added to the old ones, resulting in an increase in total consumption of alcohol. In other countries, the increase in wine drinking during the period 1975-85 has been at least partly offset by a decrease in consumption of spirits. Examples of the latter are Norway, Sweden (Systembolaget, 1986) and the USA (National Institute on Alcohol Abuse and Alcoholism, 1987).

Table 20. Consumption of commercially produced wine (in litres per head)[a]

Country	1960		Country	1981	
	Total population	Population over 14 years		Total population	Population over 14 years
France	126.9	171.5	France	90.0	116.9
Italy	108.3	144.4	Portugal	77.0	106.9
Portugal	85.0	119.7	Italy	74.0	97.4
Argentina	75.9	108.4	Argentina	73.0	101.4
Spain	50.7	70.4	Spain	60.0	83.3
Chile	46.0	76.6	Switzerland	48.5	61.3
Greece	40.8	55.9	Chile	43.7	66.2
Switzerland	36.0	48.6	Greece	42.0	55.3
Luxembourg	31.3	39.1	Luxembourg	40.2	50.2
Hungary	29.9	39.9	Austria	34.2	44.4
Romania	21.7	29.7	Hungary	33.0	41.8
Yugoslavia	21.4	31.5	Romania	28.9	38.6
Uruguay	21.0	28.8	Yugoslavia	28.2	38.1
Austria	20.7	26.9	Uruguay	25.0	34.2
Bulgaria	20.2	27.3	Bulgaria	22.0	28.2
Czechoslovakia	13.2	18.3	Belgium	21.0	26.9
Cyprus	11.5	18.3	Germany, Federal Republic of	20.2	25.3
Germany, Federal Republic of	10.8	13.8	Australia	18.3	25.1
South Africa	8.8	13.1	Denmark	16.1	20.6
Belgium	7.8	10.3	Netherlands	13.0	16.9
Australia	5.2	7.4	USSR	14.5	19.6
Poland	4.5	6.9	New Zealand	14.4	20.3
USA	3.4	5.0	Czechoslovakia	13.5	17.5
German Democratic Republic	3.3	4.2	Cyprus	10.8	14.4
Sweden	3.3	4.2	German Democratic Republic	10.2	12.6
Denmark	3.1	4.1	Sweden	9.7	12.3
Canada	2.0	3.1	South Africa	9.0	15.5
Netherlands	1.9	2.7	Canada	8.9	11.9
United Kingdom	1.6	2.1	United Kingdom	8.4	10.8
Finland	1.3	1.9	USA	8.2	10.8
Norway	1.2	1.6	Poland	7.5	9.9
Iceland	0.8	1.2	Iceland	6.3	8.9
			Finland	5.4	6.9
			Norway	4.2	5.5

[a] From Walsh & Grant (1985)

Table 21. Consumption of commercially produced wine (in litres per head) in countries where it has increased or decreased rapidly[a]

Increased consumption			Decreased consumption		
Country	1960	1981	Country	1960	1981
Germany, Federal Republic of	10.8	20.2	France	129.9	90.0
Belgium	7.8	21.0	Italy	108.3	74.0
Australia	5.2	18.3	Portugal	85.0	77.0
USA	3.4	8.2			
German Democratic Republic	3.3	10.2			
Sweden	3.3	9.7			
Denmark	3.1	16.1			
Canada	2.0	8.9			
Netherlands	1.9	13.0			
United Kingdom	1.6	8.4			
Finland	1.3	5.4			
Norway	1.2	4.2			
Iceland	0.8	6.3			

[a]From Walsh & Grant (1985)

2.4 Drinking patterns

Drinking patterns vary between regions and countries, between groups within a country, between individuals belonging to the same social and ethnic group and between different times in the life of an individual. As travel, trade, standards of living and media communication increase, drinking habits may be introduced from one country or group into another.

Societies differ substantially in the proportion of the adult population who drinks at all. Surveys in India, for instance, typically report abstention rates of 50-70% (Mohan *et al.*, 1980; Sundaram *et al.*, 1984). The variation between European and North American countries is narrower: from about one-third abstainers among adults in the USA and Ireland to fewer in many western European countries (see Table 24). Rates of abstention have fallen considerably over the last 40 years in some countries that had had strong temperance traditions; for instance, in Finland, there were 25% nondrinkers in 1968 and 13% in 1976 (Mäkelä *et al.*, 1981).

Table 22. Consumption of commercially produced spirits (in litres of ethanol per head)[a]

Country	1960		Country	1981	
	Total population	Population over 15 years		Total population	Population over 15 years
USSR	2.6	3.3	Republic of Korea	5.4	9.2
Austria	2.4	3.2	German Democratic Republic	4.8	5.9
Poland	2.4	3.6	Hungary	4.8	6.2
Sweden	2.3	2.9	Luxembourg[b]	4.5	5.5
USA	2.1	3.0	Poland	4.3	5.7
France	2.0	2.7	Czechoslovakia	4.0	5.3
Spain	2.0	2.8	USSR	3.3	4.4
Germany, Federal Republic of	1.9	2.4	Canada	3.3	4.3
Yugoslavia	1.8	2.6	Japan	3.2	4.2
Iceland	1.6	2.5	Spain	3.0	4.1
Switzerland	1.5	2.0	USA	3.0	4.1
Canada	1.5	2.3	Germany, Federal Republic of	2.9	3.5
Hungary	1.4	1.9	Finland	2.8	4.1
German Democratic Republic	1.4	1.8	Sweden	2.8	3.5
Norway	1.3	1.8	Netherlands	2.6	3.4
Finland	1.3	1.9	France	2.5	3.2
Bulgaria	1.3	1.8	Iceland	2.2	3.5
Japan[c]	1.2	1.6	Switzerland	2.1	2.6
Romania	1.1	1.5	Belgium	2.1	2.6
Netherlands	1.1	1.6	Yugoslavia	2.0	2.7
Italy	1.0	1.3	Romania	2.0	2.7
Luxembourg	1.0	1.3	Bulgaria	2.0	2.6
New Zealand	1.0	1.5	Ireland	1.9	2.8
Czechoslovakia	1.0	1.4	Italy	1.9	2.4
Australia	0.8	1.1	New Zealand	1.8	2.4
Belgium	0.8	1.1	United Kingdom	1.7	2.2
Ireland	0.8	1.2	Norway	1.6	2.0
South Africa	0.7	1.0	Denmark	1.5	1.9
United Kingdom	0.7	0.9	Austria	1.5	1.9
Republic of Korea	0.7	1.2	Peru	1.4	2.6
			South Africa	1.4	2.5
			Australia	1.1	1.5

[a] From Walsh & Grant (1985)
[b] Based on production figures
[c] 1965

Table 23. Consumption of commercially produced spirits (in litres of ethanol per head for populations aged 15 years and over) in countries where it has increased substantially[a]

Country	1960	1981
Republic of Korea	2.2[b]	9.2[c]
German Democratic Republic	1.8	5.9
Luxembourg	1.3	5.5
Czechoslovakia	1.4	5.3
Hungary	1.4	4.8
Japan	1.6[b]	4.2
Finland	1.9	4.1
Netherlands	1.6	3.4
Ireland	1.2	2.8
Belgium	1.1	2.6
South Africa	1.0	2.5
United Kingdom	0.9	2.2

[a]From Walsh & Grant (1985)
[b]1965
[c]1980

Table 24. Percentages of adults reporting current abstention from drinking alcoholic beverages in an international public opinion survey, 1985[a]

Country	%	Country	%
Israel	56	Australia	24
Philippines	44	Canada	23
Brazil	40	Colombia	23
Uruguay	33	Mexico	22
USA	33	Switzerland	20
Ireland	32	Iceland	18
Japan	31	Norway	18
Belgium	31	United Kingdom	17
Germany, Federal Republic of	29	Netherlands	16
Argentina	28	Sweden	14
Finland	26	Greece	11
Republic of Korea	24		

[a]From Gallup *et al.* (1985). The data were collected in a coordinated fashion by the Gallup Poll and its affiliates, but should be taken only as indicative, since methods were not specified, and reported proportions of abstainers are in some cases higher than reported in other surveys, particularly for several western European countries.

Surveys of drinking habits, undertaken mostly in Europe and North America, indicate that consumption of alcoholic beverages is skewed, so that the relatively small group of heavier drinkers accounts for a large proportion of alcohol consumption. Under conditions of relatively free market availability, alcohol consumption is distributed roughly log normally among drinkers, with the distribution skewed towards lighter drinkers (Skog, 1980). The proportion of heavy consumers appears to be approximately proportional to the square of the mean consumption. This empirical regularity is seen to reflect what has been termed the 'collectivity of drinking cultures': that people's drinking practices affect each other's and, indeed, that drinking is often a collective act (Skog, 1985).

Women generally more often abstain from drinking than men, and they tend to drink less than men in all age groups and socioeconomic groups. These differences are tending to become smaller for moderate consumption but not for heavier drinking (Room, 1978; National Institute on Alcohol Abuse and Alcoholism, 1987).

Age-related variations in drinking patterns are exemplified by current US and Canadian data, which show a general concentration of abstainers in the older age groups and children, while the 20-29-year age group has the lowest rate of abstainers (Room, 1978; Addiction Research Foundation, 1985; Rydberg, 1985; National Institute on Alcohol Abuse and Alcoholism, 1987). Abstention seems to be declining among teenagers in many countries, although in the 1980s there has been a decline in alcohol use by teenagers in countries such as the USA and Sweden (Rydberg, 1985; National Institute on Alcohol Abuse and Alcoholism, 1987). Among regular drinkers, the most common pattern after the age of 30 appears to be frequent, light drinking, whereas among younger consumers, it appears to be less frequent, heavier drinking (Room, 1978).

The relationship between drinking behaviour and social class is more complicated and varied. In some countries, heavy drinkers belong to lower socioeconomic classes, while in others they are of higher social status. In countries where alcoholic beverages are relatively expensive, such as the Nordic countries, there seems to be a positive correlation between income and total alcohol consumption, although different socioeconomic groups may vary in their style of drinking. 'Binge drinking' — periodic heavy drinking — tends to be more common in lower income groups and, in many instances, might be affected by traditions in specific occupational groups. Data on the relationship between specific occupations and particular drinking patterns in the general population are very sparse (Edwards *et al.*, 1972; Room, 1978; Mäkelä *et al.*, 1981; Fillmore & Caetano, 1982).

In wine-producing countries, where wine is cheap, it is drunk widely in rural areas; in nonproducing countries, where alcoholic beverages tend to be more expensive, drinking may be less common in rural areas (Péquignot *et al.*, 1988). Within a country, there may be regional variations in choice of beverage and levels of consumption (Room, 1983). Cultural and religious differences are reflected in international comparisons but can also occur within countries where there are various ethnoreligious groups. In many countries, for example, Islamists have a very low consumption of alcohol. American Indians and Alaskan natives, taking another example, appear to have very high rates of alcohol abuse and alcoholism overall, although most members of many tribes are abstainers.

3. CHEMICAL COMPOSITION OF ALCOHOLIC BEVERAGES, ADDITIVES AND CONTAMINANTS

3.1 General aspects

Ethanol and water are the main components of most alcoholic beverages, although in some very sweet liqueurs the sugar content can be higher than the ethanol content. Ethanol (CAS Reg. No. 64-17-5) is present in alcoholic beverages as a consequence of the fermentation of carbohydrates with yeast. It can also be manufactured from ethylene obtained from cracked petroleum hydrocarbons. The alcoholic beverage industry has generally agreed not to use synthetic ethanol manufactured from ethylene for the production of alcoholic beverages, due to the presence of impurities. In order to determine whether synthetic ethanol has been used to fortify products, the low ^{14}C content of synthetic ethanol, as compared to fermentation ethanol produced from carbohydrates, can be used as a marker in control analyses (McWeeny & Bates, 1980).

Some physical and chemical characteristics of anhydrous ethanol are as follows (Windholz, 1983):

Description: Clear, colourless liquid
Boiling-point: 78.5°C
Melting-point: −114.1°C
Density: d_4^{20} 0.789

It is widely used in the laboratory and in industry as a solvent for resins, fats and oils. It also finds use in the manufacture of denatured alcohol, in pharmaceuticals and cosmetics (lotions, perfumes), as a chemical intermediate and as a fuel, either alone or in mixtures with gasoline.

Beer, wine and spirits also contain volatile and nonvolatile flavour compounds. Although the term 'volatile compound' is rather diffuse, most of the compounds that occur in alcoholic beverages can be grouped according to whether they are distilled with alcohol and steam, or not. Volatile compounds include aliphatic carbonyl compounds, alcohols, monocarboxylic acids and their esters, nitrogen- and sulphur-containing compounds, hydrocarbons, terpenic compounds, and heterocyclic and aromatic compounds. Non-volatile extracts of alcoholic beverages comprise unfermented sugars, di- and tribasic carboxylic acids, colouring substances, tannic and polyphenolic substances, and inorganic salts. The flavour composition of alcoholic beverages has been described in detail in several reviews (Suomalainen & Nykänen, 1970; Amerine *et al.*, 1972; Nykänen & Suomalainen, 1983), and a recent review on the compounds occurring in distilled alcoholic beverages is available (ter Heide, 1986). The volatile compounds of alcoholic beverages and distillates generally originate from three sources: raw materials, fermentation and the wooden casks in which they are matured (Jouret & Puech, 1975).

During maturation, unpleasant flavours, probably caused by volatile sulphur compounds, disappear. Extensive investigations on the maturation of distillates in oak casks have shown that many compounds are liberated by alcohol from the walls of the casks (Jouret & Puech, 1975; Reazin, 1983; Nykänen, L., 1984; Nykänen *et al.*, 1984). Lignin plays an important role and is responsible for the occurrence of some aromatic aldehydes and phenolic compounds (Jouret & Puech, 1975; Nykänen *et al.*, 1984). These compounds are liberated from oak during the maturation process, together with monosaccharides (pentoses, quercitol), carboxylic acids and 'whisky lactone' (5-butyl-4-methyldihydro-2(3*H*)-furanone) (Nykänen, L., 1984; Nykänen *et al.*, 1984). The occurrence of aromatic compounds has been considered a manifestation of the degradation (oxidation) of oak lignin (Jouret & Puech, 1975).

The distillation procedure influences the occurrence and concentration of volatile flavour compounds in the distillate. Particularly in the manufacture of strong spirits, it is customary to improve the flavour of the distillate by stripping it of low-boiling and high-boiling compounds to a greater or lesser degree.

Certain flavoured alcoholic beverages may contain, in addition to the natural compounds of the beverages, added synthetic substances and ingredients isolated from herbs and spices. For instance, the flavour of vermouths, aperitifs, bitters, liqueurs and some flavoured vodkas is frequently composed of different essential oils or their mixtures; synthetic products and colouring substances, such as caramel (Ministry of Agriculture, Fisheries and Food, 1987), may also be added to improve the perceived flavour.

The exact compositions of many alcoholic beverages are trade secrets; however, there is extensive literature on the aroma components which are usually present at low levels, more than 1300 of which have been identified (Nykänen & Suomalainen, 1983). Information about nonaroma compounds is less extensive. A list of compounds identified in alcoholic beverages is given in Appendix 1 to this volume.

Definitions of the traditional terms for production processes and types of beverage are given by Lord (1979), Jackson (1982) and Johnson (1985). A useful glossary has been drawn up by Keller *et al.* (1982).

3.2 Compounds in beer

(*a*) *Carbonyl compounds*

Carbonyl compounds are among the most volatile substances in alcoholic beverages.

The levels of some aldehydes found in pasteurized and unpasteurized beers are given in Table 25. Acetaldehyde (see also IARC, 1985, 1987a) is the principal carbonyl compound in beer and has been found at similar ranges (0.1-16.4 mg/l) in US, German and Norwegian beers; levels as high as 37.2 mg/l were found in an unspecified beer (Nykänen & Suomalainen, 1983).

Table 25. Content (mg/l) of some aldehydes in pasteurized and unpasteurized beers[a]

Aldehyde	Pasteurized beer	Unpasteurized beer
Acetaldehyde	3.9–9.8	0.9–1.4
Pyruvaldehyde	0.119–0.293	0.040–0.046
Crotonaldehyde	0.002–0.036	≤0.001
Isobutyraldehyde	0.011–0.024	0.007–0.008
Isovaleraldehyde	0.055–0.105	0.047–0.065
Octanal	0.007–0.017	0.005–0.006
Nonanal	0.005–0.014	0.004–0.006
Decanal	0.006–0.015	0.008–0.010
Dodecanal (Lauraldehyde)	0.004–0.016	0.002–0.006

[a]Reported by Nykänen & Suomalainen (1983)

Of the minor carbonyls identified in beer, formaldehyde (see IARC, 1982a, 1987a) has been found at a level of 0.17-0.28 mg/l in a Swiss beer (Steiner *et al.*, 1969); a fresh beer was reported to contain 0.009 mg/l formaldehyde and a stale beer, 0.002 mg/l (Lau & Lindsay, 1972). Some unsaturated aldehydes have also been identified in beer. Particular attention has been paid to the occurrence of *trans*-2-nonenal, which has been shown to be responsible for the oxidized or 'cardboard' flavour of stale beer, and to that of *trans,cis*-2,6-nonadienal, which gives rise to cucumber- or melon-like odours in beer (Visser & Lindsay, 1971; Wohleb *et al.*, 1972; Withycombe & Lindsay, 1973).

Beer also contains some aliphatic ketones. Postel *et al.* (1972a) found 0.3-1.7 mg/l acetone in German beer, and Tressl *et al.* (1978) determined the following ketones: 3-hydroxy-2-butanone (0.42 mg/l), 2-pentanone (0.02 mg/l), 3-hydroxy-2-pentanone (0.05 mg/l), 3-methyl-2-pentanone (0.06 mg/l), 4-methyl-2-pentanone (0.12 mg/l), 2-heptanone

(0.11 mg/l), 6-methyl-5-hepten-2-one (0.05 mg/l), 2-octanone (0.01 mg/l), 2-nonanone (0.03 mg/l) and 2-undecanone (0.001 mg/l).

The occurrence of 2,3-butanedione (diacetyl), 2,3-pentanedione and 3-hydroxy-2-butanone in beer has been investigated. The 2,3-butanedione content of beer generally varies from 0.01 to 0.2 mg/l (Nykänen & Suomalainen, 1983), but concentrations as high as 0.63 mg/l have been determined in British beer. Slightly smaller amounts (0.01-0.16 mg/l) of 2,3-pentanedione were found in British beers (White & Wainwright, 1975).

(*b*) *Alcohols*

The glycerol content of beer varies little — generally from 1100 to 2100 mg/l (Nykänen & Suomalainen, 1983), although Drawert *et al.* (1976) found average glycerol contents ranging up to 3170 mg/l in some German beers.

According to a review (Nykänen & Suomalainen, 1983), beers produced in different countries do not differ greatly in their content of aliphatic fusel alcohol (higher alcohols formed during yeast fermentation of carbohydrates), although the amounts vary to some extent between the different beer types because their formation depends on the yeast used and, in particular, on fermentation conditions. Thus, beers have been found to contain 4-60 mg/l 1-propanol, 6-72 mg/l 2-methyl-1-propanol (isobutanol), 3-41 mg/l 2-methyl-1-butanol and 35-52 mg/l 3-methyl-1-butanol.

Phenethyl alcohol (2-phenylethyl alcohol), an aromatic fusel alcohol, has a relatively strong rose-like odour, and therefore its determination in different beers has been a central subject of many studies; concentrations in beers vary from 4 to 102 mg/l. Benzyl alcohol occurs as a minor component in beer. Tyrosol and tryptophol, which are formed during fermentation, have been found in many beers, the tyrosol content varying from 1 to 29 mg/l and the tryptophol content from 0.2 to 12 mg/l (Nykänen & Suomalainen, 1983).

(*c*) *Volatile acids*

Most of the monocarboxylic acids — from formic acid to C_{18}-acids — are present in beer but, in general, as minor components. The acidity due to volatile compounds has been found to be greater in beer than in wort, indicating that the acids are formed during fermentation. Acetic acid is the most abundant, occurring at 12-155 mg/l in ales, 22-107 mg/l in lagers and 30-35 mg/l in stouts. The levels of other short-chain acids, up to hexanoic acid, vary from 0.3 to 3.4 mg/l. The principal volatile acids in beer have been reported to be hexanoic acid (1-25 mg/l), octanoic acid (2-15.4 mg/l) and decanoic acid (0.1-5.2 mg/l) (Nykänen & Suomalainen, 1983).

(*d*) *Hydroxy and oxo acids*

The occurrence of the L(+) and D(−) forms of lactic acid, which is a major hydroxy acid in beer, indicates bacterial activity during fermentation. Mändl *et al.* (1971a,b, 1973, 1975) found levels as high as 360 mg/l L-lactic acid in a French beer and 430 mg/l D-lactic acid in an Irish porter stout; most of the beers examined contained 2-40 mg/l L-lactic acid and

25-100 mg/l D-lactic acid. Beer also contains small amounts of other short-chain hydroxy acids (see Appendix 1). Some trihydroxy acids have also been detected: German, Austrian and American beers were reported to contain 5-9 mg/l 9,12,13-trihydroxy-10-*trans*-octadecenoic acid, 1-2.4 mg/l 9,10,13-trihydroxy-11-*trans*-octadecenoic acid, and 0.4-0.7 mg/l 9,10,13-trihydroxy-12-*trans*-octadecenoic acid (Nykänen & Suomalainen, 1983).

Of the oxo acids that occur in beer, pyruvic acid is present in fairly high amounts; Mändl *et al.* (1971b, 1973) determined concentrations of 53-89 mg/l in American beers and 17-138 mg/l in European beers.

(*e*) *Nonvolatile (fixed) acids*

The occurrence of certain nonvolatile (fixed) acids in beer is well established. The oxalic acid content is small, but it is of considerable interest because the formation of calcium oxalate may contribute to the appearance of hazes and sediments in beer. Bernstein and Khan (1973) reported 9-15 mg/l oxalic acid in ales and lager beers; Fournet and Montreuil (1975) found 2-11 mg/l in French beers; and German beers were found to contain 14-28 mg/l (Drawert *et al.*, 1975, 1976).

Succinic acid has been reported to occur at concentrations of 12-166 mg/l, malic acid at 0-213 mg/l and citric acid at 5-252 mg/l (Nykänen & Suomalainen, 1983). Numerous acids that occur at concentrations of only a few milligrams per litre are listed in Appendix 1.

(*f*) *Esters*

Beer contains a great number of esters of aliphatic fatty acids. Ethyl acetate is the principal one, occurring at 10-30 mg/l (with values up to 69 mg/l), while isopentyl acetate has been found at 1-7.8 mg/l. Of the high-boiling esters, ethyl hexanoate and ethyl octanoate occur at 0.1-0.5 mg/l and 0.1-1.5 mg/l, respectively, although some beers have been shown to contain 2.4-4 mg/l ethyl octanoate. The amount of phenethyl acetate varies between 0.03 and 1.5 mg/l (Nykänen & Suomalainen, 1983).

(*g*) *Nitrogen compounds*

(i) *Amines and amides*

Amines occur in beer due to the biochemical degradation of amino acids, which may begin during malting and then continues during fermentation. They are listed in Appendix 1. The following acetamides have been found in German dark beer: *N*,*N*-dimethylformamide, 0.015 mg/l; *N*,*N*-dimethylacetamide, 0.01 mg/l; *N*-methylacetamide, traces; *N*-ethylacetamide, 0.02 mg/l; *N*-(2-methylbutyl)acetamide, 0.01 mg/l; *N*-(3-methylbutyl)-acetamide, 0.025 mg/l; *N*-(2-phenylethyl)acetamide, 0.015 mg/l; and *N*-furfurylacetamide, 0.12 mg/l (Tressl *et al.*, 1977). The occurrence of several primary, secondary and tertiary amines in different beers is summarized in Table 26. Aminoacetophenone may be responsible in part for the characteristic odour of beers.

Table 26. Content (mg/l) of some amines in beer[a]

Amine	Amount (range)
Methylamine	0.02–0.32
Ethylamine	0.11–2.12
n-Propylamine	traces–0.17
Isobutylamine	0.004–0.22
n-Butylamine	traces–0.07
Isopentylamine (isoamylamine)	traces–0.14
n-Hexylamine	0.005–0.28
N,*N*-Dimethyl-*n*-butylamine	traces–0.16
2-Aminoacetophenone[b]	0.01
Dimethylamine	0.37–0.78
Trimethylamine	0.03–0.06
para-(2-Aminoethyl) phenol (tyramine)	6.5–11.22

[a]From Palamand *et al.* (1969); Sen (1969; Canadian beer); Palamand *et al.* (1971); Slaughter & Uvgard (1971; English beer); Koike *et al.* (1972; Japanese beer); Tressl *et al.* (1977; German beer)

(ii) N-*Heterocyclic compounds*

N-Heterocyclic compounds present in malt can be detected at low levels in some beers. The amounts of pyrazines in dark Bavarian beer are given in Table 27. Tressl *et al.* (1977) assumed that the pyrroles occurring in some beers are responsible for the smoky odour resembling that of pastry and bread. A number of compounds with such an odour were found, four of which were identified as nicotinic acid esters. The pyrroles and thiazoles found in dark Bavarian beer are listed in Table 28.

(iii) *Histamine and other nonvolatile* N-*heterocyclic compounds*

Granerus *et al.* (1969) showed that the level of histamine was 0.03-0.05 mg/l in Swedish beer and 0.03-0.15 mg/l in Danish beer. Chen and Van Gheluwe (1979) found means of 0.22 mg/l in Canadian ale, 0.20 mg/l in Canadian lager, 0.38 mg/l in Canadian malt liquor, 0.41 mg/l in Canadian porter, 0.13 mg/l in Canadian light beer, 0.13 mg/l in American lager and 0.20 mg/l in European beers. A high histamine content, 1.9 mg/l, was found in a Belgian Gueuze produced by 'spontaneous' fermentation with microorganisms other than brewer's yeast.

The purine and pyrimidine contents of beer have been investigated in several studies (Saha *et al.*, 1971; Buday *et al.*, 1972; Charalambous *et al.*, 1974; Kieninger *et al.*, 1976; Ziegler & Piendl, 1976; Mändl *et al.*, 1979; Boeck & Kieninger, 1979). In most beers the amounts of uracil, cytosine, hypoxanthine, xanthine, adenine, guanine, thymine, thymidine, adenosine and inosine were found to range from 0.1 to 40 mg/l, whereas higher amounts of guanosine (30-160 mg/l), cytidine (18-70 mg/l) and uridine (15-200 mg/l) were detected.

Table 27. Content (mg/l) of pyrazines in dark Bavarian beer[a]

Pyrazine	Amount
Methyl-	0.07
2,5-Dimethyl-	0.11
2,6-Dimethyl-	0.035
2,3-Dimethyl-	0.015
Trimethyl-	0.02
Tetramethyl-	traces
Ethyl-	0.01
2-Ethyl-6-methyl-	0.035
2-Ethyl-5-methyl-	traces
2-Ethyl-3-methyl-	traces
2-Ethyl-3,5-dimethyl-	0.01
2-Ethyl-3,6-dimethyl-	0.02
2-Ethyl-5,6-dimethyl	traces
6,7-Dihydro-5*H*-cyclopenta-	0.01
5-Methyl-6,7-dihydro-5*H*-cyclopenta-	0.015
2-Methyl-6,7-dihydro-5*H*-cyclopenta-	0.01
5-Methylcyclopenta-	traces
2-Furyl-	0.025
2-(2'-Furyl)methyl-	0.01
2-(2'-Furyl)dimethyl-	traces

[a]From Tressl *et al.* (1977)

Table 28. Content (mg/l) of pyrroles, thiazoles and some other cyclic compounds determined in dark Bavarian beer[a]

Compound	Amount
Pyrrole	traces
2-Methylpyrrole	1.8
2-Formylpyrrole	0.03
2-Acetylpyrrole	1.4
2-Acetyl-5-methylpyrrole	0.01
2-Formyl-5-methylpyrrole	0.11
1-Acetylpyrrole	traces
1-Furfurylpyrrole	0.01
2-Pyrrolidone	0.01
1-Methyl-2-pyrrolidone	traces
Indole	traces
2-Acetylthiazole	traces
4-Methyl-5-hydroxyethylthiazole	traces
Methyl nicotinate	traces
Ethyl nicotinate	1.5
3-Methylbutyl nicotinate	traces
2-Phenethyl nicotinate	traces

[a]From Tressl *et al.* (1977)

(*h*) *Aromatic compounds*

(i) *Phenols*

Special attention has been paid to the occurrence of phenols in beer due to their potential influence on the flavour (Nykänen & Suomalainen, 1983). Wackerbauer *et al.* (1977) investigated the sources of the phenolic flavour of beer and found cresol (0.012 mg/l), 4-vinylphenol (0.17 mg/l), 2-methoxy-4-vinylphenol (4-vinylguaiacol; 0.074 mg/l) and 4-hydroxybenzaldehyde (0.018 mg/l) in a flawed beer. Many different phenols have been found in beers (Tressl *et al.*, 1975a, 1976; see also Appendix 1).

(ii) *Aromatic acids*

Beer contains numerous aromatic acids (Appendix 1); their occurrence in beer is summarized in Table 29.

Table 29. Content (mg/l) of aromatic acids in beer[a]

Acid	Amount
Benzoic acid	0.45
Phenyllactic acid	1.2
Salicylic acid (2-Hydroxybenzoic acid)	0.02
4-Hydroxybenzoic acid	0.13
Protocatechuic + vanillic acid	2.4
Phthalic acid	0.02
Phenylacetic acid	0.93
4-Hydroxyphenylacetic acid	0.04
Ferulic acid (4-Hydroxy-3-methoxycinnamic acid)	
,*cis*-	1.1
,*trans*-	4.6
Cinnamic acid	
,*cis*-	<0.01
,*trans*-	0.50
para-Coumaric acid (4-Hydroxycinnamic acid)	
,*cis*-	0.02
,*trans*-	1.9
Phenylpropionic acid	0.01
4-Hydroxyphenylpropionic acid	0.02

[a]From Tressl *et al.* (1975b)

3.3 Compounds in wine

(*a*) *Carbonyl compounds*

Acetaldehyde constitutes more than 90% of the total aldehyde content of wines, occurring at 50-100 mg/l (Nykänen & Suomalainen, 1983). Wucherpfennig and Semmler (1972, 1973) found 74-118 mg/l acetaldehyde in wines produced from different grapes in various vineyards in different countries, and Postel *et al.* (1972b) found 11-160 mg/l in German 'Spätlesen', 'Auslesen' and 'Beerenauslesen' white wines and in red wines; white and red wines had similar aldehyde contents. The aldehyde content is, however, low, and this may be explained by the fact that the sulphur dioxide added to wine reacts with aldehydes to form α-hydroxysulphonic acids, which reduce the free aldehyde content. Furthermore, aldehydes can be chemically bound to ethanol and higher alcohols as acetals.

Minor amounts of other aliphatic aldehydes and ketones are also present in wine (Appendix 1). Baumes *et al.* (1986) found 3-hydroxy-2-butanone (0.002-0.3 mg/l) and 3-hydroxy-2-pentanone in French white and red wines. The volatile flavour of Chardonnay and Riesling wines has been reported to include minor amounts of 2-methylbutanal, 3-methylbutanal, hexanal and 2-heptanone (Simpson & Miller, 1983, 1984). Benzaldehyde has been found in detectable amounts (0.002-0.504 mg/l) in different French wines (Baumes *et al.*, 1986), in Chardonnay and Riesling wines (Simpson & Miller, 1983, 1984) and in Pinot Noir wine (Brander *et al.*, 1980).

Two vicinal diketones, 2,3-butanedione and 2,3-pentanedione, may be of importance to the flavour nuances, although they occur at low levels. 2,3-Butanedione has been found in white wines at 0.05-3.4 mg/l and in red wines at 0.02-5.4 mg/l, whereas lower values have been reported for 2,3-pentanedione (0.007-0.4 mg/l in white wines and 0.01-0.88 mg/l in red wines; Leppänen *et al.*, 1979; Nykänen & Suomalainen, 1983).

(*b*) *Acetals*

In contrast to beers, wines contain acetal (1,1-diethoxyethane) as a major component of the volatiles. It is generally assumed that the reaction of acetaldehyde with ethanol to yield acetal may 'round' the smell of wines, which is of great importance. In the French wines investigated by Baumes *et al.* (1986), the total amounts of acetal and 2,4-dimethyl-1,3-dioxane were reported to vary from 0.18 to 9.3 mg/l in white wines and from 0.09 to 0.52 mg/l in red wines. Other acetals found at low concentrations were 2,4,5-trimethyl-1,3-dioxolane (previously identified by Brander *et al.* (1980) in Pinot Noir wine), 1,3-dimethyl-4-ethyl-1,3-dioxolane, 1-ethoxy-1-(2′-methylpropoxy)ethane, 1-ethoxy-1-(3′-methylbutoxy)ethane, 1-(3′-methylbutoxy)-1-(2′-methylbutoxy)ethane, 1,1-di-(3′-methylbutoxy)-ethane, 1-ethoxy-1-(2′-phenethoxy)ethane, 1-(3′-methylbutoxy)-1-(2′-phenethoxy)ethane, *cis*-2-methyl-4-hydroxymethyl-1,3-dioxolane and *trans*-2-methyl-4-hydroxymethyl-1,3-dioxolane (Baumes *et al.*, 1986).

An ether possibly related to the acetals, 3-ethoxypropanol, has been identifed in Pinot Noir wine (Brander *et al.*, 1980).

(*c*) *Alcohols*

(i) *Di- and trihydric alcohols*

Apart from ethanol, glycerol and 2,3-butanediol are the principal alcohols in wine. The glycerol content has been reported to range between 2000 and 36 000 mg/l in sound wines (Nykänen & Suomalainen, 1983). The contents of numerous European and American wines have been found to vary from 400 to 1100 mg/l; exceptionally high amounts of 2,3-butanediol were found in a Romanian 'Trockenbeerenauslese' (2700 mg/l) and in an 'Edelauslese' (3300 mg/l; Patschky, 1973).

(ii) *Fusel alcohols and long-chain alcohols*

Numerous investigations on the volatile components of different wines have shown that higher alcohols are ubiquitous. White and red wines produced in various countries contain 1-propanol (11-125 mg/l), 2-methyl-1-propanol (15-174 mg/l), 2-methyl-1-butanol (12-311 mg/l) and 3-methyl-1-butanol (isopentanol; 49-180 mg/l). In addition, wines contain 5-138 mg/l phenethyl alcohol. The occurrence of the aromatic alcohols, tyrosol (4-hydroxyphenethyl alcohol) and tryptophol (3-indolethanol), which are formed by biochemical mechanisms similar to those proposed for the formation of phenethyl alcohol and aliphatic fusel alcohols, has also been established; white and red wines have been reported to contain 5-45 mg/l tyrosol and 0.3-3.1 mg/l tryptophol (Nykänen & Suomalainen, 1983).

A number of long-chain alcohols, such as 1-pentanol, 4-methyl-1-pentanol, 3-methyl-1-pentanol, *Z*-2-penten-1-ol, 1-hexanol, the *E*- and *Z*-isomers of 2-hexen-1-ol and 3-hexen-1-ol, 1-heptanol, 1-octanol, 1-nonanol and 1-decanol, have been identified in wines (Brander *et al.*, 1980; Nykänen & Suomalainen, 1983; Simpson & Miller, 1983, 1984). Of these, 3-methyl-1-pentanol, 1-hexanol and *E*-3-hexen-1-ol seem to be fairly important components (Baumes *et al.*, 1986).

(*d*) *Volatile acids*

Acetic acid is the most abundant of the volatile acidic constituents of wine, although yeast is known to produce only minor amounts of acetic acid in fermentation under anaerobic conditions. Any substantial increase in the volatile acidity in wines thus seems to be due to the activity of spoilage microorganisms. Acetic acid bacteria can oxidize ethanol, first forming acetaldehyde, followed by oxidation of aldehyde to acetic acid, thus restricting volatile acidity to, for example, the permissible values of under 900 mg/l in French wines and in German white wines, under 1200 mg/l in German red wines, under 1100 mg/l in Californian white table wines and under 1200 mg/l in Californian red wines (Nykänen & Suomalainen, 1983). The volatile acidity of German wines, for instance, has been reported to be about 300 mg/l (Schmitt, 1972).

(e) *Hydroxy acids*

Wines contain fairly large amounts of L(+)- and D(−)-lactic acid. The total concentration of lactic acid in French wines that have undergone malolactic fermentation has been found to vary from 900 to 2600 mg/l, and total lactic acid contents of 100-5600 mg/l and 200-3100 mg/l have been reported. Other monohydroxy acids occur as minor components: 2,3-dihydroxy-2-methylbutyric acid has been found at 60-523 mg/l in a large number of wines, at 34-205 mg/l in Italian wines and at 70-550 mg/l in Bordeaux wines (Nykänen & Suomalainen, 1983).

(f) *'Fixed' acids*

The acidity of wines depends mainly on the presence of nonvolatile acids from the grapes. Tartaric, malic, citric and succinic acids are usually the most abundant and are of great importance, not only because they regulate the acidity of the wine but also because their acidity protects sound wine from spoilage and increases the stability of coloured substances. Their total amount is determined by a titrimetric method (Nykänen & Suomalainen, 1983).

de Smedt *et al.* (1981) found malic acid (3380 mg/l), tartaric acid (2120 mg/l), succinic acid (500 mg/l), citric acid (270 mg/l) and phosphoric acid (240 mg/l). Of the minor components, they determined shikimic acid (70 mg/l) and citramalic acid (20 mg/l) quantitatively.

(g) *Esters*

The largest group of flavour compounds in wines consists of esters of the aliphatic monocarboxylic acids. Ethyl acetate and many of the long-chain esters in wine are formed by yeast principally by enzymic reactions during fermentation and not in chemical reactions between ethanol and corresponding acids (Nykänen & Suomalainen, 1983). The acid-catalysed esterification and hydrolysis of the esters, however, may be of importance during prolonged ageing, even though the reactions proceed slowly and equilibrium concentrations are reached only after a long time.

Ethyl acetate is the principal ester component. Postel *et al.* (1972b) found 44-122 mg/l ethyl acetate in white wines and 78-257 mg/l in red wines. Higher levels were found in sound white wines produced in different countries (11-261 mg/l), and similar concentrations were found in red wines (22-232 mg/l; Shinohara & Watanabe, 1976). Late harvest wines, such as 'Spätlese', 'Auslese' and 'Beerenauslese', were found to contain 52-99 mg/l, 92-108 mg/l and 191-285 mg/l ethyl acetate, respectively (Postel *et al.*, 1972b).

Ethyl esters of short-chain acids as well as acetate esters of fusel alcohols are frequently found in white and red wines. The ethyl esters of decanoic and dodecanoic acids are usually the longest chain esters found (Nykänen & Nykänen, 1977; Nykänen *et al.*, 1977).

In addition, a number of esters originating in grapes have been identified in wines, such as methyl anthranilate, of which the odour has been reported to be characteristic of the grape variety *Vitis labrusca* and may be responsible for the 'foxy' ('rosé') character of some

American wines (Nelson *et al.*, 1978; Nykänen, 1986). The cyclic ester, 2,6,6-trimethyl-2-vinyl-4-acetoxytetrahydropyran, together with a tetrahydrofuran derivative, linalool oxide, potentially contributes to flavour in wine (Schreier & Drawert, 1974).

A number of esters of di- and tricarboxylic acids have also been identified in wine, of which diethyl succinate is ubiquitous. Baumes *et al.* (1986) found 2,3-butanediol monoacetate, methylethyl succinate, diethyl malonate, diethyl malate, diethyl 2-ketoglutarate and diethyl 2-hydroxyglutarate in French wines. DiStefano (1983) identified ethyl esters of 2-hydroxyglutaric acid and 2-hydroxyglutaric acid γ-lactone in Italian wine. Diethyl succinate has been found in Australian Chardonnay wines and ethyl 3-methylbutyl succinate in Riesling wines (Simpson & Miller, 1983, 1984). The occurrence of mono- and diethyl esters of tartaric acid in wine has been confirmed in several studies (Shimizu & Watanabe, 1978; Sponholz, 1979; Edwards *et al.*, 1985).

(*h*) *Nitrogen compounds*

(i) *Amines and some* N-*heterocyclic compounds*

Amines are probably formed mainly by bacterial decarboxylation of amino acids, but small amounts may also occur as the result of enzymic reactions of yeast. Schreier *et al.* (1975) showed that the yeast *Saccharomyces cerevisiae* can produce the corresponding *N*-acetylamines from 2-methylbutylamine, 3-methylbutylamine and 2-phenethylamine in a fermentation solution. Consequently, some amides detected in wine may be formed by yeast from amines during wine fermentation. Desser and Bandion (1985) showed that certain technological treatments and the storage of bottled wine may decrease the concentrations of biogenic amines such as 1,3-propanediamine, putrescine (1,4-butanediamine), histamine (2-(4-imidazolyl)ethylamine), cadaverine (1,5-pentanediamine), spermidine (*N*-(3-aminopropyl)-1,4-butanediamine) and spermine (*N*,*N*′-bis(3-aminopropyl)-1,4-butanediamine) in wine. Puputti and Suomalainen (1969) determined the concentrations of a number of volatile and nonvolatile compounds in white and red wines (Table 30).

The amounts of amines in different wines vary widely. Spettoli (1971) found ethylamine (traces-0.36 mg/l), isobutylamine (traces-0.7 mg/l), isopentylamine (isoamylamine; 0.04-0.7 mg/l), hexylamine (0.1-0.9 mg/l), ethanolamine (0.05-0.9 mg/l) and *para*-(2-aminoethyl)phenol (tyramine; 0.06-0.7 mg/l) in Italian white and red wines. The diamines, 1,4-butanediamine (putrescine), 1,5-pentanediamine (cadaverine) and tyramine are metabolic products of bacteria; diamines are found in greater amounts in red wines. Concentrations of 1,4-butanediamine have been reported to reach 24 mg/l in Swiss white wines and 45 mg/l in Swiss red wines, whereas the concentrations of 1,5-pentanediamine reached 2 mg/l in white wines and 4 mg/l in red wines (Mayer & Pause, 1973). Woidich *et al.* (1980) found the amines reported in Table 31 in several Austrian wines.

Other amines and *N*-heterocyclic compounds have been identified in wine (Table 32). Bosin *et al.* (1986) determined 1,2,3,4-tetrahydro-β-carboline-3-carboxylic acid and 1-methyl-1,2,3,4-tetrahydro-β-carboline-3-carboxylic acid at 0.8-1.7 and 1.3-9.1 mg/l, respectively. Some of the pyrroles, thiazoles and piperazines that occur in other beverages have also been identified in wine; these are 1-ethyl-2-formylpyrrole, *N*-methylpyrrole,

Table 30. Content (mg/l) of amines in white and red wines[a]

Amine	Burgundy red wine	Bordeaux white wine	Riesling white wine
Volatile amines			
Ethylamine	1.7	0.5	0.7
Isopropylamine	0.05	0.02	0.04
Isobutylamine	0.07	0.02	0.05
n-Butylamine	0.01	traces	traces
Isopentylamine (Isoamylamine)	2.2	1.0	4.0
Pentylamine (*n*-Amylamine)	0.01	traces	traces
Hexylamine	0.7	0.4	0.4
Nonvolatile amines			
Ethanolamine	0.3	0.08	0.08
1,4-Butanediamine (Putrescine)	0.3	traces	traces
para-(2-Aminoethyl)phenol (Tyramine)	1.0	0.1	0.2
Histamine	0.5	0.04	traces

[a]From Puputti & Suomalainen (1969)

Table 31. Content (mg/l) of some biogenic amines in Austrian wines[a]

Amine	Red wine	White wine
1,4-Butanediamine	0.51–24.2	<0.05–1.7
1,5-Pentanediamine	<0.05–3.0	<0.05–2.8
Histamine	<0.1–13.6	<0.1–3.5
4-Azaheptamethylenediamine	0.05–1.3	<0.05–2.7
Spermine	<0.1–0.4	<0.1–0.8
para-(2-Aminoethyl)phenol	<0.1–8.1	<0.1–2.7
Phenethylamine	<0.1–5.1	<0.1–3.8

[a]From Woidich *et al.* (1980)

N-ethylpyrrole, *N*-propylpyrrole, benzothiazole, *N*-methylpiperazine, 2-methylpiperazine, *trans*-2,5-dimethylpiperazine and *N*,*N*-dimethylpiperazine (Ough, 1984). The occurrence of 2-methoxypyrazines in wine has been confirmed (Heymann *et al.*, 1986). Serotonin [3-(2-aminoethyl)-1*H*-indol-5-ol] and octopamine [(4-hydroxyphenyl)ethanolamine] have been determined by a high-pressure liquid chromatographic method among the nonvolatile compounds in wine (Lehtonen, 1986).

Table 32. Content (mg/l) of amines and N-heterocyclic compounds in wine[a]

Compound	Content
Dimethylamine	0.1-0.7
Trimethylamine	0.01-0.07
Diethylamine	<0.001
Triethylamine	0.01-0.02
Pyrrolidine	traces-0.06
Piperidine	traces
Morpholine	0.07
2-Pyrrolidone	0.01
1-Methyl-2-pyrrolidone	traces
1-Pyrroline	0.01-0.5
Indole	traces
1-Methyl-1,2,3,4-tetrahydro-β-carboline	0.001-0.084
4,5-Dimethyl-1,3-dioxolan-2-propanamine	traces
2-Aminomethyl benzoate	traces
6-Hydroxy-1-methyl-1,2,3,4-tetrahydro-β-carboline	0-0.0002
Pyridine	traces
Quinoline	traces
N-Methylpiperidine	traces

[a]From Ough (1984)

(ii) *Amides*

Numerous acetamides have been identified in wines (Ough, 1984). These include *N*,*N*-dimethylformamide, *N*-3-methylbutylacetamide, *N*-*n*-pentylacetamide, *N*-ethylacetamide, *N*-*n*-hexylacetamide, *N*-*n*-propylacetamide, *N*-cyclohexylacetamide, *N*-isopropylacetamide, *N*-(3-(methylthio)propylacetamide, *N*-*n*-butylacetamide, *N*-2-phenethylacetamide, *N*-isobutylacetamide, *N*-*tert*-butylacetamide, *N*-piperidylacetamide, *N*-2-methylbutylacetamide and *N*,*N*-diethylacetamide. Only a few quantitative results have been reported; for example, *N*-2-methylbutylacetamide at 0.002-0.02 mg/l and *N*-3-methylbutylacetamide at 0.002 mg/l.

(*i*) *Terpenic compounds*

Wine contains numerous terpene hydrocarbons, terpene aldehydes and ketones, terpene alcohols, esters of terpene alcohols, and their oxidation products (see Appendix 1). The quantities of individual terpenes vary widely according to the wine. Terpene composition depends, in part, on grape varieties; varieties of white *Vitis vinifera* grapes and wines have been classified according to their terpene profiles (Schreier *et al.*, 1976a,b; Rapp *et al.*, 1984), although whether this can be generally used for classifying different grape varieties or wines produced from these grapes is not established. Since free and glycosidic derivatives of monoterpenes are uniformly distributed among the skin, pulp and juice (Wilson *et al.*, 1984; Williams *et al.*, 1985; Wilson, B. *et al.*, 1986), a fairly large proportion of terpenes are present bound to glycosides in young wine; however, when the glycosidic compounds are hydrolysed during ageing, the terpene profile changes (Rapp *et al.*, 1985).

The amounts of terpene compounds in wine have not been reported, but it has been suggested that they contribute markedly to the specific characteristics of wine flavour (Williams, 1982; Rapp *et al.*, 1984; Schreier, 1984; Strauss *et al.*, 1984; Williams *et al.*, 1985; Rapp & Mandery, 1986).

(*j*) *Phenolic compounds*

Besides phenolic alcohols, aldehydes and acids, red wines contain small amounts of phenol, *m*-cresol, guaiacol, 4-ethylphenol, 4-vinylphenol, 4-ethylguaiacol, 4-vinylguaiacol, eugenol and 2,6-dimethoxyphenol. Corbières wine has been reported to contain 0.001-0.1 mg/l phenol, *ortho*-cresol, *meta*-cresol, *para*-cresol, 2-ethylphenol, 4-ethylphenol, 4-vinylphenol, 2-methoxyphenol (guaiacol), 2-methoxy-4-ethylphenol, 2-methoxy-4-vinylphenol, acetovanillone and propiovanillone (Etiévant, 1981). The following volatile phenolic compounds were determined in sherry: 4-ethylphenol (0.35 mg/l), 2-methoxy-4-ethylphenol (4-ethylguaiacol; 0.08 mg/l), 2-ethylphenol (0.05 mg/l), 2-methoxy-4-vinylphenol (4-vinylguaiacol; 0.05 mg/l), 2,6-dimethoxy-4-ethylphenol (ethyl syringol; 0.04 mg/l), 4-vinylphenol (0.02 mg/l), *meta*-cresol (0.01 mg/l), *para*-cresol (0.01 mg/l) and 2-methoxy-4-allylphenol (eugenol; 0.01 mg/l). Phenol, *ortho*-cresol, 2-methoxy-4-methylphenol (4-methylguaiacol) and 2,6-dimethoxy-4-isopropylphenol (isopropyl syringol) were detected at trace levels (Tressl *et al.*, 1976).

Cinnamic acid derivatives, anthocyanins, flavonols and condensed tannins also occur in wine. Anthocyanins and tannins originating in grapes are the main pigments in red wine, and their presence influences the colour and organoleptic characteristics of the wine. Colour stability increases with the degree of methylation, glycosylation and acylation of the basic anthocyanin moiety (Van Buren *et al.*, 1970). Anthocyanins are water soluble and have a 4′-hydroxyflavylium structure. The individual anthocyanins differ in the number of hydroxyl and methoxyl groups in the molecule, as well as in the nature and number of glycosidically bound sugars. Furthermore, aliphatic and aromatic acids may attach to the skeleton of the aglycone; in the acylated anthocyanins, cinnamic acid and, more generally, *para*-coumaric acid is esterified with the hydroxyl group in the sixth position of a glucose molecule attached glycosidically to the aglycone (Windholz, 1983).

Five anthocyanins — delphinidin, petunidin, malvidin, cyanidin and peonidin — and their 3-monoglucosides and 3,5-diglucosides are found commonly in grapes and wines. Malvidin 3,5-diglucoside is apparently the principal pigment in wines produced from hybrid grapes, whereas malvidin monoglucoside predominates in wines made from *Vitis vinifera* grapes (Van Buren *et al.*, 1970). Quercetin-3-glucoside, quercetin-3-glucuronide and myricetin-3-glucoside (the principal flavonols), kaempferol-3-glucoside, kaempferol-3-galactoside and isorhamnetin-3-glucoside (minor compounds) and caffeoyl tartaric acid and *para*-coumaroyl tartaric acid all contribute to the pigment of grapes and wines.

Kaempferol- and myricetin-3-glucuronides and three diglycosides were also identified tentatively (Cheynier & Rigaud, 1986).

3.4 Compounds in spirits

(*a*) *Carbonyl compounds*

(i) *Aliphatic aldehydes*

Acetaldehyde (see IARC, 1985, 1987a) is frequently the major carbonyl component and generally constitutes more than 90% of the total aldehyde content. It is easily distilled together with water and alcohol and is therefore found in all spirits.

Acetal formation is a reversible reaction, with an equilibrium coefficient of about 0.9 (Misselhorn, 1975); thus, if the alcohol content is between 40% and 50% by volume, as is the case for many strong spirits, only 15-20% of the total amount of acetaldehyde combines with ethanol. Hence, acetal formation does not reduce the free aldehyde content of strong spirits markedly, even after prolonged maturation.

The total aldehyde content in alcoholic beverages has been found to vary widely; some levels are summarized in Table 33. In Scotch whisky and cognac, a number of other aldehydes are present at levels similar to that of acetaldehyde (Table 34).

According to an investigation by Marché *et al.* (1975), wine distillate and brandy contain the saturated aliphatic aldehydes from formaldehyde (C_1; see IARC, 1982a, 1987a) to dodecanal (C_{12}). Liebich *et al.* (1970) investigated the flavour compounds in Jamaican rum and found propionaldehyde (0.01 mg/l), isobutyraldehyde (0.25 mg/l), 2-methylbutyraldehyde (1.5 mg/l) and isovaleraldehyde (1.8 mg/l). Kirsch has been reported to contain the following aldehydes, calculated as mg/l ethanol: formaldehyde, 10-20; propionaldehyde, 10-30; valeraldehyde, ≤10; *n*-heptanal, ≤10; octanal, ≤10; and *n*-nonanal, ≤10 (Tuttas & Beye, 1977).

(ii) *Unsaturated aldehydes*

Of the unsaturated aldehydes, only acrolein (see IARC, 1985, 1987a) has been found in new, unaged whisky distillates. Propenal reacts with high concentrations of ethanol to form 1,1,3-triethoxypropane *via* 1,1-diethoxyprop-2-ene and 3-ethoxypropionaldehyde as intermediate products (Kahn *et al.*, 1968).

A number of unsaturated aldehydes have been identified in cognac and brandy. The occurrence of 2-buten-1-al and 2-hexen-1-al was reported in cognac by Marché *et al.* (1975). ter Heide *et al.* (1978) detected 2-methyl-2-propen-1-al in headspace and (*Z*)-2-methyl-2-buten-1-al, 3-methyl-2-buten-1-al, (*E*)-2-penten-1-al, (*E*)-2-methyl-2-penten-1-al, the (*E*)-isomers of 2-C_6, 2-C_7, 2-C_8, 2-C_9-enals and (*E,E*)-hepta-2,4-dien-1-al, nona-2,4-dien-1-al and deca-2,4-dien-1-al in extracts of cognac.

Table 33. Total aldehydes (mg/l ethanol), determined as acetaldehyde, in some brands of distilled beverages[a]

Beverage	Acetaldehyde
American bourbon whiskey	40–120
Canadian whisky	20–70
Irish whiskey	30–140
Scotch blended whisky	40–220
Scotch malt whisky	40–160
Brandy	130–600
Cognac	~210
Rum	20–150

[a]From Nykänen & Suomalainen (1983)

Table 34. Content (mg/l) of some low-boiling aldehydes in Scotch whisky and cognac[a]

Aldehyde	Whisky	Cognac
Acetaldehyde	7	10
Propionaldehyde	1.2	1
Isobutyraldehyde	20	20
2-Methylbutyraldehyde + 3-methylbutyraldehyde (Isovaleraldehyde)	6.3	4

[a]Reported by Nykänen & Suomalainen (1983)

Some unsaturated aldehydes have also been found in rum. Postel and Adam (1982) detected acrolein at 11 mg/l ethanol; ter Heide *et al.* (1981) found (*E*)-2-octen-1-al, (*E*)-2-nonen-1-al, (*E,E*)-2,4-decadien-1-al, β-cyclocitral, α-phellandral and geranial.

(iii) *Aliphatic ketones*

A large number of aliphatic ketones, from acetone to tetradecanone, have been identified in spirits; most are monoketones. In general, little attention has been paid to the determination of monoketones in spirits because of their relatively high sensory thresholds. In contrast, the occurrence of 2,3-butanedione (diacetyl) and 2,3-pentanedione in alcoholic beverages has been investigated (ter Heide, 1986).

The acetone content of spirits varies widely, and concentrations of 3-10 mg/l in whiskies, 0.25 mg/l in rums and <3-10 mg/l ethanol in cognacs and brandies have been reported (Nykänen & Suomalainen, 1983). Schreier *et al.* (1979) determined the contents of some monoketones in German and French brandies and French cognacs and found 2-pentanone (0.012-0.274 mg/l), 2-methylcyclopentanone (0.004-0.043 mg/l), 2-hexanone (0.009-0.117 mg/l), 2-heptanone (0.017-0.628 mg/l) and 2-nonanone (<0.001-0.107 mg/l). Liebich *et al.* (1970) found that a Jamaican rum contained 2-butanone (0.03 mg/l), 3-penten-2-one (7 mg/l), 2-pentanone (1.2 mg/l), 4-ethoxy-2-butanone (5 mg/l) and 4-ethoxy-2-pentanone (7.5 mg/l). Tuttas and Beye (1977) found 2-butanone and 2-heptanone at concentrations of 10 mg/l ethanol in kirsch.

(iv) *Unsaturated monoketones*

In an investigation of flavour constituents in Japanese whisky, Nishimura and Masuda (1984) identified three unsaturated ketones — tri-6-decen-2-one, penta-6-decen-2-one and hepta-6-decen-2-one. The unsaturated ketones 3-penten-2-one (Liebich *et al.*, 1970) and (*E*)-6-nonen-2-one (ter Heide *et al.*, 1981) have been identified in rum. Schreier *et al.* (1978) detected 0.05 mg/l 6-methyl-5-hepten-2-one in raw apple brandy. The unsaturated ketones (*E*)-3-penten-2-one, (*E*)-3-nonen-2-one, 6-methyl-5-hepten-2-one, (*E*)- and (*Z*)-6-methyl-hepta-3,5-diene-2-one, (*E*)-2-nonen-4-one and (*E*)-2-undecen-4-one have been found in cognac (ter Heide *et al.*, 1978).

(v) *Diketones*

The butterscotch odour of 2,3-butanedione can be recognized at very low concentrations. Diketones are marked flavour compounds in alcoholic beverages, many of which contain 2,3-butanedione and 2,3-pentanedione in detectable amounts (Nykänen & Suomalainen, 1983). 2,3-Butanedione (<0.01-4.4 mg/l) and 2,3-pentanedione (<0.003-0.57 mg/l) have been found in whisky, vodka, brandy and rum (Leppänen *et al.*, 1979).

(vi) *Aromatic aldehydes*

The simplest aromatic aldehyde, benzaldehyde, can be found in many distilled beverages. It has been detected in large amounts in brandies produced from stone fruits (Nykänen & Suomalainen, 1983). According to Bandion *et al.* (1976), the benzaldehyde content of cherry brandies is 33-75 mg/l; the highest amount, 129 mg/l, was found in an apricot brandy.

The appearance of aromatic aldehydes in spirits matured in wooden casks is associated with the degradation of wood lignin. During the maturation of whisky distillates, the amounts of aromatic aldehydes liberated depend on the type of cask; alcoholysis of lignin and extraction of the compounds with spirit give different yields when new or old charred or uncharred casks are used. It has been suggested that aromatic aldehydes produced in the free form by charring are extracted directly by the spirits. Moreover, ethanol reacts with lignin to form ethanol lignin, some of which breaks down to yield coniferyl and sinapic alcohols, which can then be oxidized into coniferaldehyde (4-hydroxy-3-methoxycinnamaldehyde) and sinapaldehyde (3,5-dimethoxy-4-hydroxycinnamaldehyde). Aldehydes with a double bond in the side chain, such as coniferaldehyde and sinapaldehyde, are further oxidized to yield vanillin (4-hydroxy-3-methoxybenzaldehyde) and syringaldehyde (3,5-dimethoxy-4-hydroxybenzaldehyde; Baldwin *et al.*, 1967; Baldwin & Andreasen, 1974; Reazin *et al.*, 1976; Nishimura *et al.*, 1983; Reazin, 1983). Concentrations of vanillin and syringaldehyde

Table 35. Content (mg/l) of vanillin and syringaldehyde in some brands of spirits[a]

Beverage	Vanillin	Syringaldehyde
Scotch whisky	0.31–2.06	0.67–4.04
Other whiskies	0.04–5.96	ND–10.2
Cognac and armagnac	0.25–1.85	0.41–3.75
Brandy	0.17–1.16	0.18–2.54
Rum	ND–3.17	ND–8.73

[a]From Lehtonen (1983); ND, not detected

in different commercial brands of distilled beverages are given in Table 35. Coniferaldehyde and sinapaldehyde were found in whisky and cognac, whereas salicylaldehyde was found only in whisky (Lehtonen, 1984).

(*b*) *Alcohols*

Some spirits, such as vodka, contain few flavour compounds and consist essentially of ethanol and water. In contrast, whiskies, cognacs, brandies and rums frequently contain large numbers of different volatile compounds.

(i) *Methanol*

Methanol is not a by-product of yeast fermentation but originates from pectins in the must and juice when grapes and fruits are macerated. In general, the methanol content of commercial alcoholic beverages is fairly small, except in those produced from grapes in prolonged contact with pectinesterase and in some brandies produced from stone fruits, such as cherries and plums. Apricot brandies have been found to contain up to 10 810 mg, plum brandies, up to 8850 mg, and cherry brandies, up to 5290 mg methanol/l pure alcohol. Cognac and grape brandies contain 103-835 mg/l and Scotch whisky 80-260 mg/l methanol (Nykänen & Suomalainen, 1983).

(ii) *Higher alcohols*

Higher alcohols and fusel alcohols (1-propanol, 2-methylpropanol, 2-methylbutanol, 3-methylbutanol and phenylethyl alcohol) are formed in biochemical reactions by yeast on amino acids and carbohydrates. The amounts in different beverages vary considerably. Scotch whisky has been reported to contain 1-propanol (70-255 mg/l), 2-methyl-1-propanol (170-410 mg/l), 2-methyl-1-butanol (74-124 mg/l) and 3-methyl-1-butanol (215-352 mg/l). Irish whiskey, Canadian whisky and Japanese whisky do not differ considerably from Scotch whiskies in concentrations of fusel alcohols, whereas American bourbon whiskeys can contain up to 1390 mg/l 2-methyl-1-butanol and up to 1465 mg/l 3-methyl-1-butanol.

Brandies and cognacs contain slightly more fusel alcohols than Scotch whiskies: 1-propanol (53-895 mg/l), 2-methyl-1-propanol (7-688 mg/l), 2-methyl-1-butanol (21-396 mg/l) and 3-methyl-1-butanol (98-2108 mg/l). The total amounts of fusel alcohols in rums correlate with the total congener content. Exceptionally high values have been reported for 1-propanol in some heavily flavoured Jamaican rums, in which the concentration of congeners was more than 9000 mg/l pure alcohol; the 1-propanol content ranged from 23 840 to 31 300 mg/l pure alcohol (Horak *et al.*, 1974a,b; Mesley *et al.*, 1975; Nykänen & Suomalainen, 1983).

The rose-like odour of phenethyl alcohol can be recognized in some whiskies, which usually contain 1-30 mg/l (ter Heide, 1986). In brandies and rums, the concentration is much lower. A very high content, 131 mg/l, was found in an American bourbon whiskey (Kahn & Conner, 1972).

A number of long-chain alcohols, up to C_{18}, have been found in distilled alcoholic beverages, but the concentrations are very small (Nykänen & Suomalainen, 1983).

(*c*) *Acids*

(i) *Aliphatic acids*

All the straight-chain monocarboxylic acids from C_2 to C_{18} and a large number of branched-chain acids have been identified in distilled alcoholic beverages (ter Heide, 1986); most are produced by yeast during fermentation. Recently, the presence of formic acid in cognac and rum has been confirmed, and it is one of the major acids in whisky (ter Heide, 1984, 1986). Saturated C_3-C_{18} straight-chain acids predominate, and acetic acid is generally the main component (ter Heide, 1986). Its relative proportion in Scotch whiskies is approximately 50% of total volatile acids, and that in other whiskies, 60-95%; cognacs and rums contain quantities of acetic acid amounting to 50-75% and 75-90% of the total volatile acids, respectively (Nykänen *et al.*, 1968).

The second largest acid component in distilled beverages is decanoic acid, followed by octanoic acid and dodecanoic acid or lauric acid. The concentration of palmitic acid and (*Z*)-hexadec-9-enoic acid (palmitoleic acid) is relatively high in Scotch whisky in particular. Of the short-chain acids, propionic, 2-methylpropionic, butyric, 3-methylbutyric and pentanoic acids are present in abundance. The concentrations of short-chain acids in rums were: acetic acid (4.5-11.7 mg/l), propionic acid (0.5-4.2 mg/l), butyric acid (0.4-2.6 mg/l), 2-ethyl-3-methylbutyric acid (0.1-2.2 mg/l) and hexanoic acid (0.3-1.3 mg/l; Nykänen & Nykänen, 1983); West Indian and Martinique rums contained 2-propenoic acid (0.1-0.2 mg/l) and dark rums, *trans*-2-butenoic acid, among others (ter Heide, 1986).

(ii) *Aromatic acids*

Small amounts of aromatic acids can be found in distilled alcoholic beverages (Nykänen & Suomalainen, 1983). Most are phenolic acids and probably originate in wooden casks used for maturation. In investigations of the nonvolatile compounds liberated by alcohol from oak chips, Nykänen, L. (1984) and Nykänen *et al.* (1984) found benzoic acid, phenylacetic acid, cinnamic acid, 2-hydroxybenzoic acid and benzenetricarboxylic acid in extracts. 3-Phenylpropanoic acid, salicylic acid and homovanillic acid ((4-hydroxy-3-methoxyphenyl)acetic acid) were identified in dark rum, and 4-hydroxybenzoic acid was identified in cognac matured for 50 years. In addition, coumaric acid (4-hydroxycinnamic acid) has been found in whisky, and gallic acid (3,4,5-trihydroxybenzoic acid), vanillic acid (4-hydroxy-3-methoxybenzoic acid), syringic acid (3,5-dimethoxy-4-hydroxybenzoic acid) and ferulic acid (4-hydroxy-3-methoxycinnamic acid) in rum (ter Heide, 1986). A prolonged maturation may increase the content of some aromatic acids, although, in armagnac, concentrations of cinnamic acid, benzoic acid, syringic acid, vanillic acid, ferulic acid, 4-hydroxybenzoic acid and 4-hydroxycinnamic acid reached their highest values after 15 years; in 30-year-old armagnac, the total amounts of these acids had decreased to approximately 30% of the maximal value (Puech, 1978).

(*d*) *Esters*

(i) *Esters of aliphatic acids*

Numerically, the largest group of flavour compounds in whisky, cognac and rum consists of esters (Nykänen & Suomalainen, 1983; ter Heide, 1986), most of which are ethyl esters of monocarboxylic acids. The straight-chain ethyl esters from C_2 up to C_{18} acids, and some ethyl esters of branched-chain acids, are present in whisky, cognac and heavily flavoured rum. The number of esters increases further by esterification of acids with fusel alcohols and with long-chain fatty alcohols as well as by the appearance of aromatic esters formed during maturation.

The total ester content varies widely in strong spirits. Esters have been found in aged Scotch malt whiskies (360 mg/l), in Scotch whiskies (550 mg/l), Irish whiskeys (1010 mg/l), Canadian whiskies (645 mg/l) and American whiskeys (269-785 mg/l). The ester contents of rums (44-643 mg/l) and brandies (300-6000 mg/l) are similar (Schoeneman *et al.*, 1971; Schoeneman & Dyer, 1973; Reazin *et al.*, 1976; Reinhard, 1977; Nykänen & Suomalainen, 1983).

Ethyl formate is a common component of spirits. Its concentration varies between 4 and 27 mg/l in whiskies and 13 and 33 mg/l in cognacs (Carroll, 1970; Nykänen & Suomalainen, 1983). Postel *et al.* (1975) reported 5-35 mg ethyl formate/l in rums. Ethyl acetate is quantitatively the most important component of the ester fraction, usually accounting for over 50%. Many short-chain esters, such as isobutyl acetate, ethyl isobutyrate, ethyl *n*-butyrate, ethyl isovalerate, 2-methylbutyl acetate and 3-methylbutyl acetate, have fairly strong odours; therefore, their occurrence in whisky, cognac and rum has been investigated extensively (Nykänen & Suomalainen, 1983).

In whisky, the concentrations of long-chain carboxylic acid esters increase from ethyl hexanoate up to ethyl decanoate and then decrease, so that C_{18} ethyl esters are usually the last components to be detected. In Scotch whisky, the ethyl esters of hexadec-9-enoic acid and hexadecanoic acid frequently occur in nearly equal amounts. In cognac, brandy and rum, the concentrations of the ethyl esters of C_{14}-C_{18} acids, and particularly of ethyl hexadec-9-enoate, are smaller than those in whisky (Suomalainen & Nykänen, 1970; ter Heide, 1986).

(ii) *Esters of aromatic acids*

The aromatic acids that occur in whisky, cognac and rum are also present as ethyl esters, although in very small amounts (Nykänen & Suomalainen, 1983). Higher amounts of ethyl benzoate have been found in plum brandies (ter Heide, 1986). Postel *et al.* (1975) found 8 mg ethyl benzoate/l alcohol in plum brandy, 10 mg/l in mirabelle brandy and 6 mg/l in kirsch. Beaud and Ramuz (1978) found 15-18 and 12-13 mg ethyl benzoate/l alcohol in kirsch and Morello cherry brandy, respectively. Schreier *et al.* (1978) reported that apple brandy contains 0.32 mg/l ethyl benzoate. Minor amounts of ethyl phenylacetate have been detected in cognac, German and French brandies and apple brandy (Schreier *et al.*, 1978, 1979).

(*e*) *Phenolic compounds*

Minor amounts of phenols, probably originating from raw materials, have been found in spirits. The phenolic compounds determined in whisky by Nishimura and Masuda (1971) and by Lehtonen and Suomalainen (1979) are listed in Table 36.

Table 36. Content (mg/l) of phenols in commercial whiskies

Compound	Malt whisky[a]	Blended Scotch whisky[a]	Scotch whisky[b]	Japanese whisky[b]
Phenol	0.1	0.19	0.003	0.012
ortho-Cresol	0.075	0.075	0.015	0.013
meta-Cresol	0.030	0.035	ND	ND
para-Cresol	0.050	0.050	0.009	0.010
2-Methoxyphenol (Guaiacol)	0.090	0.120	0.012	0.006
2,6-Xylenol	ND	ND	0.001	ND
2-Ethylphenol	ND	ND	0.002	0.002
4-Ethylphenol	0.070	0.040	0.009	0.002
2-Methoxy-4-methylphenol	ND	ND	0.005	traces
2-Methoxy-6-methylphenol	ND	ND	ND	traces
2-Methoxy-4-ethylphenol	0.100	0.030	0.035	0.002
2-Methoxy-4-allylphenol (Eugenol)	0.050	0.100	0.032	0.011

[a]From Lehtonen and Suomalainen (1979)
[b]From Nishimura and Masuda (1971)
ND, not detected

The phenolic compounds found in cognac are 2-methoxy-4-ethylphenol (0.29 mg/l), 2-methoxy-4-allylphenol (0.14 mg/l), phenol (0.03 mg/l), 4-ethylphenol (0.03 mg/l) and 2-methoxyphenol (0.03 mg/l). In addition, *ortho*-cresol, *meta*-cresol and *para*-cresol were detected as trace components. In a commercial dark Martinique rum, 4-ethylphenol (1.8 mg/l), 2-methoxy-4-ethylphenol (1.1 mg/l), 2-methoxy-4-allylphenol (0.8 mg/l), 2-methoxyphenol (0.7 mg/l), phenol (0.2 mg/l), *para*-cresol (0.08 mg/l), *ortho*-cresol (0.06 mg/l) and *meta*-cresol (0.04 mg/l) were found (Jounela-Eriksson & Lehtonen, 1981). Schreier *et al.* (1979) reported the occurrence of 4-ethylphenol and 2-methoxy-4-ethylphenol in grape brandy.

Tannins are present in spirits matured in wooden caskes. Brandies were reported to contain epicatechin, gallocatechin, catechin, flavonones and a number of other phenolic compounds (Marché *et al.*, 1975). The concentration of tannins in brandy aged for four to ten years in oak barrels ranged between 240 and 1120 mg/l (Guymon & Crowell, 1972). Bourbon whiskeys matured in charred barrels for up to 12 years contained 230-670 mg/l tannins (Baldwin & Andreasen, 1974).

3.5 Additives and contaminants

(*a*) *Flavouring additives*

Hops and hop extracts are used by breweries to improve the flavour of beers. The presence of nonvolatile, bitter and other substances — hop acids and volatile terpenes — in hops has been reviewed (Verzele, 1986) and the chemical composition of hops is summarized in Table 37.

Table 37. Chemical composition of hops[a]

Compound	Amount (%)
α-Acids	2-12
β-Acids	1-10
Essential oil	0.5-1.5
Polyphenols	2-5
Oil and fatty acids	traces-25
Protein	15
Cellulose	40-50
Water	8-12
Pectins	2
Salts (ash)	10

[a]From Verzele (1986)

Various plant extracts and essential oils are used in the manufacture of alcoholic beverages, in addition to synthetic products, to flavour liqueurs, aperitif beverages like vermouth and some vodkas. For instance, the strongly flavoured Russian vodka *subrowka* contains a blade of sweet, or holy, grass (*Hierochloe odorata*), beloved of the European bison, from which colouring matter and flavouring compounds are extracted by alcohol during storage. Many terpenic compounds, a number of ketones, alcohols, aldehydes, esters, lactones, phenols and phenol ethers, and acids have been identified as the flavour components of *H. odorata*. The principal component of the grass is coumarin, which represents about 60% of the total content of the volatile compounds (Nykänen, I., 1984).

Anethole, which has a strong aniseed-like odour, is another natural substance encountered in many beverages, and particularly in liqueurs. Natural anethole is obtained from plant materials, but it is also produced synthetically. A large number of other natural and synthetic flavourings with the same odour are used (Liddle & Bossard, 1984, 1985).

(*b*) *Other additives*

Preservatives are often added to beers and wines to prevent the activity of bacteria and moulds. In the UK, breweries are permitted to use sulphur dioxide as an antibacterial and antioxidant agent at a statutory limit of 70 mg/l. Many yeasts can form small quantities of sulphur dioxide during fermentation. However, the sulphur dioxide formed in beers is bound to naturally occurring compounds, and only small amounts can be detected. The sulphur dioxide content of German, Belgian and Dutch beers varies from none to 2.3 mg/l as free sulphur dioxide and from 0.8 to 2.4 mg/l as total sulphur dioxide (Nykänen & Suomalainen, 1983).

Sulphur dioxide is also one of the most important additives in wine making. It is added in aqueous solution or as potassium metabisulphite water solution; most is bound to aldehydes (Ough, 1987), pigments and polyphenols. In many countries, the permitted amount of free sulphur dioxide in commercial wines is 35-100 mg/l; the concentrations reported depend on the analytical method used. Most wines contain similar amounts of total sulphur dioxide (>100 mg/l; Nykänen & Suomalainen, 1983). Sulphur dioxide reacts slowly with free oxygen in wine and is therefore a poor antioxidant, unless it is added to wine at much higher levels than those generally accepted for inhibiting bacterial activity. Addition of ascorbic acid to wine just before bottling maintains a moderate level of sulphur dioxide. In the presence of oxygen, ascorbic acid reacts rapidly to yield hydrogen peroxide and dehydroascorbic acid. Sulphur dioxide then reacts with hydrogen peroxide to form sulphate ions (Ough, 1987).

The use of sorbic acid (hexa-2,4-dienoic acid) is permitted to protect wine against the activity of bacteria and moulds. At concentrations of 180-200 mg/l, it inhibits yeast growth but does not affect bacteria. Certain genera of malolactic bacteria convert sorbic acid to 2-ethoxy-3,5-hexadiene (Ough, 1987).

A number of spirits contain added colouring agents on which little data have been published. Sunset yellow FCF (FD & C yellow 6; see IARC, 1975, 1987a) has been reported to be present in cocktails and liqueurs (Anon., 1987).

(*c*) *Trace elements*

Most of the published literature on trace elements in alcoholic beverages concerns wine.

Concentrations of trace elements found in wines and some other alcoholic beverages are presented in Table 38.

Table 38. Content (mg/l) of trace elements in some alcoholic beverages[a]

Trace element	Light beer	White wine	Red wine	Whisky
Calcium	20-50	80-110	34-140	11-17
Chloride	-	20-80	18-390	-
Cobalt	-	0-0.012	0-0.012	-
Copper	0.2-0.5	0.4-1.0	-	-
Fluoride	-	0.2-0.5	0.06-0.40	-
Iodide	-	0.1-0.6	0.1-0.6	-
Iron	-	4-10	-	-
Magnesium	-	60-150	65-110	1.9-2.8
Manganese	-	0-3.0	0-2	-
Phosphorus	250-300	100-200	150-400	-
Potassium	320-440	660-920	750-1160	26-30
Sodium	20-60	5-40	10-140	1-3
Zinc	0.1-0.2	1.0-3.4	1-3	-

[a]From Hoofdproduktschap voor Akkerbouwprodukten (1984)

Trace elements from grapes are transferred during crushing into the must and eventually into wine (Eschnauer, 1982). The total concentration of mineral constituents in wine may be as high as 1000 mg/l and more (Eschnauer, 1967). The main trace elements are potassium, magnesium, calcium and sodium (see Table 38), but iron, copper, manganese and zinc are also present. In most wines, the iron content varies from 1 to 5 mg/l and copper from 0.1 to 1 mg/l.

A concentration of 0.0002-0.003 mg/l cadmium has been reported in European wines, the majority of levels being in the range 0.0002-0.0015 mg/l (Golimowski *et al.*, 1979a,b). The natural lead content of German wines has been reported to be 0.01-0.03 mg/l, and the average chromium content is 0.065 mg/l. It has been suggested that in younger wines the chromium content may be slightly higher (0.18 mg/l) than in old wines because they are more frequently in contact with stainless steel (Eschnauer, 1982). Interesse *et al.* (1984) determined 14 trace elements in 51 southern Italian wines; the chromium content was found to range from 0.01 to 0.81 mg/l and that of nickel from <0.01 to 0.09 mg/l.

In the 1960s, an epidemic of cardiomyopathy in Québec was seen after the introduction of cobalt to enhance the 'head' of foam on commercially produced beer (Morin & Daniel, 1967; Milon *et al.*, 1968; Dölle, 1969).

(*d*) *Contaminants*

For the purposes of this section of the monograph, the term 'contaminants' refers to those minor constituents sometimes present in alcoholic beverages which are not essential to the flavour and properties of the product. Some of these contaminants have known toxicological and, in some cases, carcinogenic effects.

(i) N-*Nitrosamines*

The occurrence of nitrosamines (see IARC, 1978) in alcoholic beverages has been well established in many investigations despite analytical difficulties (McGlashan *et al.*, 1968, 1970; Collis *et al.*, 1971; Bassir & Maduagwu, 1978). Reviews on the chemistry of formation of nitrosamines, with special reference to malting, are available, which report that the most important source of *N*-nitrosodimethylamine (NDMA) in beer is malt kilning by reactions involving nitrogen oxides (Wainwright, 1986a,b); a number of other kilning practices have been tested to reduce the quantities of *N*-nitrosamines in malt. The mechanism of formation suggests that small amounts of NDMA may occur in whisky (Klein, 1981). The concentrations found in various alcoholic beverages are given in Table 39. Leppänen and Ronkainen (1982) reported NDMA levels in Scotch whisky of 0.6-1.1 μg/l, an average of 0.3 μg/l in Irish whisky, of <0.1 μg/l in Bourbon whiskey and <0.05-1.7 μg/l in beer. Of 158 samples of beer, 70% were found to contain NDMA; the mean concentration in all samples was 2.7 μg/l; the highest value, 68 μg/l, was found in a so-called 'Rauchbier' which is made from smoked malt to give a smokey taste (Spiegelhalder *et al.*, 1979).

Other nitrosamines that have been identified in beer include *N*-nitrosopyrrolidine (Klein, 1981) and *N*-nitrosoproline (Massey *et al.*, 1982).

Table 39. Average amounts of N-nitrosamines in alcoholic beverages[a]

Beverage	No. of samples	NDMA (μg/l)	NDEA (μg/l)	NDPA (μg/l)
Cider distillate	120	<0.05-10	<0.05-2	<0.05-2.6
Cider	21	<0.05-1.8	<0.05-2.2	<0.05-1.1
White alcohol[b]	9	<0.05-2.2	<0.05-4.8	ND
Whisky	8	<0.05-0.7	<0.05-0.4	<0.05-0.4
Rum	8	<0.05-0.3	<0.05-0.2	<0.05-0.2
Cognac and armagnac	12	<0.05-1.6	<0.05-0.15	<0.05-0.3
Wine	33	<0.05-0.6	0.3 (one sample)	ND
Beer	40	<0.05-8.6	<0.05-0.8	ND

[a]From Klein (1981); NDMA, N-nitrosodimethylamine; NDEA, N-nitrosodiethylamine; NDPA, N-nitrosodipropylamine; ND, not detected

[b]From fruit or grains

(ii) *Mycotoxins*

A wide variety of moulds is found on grapes; *Aspergillus flavus* may be among them, and hence aflatoxins may occur exceptionally in wines. In an investigation by Schuller *et al.* (1967), aflatoxin B_1 was found to be present in two (Ruländer 1964 and Gewürztraminer 1964) of 33 German wines analysed at amounts of <1 μg/l. Lehtonen (1973) investigated the occurrence of aflatoxins in 22 wines from different countries by a thin-layer chromatographic method and reported <1 μg/l in 11 samples and 1.2-2.6 μg/l in five samples; six samples were aflatoxin-free. Takahashi (1974) increased the sensitivity of the method and was able to determine aflatoxins B_1, B_2, G_1 and G_2 at concentrations of 0.25 μg/l wine; aflatoxins were not determined in 11 samples of French red wine, Spanish sherry, madeira and port wine. French wines and German wines investigated using improved methods have also been found to be free of aflatoxins (Drawert & Barton, 1973, 1974; Lemperle *et al.*, 1975).

Aflatoxins were found by Peers and Linsell (1973) in 16 of 304 Kenyan beer samples at concentrations of 1-2.5 μg/l. The probable source was rejected maize, which is often used in the production of local beers. In a study in the Philippines, 47% of 55 samples of [unspecified] alcoholic beverages contained aflatoxins at an average concentration of 1.9 μg/l (Bulatao-Jayme *et al.*, 1982).

Two other mycotoxins, ochratoxin A (see IARC, 1983a, 1987a) and zearalenone (see IARC, 1983a), have been found in beer made from contaminated barley. Krogh *et al.* (1974) reported that the malting process degraded ochratoxin A in moderately contaminated (830 μg/kg and 420 μg/kg) barley lots; however, small amounts of ochratoxin A (11 μg/l and 20 μg/l) were left in beer produced from heavily contaminated barley (2060 μg/kg and 27 500 μg/kg). Commercial and home-made Zambian beer brewed from maize contained zearalenone at concentrations ranging from no detectable amount to 2470 μg/l. The concentration of zearalenone in 12% of 140 beer samples in Lesotho was 300-2000 μg/l (Food and Agricultural Organization, 1979).

(iii) *Ethyl carbamate (urethane)*

Urethane (see IARC, 1974, 1987a) is formed by the reaction of carbamyl phosphate with ethanol (Ough, 1976a, 1984) and is, therefore, present in most fermented beverages. Ough (1976b, 1984) found urethane in commercial ales (0.5-4 25g/l), in saké (0.1-0.6 mg/l) and in some experimental (0.6-4.3 μg/l) and commercial wines (0.3-5.4 μg/l).

Numerous samples of distilled alcoholic beverages have been analysed for their urethane content, probably because of the high amounts found in stone fruit brandies. Christoph *et al.* (1986) reported urethane in Yugoslavian plum brandy (1.2-7 mg/l), in Hungarian apricot brandy (0.3-1.5 mg/l), in various plum brandies (0.4-10 mg/l), in kirsch (2-7 mg/l), in fruit brandy (0.1-5 mg/l), in Scotch, American bourbon, Canadian and Irish whiskies (0.03-0.3 mg/l) and in cognac and armagnac (0.2-0.6 mg/l). Urethane contents of alcoholic beverages reported by Mildau *et al.* (1987) are given in Table 40. Adam and Postel (1987) reported the following average urethane contents in some fruit brandies: kirsch (1.8 mg/l), plum brandy (1.7 mg/l), mirabelle plum brandy (4.3 mg/l), Williams pear brandy (0.18 mg/l), apple brandy (0.5 mg/l), Jerusalem artichoke brandy (0.7 mg/l) and tequila (0.1 mg/l).

Table 40. Content (mg/l) of urethane in some alcoholic beverages[a]

Beverage	Number of samples	Content
Kirsch	67	0.2–5.5
Plum brandy	27	0.1–7.0
Mirabelle plum brandy	8	0.2–2.3
Stone fruit brandy	2	0.2–0.3
Grain spirit	1	ND
Wine distillate	2	ND–0.05
Cognac	1	0.04
Rum	4	ND–0.06
Whisky	2	0.04–0.08
Liqueur	9	ND–0.16
Sherry	5	0.02–0.07
White wine	10	ND–0.02
Red wine	7	ND–0.05

[a]From Mildau et al. (1987); ND, not detected (<0.01 mg/l)

(iv) *Asbestos*

Asbestos (see IARC, 1977a, 1987a) fibres have been identified in some alcoholic beverages, possibly arising from the filters used for clarifying beverages, from water used during the production processes and from asbestos-cement water pipes. Biles and Emerson (1968) detected fibres of chrysotile asbestos in British beers by electron microscopy followed by electron diffraction examination. Cunningham and Pontefract (1971) found asbestos fibres in Canadian and US beers (1.1-6.6 million fibres/l), in South African, Spanish and Canadian sherries (2.0-4.1 million fibres/l), in Canadian port (2.1 million fibres/l), in French and Italian vermouth (1.8 and 11.7 million fibres/l), and in European and Canadian wine [concentrations not reported]. The asbestos fibres in Canadian beer and sherry were identified as chrysotile, while some of the European samples contained amphibole asbestos. Fibres of chrysotile asbestos were also found by electron microscopy in three of nine samples of US gin (estimated maximal concentrations, 13-24 million fibres/l; Wehman & Plantholt, 1974).

In some European countries, the use of asbestos to filter alimentary fluids has been prohibited (e.g., Ministère de l'Agriculture, 1980).

(v) *Arsenic compounds, pesticides and adulterants*

The use of arsenic-containing fungicides in vineyards may lead to elevated levels of arsenic in grapes and wines (see IARC, 1980, 1987a). Crecelius (1977) analysed 19 samples of red and white wines and found arsenite (As^{+3}) at <0.001-0.42 mg/l and arsenate (As^{+5}) at 0.001-0.11 mg/l. Four samples were further analysed for total arsenic content by X-ray fluorescence (diffractometry), which confirmed these results. A review of older studies by Noble *et al.* (1976) reported concentrations ranging from 0.02 to 0.11 mg/l in nine US wines.

Aguilar *et al.* (1987) have investigated the occurrence of arsenic in Spanish wines. They found that crushing, pressing, cloud removal and yeast removal after fermentation and finally clarification and ageing markedly reduced the arsenic content of wine. Arsenic contamination of German wines has been reported to have decreased since 1940, levelling out at 0.009 mg/l in wines after 1970. The natural arsenic content has been assumed to be 0.003 mg/l, with earlier arsenic contents reaching the level of 1.0 mg/l due to use of arsenic-containing pesticides and insecticides (Eschnauer, 1982).

The fungicides used in vineyards include zineb (see IARC, 1976a, 1987a), maneb (see IARC, 1976a, 1987a), mancozeb, nabam, metalaxyl, furalaxyl, benalaxyl, cymoxanil, triadimefon, dichlofluanid, captan (see IARC, 1983b, 1987a), captafol, folpet, benomyl, carbendazim, thiophanate, methyl thiophanate, iprodione, procymidone, vinclozolin, chlozolinate (Cabras *et al.*, 1987) and simazine (Anon., 1980). Residues of metalaxyl, carbendazim, vinclozolin, iprodione and procymidone may be found in wine. In addition, ethylenethiourea (see IARC, 1974, 1987a), an impurity and a degradation product of ethylene bisdithiocarbamates (zineb, maneb, mancozeb, nabam), has been reported to be present at trace levels in wine (Cabras *et al.*, 1987). Hiramatsu and Furutani (1978) reported that the concentrations of trichlorfon and its metabolite, dichlorvos (see IARC, 1979b, 1987a), are higher in wine than in berries, indicating that they may be accumulated in wine.

Fungicides that are prohibited in most European countries, Australia and the USA but may be used in other countries include diethyl dicarbonate, dimethyl dicarbonate, pimaricin, 5-nitrofurylacrylic acid and *n*-alkyl esters of 4-hydroxybenzoate (Ough, 1987).

Occasionally, illegal additives, which may be very toxic and which are not permitted for use in commercial production in most countries, have been identified in alcoholic beverages. These include methanol, diethylene glycol (used as a sweetener), chloroacetic acid or its bromine analogue, sodium azide and salicylic acid, used as fungicides or bactericides (Ough, 1987).

4. BIOLOGICAL DATA RELEVANT TO THE EVALUATION OF CARCINOGENIC RISK TO HUMANS

Imbalances in caloric and micronutrient intake are known to influence the incidence of spontaneous and experimentally induced tumours and most aspects of reproduction. In experiments evaluated in this section on the carcinogenicity and reproductive effects of ethanol in animals, including the modifying effects of ethanol, the controls and treated groups were not always maintained on isocaloric diets and no experiment involved isonutrient diets.

Some of the minor components of alcoholic beverages have carcinogenic, mutagenic and teratogenic activity; however, only studies referring to ethanol and alcoholic beverages are covered in this monograph.

Unless otherwise mentioned, the purity of the ethanol used in the carcinogenicity experiments described below was not specified. Similarly, when ethanol was given as a percentage in drinking-water, unless mentioned, it was not specified whether the percentage was calculated on a weight or volume basis.

4.1 Carcinogenicity studies in animals

(*a*) *Ethanol and alcoholic beverages*

The Working Group was aware of some early studies in which ethanol was administered to mice (Krebs, 1928; Ketcham *et al.*, 1963; Horie *et al.*, 1965) and to hamsters (Elzay, 1966; Henefer, 1966; Elzay, 1969; Freedman & Schklar, 1978) using various protocols, but these were found to be inadequate for evaluation.

(i) *Oral administration*

Mouse: A group of 108 male and 42 female CF1 mice, 75-120 days old, was given 43% ethanol in water as the drinking fluid intermittently (five days a week; Horie *et al.*, 1965) for periods of up to 1020 days. A group of 44 male CF1 mice, 65 days old, was given 14% ethanol similarly for up to 735 days. Two mice given 43% ethanol developed papillomas of the forestomach; a few other tumours, malignant lymphomas (four) and lung adenomas (three) were also found in the high-dose group. A further group of 100 male ddN mice, 130 days old, was given 19.5% as the drinking fluid intermittently for a maximum of 664 days; one mouse developed a papilloma of the forestomach. Groups of 42-69 male or female CF1 mice, 65-120 days old, were given Japanese whisky, Scotch whisky or saké as the drinking fluid intermittently for periods of up to 978 days. Three mice treated with Japanese whisky developed malignant lymphomas; one mouse treated with Scotch whisky developed a forestomach papilloma; and three malignant lymphomas and one forestomach papilloma were observed in the group treated with saké. A further group of 100 male ddN mice, 130 days old, was given sherry as the drinking fluid for periods of up to 536 days; papillomas of the forestomach were found in three mice (Kuratsune *et al.*, 1971). [The Working Group noted the absence of untreated control groups and the inadequate reporting of the data, such as survival rates.]

A group of 15 female C3H/St mice, 20-35 days old, received 12% ethanol (v/v) in water as the drinking fluid for 80 weeks. A control group of 30 females was maintained on deionized water. Mammary tumours developed between six and 11 months of age in 8/11 (73%) mice in the ethanol-treated group and between 12 and 16 months of age in 22/27 (82%) control mice. The tumour incidence in ethanol-treated mice was not statistically different from that in controls, but the shorter median time to tumour appearance in the ethanol-treated group (eight months *versus* 14.2 months of age) was significant ($p < 0.001$; Schrauzer *et al.*, 1979). [The Working Group noted the small number of animals used and the absence of histopathological examination of the tumours.]

A group of 16 female C3H/St weanling mice received decarbonated light beer (6% ethanol v/v) as the drinking fluid for life after weaning. A control group of 16 mice was maintained on deionized water. The incidence of 'mammary adenocarcinomas' (58.3% and 64%) and tumour latency (16.8 and 14.5 months of age) were similar in the two groups. Both groups reached 50% survival at about 15.5 months (Schrauzer *et al.*, 1982). [The Working Group noted the small number of animals and absence of histopathological examination of the tumours.]

As part of a study on modifying effects (see pp. 105-106, 108), 36 male and 32 female C57Bl mice, eight weeks of age, were administered 0.2 ml 40% ethanol by intragastric intubation twice a week for 50 weeks (total dose, 20 ml). All 68 surviving mice were killed at 80 weeks of age, at which time no treatment-related tumour was observed (Griciute *et al.*, 1981, 1982, 1984). [The Working Group noted the absence of an untreated control group and the limited dose of ethanol administered.]

Three groups of 100 male C57Bl/10J mice, 14 weeks old, were housed individually and given 3.5-15% ethanol solution for five weeks and subsequently 3.5, 7.5 or 12% v/v ethanol in distilled water as the drinking fluid *ad libitum* for their lifespan. A control group of 100 male mice received distilled water *ad libitum*. All groups were treated for up to 160 weeks. No difference in survival was noted between the group fed 3.5% ethanol and the controls (mean survival, 742 days); the longest survival time was in the group given 7.5% ethanol (792 days), and the group receiving 12% ethanol had a mean survival time of 760 days. Increased incidences of liver sarcomas [probably lymphomas], but not of hepatocellular carcinomas, were observed in mice given 7.5 and 12% ethanol (13/87 and 10/72) compared with 4/79 in the controls and 6/77 in the group given 3.5% ethanol, but not all mice were necropsied (Schmidt *et al.*, 1987). [The Working Group noted that many mice in each group were autolysed and could therefore not be used for pathological examination, and the inadequate reporting of the histopathological findings.]

Rat: In a study on modifying effects (see pp. 106-107), 40 albino (similar to BDII) rats [sex distribution unspecified], 10-12 weeks of age, were given a commercial brandy (38% ethanol) *ad libitum* as the drinking fluid. The rats failed to gain weight during the experiment and more than half had died by week 32. No liver tumour was reported in animals that had died by 56 weeks or in 20 controls given tap-water (Schmähl *et al.*, 1965). [The Working Group noted the short duration of the study and the short survival.]

As part of a study on modifying effects (see pp. 107, 109), groups of 40 Sprague-Dawley rats [sex distribution unspecified], three months old, were given 0.5 ml of 30% or 50% ethanol (v/v) daily by gavage for life. The average lifespan of rats treated with 30% ethanol was 500 days, and that of the group given 50% ethanol was 396 days. A group of ten rats given 1 ml saline orally served as controls. No oesophageal, stomach or hepatic tumour was found in any of these groups (Gibel, 1967). [The Working Group noted the limited extent of pathological examination.]

As part of a study on modifying effects (see p. 109), 48 Sprague-Dawley rats [sex distribution unspecified], three months old, were given 25% ethanol as the drinking fluid five times a week until their natural death. Another group of 48 rats was untreated and served as controls. Mean survival was 780 and 730 days in the two groups, respectively. No statistically significant increase in tumour incidence was observed (Schmähl, 1976). [The Working Group noted the inadequate reporting of the data.]

A group of 15 male Holtzman rats, weighing 80-100 g, was fed a synthetic diet containing ethanol (contributing 35% of total calories; mean ethanol consumption, 5 g/kg bw per day) for up to 370 days. A group of 15 males served as pair-fed controls. When animals were killed at 14 months, no liver tumour was found in either the ethanol-treated or control group (Mendenhall & Chedid, 1980). [The Working Group noted the short duration of the study, the small group size and that pathological examination was limited to the liver.]

Groups of 20-25 male and 20-25 female Wistar rats, six weeks of age, were given 15 or 55% ethanol, 15 or 55% farm apple brandy or 15 or 40% industrial apple brandy as the drinking fluid for up to 23 months. The higher concentrations were given on alternate days. Groups of 20 male and 20 female rats given water alone served as controls. After 23 months, survivors (80-93% of animals) were killed. No excess of tumours of any kind was found in any of the groups (Mandard *et al.*, 1981). [The Working Group noted that the daily intake of ethanol was lower at the higher concentrations.]

As part of a study on modifying effects (see p. 114), 80 male Sprague-Dawley rats [age unspecified] were given 5% ethanol (v/v) in water as the drinking fluid for up to 30 months. A group of 80 male rats given water alone served as controls. About 70% of animals in both groups were still alive at 18 months. Hepatocellular carcinomas were found in 8/79 ethanol-treated and in 1/80 control animals [$p = 0.016$]. Hyperplastic nodules [inadequately described] occurred in the livers of ten controls and 29 ethanol-treated animals. Endocrine tumours (benign and malignant) developed in 57/79 ethanol-treated animals (26 of the pituitary [$p = 0.0004$], 14 of the adrenal, 14 of the pancreas and three of the testis) and in

8/80 control animals (in the pituitary) (Radike *et al.*, 1981). [The Working Group noted that isocaloric and isonutrient intakes were not controlled in either treated or control groups.]

As part of a study on modifying effects (see pp. 109-110), groups of 26 male Fischer 344 rats, nine weeks old, were fed a liquid diet containing 6% ethanol (w/v; corresponding to 35% of the total caloric content) or control liquid diet for 26 weeks, after which they were returned to normal laboratory diet. All surviving rats were killed at 98 weeks of age. No statistically significant difference in tumour incidence was found between the treated group and controls (Castonguay *et al.*, 1984). [The Working Group noted the short period of exposure to ethanol.]

As part of a study on modifying effects (see p. 110), 25 male and 25 female young adult BDVI rats were given 40% ethanol [amount unspecified] by intragastric instillation twice a week for 78 weeks. A group of 25 males and 25 females served as untreated controls. Average lifespan was 98 weeks in male and 105 weeks in female treated animals and 107 and 113 weeks in controls; all surviving animals were killed at 120 weeks of age. No tumour that could be related to ethanol treatment was observed in these animals (Griciute *et al.*, 1986). [The Working Group noted that the dose of ethanol administered was not specified.]

As part of a study on modifying effects (see p. 112), groups of ten male Wistar rats [age unspecified] were given either 10% ethanol in water as the drinking fluid or water alone for up to 40 weeks, at which time they were killed. No tumour was found in either group (Takahashi *et al.*, 1986). [The Working Group noted the small sizes of the groups and the short duration of the experiment.]

Hamster: Groups of 58 male and six female or seven male and three female golden hamsters, 75 days old, were given sherry or 19.5% ethanol in water intermittently (on five days per week; Horie *et al.*, 1965) as the drinking fluid for up to 807 days. One hamster given sherry developed a papilloma of the forestomach (Kuratsune *et al.*, 1971). [The Working Group noted the absence of untreated control groups, the unusual group sizes and the inadequate reporting of the experiment.]

As part of a study on modifying effects (see pp. 110-111), 19 male outbred Syrian golden hamsters, nine weeks of age, were maintained on a liquid diet containing 6% (w/v) ethanol (35% of total caloric content) for a total of 29 weeks, with a four-week interruption after the first 20 weeks of the experiment. A group of 21 male hamsters served as controls. The animals were followed for up to a total of 19 months. No statistically significant difference in tumour incidence was found (McCoy *et al.*, 1981). [The Working Group noted the limited number of animals and the short duration of ethanol treatment.]

As part of a study on modifying effects (see p. 111), 20 male and 20 female outbred Syrian golden hamsters, eight weeks old, were given 5% (w/v) ethanol in water as the drinking fluid for up to 46 weeks, at which time all surviving animals were killed. No pancreatic tumour was observed (Pour *et al.*, 1983). [The Working Group noted the short duration of the experiment and that histological examination was limited to the pancreas, common duct and gall-bladder.]

As part of a study on modifying effects (see p. 111), groups of 27 male outbred Syrian golden hamsters, nine weeks old, were given 7.4% or 18.5% ethanol in water as the drinking fluid for 29 weeks, after which they were given tap-water only. A group of 27 male hamsters given tap-water served as controls. All surviving animals were killed 18 months after the beginning of the experiment. No statistically significant difference in tumour incidence was found (McCoy *et al.*, 1986). [The Working Group noted the short duration of ethanol treatment.]

(ii) *Skin application*

Mouse: A group of 29 female and 36 male C57Bl mice, 95-125 days old, received skin applications of a distillation residue of a saké (33% residue in 50% ethanol) three times a week for up to 829 days. A control group of 31 females and 33 males was painted on the skin with 50% ethanol and observed for up to 830 days. A skin papilloma developed in one mouse in the control group, but in none of the saké-treated group. A further group of 58 male CF1 mice, about 100 days old, received skin applications of a distillation residue of a Japanese whisky (33% residue in 50% ethanol) three times a week for up to 814 days. A control group of 57 males received applications of 50% ethanol for up to 802 days. No skin tumour was found in either group (Kuratsune *et al.*, 1971). [The Working Group noted the limited reporting of the experiment, such as on survival rates.]

(iii) *Transplacental and neonatal administration*

Mouse: Two groups of female C3H mice [age not specified] were given 0.5 or 5% ethanol (v/v) as the drinking fluid during pregnancy and their male offspring were observed for 15 months. Two additional groups were given water during pregnancy and 0.5 or 5% ethanol for one week beginning when their pups were one week old; male offspring were followed for 15 months after weaning. In offspring exposed to ethanol during embryogenesis, liver tumours (diagnosed grossly and described as hepatomas) developed in 3/25 exposed to 0.5% and in 1/10 exposed to 5% ethanol. In those exposed to ethanol *via* the milk for one week, liver tumours developed in 5/31 exposed to 0.5% and 5/45 exposed to 5%. The incidence of hepatomas in pooled control males was 27/62. The lower incidence of hepatomas in male mice exposed to ethanol during embryogenesis or for one week during suckling was statistically significant ($p < 0.005$ for combined experiments; Kahn, 1968). [The Working Group noted the short duration of treatment, the absence of information on initial group sizes and the lack of histopathological examination of the liver tumours.]

(*b*) *Modifying effects of ethanol on the activity of known carcinogens*

(i) N-*Nitrosodimethylamine* (NDMA)

Groups of 31-32 female and 37-38 male C57Bl *mice*, eight weeks of age, received gastric intubations of 0.03 mg NDMA in 0.2 ml water (total dose, 3 mg) or 0.03 mg NDMA in 0.2 ml 40% ethanol (total doses, 3 mg NDMA and 20 ml 40% ethanol [6.4 g 100% ethanol]) twice a week for 50 weeks. The experiment was terminated 72 weeks after the start of treatment, at which time all survivors were sacrificed. At that time, 25/68 mice given NDMA and 3/70 given NDMA plus ethanol were still alive. In animals given NDMA plus ethanol, 12/36 males and 12/30 females developed aesthesioneuroepitheliomas (olfactory tumours that infiltrate the frontal lobe of the brain); no such tumour was observed in animals given

NDMA. No significant difference in the incidence of other tumours was observed (Griciute *et al.*, 1981).

A group of 50 hybrid CBA × C57Bl/6 female *mice*, weighing 10-12 g, received NDMA (10 mg/l) in the drinking-water; another group of 100 mice received NDMA (10 mg/l) in combination with ethanol (6000 mg/l) in water as the drinking fluid. At nine months, all survivors were killed. There was no significant difference in the incidences of liver, lung or kidney tumours between the two groups (Litvinov *et al.*, 1986a). [The Working Group noted the short duration of the study.]

Two groups of 17 female Sprague-Dawley *rats*, weighing 130 g, were pair-fed for three weeks on a nutritionally adequate liquid diet containing either ethanol (36% of total calories) or isocalorically substituted carbohydrates (control diet) and were then maintained on laboratory chow and tap-water *ad libitum* for two weeks, during the first week of which they each received five daily intraperitoneal injections of 1.5 mg NDMA. This five-week cycle was repeated four times (total dose of NDMA, 30 mg/animal), after which time the animals were fed laboratory chow and observed for life. Survival in the group receiving NDMA plus ethanol was significantly longer than in the group receiving NDMA alone. The total number of tumours, the histological type and the target organs (liver, kidney, lung and thyroid gland; subcutaneous sarcomas) were similar in the two groups (Teschke *et al.*, 1983). [The Working Group noted the limited number of animals used and the short duration of exposure to ethanol.]

(ii) N-*Nitrosodiethylamine* (NDEA)

Groups of 38 male and 32 female C57Bl *mice*, eight weeks of age, received gastric intubations of 0.03 mg/animal NDEA in 0.2 ml tap-water (total dose, 3 mg/animal) or 0.03 mg/animal NDEA in 0.2 ml 40% aqueous ethanol (total doses, 3 mg/animal NDEA and 20 ml 40% ethanol [6.4 g 100% ethanol]) twice a week for 50 weeks. Animals were held for a further 28 weeks, at which time all survivors were sacrificed. A higher incidence of lymphomas was observed in the group given NDEA (45/70) than in mice given NDEA plus ethanol (21/69). The incidence of malignant oesophageal/forestomach tumours (mainly spinocellular [squamous-cell] carcinomas) was higher in the NDEA plus ethanol group (13/38 males, 19/31 females) than in the NDEA group (4/38 males, 3/32 females; Griciute *et al.*, 1984).

Groups of 100 female hybrid CBA × C57Bl/6 *mice*, weighing 10-12 g, received NDEA (10 mg/l) or NDEA in combination with ethanol (6000 g/l) in the drinking-water for 12 months, at which time all survivors were killed. The incidence of pulmonary tumours (mainly adenomas) was 49/86 in the group that received NDEA plus ethanol as compared to 22/79 in mice treated with NDEA only [$p = 0.0002$]. No difference in the incidences of other tumours was observed (Litvinov *et al.*, 1986b).

Groups of albino (similar to BDII) *rats* [sex distribution unspecified], 10-12 weeks of age, received 3 mg/kg bw NDEA in the drinking-water daily (28 rats; total dose, 700 ± 71 mg/kg bw), or 3 mg/kg bw NDEA as well as 40 ml of a commercial brandy (38% alcohol) as the drinking fluid (20 rats; total dose of brandy, 8100 ml/kg bw) [exact length of survival and of the experiment unspecified]. Hepatocellular carcinomas developed in 28/28 animals given NDEA and in 16/20 animals given NDEA plus brandy (Schmähl *et al.*, 1965). [The Working Group noted the inadequate reporting of the experiment.]

Groups of 13-27 male and female Sprague-Dawley *rats* [sex distribution unspecified], three months of age, received daily intragastric intubations of 2.5 mg/kg bw NDEA (total dose, 607 mg/kg bw), 2.5 mg/kg bw NDEA in 0.5 ml 30% (v/v) ethanol (total doses, 529 mg/kg bw NDEA and 106 ml/kg bw ethanol), 10 mg/kg bw NDEA (total dose, 1867 mg/kg bw) or 10 mg/kg bw NDEA in 0.5 ml 30% ethanol (total doses, 1806 mg/kg bw NDEA and 90 ml/kg bw ethanol) for life [duration of the study unspecified]. Mean times to tumour appearance in these groups were 242, 211, 186 and 180 days, respectively. The combination of NDEA plus ethanol increased the incidence of papillomas in the oesophagus and/or forestomach [sites not clearly specified]: 2.5 mg/kg bw NDEA, 5/23; 2.5 mg/kg bw NDEA plus ethanol, 17/27; 10 mg/kg bw NDEA, 10/23; 10 mg/kg bw NDEA plus ethanol, 13/13. In contrast, the incidence of epidermoid carcinomas of the oesophagus and/or forestomach [sites not clearly specified] was increased only in the high-dose group: 10 mg/kg bw NDEA, 3/23; 10 mg/kg bw NDEA plus ethanol, 7/13 [$p = 0.013$] (Gibel, 1967). [The Working Group noted inconsistencies in the reporting.]

Two groups of 90 male Sprague-Dawley *rats*, 14 weeks of age, received daily administrations of 0.1 mg/kg bw NDEA in the drinking-water on five days per week for life or the same NDEA treatment and subsequent daily administration of 5 ml 25% ethanol in water as the drinking fluid on five days per week for life. Average survival times were 116 weeks in the group receiving NDEA alone and 104 weeks in the group receiving NDEA plus ethanol; in the latter group, 31 animals died prior to the appearance of the first tumours. The incidence of liver tumours (described as malignant hepatomas) was lower in the group receiving both NDEA and ethanol (4/59; 7%) than in animals treated only with NDEA (36/80; 45%; $p < 0.01$). There was also a decrease in the incidence of squamous-cell carcinomas and/or papillomas of the oesophagus in animals treated with both NDEA and ethanol (18/59; 31%) as compared to the NDEA-treated group (33/80; 41%; Habs & Schmähl, 1981). [The Working Group noted the high mortality of animals in the group treated with both agents which precludes a meaningful evaluation of the study.]

Two groups of 19 female Sprague-Dawley *rats* weighing 100 g were fed semisynthetic choline-deficient or choline-supplemented diets and 25% sucrose plus 32% (w/v) ethanol (decreased to 25% during the first five days) as the drinking fluid for up to ten months. One day prior to the start of the experiment and two months later, the rats were given an intraperitoneal injection of 100 mg/kg bw NDEA. Two additional groups of 12 female rats were fed the same isocaloric diets without ethanol and received the two doses of NDEA. A further group of ten rats were pair-fed a choline-deficient diet but not treated with NDEA, and served as controls. Seven months after the initiation of the experiment, 12, 11, six, six and four rats in the different groups, respectively, were killed; the remaining animals were killed at the end of the tenth month. No tumour of the liver or kidney was found in any of the rats killed at seven months. At termination of the experiment at ten months, hepatocellular carcinomas and renal 'adenomas' were found in 3/6 and 2/6 rats given NDEA and fed the choline-deficient diet, but in none of the other groups (Porta *et al.*, 1985). [The Working

Group noted the short duration of the study and the small number of animals left after the interim kill.]

Male Wistar *rats* weighing 80-120 g received a single intraperitoneal injection of 30 mg/kg bw NDEA, and, one week later, received either tap-water or 5% ethanol in water as the drinking fluid, and were observed for 18 months. Hepatocellular carcinomas developed in 2/8 animals given NDEA plus ethanol and in 0/18 controls (Driver & McLean, 1986). [The Working Group noted the small number of animals used.]

Either tap-water or 20% ethanol plus 10% sucrose in water was given as the drinking fluid to male Wistar *rats* that had been subjected to a 70% partial hepatectomy, followed by an intraperitoneal injection of 10 mg/kg bw NDEA 24 h after surgery. The group that received ethanol plus sucrose as the drinking fluid was placed on this regimen eight weeks after surgery and consumed an average of 110 ml/kg bw (15.4 g/kg bw ethanol) daily. All rats were killed 40 weeks after NDEA treatment. In five rats given NDEA alone, two hepatocellular nodules [adenomas] less than 2 mm in diameter were found; in ten rats given NDEA followed by ethanol, 15 nodules ranging in diameter from less than 2 mm (11 nodules) to 6 mm were found and confirmed histologically ($p < 0.05$; Takada *et al.*, 1986). [The Working Group noted the small number of animals used and the short duration of the study.]

(iii) N-*Nitrosodi*-n-*propylamine* (NDPA)

Groups of 38 male and 32 female C57Bl *mice*, eight weeks of age, received intragastric intubations of 0.03 mg NDPA in 0.2 ml water (total dose, 3 mg) or 0.03 mg NDPA in 0.2 ml 40% ethanol (v/v) in water (total doses, 3 mg NDPA; 20 ml 40% ethanol [6.4 g 100% ethanol]) twice a week for 50 weeks. At 72 weeks after the beginning of the experiment, all survivors were killed. A statistically significant increase in the incidence of spinocellular [squamous-cell] carcinoma of the oesophagus/forestomach was observed in the group give NDPA plus ethanol (36/70; $p < 0.00005$) as compared to the group given NDPA alone (7/70) (Griciute *et al.*, 1982).

Groups of 70 C57Bl *mice* [sex distribution and age unspecified] received intragastric instillations of a mixture of 0.01 mg NDMA plus 0.01 mg NDEA plus 0.01 mg NDPA in 40% ethanol [volume unspecified] or in water twice a week for 50 weeks. All surviving animals were killed after 79 weeks. Tumour incidences in the two groups were: malignant forestomach/oesophageal tumours, 35/70 and 8/70; pulmonary adenomas, 55/70 and 34/70; and aesthesioneuroepitheliomas infiltrating the brain, 2/70 and 0/70, respectively (Griciute *et al.*, 1987).

(iv) N-*Nitrosomethylbenzylamine* (NMBzA)

Two groups of 40 male weanling Sprague-Dawley *rats* were fed a zinc-deficient diet containing 7 mg/kg zinc and were given either deionized water or 4% ethanol in deionized water as the drinking fluid. After four weeks, NMBzA was administered intragastrically to both groups at a dose of 2 mg/kg bw twice weekly for four weeks and the dietary regimes were maintained for a further 29 weeks. Oesophageal tumours were observed in 25/33 rats fed the diet without ethanol as drinking fluid and in 29/34 rats fed the diet with 4% ethanol in water as the drinking fluid (Gabrial *et al.*, 1982).

(v) N-*Nitrosomethylphenylamine* (NMPhA)

Groups of 48 Sprague-Dawley *rats* [sex distribution unspecified], 13 weeks of age, received either weekly subcutaneous injections of 10.0 mg/kg bw NMPhA for 24 weeks (group 1); weekly subcutaneous injections of 2.0 mg/kg bw NMPhA for 39 weeks (group 2); daily administration of 1.5 [presumably mg/kg bw] NMPhA in the drinking-water for 22 weeks (group 3); or daily administration of 0.3 [presumably mg/kg bw] NMPhA in the drinking-water for 29 weeks (group 4). Four other groups received the same treatments in combination with administration of 25% ethanol (about 30 ml/kg bw) in water five times per week. The animals were observed until natural death; the mean life expectancy was 780 ± 120 days for all treated groups. The incidences of oesophageal tumours (squamous-cell carcinomas, transition from papilloma to carcinoma often seen) were group 1, 41/48 (84%); group 2, 22/48 (46%); group 3, 42/48 (87%); and group 4, 39/48 (80%); administration of ethanol did not alter these incidences (Schmähl, 1976). [The Working Group noted limitations in the experimental design and reporting.]

(vi) N-*Nitrosopiperidine* (NPIP)

Groups of about 28 male Fischer 344 *rats* weighing 160 g received either 0.06% NPIP in the basal diet for eight weeks; 0.06% NPIP in the basal diet for eight weeks followed by 10% ethanol in water as the drinking fluid for 12 weeks; 0.06% NPIP in the basal diet plus administration of 1 ml 50% ethanol through a tube inserted into the pharynx once every two days for eight weeks followed by no further treatment or followed by 10% ethanol as the drinking fluid for 12 weeks. The study was terminated 20 weeks after the start of the experiment. No significant difference in the incidence of oesophageal carcinomas was found (Konishi *et al.*, 1986). [The Working Group noted the relatively short duration of the experiment.]

(vii) N,N′-*Dinitrosopiperazine* (DNPIP)

Groups of 20 Sprague-Dawley *rats* [sex distribution unspecified], three months of age, received daily administration of 5 mg/kg bw DNPIP (total dose, 2605 mg) or 5 mg/kg bw DNPIP plus 0.5 ml 30% (v/v) ethanol (total doses: DNPIP, 2250 mg; ethanol, unspecified) by gastric intubation for life [duration unspecified]. The numbers of oesophageal and/or forestomach tumours [sites not clearly specified] induced by DNPIP were 11 papillomas and one carcinoma in DNPIP-treated animals and 16 papillomas and one carcinoma in those given DNPIP plus ethanol. Time to appearance of tumours was 521 days in the groups given DNPIP compared with 450 days in the group given DNPIP plus ethanol (Gibel, 1967). [The Working Group noted inconsistencies in the reporting.]

(viii) N′-*Nitrosonornicotine* (NNN)

Groups of 26 or 30 male Fischer 344 *rats*, nine weeks of age, were maintained on either a control liquid diet (groups 1 and 3) or a liquid diet containing 6.6% w/v ethanol (35% of calories; groups 2 and 4). At 13 weeks of age, rats in groups 1 and 2 were given a subcutaneous injection of 10 mg/kg bw NNN in saline on three alternate days per week (56-66 injections; total dose, 177 mg/rat); the liquid diets were replaced with basal diet 24 h after the last injection. At 13 weeks of age, rats from groups 3 and 4 received addition of 17.5 mg/l NNN to their respective liquid diets for 27 weeks (total dose, 177 mg/rat), after which time they were placed on basal diets during the observation period. The study was terminated when rats were 98 weeks of age. No significant difference was observed in the incidence of nasal cavity tumours between animals receiving subcutaneous injections of NNN (group 1, 24/30; group 2, 22/30); however, in rats administered NNN in the liquid diet, nasal cavity tumours developed in 18/30 rats in group 3 (NNN; 11 benign and seven malignant) and in 26/30 rats in group 4 (NNN plus ethanol; 20 benign and six malignant; $p < 0.05$). The incidence of oesophageal tumours was 25/30 in rats in group 3 (16 benign and nine malignant) and 20/30 in group 4 (13 benign and seven malignant; Castonguay *et al.*, 1984).

Groups of 25 male and 25 female young adult BDVI *rats* received gastric instillations of 0.3, 1.0 or 3.0 mg/rat NNN in water, or 0.3, 1.0 or 3.0 mg/rat NNN in a 40% aqueous ethanol solution [volume unspecified] twice a week for 78 weeks (total doses of NNN, 46.8, 156 and 468 mg/rat). Animals were held for observation until 120 weeks of age, at which time survivors were killed. Only seven rats receiving 3.0 mg NNN in water and none receiving 3.0 mg NNN in ethanol survived for more than 78 weeks. The time to appearance of the first tumour of the nasal cavity was shorter in all rats given NNN in ethanol solution. The incidences of malignant nasal cavity tumours (mainly aesthesioneuroepitheliomas [neuroblastomas]) were slightly elevated in ethanol-treated rats: males — 0/25, 2/25 and 20/25 given NNN in water; 0/25, 5/25 and 24/25 given NNN in ethanol; and females — 1/25, 3/25 and 22/25 given NNN in water; 0/25, 2/25 and 25/25 given NNN in ethanol. No difference in the incidence of tumours at other sites was noted (Griciute *et al.*, 1986). [The Working Group noted that animals were given the same amount of NNN irrespective of body weight, that few animals received the total dose of NNN, and that the volume of ethanol given was not stated.]

Groups of 21 male outbred Syrian golden *hamsters*, nine weeks of age, were fed control liquid diets or liquid diets containing 6% (w/v) ethanol (35% of caloric intake). At 13 weeks of age, the animals received 0.5-ml intraperitoneal injections of 2.37 or 4.74 mg/animal NNN three times a week for 25 weeks (total dose, 177 or 354 mg) and were maintained on their respective diets. Treatment was suspended during weeks 17-21 because of weight loss. At the end of the treatment, animals in both groups were returned to a diet of laboratory chow and water. Animals were sacrificed when moribund, and survivors were sacrificed 18 months after the beginning of carcinogen administration. There was no significant difference in the incidence of nasal cavity or tracheal tumours in the two treated groups (McCoy *et al.*, 1981). [The Working Group noted the short duration of exposure to ethanol and that animals were given the same amount of NNN, irrespective of body weight.]

(ix) N-*Nitrosopyrrolidine* (NPYR)

Groups of 21 male outbred Syrian golden *hamsters*, nine weeks of age, were fed control liquid diets or liquid diets containing 6% (w/v) ethanol (35% of caloric intake). At 13 weeks of age, the animals received 0.5-ml intraperitoneal injections of 1.33 or 2.67 mg/animal NPYR three times a week for 25 weeks (total dose, 100 or 200 mg) and were maintained on their respective diets. Treatment was suspended during weeks 17-21 because of weight loss. At the end of the treatment, animals in both groups were returned to a diet of laboratory chow and water. All survivors were killed 15 months after the beginning of carcinogen administration. The incidences of nasal cavity tumours were: low-dose NPYR, 1/20; low-dose NPYR plus ethanol, 8/18 ($p < 0.05$); high-dose NPYR, 14/21; and high-dose NPYR plus ethanol, 16/17 ($p < 0.05$). The incidences of tracheal tumours were: low-dose NPYR, 4/20; low-dose NPYR plus ethanol, 9/18 ($p < 0.05$); high-dose NPYR, 8/21; and high-dose NPYR plus ethanol, 11/17 (McCoy *et al.*, 1981). [The Working Group noted that animals were given the same amount of NPYR, irrespective of body weight.]

In a subsequent experiment, the effect of changes in the amount of ethanol consumed on the carcinogenicity of NPYR was determined. Groups of 27 male outbred Syrian golden *hamsters*, nine weeks of age, were administered tap-water, 7.4% ethanol or 18.5% ethanol in water as the drinking fluid for four weeks, followed by 0.5-ml intraperitoneal injections of 1.33 mg/animal NPYR three times a week for 25 weeks (total dose, 100 mg/animal), after which ethanol-treated animals were administered tap-water only. Animals were killed 17 months after the beginning of carcinogen administration. The incidences of tracheal papillomas were: tap-water plus NPYR, 3/26; low-dose ethanol plus NPYR, 6/26; and high-dose ethanol plus NPYR, 4/26. The incidences of hepatic neoplastic nodules were 6/26, 17/26 ($p < 0.01$) and 17/26 ($p < 0.01$), respectively (McCoy *et al.*, 1986). [The Working Group noted that animals were given the same amount of NPYR, irrespective of body weight.]

(x) N-*Nitrosobis(2-oxopropyl)amine* (NDOPA)

Two groups of 15 male Syrian *hamsters*, six weeks old, received either a single subcutaneous injection of 20 mg/kg bw NDOPA alone or 25% ethanol in water (w/v) as the drinking fluid; two weeks after the start of ethanol treatment, animals were given a single subcutaneous injection of 20 mg/kg bw NDOPA. Treatment continued for 24 weeks, at which time the hamsters were killed. Histopathological examination of the exocrine pancreas showed fewer neoplastic lesions [details not given] in animals treated with NDOPA plus ethanol (0/13) than in those treated with NDOPA alone (11/14; Tweedie *et al.*, 1981). [The Working Group noted the small number of animals used, the short duration of the study and the inadequate reporting.]

Groups of 20 male and 20 female outbred Syrian golden *hamsters*, eight weeks old, received 5% (w/v) ethanol in water as the drinking fluid for 46 weeks. Then, one group received a single subcutaneous injection of 20 mg/kg bw NDOPA prior to ethanol treatment, and the other received a subcutaneous injection of 20 mg/kg NDOPA four weeks after the beginning of ethanol treatment. A further group of 20 males and 20 females received the injection of NDOPA and were maintained on tap-water. All survivors were killed at the end of 46 weeks. No significant different in the incidence of pancreatic tumours was noted (Pour *et al.*, 1983).

(xi) N-*Methyl*-N′-*nitro*-N-*nitrosoguanidine* (MNNG)

Two groups of male Wistar *rats*, seven weeks of age, received 100 mg/l MNNG continuously in their drinking-water simultaneously with a 10% sodium chloride supplemented diet for eight weeks, after which time they were returned to nonsupplemented diets and either tap-water (30 rats) or 10% ethanol in water as the drinking fluid (21 rats). At the end of 40 weeks, all survivors were killed. Adenocarcinomas of the glandular stomach or duodenum occurred in 4/30 and 2/21 rats given tap-water and 10% ethanol, respectively (Takahashi *et al.*, 1986).

(xii) N-*Hydroxy-2-acetylaminofluorene* (OH-AAF)

Groups of four to ten male and six to 12 female inbred Fischer *rats*, four to 16 weeks of age, were fed a semisynthetic diet with or without 160 mg/kg OH-AAF for 12-20 weeks, after which they were maintained on basal diet for up to 20 weeks. Groups also received 10 or 20% (by volume) ethanol in water as the drinking fluid or water alone, simultaneously with the OH-AAF diet. Other groups were given the OH-AAF treatment and water in the first experimental period followed by control diet and ethanol in the second period. In a second series, groups of 20 male and 20 female weanling random-bred NIH black rats were fed a diet containing 80 mg/kg OH-AAF for 64 weeks and received either water alone or 10% ethanol in water as the drinking fluid. No significant treatment-related increase in the incidence of hepatocellular adenomas was observed in any of the groups of either strain (Yamamoto *et al.*, 1967). [The Working Group noted the small numbers of animals per group and the large variations in age at the start of treatment.]

(xiii) *Azoxymethane*

Groups of 26 male Fischer 344 *rats*, ten weeks of age, were pair-fed isocaloric liquid diets containing 12 or 23% of calories as beer or 9 or 18% as ethanol. Three weeks after the start of treatment, the rats received ten weekly subcutaneous injections of 7 mg/kg bw azoxymethane in sterile water and were maintained on the same diets until sacrifice at week 26. The high-dose ethanol group showed a trend towards reduced number of tumours in the right colon but not in the left. The number of right colonic tumours was inversely correlated with ethanol consumption in all animals (Spearman's rank correlation coefficient: r, −0.350; $p < 0.001$), but there was no correlation with left colonic tumours. The total number of colonic tumours in the high-dose ethanol group was markedly reduced in comparison with controls (18 tumours *versus* 45) but not in the low-dose ethanol group (37 tumours *versus* 45). Similar effects were found in the group given 23% calories as beer (Hamilton *et al.*, 1987a). [The Working Group noted that the exact incidences and the histopathological nature of the tumours were not reported.]

In a further study, groups of 35 male ten-week-old Fischer 344 *rats* were given liquid diets providing 11, 22 or 33% of calories from ethanol. All rats were given ten weekly subcutaneous injections of 7 mg/kg bw azoxymethane, and the liquid-ethanol diets were given either three weeks prior to and during treatment or for 16 weeks after treatment with azoxymethane, at which time all animals were killed. Administration of the liquid-ethanol diet after injection of the carcinogen had no effect on the incidence of tumours of the right and transverse colon or of the left colon. The incidence of tumours of the left colon was significantly reduced by the 22 and 33% liquid-ethanol diets, as was that of tumours of the right and transverse colon by the 33% liquid-ethanol diet given prior to and during administration of the carcinogen (Hamilton *et al.*, 1987b). [The Working Group noted the absence of data on the histopathological nature of the tumours.]

(xiv) *7,12-Dimethylbenz[a]anthracene* (DMBA)

Two groups of 30 or 20 female NMRI *mice* [age unspecified] received skin applications of 0.02 ml of a 1% solution (v/w) of DMBA in acetone or ethanol (purity, 99.5%) three times a week for 20 weeks. Skin tumours, including some squamous-cell carcinomas, occurred in 4/30 mice treated with DMBA in acetone (11 tumours; latency, nine weeks) compared with 11/20 [$p = 0.002$] mice treated with DMBA in ethanol (48 tumours; latency, six weeks; Stenbäck, 1969).

Two groups of 72 or 70 male CF1 *mice*, two months of age, received a single skin application of 0.02 ml of a 1.5% DMBA solution in acetone. One group received no further treatment, but, one month later, the second group received applications of 0.04 ml of a 50% aqueous ethanol solution on the same region twice a week for 40 weeks. At the end of the treatment period, the number of tumour-bearing animals in the ethanol-treated group (25/59; papillomas and one squamous-cell carcinoma) was not significantly different from that in controls (15/46; all papillomas). In a second experiment, groups of mice received a single application of 0.025 ml DMBA (1.5%) in acetone. One month later, animals received applications to the skin of 0, 12 or 43% ethanol twice a week for 40 weeks. There was no statistically significant difference in tumour yield between mice treated with 12% ethanol (6/55; one squamous-cell carcinoma) or with 43% ethanol (9/56; all papillomas) or controls (5/46; Kuratsune *et al.*, 1971).

(xv) *1,2-Dimethylhydrazine* (DMH)

Two groups of 16 male Sprague-Dawley *rats*, 60 days of age, were fed a liquid diet containing 36% of total calories as ethanol (concentration, 6.6% v/v) or as isocaloric carbohydrates. After four weeks of treatment, the animals were fed a standard laboratory diet for three weeks and received four weekly subcutaneous injections of 30 mg/kg bw DMH. This feeding schedule was repeated for a total of four cycles. After 32 weeks, the 28 survivors were killed; all had intestinal tumours. A higher number of rectal tumours (17 *versus* 6) was seen in rats treated with DMH and ethanol than in rats treated with DMH and an isocaloric diet, but no difference was seen in tumour incidences at other sites in the intestine (Seitz *et al.*, 1984, 1985).

Four groups of 20 male inbred D/A *rats*, four to six weeks of age, were fed a low-fat diet (5%, w/w; standard diet), and four other groups were fed a high-fat diet (33.5%, w/w). Both diets had a ratio of polyunsaturated:saturated fat of 3:2. One group on each diet received commercially available beer, and another received 4.8% ethanol (v/v) in water as the drinking fluid. All of these groups received 20 weekly subcutaneous injections of 20 mg/kg bw DMH. The other four groups served as low- or high-fat untreated or DMH-treated controls and received tap-water. Animals were killed 28 weeks after the first injection. The number of tumours per animal in both the small and large intestines was significantly greater in DMH-treated rats receiving the high-fat as compared to those receiving the low-fat diet. However, no significant difference in the incidence of intestinal cancer was noted in the groups given ethanol or beer as compared to those given water (Howarth & Pihl, 1985).

Two groups of 22 male Sprague-Dawley *rats*, five weeks of age, received either tap-water alone or 95% laboratory-grade ethanol diluted to 5% (v/v) in tap-water as the drinking fluid. After three weeks, both groups also received 16 weekly subcutaneous injections of 15 mg/kg bw DMH. A third control group of 22 rats received neither ethanol nor DMH. Animals were killed 22 weeks after the first injection of DMH. All animals given DMH had colonic cancers; ethanol did not affect the number of tumours per rat (3.9 ± 0.45 without DMH *versus* 3.5 ± 0.45 with DMH) (Nelson & Samelson, 1985).

In the same study, two groups of 12 male Sprague-Dawley *rats*, five weeks of age, received either tap-water alone or a commercially available beer as the drinking fluid. After three weeks, both groups also received ten weekly [presumably subcutaneous] injections of 20 mg/kg bw DMH. Animals were killed 14 weeks after the last injection of DMH. All 12 rats given DMH alone developed gastrointestinal tumours, compared to 8/12 rats given DMH plus beer, and there were fewer of these tumours per rat compared with rats treated with DMH alone (1.33 ± 0.43 *versus* 2.91 ± 0.52; $p = 0.043$; Nelson & Samelson, 1985). [The Working Group noted the small number of animals used and the absence of histological diagnosis of the tumours.]

(xvi) *Vinyl chloride* (VC)

Groups of 80 male Sprague-Dawley *rats* [age unspecified] received 5% ethanol in water or water alone as the drinking fluid for life. Four weeks after the start of treatment, one ethanol-treated and one untreated group were exposed by inhalation to 600 ppm (1560 mg/m³) VC for 4 h per day on five days per week for one year. At 18 months, survival was 40% in rats exposed to VC and 18% in animals exposed to VC plus ethanol. All survivors were killed 30 months after the first exposure to VC. Of the rats exposed to VC and to VC plus ethanol, 35/80 and 48/80 [$p = 0.028$] had hepatocellular carcinomas and 18/80 and 40/80 [$p = 0.002$] had liver angiosarcomas, respectively (Radike *et al.*, 1981).

(xvii) *Urethane*

In a study reported as an abstract, three groups of 30 male C3H *mice*, eight weeks of age, received gastric intubations of 2 mg/animal urethane in 0.2 ml water, 2 mg/animal urethane in 0.2 ml 40% ethanol or 2 mg/animal urethane in 0.2 ml water followed 24 h later by 0.2 ml 40% ethanol twice a week for five treatments. They were then given basal diet and tap-water for six months, at which time all survivors were killed. The presence of ethanol as a solvent enhanced pulmonary adenoma development; subsequent administration of ethanol had no influence on the carcinogenicity of urethane (Barauskaite, 1985).

In a study reported as an abstract, groups of 12-14 white outbred male and female *mice* [strain unspecified], eight weeks of age, received intraperitoneal injections of 10 mg urethane in 0.2 ml saline or in 0.2 ml 40% ethanol solution twice weekly for five weeks. Mice were held for 12 weeks, at which time all survivors were killed. All animals given urethane developed pulmonary tumours; the average number of pulmonary adenomas per animal was 30 in the group given urethane in ethanol and 13 in the group given urethane in saline ($p = 0.002$; Griciute, 1981).

(*c*) *Carcinogenicity of metabolites*

Acetaldehyde, the major intermediary metabolite of ethanol, was tested for carcinogenicity in rats by inhalation exposure and in hamsters by inhalation and by intratracheal instillation. It produced tumours of the respiratory tract following its inhalation, particularly adenocarcinomas and squamous-cell carcinomas of the nasal mucosa in rats and laryngeal carcinomas in hamsters. In hamsters, it did not result in an increased incidence of tumours following intratracheal instillation. Inhalation of acetaldehyde enhanced the incidence of respiratory-tract tumours induced by intratracheal instillation of benzo[*a*]pyrene in hamsters. Previous IARC working groups have concluded that there is *sufficient evidence* for the carcinogenicity of acetaldehyde in experimental animals (IARC, 1985, 1987a).

4.2 Other relevant data from experimental systems

(*a*) *Absorption, distribution and excretion*

The absorption, distribution, excretion and metabolism of ethanol have been reviewed extensively (Wallgren & Barry, 1970; Kalant, 1971; Hawkins & Kalant, 1972; Khanna & Israel, 1980; Lieber, 1982, 1983, 1984a, 1985a,b).

Ethanol is absorbed from the gastrointestinal tract by simple diffusion. The rate of absorption is decreased by delayed gastric emptying and by the intestinal contents. It has been demonstrated in several animal species that food delays absorption, producing a slower rise and lower peak value of the blood ethanol in fed than in fasting animals. The absorption of ethanol was slower from beer and wine than from distilled beverages. High ethanol concentrations may delay gastric emptying (Rasmussen, 1940; Wallgren & Barry, 1970) as does intraperitoneal administration of glucose (Wallgren & Hillbom, 1969). In contrast, carbohydrates (Broitman *et al.*, 1976), amino acids and dipeptides (Hajjar *et al.*, 1981) have been shown to enhance ethanol absorption in perfused rat jejunum *in vivo*.

The diffusion of ethanol through cell boundaries is slow and is affected by blood flow. Ethanol in the blood passes almost immediately into brain tissue (Harger *et al.*, 1937; Hulpieu & Cole, 1946; Crone, 1965). In contrast, the distribution of ethanol to resting skeletal muscle is particularly slow (Harger & Hulpieu, 1956).

After oral dosage, ethanol disappeared from the blood of dogs linearly in the post-absorption phase, irrespective of the concentration of ethanol in the body; zero-order kinetics was also found in dogs, cats, rabbits, pigeons and chicken after intravenous administration (Newman & Lehman, 1937).

(*b*) *Metabolism*

Ethanol is eliminated from the body mainly by metabolism in the liver and only minimally by urinary excretion and pulmonary exhalation (Wallgren & Barry, 1970). Other tissues such as kidney (Leloir & Muñoz, 1938), stomach and intestine oxidize ethanol to a small extent (Carter & Isselbacher, 1971; Lamboeuf *et al.*, 1981).

The hepatic metabolism of ethanol proceeds in three basic steps. First, ethanol is oxidized within the cytosol of hepatocytes to acetaldehyde; second, acetaldehyde is converted to acetate, mainly in the mitochondria; and third, acetate produced in the liver is released into the blood and is oxidized by peripheral tissues to carbon dioxide, fatty acids and water. The main pathway for ethanol metabolism proceeds *via* alcohol dehydrogenase (ADH). However, alternative pathways for ethanol oxidation have been described, which are situated in other subcellular compartments.

(i) *Alcohol dehydrogenase (ADH)*

ADH occurs in the soluble fraction of the liver and is also found in other tissues in the body, such as gastrointestinal mucosa, kidney, lung and possibly brain (Mistilis & Garske, 1969; Hawkins & Kalant, 1972). It catalyses the oxidation of alcohols, including ethanol, to their corresponding aldehydes in the presence of NAD, according to the following scheme:

$$CH_3CH_2OH + NAD^+ \dashrightarrow CH_3CHO + NADH + H^+$$

(Hawkins & Kalant, 1972). The optimal pH for ADH-mediated oxidation of ethanol is 10-11 (von Wartburg *et al.*, 1965; Lieber, 1970). Several factors affect the pathway, including the activity of ADH, the intracellular acetaldehyde concentration, the activity of the shuttle mechanisms that transport reducing equivalents into the mitochondria and the rate of oxidation of reducing equivalents *via* the mitochondrial respiratory chain. The rate-limiting step in the ADH pathway can therefore vary depending on the experimental conditions (Thurman, 1977).

The rate of elimination of ethanol *in vivo* correlates with the basal metabolic rate, indicating that the rate of mitochondrial NADH oxidation is a major rate-limiting step in the ADH pathway. Horse liver, for example, contains large amounts of ADH, yet the rate of ethanol metabolism is relatively low, reflecting the animal's basal metabolic rate (Lester & Keokosky, 1967). In smaller animals, such as rats, although a greater proportion of total ADH activity (50-85%) may be used for ethanol oxidation, the theoretical capacity of ADH to metabolize ethanol still exceeds the actual rate *in vivo* (Crow *et al.*, 1977). This conclusion is supported by studies demonstrating an increase in ethanol elimination following administration of fructose (Thieden & Lundquist, 1967). The effect of fructose in both fasting and fed animals is due to the fact that ATP is consumed during its phosphorylation, thus increasing the capacity of the respiratory chain to oxidize NADH derived from the oxidation of ethanol and acetaldehyde (Thieden *et al.*, 1972; Scholz & Nohl, 1976).

ADH activity is under hormonal control. Thus, castration of rats increases ADH activity in liver (Mezey *et al.*, 1980; Lumeng & Crabb, 1984); and chronic administration of testosterone to male rats castrated before puberty and to female rats decreases both the metabolic rate of ethanol and ADH activity to values similar to those found in mature males (Rachamin *et al.*, 1980).

Decreased activity of hepatic ADH, leading to a corresponding reduction in the rate of ethanol elimination, is observed in rats with advancing age (Hahn & Burch, 1983), with protein deficiency (Horn & Manthei, 1965; Bode *et al.*, 1970; Wilson, J.S. *et al.*, 1986) and in spontaneously hypertensive animals (Rachamin *et al.*, 1980). Numerous studies support the conclusion that, while increased ADH activity is not associated with increased rates of ethanol oxidation, reduction in ADH activity does lead to a decrease in ethanol elimination (Lieber, 1983).

(ii) *Cytochrome P450*

In 1965, a NADPH-dependent ethanol oxidase was found in microsomes from pig's liver which catalyses the oxidation of methanol to formaldehyde and that of ethanol to acetaldehyde (Orme-Johnson & Ziegler, 1965). This system, which was subsequently designated the microsomal ethanol-oxidizing system (MEOS; Lieber & DeCarli, 1968), carries out the following reaction:

$$CH_3CH_2OH + NADPH + O_2 + H^+ \dashrightarrow CH_3CHO + NADP^+ + 2H_2O$$

(Lieber, 1970).

Ethanol binds to hepatic cytochrome P450 and gives a modified type-II binding spectrum (Rubin *et al.*, 1971). The K_m of cytochrome P450 for ethanol (about 8 mM) is greater than that for ADH (Lieber & DeCarli, 1970; Lindros *et al.*, 1974). An isozyme of cytochrome P450 that is induced by ethanol, IIE1 (previously described as $P450_{3a}$, $P450_{ALC}$ or P450j; Nebert *et al.*, 1987) has been purified from the liver of rabbits (Koop *et al.*, 1982), rats (Peng *et al.*, 1982), hamsters, deermice (*Peromyscus maniculatus*) and baboons (Lasker *et al.*, 1986a); and its presence has been demonstrated in rabbit kidney and nasal mucosa (Ding *et al.*, 1986; Ueng *et al.*, 1987) and rat kidney (Thomas *et al.*, 1987), but not in microsomes from a variety of other tissues (Ding *et al.*, 1986). Cytochrome P450-dependent ethanol oxidizing capacity has also been demonstrated in mucosal cells from the upper gastrointestinal tract and colon of rats (Seitz *et al.*, 1979, 1982) and in macrophages from a variety of tissues in mice (Wickramasinghe *et al.*, 1987).

(iii) *Catalase*

Catalase is a haemoprotein located in the peroxisomes of many tissues (de Duve & Baudhuin, 1966). An early suggestion that catalase might play a role in the metabolism of ethanol (Keilin & Hartree, 1936) was later confirmed by Laser (1955), who showed that ethanol could be oxidized effectively in the presence of hydrogen peroxide and catalase. The scheme of the reaction is as follows:

$$\text{Catalase} + H_2O_2 \dashrightarrow \text{Cat-}H_2O_2$$

$$\text{Cat-}H_2O_2 + CH_3CH_2OH \dashrightarrow CH_3CHO + 2H_2O + \text{catalase}$$

(Thurman *et al.*, 1988).

Catalase can oxidize ethanol *in vitro* only in the presence of a hydrogen peroxide generating system (Keilin & Hartree, 1945); however, the reaction is limited by the rate of hydrogen peroxide generation rather than by the amount of catalase haem (Oshino *et al.*, 1973). It had been thought previously that the rate of hydrogen peroxide production represented only a small fraction of the rate of ethanol oxidation *in vivo* (Boveris *et al.*, 1972; Sies, 1974), but more recent experiments with physiological concentrations of fatty acid bound to albumin indicate that the role of catalase may be more important (Handler & Thurman, 1987).

(iv) *Aldehyde dehydrogenases* (ALDH)

A NAD-dependent ALDH with a broad substrate specificity for aldehydes was described in 1949 (Racker, 1949), and reviews on ALDH are available (e.g., Lindros, 1978). The enzyme has very low K_m values and a high reaction rate (Grunnet, 1973); therefore, under normal circumstances, only low concentrations of acetaldehyde are found outside the liver (Jacobsen, 1952; Kiessling, 1962). The metabolism of acetaldehyde has been reviewed (IARC, 1985). At low concentrations of acetaldehyde (<50 μM) during ethanol oxidation, acetaldehyde oxidation is predominantly a mitochondrial process (Grunnet, 1973; Marjanen, 1973; Lindros *et al.*, 1974; Parrilla *et al.*, 1974). Several isozymes of ALDH have been identified (for reviews, see Lindros, 1978; Salaspuro & Lindros, 1985). Tissues other than the liver may also produce acetaldehyde after ethanol administration (Baraona *et al.*, 1985), and intestinal bacteria have been shown to produce small amounts (Baraona *et al.*, 1986).

(v) *Ethanol acyltransferase*

Ethanol acyltransferase activity has been described in rat liver microsomes (Grigor & Bell, 1973; Bakken *et al.*, 1979) and in the pancreas (Estival *et al.*, 1981). The enzyme is responsible for esterification of fatty acids with ethanol.

(vi) *Modifying effects of repeated ethanol consumption on the metabolism of ethanol and acetaldehyde*

Most studies show that repeated or long-term consumption of ethanol enhances its clearance (e.g., Lieber & DeCarli, 1970; Misra *et al.*, 1971; Feinman *et al.*, 1978; Yuki & Thurman, 1980; for review, see Eriksson & Deitrich, 1983).

Feeding of ethanol (36% of total calories for 24 days) to rats enhanced its metabolism in microsomes (Lieber & DeCarli, 1968; Rubin & Lieber, 1968) and in isolated hepatocytes (Cederbaum *et al.*, 1978) and increased the rate of its disappearance from the blood (Tobon & Mezey, 1971; Lieber & DeCarli, 1972; Bleyman & Thurman, 1979; Wendell & Thurman, 1979). Enhanced clearance of ethanol from the blood has also been demonstrated *in vivo* in deermice (*Peromyscus maniculatus*; Shigeta *et al.*, 1984), in chimpanzees, in rhesus monkeys (Pieper & Skeen, 1973) and in baboons (Pikkarainen & Lieber, 1980; Nomura *et al.*, 1983). Further examples are listed in Table 41. The biochemical background for this phenomenon has been attributed to a hypermetabolic state in the liver (Israel *et al.*, 1975) or to increased ethanol oxidation *via* cytochrome P450 (Lieber & DeCarli, 1970).

Blood concentrations of acetaldehyde in baboons were increased following chronic ethanol consumption; these correlated positively with rates of ethanol elimination and negatively with liver mitochondrial ALDH activity (Pikkarainen *et al.*, 1981).

Table 41. Enhanced xenobiotic metabolism in the liver due to prior ethanol treatment

Substrate tested	Species examined	Reference
Alcohols and ketones		
Ethanol	Rat	Lieber & DeCarli (1968)
	Rabbit	Morgan *et al*. (1981)
	Hamster	McCoy (1980)
	Deermouse (*Peromyscus maniculatus*)	Burnett & Felder (1980)
	Rabbit	Koop & Casazza (1985)
Acetone	Rat	Casazza & Veech (1985)
2-Butanol	Rat	Krikun & Cederbaum (1984)
Halogenated alkanes, alkenes and ethers		
Carbon tetrachloride	Rat	Johansson & Ingelman-Sundberg (1985)
Chloroform	Rat	Sato, A. *et al*. (1981); Sato & Nakajima (1985)
Trichloroethylene	Rat	Sato, A. *et al*. (1981); Sato & Nakajima (1985)
1,1-Dichloroethylene	Rat	Sato, A. *et al*. (1981); Sato & Nakajima (1985)
Enflurane	Rat	Pantuck *et al*. (1985)
Aromatic compounds		
Benzene	Rat	Sato, A. *et al*. (1981); Sato & Nakajima (1985)
Toluene	Rat	Sato, A. *et al*. (1981); Sato & Nakajima (1985)
para-Nitrophenol	Rat	Reinke & Moyer (1985)
Acetaminophen	Rat	Sato, C. *et al*. (1981)
	Mouse	Walker *et al*. (1983)
	Hamster	Elliott *et al*. (1985)
Benzo[*a*]pyrene	Rat	Seitz *et al*. (1978)
	Hamster	Murphy & Hecht (1986)
	Rabbit	Koop & Casazza (1985)
Aflatoxin B_1	Rat	Toskulkao & Glinsukon (1986)
Aromatic amines		
Benzidine	Rat	Neis *et al*. (1985)
para-Aminobenzoic acid	Rat	Neis *et al*. (1985)
2-Acetylaminofluorene	Rat	Smith & Gutmann (1984)
Nitrosamines		
N-Nitrosodimethylamine	Rat	Garro *et al*. (1981)
	Rabbit	Yang *et al*. (1985b)
N-Nitrosopyrrolidine	Rat	Farinati *et al*. (1985)
	Hamster	McCoy *et al*. (1979)
N′-Nitrosonornicotine	Rat	Castonguay *et al*. (1984)
Azoxymethane	Rat	Sohn *et al*. (1987)
Testosterone	Rat	Rubin *et al*. (1976)
Vitamin D	Rat	Gascon-Barré & Joly (1981); Gascon-Barré (1982)

Following repeated alcohol consumption, ALDH activity has been reported to decrease (Koivula & Lindros, 1975; Greenfield *et al.*, 1976; Lebsack *et al.*, 1981), to remain the same (Redmond & Cohen, 1971; Tottmar *et al.*, 1974) and to increase (Horton, 1971; Greenfield *et al.*, 1976; Väänänen *et al.*, 1984), depending mainly on the acetaldehyde concentrations used.

Chronic alcohol consumption has been shown to increase ADH activity in the distal colon of rats (Seitz, 1985).

(*c*) *Modifying effects of ethanol on the metabolism of xenobiotics*

Pretreatment of animals with ethanol enhances the hepatic metabolism of a variety of agents, such as volatile hydrocarbons, alcohols and ketones, aromatic amines and nitrosamines (for examples, see Table 41).

Long-term ethanol consumption results in proliferation of smooth hepatic endoplasmic reticulum and an increase in the level of cytochrome P450 (Iseri *et al.*, 1966; Rubin *et al.*, 1968; Joly *et al.*, 1973). The induction of cytochrome P450 by ethanol is associated with an increase in metabolism (see Table 41) and, in some instances, in the toxicity of many compounds, including *N*-nitrosodimethylamine (Garro *et al.*, 1981; Olson *et al.*, 1984), acetaminophen (paracetamol; Strubelt *et al.*, 1978; Sato, C. *et al.*, 1981; Walker *et al.*, 1983), carbon tetrachloride (Traiger & Plaa, 1971; Hasumura *et al.*, 1974), aflatoxin B_1 (Glinsukon *et al.*, 1978) and benzene (Nakajima *et al.*, 1985). It increases the hydroxylation of aniline (Morgan *et al.*, 1981; Villeneuve *et al.*, 1976). The unique cytochrome P450 isozyme (IIE1) induced by ethanol catalyses the oxidation of some other alcohols, aniline (Morgan *et al.*, 1982) and *N*-nitrosodimethylamine (Yang *et al.*, 1985a,b).

In contrast, ethanol inhibited the metabolism of xenobiotics *in vitro* (for examples, see Table 42). Acute administration of ethanol also inhibited the metabolism of some drugs *in vivo* (see Rubin *et al.*, 1970; Mezey, 1976; Sato *et al.*, 1985). There are two possible explanations for this phenomenon: direct competition for cytochrome P450 (Sato, A. *et al.*, 1981) or a decrease in the supply of a cofactor for the monooxygenase system (Reinke *et al.*, 1980).

The hepatic enzymes that catalyse conjugation of xenobiotics, such as UDP-glucuronyltransferase (Dioguardi *et al.*, 1970; Idéo *et al.*, 1971; Yost & Finley, 1983; Reinke *et al.*, 1986; Sweeny & Reinke, 1987) and glutathione-*S*-transferases (Younes *et al.*, 1980; Hétu *et al.*, 1982; David & Nerland, 1983; Schnellmann *et al.*, 1984), are similarly induced by feeding ethanol.

Conjugation reactions have also been found to be inhibited by concomitant ethanol administration; for example, glucuronidation was inhibited in isolated hepatocytes (Moldéus *et al.*, 1978; Sundheimer & Brendel, 1984) and in rat liver microsomes (Marniemi *et al.*, 1975), and glucuronidation and sulphation were inhibited in perfused rat liver (Reinke *et al.*, 1986).

Pretreatment of rats with ethanol increases the metabolism of *N*-nitrosamines in the lung, oesophagus (Farinati *et al.*, 1985) and nasal mucosa (Castonguay *et al.*, 1984). When ethanol was given concomitantly with NDMA, concentrations of the nitrosamine in brain,

Table 42. Inhibition of cytochrome P450-dependent metabolism by ethanol in the liver *in vitro*

Substrate tested	Species examined	Reference
Halogenated alkanes and alkenes		
Chloroform	Rat	Sato, A. *et al.* (1981)
1,2-Dichloroethane	Rat	Sato, A. *et al.* (1981)
Trichloroethylene	Rat	Sato, A. *et al.* (1981)
Aromatic compounds		
Aniline	Rat	Rubin & Lieber (1968)
Benzene	Rat	Sato, A. *et al.* (1981)
Styrene	Rat	Sato, A. *et al.* (1981)
Toluene	Rat	Sato, A. *et al.* (1981)
Polycyclic aromatic compound		
Benzo[*a*]pyrene	Rat	Rubin & Leiber (1968)
Nitrosamines		
N-Nitrosodimethylamine	Rat	Swann *et al.* (1984); Tomera *et al.* (1984)
N-Nitrosoethylmethylamine	Rat	Peng *et al.* (1982)
Drugs		
Meprobamate	Rat	Rubin *et al.* (1970)
Pentobarbital	Rat	Rubin *et al.* (1968)

lung, liver, kidney and blood were increased markedly (Anderson *et al.*, 1986). First-pass clearance of NDMA by the liver in rats was prevented when it was administered in ethanol (1 ml, 5% v/v) instead of in water. The prevention of first-pass clearance has a dramatic effect on alkylation of kidney and oesophageal DNA: at dose levels of 30 μg/kg bw NDMA, methylation of kidney DNA of ethanol-treated rats was five times that in controls; lower doses of NDMA induced methylation in the kidneys of ethanol-treated rats but not in controls (Swann, 1984). Similarly, administration of *N*-nitrosodiethylamine (NDEA; 20 μg/kg bw) in ethanol (1 ml; 5% v/v) led to a five-fold increase in *N*7 ethylation of guanine in oesophageal DNA over that seen with a similar dose of NDEA alone (Swann *et al.*, 1984).

(*d*) *Modifying effects of ethanol on intermediary metabolism*

As described above, when ethanol is oxidized to acetaldehyde *via* ADH, NAD is required as a cofactor and is reduced to NADH during the reaction. Under normal conditions, the rate of NADH production exceeds its rate of reoxidation, resulting in an increase in the ratio of NADH:NAD in the liver. Oxidation of ethanol *via* acetaldehyde to acetate also results in the reduction of both cytosolic and mitochondrial redox states

(Lieber, 1983, 1984a), reflected in increases in the ratios of lactate to pyruvate and β-hydroxybutyrate to acetoacetate (Forsander, 1970). These changes are used widely as markers of cytosolic and mitochondrial redox states (Bücher & Klingenberg, 1958; Hohorst *et al.*, 1959) and of ethanol-induced changes in the redox balance of the liver (Forsander *et al.*, 1965; Salaspuro & Mäenpää, 1966). Most of the acute metabolic effects of ethanol, such as inhibition of hepatic gluconeogenesis (Krebs *et al.*, 1969), decreases in citric acid cycle activity (Thurman, 1977) and impairment of fatty acid oxidation (Lieber & Schmid, 1961), are due to this major effect on the intermediary metabolism of the liver (see Table 43).

Table 43. Effects of ethanol on intermediary metabolism in the liver

Metabolic effect	Reference
Redox change in liver	Lieber (1983, 1984a)
NADH:NAD ratio increases	Smith & Newman (1959); Räihä & Oura (1962)
Lactic:pyruvic acid ratio increases	Forsander et al. (1965)
β-Hydroxybutyrate:acetoacetate ratio increases	Forsander et al. (1965)
Inhibition of citric acid cycle in liver	Thurman (1977)
Inhibition of glycolysis in liver	Thurman (1977)
Inhibition of gluconeogenesis in liver	Krebs et al. (1969)
Inhibition of fatty acid oxidation and accumulation of triglycerides in liver	Lieber & Davidson (1962); Rebouças & Isselbacher (1961); Mallov & Bloch (1956)
Inhibition of protein synthesis and secretion in liver	Perin et al. (1974); Baraona et al. (1980)
Accumulation of protein in liver	Baraona et al. (1977)
Inhibition of glycoprotein secretion in liver	Tuma et al. (1980)
Potentiation of hepatic lipid peroxidation	Shaw et al. (1981)
Inhibition of intestinal amino acid transport	Mezey (1985)
Elevation of blood lipoproteins	Baraona (1985)
Increase in peripheral fat mobilization	Mallov & Bloch (1956); Lieber (1985b)
Increased formation and decreased urinary excretion of urates	Lieber (1985b)

In rats, administration of ethanol lowers the levels of vitamin A in the liver (Sato & Lieber, 1981), an effect which is potentiated by, e.g., phenobarbital and butylated hydroxytoluene (Leo *et al.*, 1987).

(*e*) *Major toxic effects*

The single-dose acute oral toxicity (LD_{50}) of ethanol has been reported to be 6.2-17.8 g/kg bw in rats (Smyth *et al.*, 1941; Kimura *et al.*, 1971; Bartsch *et al.*, 1976), 8.3-9.5 g/kg bw in mice (Spector, 1956; Bartsch *et al.*, 1976), 5.6 g/kg bw in guinea-pigs (Smyth *et al.*, 1941), 6.3-9.5 g/kg bw in rabbits and 5.5-6.5 g/kg bw in dogs (Spector, 1956). The LD_{50} after a single intraperitoneal administration of ethanol was 4.3 g/kg bw in bats (Greenwald *et al.*, 1968) and 8.6 g/kg bw in mice (Forney *et al.*, 1963); 29-38% of mice given a single intraperitoneal injection of 6.5 g/kg ethanol survived over 24 h (Macdonald *et al.*, 1977). An intraperitoneal LD_{50} of 5.0 g/kg was reported in rats (Barlow *et al.*, 1936; Bartsch *et al.*, 1976); however, it was reported that LD_{50} values decrease in male Wistar rats with age: the oral LD_{50} was 10.6 g/kg bw in three- to four-month-old rats and 7.06 g/kg bw in 10- to 12-month-old animals; the intraperitoneal LD_{50} was 6.71 g/kg bw and 5.10 g/kg bw at the two ages, respectively (Wiberg *et al.*, 1970).

(i) *Alterations in the liver*

Liver injury due to ethanol ingestion was initially attributed to malnutrition rather than to toxicity (Best *et al.*, 1949). Later, many experimental studies showed that ethanol can cause morphological alterations and effects on liver metabolism in well-fed animals (Lieber & DeCarli, 1974; Lieber *et al.*, 1975). [The Working Group noted that since ethanol interferes with the uptake of some vitamins from the gut in humans (see section 4.3(*e*)), it is unlikely that nutritional effects can be distinguished from the effects of ethanol *per se*.]

The degree and type of liver injury depend on a number of factors, including ethanol concentration, nutritional state, time of administration and type of animal. Liver changes may occur in several steps, from hepatomegaly, fatty liver, necrosis and fibrosis to cirrhosis.

Hepatomegaly and the accumulation of lipids in hepatocytes (steatosis) are the earliest manifestations of acute administration of ethanol. A significant increase in the lipid content of the liver of rats may be produced by a single dose of ethanol (Mallov & Bloch, 1956). The fatty acid composition of the lipids which accumulate resembles that of adipose tissue (Brodie *et al.*, 1961), which indicates that they are derived from extrahepatic tissue. Other possible mechanisms behind the acute fatty infiltration of the liver are related to the ethanol-induced increase in the ratio of NADH:NAD in the liver, which inhibits fatty acid oxidation (Lieber & Schmid, 1961; see Baraona, 1985) and may enhance the synthesis of glycerolipids (Nikkila & Ojala, 1963).

Subchronic and chronic administration of ethanol to rats also causes fatty liver (Lieber *et al.*, 1963), hepatocellular enlargement and a decrease in total liver tubulin (Baraona *et al.*, 1975, 1977, 1984). The latter result has been shown to be associated with the inhibition of tubulin polymerization and decreased formation of microtubules (Baraona *et al.*, 1977, 1981a; Matsuda *et al.*, 1979; Okanoue *et al.*, 1984), a phenomenon which may be mediated *via* acetaldehyde (Matsuda *et al.*, 1979). This conclusion is supported by the demonstration that disulfiram, which inhibits acetaldehyde oxidation, produces a further decrease in microtubules (Baraona *et al.*, 1981a).

Subchronic administration of ethanol to rats in a liquid diet was reported in one study to cause dose-related acidophilic degeneration, necrosis, formation of Mallory bodies and centrolobular steatosis (Holmberg *et al.*, 1986). The production of necrosis, inflammation and fibrosis is enhanced in rats when the ethanol-containing liquid diet is supplemented with either vitamin A (Leo & Lieber, 1983) or 4-methylpyrazole (Lindros *et al.*, 1983).

When rats were given ethanol by an intragastric intubation at levels rising from 8 to 15 g/kg bw per day (32-47% of total calories) over four months, together with a diet containing 25% of total calories as fat, focal necrosis, inflammation and fibrosis were observed in the liver. Serum levels of transaminases were also elevated. Alcoholic hepatitis and Mallory bodies were not detected (Tsukamoto *et al.*, 1986). When ethanol was given to rats continuously by intragastric intubation at doses which resulted in blood concentrations of 2.16 ± 1.2 g/l, together with a low-fat diet (4.9% of total calories), progressive fatty infiltration of the liver was detected; after 30 days, one-third of the animals also showed focal necrosis with infiltration of macrophages in the liver (Tsukamoto *et al.*, 1985).

It has not been possible to reproduce hepatitis or cirrhosis by feeding ethanol to rats (Salaspuro & Lieber, 1980). A high-fat diet together with alcohol has been shown to produce fatty liver in dogs, and four of 16 animals developed cirrhosis (Connor & Chaikoff, 1938).

Advanced alcoholic liver injury has also been produced in primates. All of nine baboons fed ethanol at 50% of total calories developed fatty liver, and four animals developed hepatitis within nine to 12 months (Lieber *et al.*, 1975). Of 18 baboons fed ethanol, 15 developed focal fibrous septa, five with diffuse septal fibrosis, of which four proceeded to septal cirrhosis and one each to micronodular and to mixed micro-macronodular cirrhosis; cirrhosis can occur in baboons without the polymorphonuclear inflammation characteristic of human alcoholic hepatitis (Popper & Lieber, 1980). The production of liver fibrosis in baboons fed ethanol has been confirmed, even in studies in which choline was given in excess (Nakano & Lieber, 1982; Lieber *et al.*, 1985; Miyakawa *et al.*, 1985); however, long-term feeding of ethanol produced fatty infiltration but not liver fibrosis in monkeys (Mezey *et al.*, 1983).

In rats, large single or multiple doses of ethanol (5-6 g/kg bw) produced lipid peroxidation in the liver, as measured by malonaldehyde production (Di Luzio & Hartman, 1967; Macdonald, 1973; Valenzuela *et al.*, 1980; Videla *et al.*, 1980), whereas smaller single doses (≤3 g/kg) had no effect (Hashimoto & Recknagel, 1968). However, after long-term administration of ethanol (36% of total calories for five to six weeks) to rats, a single 3-g/kg bw dose of ethanol caused increased hepatic diene conjugation; diene conjugation could be prevented, in part, by the administration of methionine (Shaw *et al.*, 1981).

(ii) *Alterations at other sites*

Ethanol can, depending on dose, irritate the oral cavity, oesophagus and gastric mucosa in experimental animals. Tissue damage has been observed in the gastric epithelium of mice (Eastwood & Kirchner, 1974) and in the small intestinal mucosa of rats (Baraona *et al.*, 1974). An increase in cell proliferation in rat oesophageal epithelium was found after ethanol had been fed in a liquid diet (Mak *et al.*, 1987). Cellular proliferation has also been observed in the gastrointestinal tract of rats and dogs after repeated administration of ethanol (Willems *et al.*, 1971; Baraona *et al.*, 1974).

A significant enhancement of rectal-cell production and an extension of the proliferative compartment in rectal crypts following chronic ethanol ingestion has been demonstrated in rats (Simanowski *et al.*, 1986).

(iii) *Effect of vitamins*

Consumption of ethanol under conditions of vitamin A deficiency increased the incidence of squamous metaplasia in rat trachea. Abnormal cilia and increased numbers of lysosomes in ciliated cells were also observed in rats depleted of vitamin A and administered ethanol (Mak *et al.*, 1984).

(iv) *Effect on hormones*

In male rats, plasma testosterone and luteinizing hormone levels fell following ethanol administration (Cicero *et al.*, 1977, 1979). Chronic ethanol ingestion produced testicular atrophy in rats (see Gavaler & Van Thiel, 1987); in addition, ethanol reduced the levels of luteinizing hormone as well as the receptor for the hormone on the Leydig cells of rat testis (Bhalla *et al.*, 1979).

In female mice, rats, rabbits and monkeys, subchronic and chronic administration of ethanol results in significant disturbances of the oestrous cycle, ovulatory function and fertility (see Gavaler & Van Thiel, 1987 and below).

(v) *Hepatic and pancreatic foci*

Effects on ATPase-deficient foci were investigated in six-week-old female Wistar rats administered 10% ethanol in water as the drinking fluid (daily intake, 8 g/kg bw) either continuously during intragastric administration of NDEA (3 mg/kg bw) or *N*-nitrosomorpholine (NMOR; 40 mg/l in the drinking-water; daily intake, 5 mg/kg bw) on four days per week, or alternately with the carcinogens (on the remaining three days per week), for 11 or 15 weeks, respectively. Another group of 12-week-old rats received 3 mg/kg bw NDEA in a 3-ml aqueous solution by stomach tube three times a week for nine weeks, followed subsequently by 10% ethanol in water as the drinking fluid continuously or intermittently (at weekly intervals) for 16 weeks. Fourteen days after the termination of treatment, both the size and number of ATPase-deficient foci in the liver were increased in animals that had received ethanol continuously or intermittently during NDEA or NMOR administration, but no such enhancement was obtained in animals that had received ethanol after the cessation of carcinogen treatment (Schwarz *et al.*, 1983, 1984). [The Working Group noted that a single marker was used for preneoplastic foci.]

In male Sprague-Dawley rats that received ten intragastric intubations of 0.38 mg/kg bw aflatoxin B_1, followed five days later by a low-fat (11% of calories as corn oil) or high-fat (35% of calories as corn oil) diet containing ethanol (35% of calories) for 12 weeks, no difference in the incidence of γ-glutamyl transferase-positive foci was observed in rats in either group (Misslbeck *et al.*, 1984). [The Working Group noted that a single marker was used for preneoplastic foci.]

A significant increase in the number of acidophilic and basophilic acinar-cell foci was observed in the exocrine pancreas of male weanling SPF Wistar rats that received 15% ethanol (v/v) in the drinking-water for 17 weeks, as compared to controls not receiving ethanol, after a single intraperitoneal injection of 30 mg/kg bw azaserine followed by a low-fat (5% corn oil) or high-fat (25% corn oil) diet. There was a positive interaction between dietary fat and ethanol in terms of the size of basophilic foci (Woutersen *et al.*, 1986).

No modulating effect of ethanol was observed after 17 weeks on the number or size of putative preneoplastic cystic or ductular exocrine pancreatic lesions in male, weanling

Syrian golden hamsters that received subcutaneous injections of 20 mg/kg bw *N*-nitrosobis(2-oxopropyl)amine at six and seven weeks of age and were fed low-fat (5% corn oil) or high-fat (25% corn oil) diets with or without 15% ethanol (v/v) in water as the drinking fluid (Woutersen *et al.*, 1986).

(*f*) *Effects on reproduction and prenatal toxicity*

The effects of acetaldehyde, a metabolite of ethanol, on reproduction and prenatal toxicity have been reviewed. Fetal malformations and resorptions were found in rats and fetal malformations were found in mice treated with acetaldehyde (IARC, 1985).

(i) *Reproductive effects*

The effects of ethanol on reproduction have been reviewed recently (Gavaler & Van Thiel, 1987). Studies in mice and rats have shown effects on the testis and on other reproductive tissues but generally have not shown an effect on reproductive performance.

When female C57Bl/Crgl *mice* were given 10% ethanol (v/v) in water as the drinking fluid before mating, throughout gestation and lactation, no significant effect on reproductive capacity or pup development or behaviour was seen (Thiessen *et al.*, 1966).

When female Wistar *rats* were given 20-25% of the calories consumed as 12% ethanol in a sucrose solution as the drinking fluid before mating and throughout gestation and lactation, there was no effect on reproductive performance or on development of offspring (Oisund *et al.*, 1978). Offspring of female Sprague-Dawley rats that were administered ethanol in water as the drinking fluid at a concentration of 20% v/v for four weeks before mating and at a concentration of 30% v/v during gestation were physically and developmentally retarded and failed to catch up with control offspring during the first four weeks postpartum (Leichter & Lee, 1979).

In a study in which male C57Bl/6J *mice* were given 5 or 6% (v/v) ethanol in a liquid diet for 70 days or 35 days, respectively, there was a significant decrease in testicular weight and in seminal vesicle/prostate weight, an increase in the frequency of germ-cell desquamation, inactive seminiferous tubules, inhibition of in-vitro fertilization of mouse oocytes by epididymal spermatozoa, as well as a significant decrease in the total number of motile sperm. During a ten-week recovery period, improvement was greater in the group given 5% than in those given 6% ethanol (Anderson *et al.*, 1985). Preparation of sperm from the cauda epididymis five weeks after oral administration of ethanol (1, 2 or 4.0 ml/kg bw) to male (CBA × Balb/c) F_1 mice five times daily did not show sperm anomalies (Topham, 1980, 1983). Addition of ethanol to ram spermatozoa (0.62 M; 15 μl in 0.4 ml semen samples containing 2-dioxy-D-glucose) inhibited sperm motility (Mayevsky *et al.*, 1983).

There is evidence *in vitro* and *in vivo* that ethanol is toxic to animal and human Leydig cells and seminiferous tubules (Gavaler & Van Thiel, 1987; Van Thiel *et al.*, 1983). Male Sprague-Dawley *rats* maintained on a liquid diet containing 6% ethanol (95% v/v) for one week followed by four weeks on a 10% ethanol liquid diet showed adverse effects on sex organs (testes, seminal vesicles, ductules) as well as a significant decrease in serum testosterone levels (Klassen & Persaud, 1978). Male Sprague-Dawley rats that received an intraperitoneal injection of 2.5 g/kg bw ethanol showed a significant decrease in the levels of luteinizing hormone and testosterone and marked attenuation of testicular steroidogenesis (Cicero *et al.*, 1979).

Exposure of male *rats* [strain unspecified] to ethanol *in utero* or as neonates by administration of a liquid diet containing ethanol (36% of total calories) resulted in adverse effects on gonadal growth and development and disturbances in their sexual behaviour and performance when adult (Parker *et al.*, 1984). Subcutaneous administration of 7.9 g/kg bw ethanol to female CD rats inhibited ovulation, primarily by blocking ovulatory surges of luteinizing hormone (Kieffer & Ketchel, 1970). Blood levels of luteinizing hormone varied with dose and timing of treatment, but ethanol administered by intraperitoneal injection increased the secretion of prolactin by female Wistar rats (Alfonso *et al.*, 1985). Exposure of Sprague-Dawley rats to ethanol (average, 11.6 g/kg bw) *in utero* altered the adult patterns of luteinizing hormone secretion in male and female offspring, indicating an effect on the central mechanisms that control secretion of pituitary luteinizing hormone (Handa *et al.*, 1985). Administration of 5% ethanol (36% of total calories) in a liquid diet to female Wistar rats for 49 days decreased ovarian weight by 60% and significantly decreased plasma oestradiol-17β levels and the development of oestrogen target organs (Van Thiel *et al.*, 1978). Ovarian function in female Holtzman rats, 20 days of age, was suppressed by feeding of liquid diets containing 5% ethanol (36% of total caloric intake) for up to 55 days, in which blood ethanol concentrations averaged 2.5 g/l, but not by 2.5% ethanol (Bo *et al.*, 1982).

Vaginal opening was delayed in female Holtzman rats fed a liquid diet containing 5% ethanol for eight or 16 weeks. Among rats treated for 16 weeks, irregular oestrous cycles and cycles longer than those in controls were observed. Mating of these females with untreated males resulted in no adverse effect on fertility, litter size or neonatal body weight (Krueger *et al.*, 1982).

In female macaque *monkeys* that administered ethanol to themselves intravenously on a schedule of reinforcement used for food acquisition, providing 2.9-4.4 g/kg bw ethanol per day for three to 6.5 months, amenorrhoea, atrophy of the uterus, decreased ovarian mass and significant decreases in luteinizing hormone levels were observed (Mello *et al.*, 1983). In female rhesus monkeys infused intravenously with 2-4 g/kg bw ethanol after spontaneous onset of labour or following the induction of labour by infusion of oxytocin, partial suppression of labour was observed only in preterm animals with irregular uterine contractions (Horiguchi *et al.*, 1971).

(ii) *Male-mediated developmental effects*

Male C3H *mice* were fed ethanol (20 or 30% of total calories) in a liquid diet and, after four weeks of treatment, were mated to untreated females. The resulting litters showed no change in the number of implants, prenatal mortality, fetal weight, sex ratio or soft-tissue malformations (Randall *et al.*, 1982).

Male Sprague-Dawley *rats* maintained for six weeks on a liquid diet containing 10% ethanol were paired with untreated females. There was body weight loss and central nervous system impairment, and only half of the treated animals had successful matings, compared to all of the controls. There was a decrease in litter size and an increase in prenatal mortality among the litters (Klassen & Persaud, 1976). When 20% ethanol in water (v/v) was given as the drinking fluid for 60 days to male Long-Evans rats, which were mated with untreated females one to three weeks after cessation of treatment, the incidence of congenital malformations in the offspring was increased (Mankes *et al.*, 1982).

(iii) *Placental transfer*

CD-1 *mice* received intraperitoneal injections of 4, 6 or 7 g/kg bw ethanol on gestation day 10. Ethanol crossed the placenta rapidly and was found in the embryo 5 min after dosage. The blood ethanol concentrations in maternal blood and liver were dose dependent; acetaldehyde was detectable in maternal blood at all dose levels and in maternal liver and embryos after administration of 7 g/kg. Within 5 min after intraperitoneal injection of pregnant dams with 200 mg/kg bw acetaldehyde on gestation day 10, acetaldehyde was detectable in the embryos. Thus, both ethanol and acetaldehyde were found to be accessible to the embryo during a sensitive period of organogenesis (Blakley & Scott, 1984a).

Sprague-Dawley *rats* received an intraperitoneal dose of 2 g/kg bw ethanol four to five days before term. Maternal and fetal ethanol levels were similar; the concentration of acetaldehyde in maternal blood was four times that in the placenta, and none was found in fetal tissues (Kesäniemi & Sippel, 1975). With similar analytical techniques, acetaldehyde was found in fetal blood 150 min after intravenous or oral administration of 2.5 g/kg bw ethanol to pregnant Wistar rats on gestation day 21. Ethanol concentrations in the fetal compartment were found to be similar to those in the mother's blood 150 min after dosage. The authors concluded that, since ADH activity is very low in the fetus, the acetaldehyde was probably transported across the placenta (Espinet & Argilés, 1984). In a subsequent study with improved methods of analysis, the acetaldehyde levels were much higher (~five fold) in maternal blood than in either umbilical or fetal blood of rats (Gordon *et al.*, 1985).

Intraperitoneal injection of golden *hamsters* with 1.5 g/kg bw ^{14}C-labelled ethanol on gestation days 6 or 15 or intravenous administration of 0.5 g/kg bw ^{14}C-labelled ethanol to cynomolgus *monkeys* during the last 30 days of pregnancy resulted in transfer of ^{14}C-labelled ethanol to the fetus in both species (Ho *et al.*, 1972).

Dorset *ewes* were infused intravenously with a total dose of 15 ml/kg bw of 9.75% ethanol over a period of 1-2 h on gestation days 121-138. Diffusion across the placenta was rapid, and blood ethanol concentrations in the maternal and fetal compartments reached about 2.3 g/l (Mann *et al.*, 1975).

Ewes were given six doses of 0.8 ml/kg bw ethanol intravenously between days 125 and 135 of gestation. At dose levels of ethanol sufficient to cause about 2 g/l maternal and fetal blood ethanol, there was rapid depression of fetal myocardial contractility, which was maintained for several hours after cessation of ethanol administration (Lafond *et al.*, 1985).

Cynomolgus and rhesus *monkeys* were administered 0.8-1.5 g/kg bw ethanol intravenously over a period of 30 min on days 106-160 of gestation. The rate of clearance from the fetus paralleled that of the mother and was determined by the rate of elimination from the mother (Hill *et al.*, 1983). Similar findings were reported by Horiguchi *et al.* (1971).

(iv) *Preimplantation effects*

In a study on the effects of preimplantation exposure, RAP strain *mice* were given ethanol intravenously on days 3 and 4 of pregnancy and offspring were examined on day 19 of pregnancy. Mean fetal and placental weights were significantly lowered, but there was no effect on skeletal development (Checiu & Sandor, 1986).

Treatment of $(C_3H \times C57Bl)F_1$ female *mice* with a single dose of 1 ml of 12.5% ethanol by gavage 2 h after a 30-min mating period produced an increase in late (after day 11) fetal deaths. The same treatment given 1 h after mating did not produce this effect. The authors proposed that the effect was due to a specific action on the fertilized ovum at the time of second meiotic division, causing aneuploidy (see also pp. 138-139), but the numbers of embryos available for examination in this study were inadequate to confirm this hypothesis (Washington *et al.*, 1985).

Preimplantation effects were studied by the examination of uterine contents of albino *rats* following consumption of plum brandy (reported as 24% ethanol) or cognac (reported as 20% ethanol) for 40-45 days before mating and during pregnancy until the rats were killed on day 5. Development was retarded, and there was an increased number of pathological morulae and blastocysts (Fazakas-Todea *et al.*, 1985).

(v) *Fetotoxicity and structural teratology*

Adverse development and teratogenic effects caused by ethanol have been reviewed (Chernoff, 1979; Abel, 1980; Streissguth *et al.*, 1980; Abel, 1985a).

Groups of C3H *mice* were given a liquid diet or a fortified liquid diet, each either alone or with 4.1% w/v ethanol, from days 0-17 of pregnancy; a further group was given an amount of liquid diet equal to that consumed by the group given liquid diet plus ethanol. Ethanol consumption inhibited fetal growth and development but did not affect litter size, irrespective of the diet used (Goad *et al.*, 1984). Retardation of muscle growth was seen in offspring killed at 12 weeks of age of inbred mice [strain unspecified] given 10-20% ethanol in the drinking-water for 11 weeks before mating and 30% ethanol after breeding until delivery. Prenatally, there was suppression of hyperplasia of muscle fibres during myogenesis; postnatally, there was suppression of normal hypertrophy of individual muscle fibres (Ihemelandu, 1984).

Some studies in several *mouse* strains have shown no teratogenic effect, even at dose levels providing blood ethanol concentrations of 2 g/l or higher. CF-1 (Schwetz *et al.*, 1978), CD-1 (Hood *et al.*, 1979) and C3H (Lochry *et al.*, 1982) mice given ethanol orally or in the drinking fluid had pups with minor skeletal variants or decreased fetal body weight, but there was no increase in resorptions or malformations. Other studies in *mice* showed teratogenic effects and resorptions, typically at blood ethanol concentrations in excess of 2 g/l. The effects, such as fetal resorptions, intrauterine growth retardation, cleft palate, altered craniofacial development and exencephaly, limb defects and heart defects, varied with the strain of mice, mode of administration and stage of gestation at which ethanol was administered (Kronick, 1976; Chernoff, 1977; Randall *et al.*, 1977; Boggan *et al.*, 1979; Randall & Taylor, 1979; Chernoff, 1980; Giknis *et al.*, 1980; Rasmussen & Christensen, 1980; Webster *et al.*, 1980; Sulik *et al.*, 1981; Bannigan & Burke, 1982; Checiu & Sandor,

1982; Sulik & Johnston, 1983; Padmanabhan *et al.*, 1984; Stuckey & Berry, 1984; Webster *et al.*, 1984; Martinez *et al.*, 1985; Padmanabhan & Muawad, 1985; Daft *et al.*, 1986).

In a study to evaluate the role of zinc deficiency in the developmental toxicity of ethanol, CBA/J *mice* were given a liquid diet, either fortified with zinc or deficient in zinc, and ethanol (15 or 20% of total calories). Zinc deficiency potentiated the ethanol-induced increase in resorptions and external malformations and the decrease in fetal weight (Keppen *et al.*, 1985). Similarly there was an increase in the incidence of both external and internal malformations in C57Bl/6 mice given a marginally zinc-deficient diet and ethanol during gestation, in comparison with mice given a control diet and with mice treated with ethanol alone (Miller, S.I. *et al.*, 1983).

Long-Evans *rats* administered 6 g/kg bw ethanol orally on gestation days 5-19 had blood ethanol concentrations of over 2.6 g/l. Fetuses had decreased body weight, increased body water and sodium content and decreased lipid-free solid content (Abel & Greizerstein, 1979).

Sprague-Dawley *rats* were given 15 or 25% ethanol-derived calories in liquid diets 20 days before mating, throughout mating and until gestation day 19; additional groups were pair-fed an isocaloric diet. There was decreased caloric intake in the group given 25% ethanol-derived calories and in the pair-fed controls, and in both of these groups there were associated decreases in fetal body weight, organ weights and DNA and protein contents compared to the pair-fed controls of the group given 15% ethanol-derived calories. The effects of 15% ethanol-derived calories were attributed to ethanol, while the effects of 25% ethanol-derived calories were attributed partly to decreased caloric intake (Sorette *et al.*, 1980).

Sprague-Dawley *rats* were provided with 18, 25 and 32% protein-derived calories and 36% ethanol-derived calories in a liquid diet on gestation days 1-21. The maternal ethanol blood levels were 1.5-2 g/l. Ethanol caused a significant decrease in fetal body weight and brain weight but an increase in relative brain weight, irrespective of the protein content of the diet (Weinberg, 1985).

Sprague-Dawley *rats* received 15% ethanol in drinking-water on days 6-15 of gestation. Decreased maternal weight gain and fetal growth retardation but no teratogenic effect were observed. The maximal blood ethanol concentration was about 400 mg/l (Schwetz *et al.*, 1978). The offspring of Sprague-Dawley rats given 20% ethanol in the drinking-water four weeks before mating and 30% ethanol in drinking-water until gestation day 20 had retarded skeletal development and decreased body weight but no gross malformation (Lee & Leichter, 1983). Following oral administration of 4 g/kg bw ethanol to Sprague-Dawley rats twice daily for three-day periods between days 7 and 15 of gestation, an increased incidence of resorptions and a marginal effect on fetal body weight but no teratogenic effect were observed (Fernandez *et al.*, 1983). Long-Evans rats were administered 5% ethanol in drinking-water for 90 days prior to mating and during gestation or during gestation only. The effects were similar. No gross malformation was observed, but there was a significant decrease in fetal body weight (Samson, 1981).

In contrast to studies in which gross malformations were not observed, polydactyly and polysyndactyly were reported in the offspring of Sprague-Dawley *rats* given 5 g/kg bw (but not in those given 6 g/kg bw) per day ethanol orally on gestation days 1-15 or 1-20. Maximal blood ethanol concentrations of 2.5-3.25 g/l were reported with the two doses (West *et al.*, 1981a). In Long-Evans rats given 4 ml/kg bw ethanol as a single oral dose between days 6 and 15 of gestation, a variety of gross malformations was reported in 72-100% offspring compared to 12% of controls (Mankes *et al.*, 1983). Prenatal treatment of Long-Evans *rats* with 35% ethanol-derived calories in a liquid diet shortened the umbilical cord (Barron *et al.*, 1986).

When Sprague-Dawley *rats* were given ethanol as 35% of total calories in a liquid diet on gestation days 1-21, offspring had abnormal distribution of nerve fibres in the temporal regions of the hippocampus, which persisted to maturity (West *et al.*, 1981b). Sprague-Dawley rats were exposed *in utero* and/or postnatally to ethanol as 36% of total calories in a liquid diet from gestation day 16 until postnatal day 14 or from birth until postnatal day 14. The sexually dimorphic nucleus in the preoptic area of the brain of adult male offspring was significantly decreased in volume (Rudeen *et al.*, 1986). In hooded rats given a liquid diet containing 37% ethanol-derived calories from day 6 of gestation to time of birth (gestation day 23 for ethanol-exposed rats; day 22 for controls), delayed and extended period of cortical neuron generation, reduced number of neurons and altered distribution of neurons were seen (Miller, 1986).

Sprague-Dawley *rats* were exposed by inhalation to concentrations of up to 20 000 ppm (37 800 mg/m^3) ethanol for 7 h per day on gestation days 1-19; blood levels as high as 1.5-2 g/l were reported. At 20 000 ppm, the dams showed signs of narcosis and had decreased food consumption; the incidence of malformations in the offspring was of borderline significance. At 16 000 and 10 000 ppm (30 240 and 19 000 mg/m^3), corresponding to blood levels of 40-80 mg/100 ml and 3 mg/100 ml, respectively, there was no increase in malformations (Nelson *et al.*, 1985a).

The fetuses of New Zealand white *rabbits* given 15% ethanol in the drinking-water on gestation days 6-18 showed no adverse effect. The maximal blood ethanol concentration in the mothers was 250 mg/l (Schwetz *et al.*, 1978).

When *ferrets* were administered 1.5 g/kg bw ethanol daily as a 25% solution orally on days 15-35 of gestation, there was a significant increase in the number of fetuses and litters with malformations but no effect on fetal weight or resorptions. The peak blood ethanol concentration was 2 g/l (McLain & Roe, 1984).

Dogs were administered 1.8 g/kg bw ethanol as a 25% solution by gavage twice daily and were given either a normal-protein or low-protein diet throughout gestation. Ethanol consumption and low dietary protein intake, independently of each other, significantly decreased maternal weight gain as well as the weight of the neonates (Switzer *et al.*, 1986).

Oral administration of 3 or 3.6 g/kg bw ethanol to *dogs* by gavage throughout gestation resulted in no gross or histological abnormality, a slight decrease in the number of offsprings per litter and in pup weight, and an increase in the number of still births. Blood ethanol concentrations were 1.3-1.75 g/l (Ellis *et al.*, 1977).

In miniature *swine* given 20% ethanol in drinking-water (>3 g/kg bw/day) as gilts (18 months old) or sows (three years old), there was a significant decrease in mean litter size and in the birth weight of piglets and a significant increase in the incidence of multiple malformations (Dexter *et al.*, 1980).

Cynomolgus *monkeys* administered up to 5 g/kg bw ethanol daily on gestation days 20-150 revealed an increase in pregnancy wastage (abortions and still births) but no structural malformation or facial change (Scott & Fradkin, 1984). Pregnant pigtailed macaque monkeys were administered 0.3-4.1 g/kg bw ethanol by gavage once a week throughout gestation starting either before day 10 or on day 40. Spontaneous abortion frequency increased at peak plasma ethanol concentrations above 2 g/l. Developmental alterations were observed consistently in offspring of monkeys with blood levels greater than 1.5 g/l when treatment was initiated at the start of gestation; infants exposed only after gestation day 40 were less consistently abnormal despite higher blood ethanol levels (5.5 g/l; Clarren *et al.*, 1987a,b). In rhesus and cynomolgus monkeys given 3 g/kg bw ethanol intravenously over 1-2 min on gestation days 120-147, transient but marked collapse of umbilical vasculature was observed within 15 min. This resulted in severe hypoxia and acidosis in the fetus, but recovery occurred during the succeeding hour (Mukherjee & Hodgen, 1982).

When ethanol is given in combination with other chemicals which tend to increase the blood level of ethanol by reducing its metabolism, e.g., 4-methylpyrazole (Blakley & Scott, 1984b) and pyrazole (Varma & Persaud, 1979), the teratogenic and fetotoxic effects are increased. Administration of ethanol with chemicals that tend to increase the acetaldehyde level, however, e.g., disulfuram (Webster, W.S. *et al.*, 1983), does not increase the teratogenicity of ethanol.

Combined administration of ethanol and metronidazole to Swiss-Webster *mice* increased the number of resorptions, decreased fetal body weight and had a marginal effect on the incidence of malformations (Giknis & Damjanov, 1983).

Administration of ethanol in combination with an unspecified extract of marijuana containing Δ^9-tetrahydrocanabinol to Swiss-Webster *mice* by subcutaneous injection on days 1-15 of gestation and to Long-Evans *rats* intragastrically on days 7-15 of gestation produced a significant decrease in maternal weight gain and an increased incidence of resorptions. In both species, the incidence of resorptions was increased with marijuana alone, but the increase was more than additive with the combination of marijuana and ethanol (Abel, 1985b).

Ethanol increased the incidence of cleft palate in Swiss *mice* administered methylmercuric chloride and retinyl acetate (Lee, 1985). Ethanol in combination with lithium carbonate had a synergistic effect on the induction of fetal abnormalities in albino rats (Sharma & Rawat, 1986).

(vi) *Behavioural and functional teratology*

Male and female Sprague-Dawley *rats* were exposed by inhalation to concentrations of 10 000 or 16 000 ppm (19 000 or 30 240 mg/m^3) ethanol for 7 h per day; males were exposed for six weeks before mating and females throughout gestation. With 16 000 ppm, the blood ethanol concentration was about 500 mg/1. There was no physical or behavioural difference among offspring of treated and control animals. Behavioural testing included rotorod, open-field and wheel activity and avoidance conditioning tests (Nelson *et al.*, 1985b).

In a study of Long-Evans hooded *rats* gives daily doses of 1 or 2 g/kg bw ethanol orally throughout gestation, there were decreases in litter size, litter weight and mean pup weight, but no gross malformation or evidence of behavioural teratogenic effects (Abel, 1978).

In other studies, the most frequently reported behavioural teratogenic effect was alteration in motor activity. When Long-Evans hooded *rats* were administered 4 or 6 g/kg bw ethanol daily througout gestation, there was decreased litter weight but not litter size at birth and increased postnatal mortality. Motor activity of neonates raised by surrogate mothers was impaired at 16 and 20 days of age (Abel & Dintcheff, 1978). Increased motor activity was also reported in offspring of Long-Evans hooded rats given liquid diets containing ethanol (35% of total calories) on gestation days 6-20 (Zimmerberg *et al.*, 1986). A significant increase in motor activity was reported at 16 days of age among offspring of Wistar rats given liquid diets containing 5% ethanol on days 6-19 of gestation. There was no significant effect on length of gestation, litter size at birth or pup weight from birth up to 28 days of age (Bond, 1986).

Offspring of pregnant Long-Evans *rats* administered liquid diets containing ethanol (35% of total calories) during days 6-20 of gestation exerted a lower maximal suckling pressure, spent less time suckling during test sessions and displayed an altered suckling pattern (Rockwood & Riley, 1986).

Confirming evidence of behavioural teratogenic effects has been reported in rats (Viirre *et al.*, 1986; Vorhees & Fernandez, 1986) and mice (Yanai & Ginsburg, 1976; Randall *et al.*, 1986).

Open-field activity was significantly increased in the offspring of ethanol-treated miniature *swine* treated as described on p. 132 (Dexter *et al.*, 1980).

(vii) *In-vitro studies*

In studies with explanted cultured embryos from rats and mice, demonstrating the effect of ethanol on embryonal development independent of maternal metabolism, growth retardation and malformations were seen following exposure to ethanol in the culture medium. Adverse effects were generally found at concentrations of 1.5 g ethanol/1 medium or greater (Brown *et al.*, 1979; Sandor *et al.*, 1980; Priscott, 1982; Wynter *et al.*, 1983). Acetaldehyde has been shown to have similar effects (IARC, 1985).

(viii) *Other effects*

In Sprague-Dawley *rats* given 30% ethanol-derived calories in a liquid diet throughout gestation, reduced placental transfer of the glucose analogue 2-deoxyglucose was observed (Snyder *et al.*, 1986). There is also evidence that administration of ethanol to rats during gestation decreases placental transport of amino acids (Henderson *et al.*, 1981; Snyder *et al.*, 1986) and sodium-potassium ATPase activity (Fisher *et al.*, 1986).

In Sprague-Dawley *rats* exposed to increasing concentrations of ethanol in a liquid diet (up to 36% of ethanol-derived calories) before and during gestation, there was a significant increase in placental weight and a decrease in membrane-associated placental folate receptor activity. The authors considered this to be evidence for the role of placental toxicity in ethanol-associated intrauterine growth retardation (Fisher *et al.*, 1985).

(ix) *Effects on sexual differentiation*

When Long-Evans *rats* were given 10% ethanol in drinking-water from gestation day 7 to delivery, gestation was prolonged, and offspring of each sex showed decreased anogenital distances at birth. Pups nursed by ethanol-drinking mothers had a significantly earlier preputial separation, but there was no effect on adult masculine sex behaviour, plasma testosterone or weights of accessory sex glands (Chen & Smith, 1979).

When Sprague-Dawley *rats* were given liquid diets containing ethanol (35% of total calories) on day 7 of gestation through parturition, absence of sexual dimorphism (saccharin preference and maze learning) was seen among offspring, suggesting disrupted perinatal androgen status (McGivern *et al.*, 1984). In the offspring of Long-Evans hooded rats given a liquid diet containing 35% ethanol-derived calories on gestation days 6-20, males showed feminized behaviour and females showed masculinized behaviour, suggesting disruption of the hormonal environment prenatally (Meyer & Riley, 1986). No evidence of altered sexual dimorphism in saccharin preference was found among offspring of Long-Evans hooded rats administered 3.5 g/kg bw ethanol twice daily intragastrically on gestation days 11-21 (Abel & Dintcheff, 1986).

Among offspring of Long-Evans *rats* fed liquid diets containing 35% ethanol-derived calories during gestation days 6-20, there was evidence of behavioural deficits, which persisted until adulthood. Female offspring showed a variety of deficits in maternal behaviour when adult, which may have been related to prenatal hormonal alterations (Barron & Riley, 1985).

In male progeny of Wistar *rats* given ethanol in a liquid diet (36% of total calories) from gestation day 12 to ten days postpartum, there was decreased anogenital distance; the weights of the testes and seminal vesicles/prostate were decreased 55 and 110 days postpartum; serum testosterone and luteinizing hormone levels were decreased on day 55 but not on day 110; and sexual motivation and performance were reduced. The authors concluded that there was less phenotypic masculinization at birth in the treated offspring (Udani *et al.*, 1985).

(x) *Lactational and postnatal effects*

Ethanol and acetaldehyde were measured in milk and peripheral blood of Wistar *rats* given ethanol as 36% of total calories in a liquid diet. Ethanol levels in the blood increased slightly (26-29 mmol/l; 1.2-1.3 g/l) from day 5 to day 15 of lactation, and levels of acetaldehyde increased from 41 to 53 μM/l (1.9-2.4 mg/l). The concentration of acetaldehyde in milk was 50% of that in the blood, while the concentration of ethanol was 44-80% of the blood level. Blood ethanol concentrations in suckling pups (around 0.3 μM/l, 14 mg/l) were much lower than those in maternal blood but increased after day 15; by the end of lactation, some pups had started to consume the liquid diet (Guerri & Sanchis, 1986). Increases in pH, protein and lipids and a decrease in lactose were seen in milk from ethanol-treated Wistar rats (Sanchis & Guerri, 1986). Sprague-Dawley rats receiving 5% ethanol in drinking-water during the second half of pregnancy showed decreased mammary gland development; when they were treated after parturition, no effect was observed (Jones & Stewart, 1984).

Pups of Sprague-Dawley *rats* were given feed containing ethanol (6.6-9.8 g/kg bw per day) by gavage on postnatal days 4-10. An oral dose of 7.4 g/kg bw gave a blood ethanol concentration of 1.6 g/l. At dose levels of 7.4 g/kg bw and above, microencephaly was observed on day 10 (Pierce & West, 1986). In Sprague-Dawley rats administered 6 and 10% ethanol in the drinking-water during lactation, blood ethanol concentrations were about 190 and 410 mg/l, respectively. A significant decrease in neonatal body weight gain was observed. However, when neonates were given ethanol directly by exposure to vapour at concentrations of 3.5-4.2% v/v, providing blood ethanol concentrations of more than 2.5 g/l, there was only minimal growth retardation (Swiatek *et al.*, 1986).

Sprague-Dawley *rats* administered 4 g/kg bw ethanol per day orally on days 6-16 of age or 6 g/kg bw ethanol on day 6 showed significant decreases in whole brain weight, in cerebellar weight and in the number of cerebellar cells, and altered balancing ability on days 17 and 70 postnatally (Burns *et al.*, 1986). Exposure of Sprague-Dawley rats to high levels of ethanol (7.2-12.0 g/kg bw per day) during days 4-8 of age decreased the weights of the brain, cerebral cortex and cerebellum, increased receptor affinity and decreased the number of neurotransmitter receptors (Serbus *et al.*, 1986).

(g) *Genetic and related effects*

Ethanol

The genetic effects of ethanol were reviewed recently (Obe & Anderson, 1987).

(i) *Prokaryotes*

In the *rec*-type repair test with *Proteus mirabilis*, ethanol (0.1 ml per plate) was inactive in the absence of an exogenous metabolic system (Braun *et al.*, 1982). Rapid lysis mutants in bacteriophage T4D were not induced by ethanol (up to 130.4 μl/ml) in the absence of an exogenous metabolic system, but the yield of phages was reduced by concentrations of ethanol greater than 69.7 μl/ml (Kvelland, 1983). In DNA repair tests with different strains of *Escherichia coli* WP2, ethanol gave very weak positive results at 5 mg/well (De Flora *et al.*, 1984a,b). It was not mutagenic in the presence or absence of an exogenous metabolic system in *Salmonella typhimurium* strains TA97, TA98, TA100, TA1535, TA1537 or TA1538 (McCann *et al.*, 1975; Cotruvo *et al.*, 1977; Arimoto *et al.*, 1982; Blevins & Taylor, 1982; Blevins & Shelton, 1983; De Flora *et al.*, 1984a,b).

In the presence of an exogenous metabolic system, De Flora *et al.* (1984a,b) consistently found a small (approximately two-fold) increase in the number of revertants in *S. typhimurium* strain TA102 in the presence of 200 and 300 μl ethanol (160 and 240 mg/plate). [The Working Group noted that *S. typhimurium* strain TA102 is considered to respond to the presence of oxygen radicals.]

(ii) *Plants*

Ethanol (up to 0.5 M) produced chromosomal aberrations in root-tip meristems of *Vicia faba* (Michaelis *et al.*, 1959; Rieger & Michaelis, 1960, 1961, 1970, 1972; Schubert *et al.*, 1979; Rieger *et al.*, 1982, 1985); exclusively chromatid-type aberrations were induced dose-dependently. Treatment of roots with ethanol (0.2 M) led to a significant elevation of sister chromatid exchange frequencies (Schubert *et al.*, 1979). Anomalies of anaphases and micronuclei were not observed when *Allium cepa* root-tip cells were exposed to up to 0.17 M ethanol, but sister chromatid exchanges were induced dose-dependently following exposure of roots (Cortés *et al.*, 1986). Exposure of cuttings of *Tradescantia paludosa* to ethanol (5-12.5%) for 6 h in a nutrient solution led to micronuclei in tetrads 24 h after exposure (Ma *et al.*, 1984).

(iii) *Fungi*

In *Saccharomyces cerevisiae*, ethanol produced respiration-deficient (or petite) mutants (Bandas & Zakharov, 1980; Bandas, 1982; Cabeça-Silva *et al.*, 1982; Hamada *et al.*, 1985). When cells were treated and held at 4°C in water instead of at 30°C in complete medium, ethanol was no longer mutagenic, showing that metabolic processes are necessary for its activity in this system (Bandas, 1982). Ethanol (5%) had no effect on the frequencies of gene conversions in *S. cerevisiae* in the absence of an exogenous metabolic system (Barale *et al.*, 1983).

In *Aspergillus nidulans*, ethanol (approximately 5%) led to nondisjunction (Käfer, 1984) and to nondisjunction and mitotic crossing-over (Harsanyi *et al.*, 1977). Treatment of germinating but not of quiescent conidia of *A. nidulans* with ethanol (6 and 7%) led to induction of nondisjunction; point mutations were not induced in this test (Morpurgo *et al.*, 1979; Gualandi & Bellincampi, 1981).

(iv) *Insects*

When ethanol (10%) was fed to *Drosophila melanogaster* larvae for 2-96 h, neither somatic mutation nor recombination was induced (Graf *et al.*, 1984).

Feeding of ethanol to male *Drosophila* larvae (9-11 days, 4% ethanol in the food; Vogel *et al.*, 1983) or adults (three days, 5% ethanol in fluid; Vogel, 1972; Vogel & Chandler, 1974) did not lead to sex-linked recessive lethal mutation. When *Drosophila* eggs were seeded in medium containing 1 ml ethanol in 25 ml food and allowed to grow until hatching (Creus *et al.*, 1983), or when adult flies were fed with 5% aqueous sucrose containing up to 30% ethanol (Woodruff *et al.*, 1984), no sex-linked recessive lethal mutation was induced.

(v) *Mammalian cells* in vitro

Treatment of primary cultures of rat hepatocytes for 3 h with 1% ethanol did not induce DNA damage as measured by the alkaline elution technique (Sina *et al.*, 1983). Ethanol (up to 0.78 M) did not induce mutations in mouse lymphoma L5178Y $TK^{+/-}$ cells (Amacher *et al.*, 1980).

In the absence of an exogenous metabolic system, ethanol (0.1% for 44 h) did not induce sister chromatid exchanges in mouse kidney fibroblasts (Garcia Heras *et al.*, 1982). In the absence of an exogenous metabolic system, ethanol (50 μl/ml for 1 h) did not induce micronuclei in Chinese hamster V79 cells (Lasne *et al.*, 1984). In Chinese hamster ovary cells, it did not induce sister chromatid exchanges (Obe & Ristow, 1977 — 0.1% one application per day for 8 days; Schwartz *et al.*, 1982 — 1% for 28 h; Darroudi & Natarajan, 1987 — 0.16 M for 30 min) or chromosomal aberrations (Darroudi & Natarajan, 1987 — 0.16 M for 30 min) in the absence of an exogenous metabolic system, although a slight increase in sister chromatid exchange frequencies was reported in one study (de Raat *et al.*, 1983 — 31.6 g/l, 1 h treatment). The frequencies were higher in the presence of an exogenous metabolic system (de Raat *et al.*, 1983). In another study, also in the presence of an exogenous metabolic system, up to 0.1 M for 3 h induced exchanges (Takehisa & Kanaya, 1983). Sister chromatid exchanges (Takehisa & Kanaya, 1983; Darroudi & Natarajan, 1987) and chromosomal aberrations (Darroudi & Natarajan, 1987) were also induced in the presence of extracts from plants. These are unusual exogenous metabolic systems.

Treatment of primary cultures of Syrian golden hamster embryo cells (ELa/ENG strain) with 0.5% ethanol did not lead to transformed cell colonies (Bokkenheuser *et al.*, 1983). As reported in an abstract, treatment of mouse C3H/10T1/2 cells with 4-32 mg/ml ethanol for 24 h led to a small fraction (1.2-2.6%) of dishes with transformed foci (Abernethy *et al.*, 1982). Ethanol inhibited intercellular communication in a dose-dependent manner (up to 200 μl/5 ml [32 mg/ml]), as measured by metabolic cooperation between cultured $6TG^s$ and $6TG^r$ Chinese hamster V79 cells (Chen *et al.*, 1984).

(vi) *Human cells* in vitro

Treatment of HeLa cells with 0.1% ethanol (one application per day for nine days) did not lead to an elevation of exchange-type aberrations or of micronuclei in the absence of an exogenous metabolic system (Obe & Ristow, 1979). Ethanol (0.1%) did not produce sister chromatid exchanges in human lymphoid cells in the presence (1-h treatment) or in the absence (48-h treatment) of an exogenous metabolic system (Sobti *et al.*, 1982, 1983).

In human lymphocyte cultures, both chromosome- and chromatid-type aberrations were found with different doses of ethanol (up to 3.5 mg/ml for 50 h) in the absence of an exogenous metabolic system (Badr *et al.*, 1977). Treatment of human lymphocytes in culture with ethanol (up to 0.5% for 72 h) led to a dose-related elevation of sister chromatid exchange frequencies in the absence of an exogenous metabolic system (Alvarez *et al.*, 1980a). In other analyses in lymphocytes, ethanol in the absence of an exogenous metabolic system did not induce chromosomal aberrations (Cadotte *et al.*, 1973 — up to 500 mg/100 ml [0.6%] for 72 h; Obe *et al.*, 1977 — 0.5% for 24 h; Königstein *et al.*, 1984 — up to 1 % for 24 h; Banduhn & Obe, 1985 — 1% for 24 or 48 h; Kuwano & Kajii, 1987 — up to 1% for 26 h) or sister chromatid exchanges (Obe *et al.*, 1977 — 0.5% for 72 h; Véghelyi & Osztovics, 1978 — 0.5% for 72 h; Athanasiou & Bartsocas, 1980 — 0.2% for 72 h; Jansson, 1982 — up to 2% for up to 68 h; Hill & Wolff, 1983 — 20 μl/5 ml [0.4%] for 70 h; Königstein *et al.*, 1984 — up to 1% for up to 48 h).

In human lymphocytes, ethanol (1%) alone had no effect on the frequencies of sister chromatid exchanges. When alcohol dehydrogenase (ADH) was added together with ethanol, the sister chromatid exchange frequencies were elevated; exposure of cells to ethanol, ADH and aldehyde dehydrogenase led to fewer sister chromatid exchanges than in cells treated with ethanol and ADH alone (Obe *et al.*, 1986).

(vii) *Mammals* in vivo

Oral or subcutaneous administration of 0.05 ml of 95% ethanol to male ddY mice or up to 40% ethanol given in water as the drinking fluid to male Swiss mice for 26 days did not increase the frequency of micronuclei in the polychromatic erythrocytes of the bone marrow (Chaubey *et al.*, 1977; Watanabe *et al.*, 1982). Giving male CBA mice 10 and 20% ethanol as their only liquid supply for up to 16 weeks led to an elevation in the frequencies of sister chromatid exchanges in the bone-marrow cells (Obe *et al.*, 1979), but oral administration of 10% ethanol to male Swiss Webster mice once a day for four days did not (Nayak & Buttar, 1986).

Feeding male CD rats for six weeks with a liquid diet containing 36% of the calories as ethanol led to an elevation in the frequencies of micronuclei in the erythrocytes of the bone marrow (Baraona *et al.*, 1981b), but male Wistar rats receiving 10 and 20% ethanol as the only liquid supply for three or six weeks did not show an increase in the frequency of micronuclei in the erythrocytes of the bone marrow or in hepatocytes. Nor did the treatment lead to chromosomal aberrations in bone-marrow cells or in lymphocytes; the frequencies of sister chromatid exchanges were elevated in the peripheral lymphocytes but not in bone-marrow cells (Tates *et al.*, 1980).

Giving Chinese hamsters 10% ethanol as their only liquid supply for nine weeks did not lead to an elevation in the frequencies of chromosomal aberrations in the bone marrow (Korte *et al.*, 1979); the same treatment for 46 weeks did not lead to an increase in the frequency of sister chromatid exchanges in bone-marrow cells or chromosomal aberrations in lymphocytes (Korte & Obe, 1981). Treatment of Chinese hamsters with ethanol *via* the drinking-water (10% in week 1, 15% in weeks 2 and 3, 20% in weeks 4-12) did not lead to an elevation in the frequencies of chromosomal aberrations or sister chromatid exchanges in bone-marrow cells (Korte *et al.*, 1981).

Intubation of pregnant ICR mice with ethanol in such a way that the total dose was 4-8 g/kg bw led to a dose-dependent elevation of the frequencies of sister chromatid exchanges in embryonal liver cells (Alvarez *et al.*, 1980b). A single intraperitoneal injection of 4 g/kg bw 10% ethanol to ICR mice on day 10 of pregnancy induced sister chromatid exchanges in embryonal cells (Czajka *et al.*, 1980).

Intragastric administration to Wistar rats of 2 ml 40% ethanol daily on days 10-25 of pregnancy led to an elevation in the number of anaphases with bridges and fragments in embryonic liver cells (Kozachuk & Barilyak, 1982).

Intra-amniotic injection of 0.02 ml of a 40% ethanol solution to 13-day-old embryos of Wistar rats did not lead to chromosomal aberrations or aneuploidy (Barilyak & Kozachuk, 1983).

No elevation in the frequency of chromosomal aberrations was seen in spermatogonia of male Wistar rats given 10% ethanol *via* the drinking-water (Kohila *et al.*, 1976) or of male Sprague-Dawley rats given ethanol as their only liquid supply (7% in weeks 1-2, 10% in weeks 3-4, 15% in weeks 5-6, 20% in weeks 7-36; Halkka & Eriksson, 1977). Oral administration of 0.8 ml of 12.5 or 15% ethanol to CBA/CA or MF1 mice with analysis of second meiotic metaphases in the testes 2-6 h later, significantly increased the frequencies of hypo- and hyperploidies (2.99 and 4.2%, respectively, compared to a control frequency of 0.5%; Hunt, 1987). Intubation of ethanol (1.5 ml of 12.5%) in male Chinese hamsters was reported not to induce aneuploidies in spermatogonia or in spermatocytes I and II (Daniel & Roane, 1987).

A high incidence of aneuploid female pronuclei was found in fertilized eggs of female (C57Bl × CBA) F1 mice given ethanol orally (1 ml of 10-15%, 1.5-2.5 h after the predicted time of ovulation; Kaufman, 1983). Intragastric administration of ethanol to female CFLP mice (1.5 ml of a 12.5% solution) 1.5 h before, or 1.75 h, 4 h, 13.5 h or 17 h after treatment with human chorionic gonadotrophin (given to induce superovulation) led to high frequencies of aneuploid (hypo- and hyperploid) first-cleavage mitoses (15.3-25.0%) of the female pronuclear set in fertilized eggs, which was independent of the treatment schedule. Essentially the same result was found when female MF1 mice were treated with ethanol (15.7-24.0% aneuploid first-cleavage mitoses; Kaufman & Bain, 1984a). In another analysis, female CFLP mice were intubated with 1.5 ml of a 12.5% ethanol solution in distilled water 4 h, 13.5 h or 17 h after injection of human chorionic gonadotrophin. The animals were sacrificed 20-21 h after the injection (one-cell-stage embryos), three days later (morula stage) or 10-11 days later. The first-cleavage metaphases showed a high incidence of aneuploidy (15.3-22.8%), and aneuploidy was also found in the morula stages (11.1-15.4%). The time of administration of ethanol did not influence the frequencies of aneuploidies considerably. At the 10th or 11th day following ethanol administration, morphologically abnormal conceptuses were seen, and triploid and trisomic embryos were found (Kaufman & Bain, 1984b). [The Working Group noted that the effects of ethanol and acetaldehyde on the formation of microtubules (see p. 123) could explain the ability of ethanol to induce aneuploidy in various test systems.]

Genetic effects of ethanol in the male germ line have been reviewed (Anderson, 1982).

Administration of up to 30% ethanol as the only liquid supply for 35 days to male Wistar rats did not lead to dominant lethal mutations (Chauhan *et al.*, 1980). Feeding male Sprague-Dawley rats a liquid diet containing 6% ethanol for one week, followed by 10% ethanol for four weeks (Klassen & Persaud, 1976) and administration of 20% ethanol in water as the drinking fluid to male Long-Evans rats for 60 days led to the induction of dominant lethal mutations (Mankes *et al.*, 1982). Dominant lethal mutations have been reported in male CBA mice after intubation on three consecutive days with 0.1 ml 40-60% ethanol (Badr & Badr, 1975). Conflicting results were obtained in CFLP mice after oral administration of 2 ml/kg bw 40% ethanol on five consecutive days (James & Smith, 1982; Smith & James, 1984).

[The Working Group noted that chromosomal aberrations, sister chromatid exchanges and point mutations are induced by ethanol in test systems in which ethanol can be metabolized. This may indicate that acetaldehyde rather than ethanol is the mutagen in these systems.]

The activity profile for ethanol in short-term tests is shown in Appendix 2.

Alcoholic beverages

The mutagenicity of several components of alcoholic beverages has been discussed in various volumes of *IARC Monographs*: formaldehyde (IARC, 1987b), acetaldehyde (IARC, 1987b), acrolein (IARC, 1987b), *N*-nitrosamines (IARC, 1978), benzene (IARC, 1987b), styrene (IARC, 1987b), benzo[*a*]pyrene (IARC, 1983c) and tannins (IARC, 1976b).

Different alcoholic beverages (30 home-made apple brandies, 18 commercial apple brandies and 28 other commercial alcoholic beverages: eight whiskies, eight rums, eight cognacs, four armagnacs) were not mutagenic to *S. typhimurium* TA98 or TA100 either in the presence or absence of an exogenous metabolic system when 200-μl samples were tested. Alcoholic fractions of some of these beverages were mutagenic in the presence or absence of an exogenous metabolic system in TA98 and TA100 (Loquet *et al.*, 1981).

Alcohol-free extracts prepared from alcoholic beverages have generally been found to be mutagenic in the presence and absence of an exogenous metabolic system (Table 44). Extracted residues of pooled and concentrated Canadian beers were not mutagenic to *S. typhimurium* TA98, TA100 or TA102 in the presence or absence of an exogenous metabolic system (Brusick *et al.*, 1988).

Treatment of Chinese hamster ovary cells with geneva (15.8 and 32.6 g/l), rum (15.8 and 32.6 g/l) or port (15.8 g/l) led to the induction of sister chromatid exchanges in the presence but not in the absence of an exogenous metabolic system. Port (32.6 g/l) and sherry (15.8 g/l) also induced sister chromatid exchanges in the absence of an exogenous metabolic system (de Raat *et al.*, 1983).

Treatment of human lymphocytes *in vitro* with different types of alcoholic beverages for 24 h, such that the final ethanol concentration was always 0.5%, did not lead to the induction of chromosomal aberrations (Obe *et al.*, 1977). Alcohol-free extracts of whisky, rum, brandy (Hoeft & Obe, 1983) and red wine (Rueff *et al.*, 1986) induced sister chromatid exchanges in human lymphocytes *in vitro* in the absence of an exogenous metabolic system.

When tested with *S. typhimurium* strains, microsomes from liver, lung, intestine and oesophagus of ethanol-treated animals more effectively transformed indirect mutagens to mutagenic compounds than did microsomes from control animals. These effects were specific to the organs from which the microsomes were prepared and to the mutagens tested (Seitz *et al.*, 1978; McCoy *et al.*, 1979; Garro *et al.*, 1981; Seitz *et al.*, 1981a,b; Lieber, 1982; Olson *et al.*, 1984; Smith & Gutmann, 1984; Farinati *et al.*, 1985; Neis *et al.*, 1985; Sato *et al.*, 1986; Steele & Ioannides, 1986; Lieber *et al.*, 1987).

Genetic and related effects of metabolites

Acetaldehyde increased the incidence of sister chromatid exchanges in bone-marrow cells of mice and hamsters treated *in vivo* and induced chromosomal aberrations in rat embryos exposed *in vivo*. It induced DNA cross-links, chromosomal aberrations and sister chromatid exchanges in human cells *in vitro* and chromosomal aberrations, micronuclei and sister chromatid exchanges in cultured rodent cells. It induced chromosomal aberrations, micronuclei and sister chromatid exchanges in plants and DNA damage and mutation in bacteria. Acetaldehyde induced cross-links in isolated DNA (IARC, 1987b). The activity profile for acetaldehyde is given in Appendix 2.

Table 44. Mutagenicity of alcohol-free extracts of alcoholic beverages

Beverage	Test system[a]	Comment	Reference
17 Chinese spirits	TA98, TA100, TA1535; +/−	− in some cases only	Lee & Fong (1979)
Chinese wine treated with nitrite	TA98, TA100, TA1535, TA1538; +/−	No effect when not treated with nitrite	Lin & Tai (1980)
Home-made and commercial apple brandies, whiskies, cognacs, armagnacs, rums	TA98, TA100; +/−	Not always congruent	Loquet *et al*. (1980, 1981)
Red wine	TA98; +/−		Tamura *et al*. (1980)
White wine	TA98; +/−	Slight effect	Tamura *et al*. (1980)
Apple cider-based drinks, commercially available beverages	TA98, TA100; +/−		Tuyns *et al*. (1980)
Whiskies, brandies	TA100; −		Nagao *et al*. (1981)
Red wine	TA98, TA100; +/−	+ more effective	Stoltz *et al*. (1982a)
Red wine, white wine, light beer	TA98, TA100; +	Dark beer, gin, liqueur no effect	Stoltz *et al*. (1982b)
Red wine	TA98; +	White wine, one rosé wine no effect	Stavric *et al*. (1983)
Red wine	TA98, TA100; +		Subden *et al*. (1984)
Red wine	TA98; +	Beer, saké, whisky no effect	Kikugawa *et al*. (1985)
Red wine	TA98, TA100; +/−	+ more effective	Sousa *et al*. (1985)
Red wine	TA98; +		Ong *et al*. (1986)
Red wine	TA98; +; SOS chromotest with *E. coli* PQ37		Rueff *et al*. (1986)
Red wine	TA98, TA100; +		Yu *et al*. (1986)
Chilean commercial and home-made red and white wines, European red wines	TA98, TA100; +/−		Bull *et al*. (1987)

[a] +, with exogenous metabolic system; −, without

4.3 Other relevant data in humans

The term 'alcoholics' is used in this monograph in a broad sense to indicate persons who have a high alcohol consumption or who are considered to be alcohol-dependent. Information that would allow a more precise categorization was usually not given in the reports reviewed.

(a) Absorption, distribution and excretion

Ethanol occurs at concentrations similar to those of alcoholic beverages in the stomach and upper jejunum after ingestion (Halsted *et al.*, 1973). Absorption of ethanol from the gastrointestinal tract occurs by simple diffusion (Wallgren & Barry, 1970). Most ingested ethanol is absorbed within the first hour from the stomach and upper intestine, resulting in ethanol concentrations in the ileum and colon similar to that of the vascular space (Halsted *et al.*, 1973).

(b) Metabolism

(i) *Ethanol metabolism*

The rate of ethanol metabolism varies among individuals, and studies of twins indicate that interindividual variability in the rate of ethanol metabolism is under genetic control (Vesell *et al.*, 1971; Kopun & Propping, 1977).

The disappearance of ethanol from the blood follows zero-order kinetics; the elimination rate is approximately 0.1 g/kg bw per h (Newman & Lehman, 1937).

It is generally accepted that the main pathway for ethanol oxidation in man is *via* the ADH pathway. Human ADH is coded by three structural gene loci, the corresponding products of which, α, β- and γ-polypeptides, combine to form active dimeric isozymes. The ADH molecule may appear in at least nine electrophoretically different isozyme forms (Smith *et al.*, 1971, 1973).

An 'atypical' ADH has been described which differs from the usual enzyme in its catalytic activity, pH optimum, kinetic parameters and molecular structure (von Wartburg *et al.*, 1965; von Wartburg & Schürch, 1968; Yoshida *et al.*, 1981). In European countries, the incidence of atypical ADH ranges from 4 to 20% (von Wartburg & Schürch, 1968). In Japan, however, 85-98% of the population carries the atypical ADH (Fukui & Wakasugi, 1972; Agarwal *et al.*, 1981; Agarwal & Goedde, 1986). In spite of the presence of highly active atypical ADH, however, the rate of ethanol metabolism in normal and atypical ADH phenotype carriers is not significantly different (see p. 145; Edwards & Price Evans, 1967). Other isozyme forms found in human liver include π-ADH (Li & Magnes, 1975; Li *et al.*, 1977) and ADH-Indianapolis (Bosron *et al.*, 1980).

Human hepatic ADH catalyses the oxidation of not only alcohols but also endogenous and exogenous sterols (Frey & Vallee, 1980).

A cytochrome P450 isozyme immunologically identical to the ethanol-inducible forms from rats and rabbits, P450 IIE1, has also been isolated from human liver (Lasker *et al.*, 1986b; Song *et al.*, 1986; Lasker *et al.*, 1987).

A nonoxidative pathway of ethanol metabolism — esterification of ethanol with fatty acids — has been described in many human organs (Lange, 1982; Laposata & Lange, 1986); its importance remains to be determined.

(ii) *Acetaldehyde metabolism*

Acetaldehyde is oxidized further to acetate by aldehyde dehydrogenase (ALDH), which also occurs in several isoenzyme forms (Agarwal *et al.*, 1981). Acetaldehyde concentrations during ethanol oxidation in the blood following ingestion of 0.8 g/kg bw were low in healthy male Caucasians: 2-20 μM (0.1-1 mg/l) in hepatic venous blood; less than 2 μM (0.1 mg/l) in peripheral venous blood (Nuutinen *et al.*, 1984). In contrast, alcohol ingestion by Orientals resulted in marked elevations of blood acetaldehyde levels concentrations ranging from 0.4 to 3 mg/l (Ijiri, 1974); and individuals developed facial flushing and tachycardia as a direct consequence of elevated blood acetaldehyde levels (Ijiri, 1974; Mizoi *et al.*, 1979; Inoue *et al.*, 1980). Acetaldehyde-mediated facial flushing occurs in individuals in whom one of the ALDH isoenzymes, ALDH2, occurs in low concentrations or is absent (Agarwal *et al.*, 1981; Ikawa *et al.*, 1983).

In one study of volunteers, it was found that infusion of fructose caused a marked elevation of acetaldehyde in the blood of four nonalcoholic control subjects but not in four alcoholics. The oxidation of acetaldehyde in blood *in vivo* and *in vitro* was similar in alcoholics and nonalcoholics (Nuutinen *et al.*, 1984).

(iii) *Modifying effects of chronic ethanol consumption on the metabolism of ethanol*

A 30-80% increase in the metabolism of ethanol in alcoholics who consume 100 g or more ethanol per day has been described in several studies (Bernhard & Goldberg, 1935; Kater *et al.*, 1969; Ugarte *et al.*, 1972; Salaspuro & Lieber, 1979; Keiding *et al.*, 1983; Nuutinen *et al.*, 1983, 1984). Consumption of smaller amounts of ethanol (45 g per day) for three weeks did not affect the rate of its disappearance in volunteers of either sex (Holtzman *et al.*, 1985).

Cirrhotic patients with jaundice who had not taken alcohol for more than four weeks showed decreased rates of ethanol elimination due to liver injury (Lieberman, 1963). In contrast, ethanol elimination rates were elevated even in the presence of relatively severe liver damage when measurements were taken during the first month of abstinence (Ugarte *et al.*, 1977).

(iv) *Modifying effects of chronic ethanol consumption on the metabolism of acetaldehyde*

Early studies of the concentration of acetaldehyde in the blood of alcoholics may have been limited by methodological difficulties (Majchrowicz & Mendelson, 1970; Truitt, 1971; Magrinat *et al.*, 1973), as pointed out by Stowell *et al.* (1977). Following intravenous alcohol administration, blood acetaldehyde concentrations were demonstrated to be higher in alcoholic than in nonalcoholic subjects (Korsten *et al.*, 1975). More recent studies with better methods have confirmed that blood acetaldehyde concentrations increase following chronic alcohol consumption (Lindros *et al.*, 1980; Palmer & Jenkins, 1982). In alcoholic patients, peak blood acetaldehyde concentrations were higher at high than at low ethanol blood levels (Nuutinen *et al.*, 1983). Blood acetaldehyde values correlated positively with rates of ethanol elimination (Lindros *et al.*, 1980) and negatively with liver ALDH activity (Jenkins & Peters, 1980; Nuutinen *et al.*, 1983; Jenkins *et al.*, 1984; Matthewson *et al.*, 1986).

Several factors, such as hepatomegaly (Pelkonen & Sotaniemi, 1982), increased reoxidation of NADH (Thurman *et al.*, 1988) and increased cytochrome P450 levels (Pelkonen & Sotaniemi, 1982), may be responsible for the enhanced elimination rates of ethanol by alcoholics.

Sera of alcoholic patients were found to contain antibodies to acetaldehyde-protein adducts. Anti-acetaldehyde adduct immunoglobulin titres in 21 healthy nondrinking individuals ranged from 10 to 80, whereas 25 of 34 alcoholics had titres of 160 or above ($p < 0.001$). These results suggest that acetaldehyde-induced immunogenic determinants can initiate an immune response which may be used to differentiate alcoholics from nonalcoholics (Hoerner *et al.*, 1986).

(*c*) *Modifying effects of ethanol on the metabolism of xenobiotics*

In both alcoholics and nonalcoholics, acute drinking of alcohol results in inhibition of xenobiotic metabolism as observed in experimental systems (see Table 42). For example, the metabolism of meprobamate and pentobarbital is inhibited by acute administration of ethanol (Rubin *et al.*, 1970). After ethanol intake, blood xylene levels in volunteers exposed to xylene by inhalation were increased 1.5-2.0 fold, while urinary excretion of methylhippuric acid, a xylene metabolite, declined by about 50% (Riihimäki *et al.*, 1982). During exposure to toluene by inhalation (3.2 mmol/m^3) for 4.5 h, moderate doses of ethanol (15 mmol/kg bw) given orally to volunteers almost doubled the maximum toluene concentration in blood and decreased the blood clearance of toluene by approximately 44% (Wallén *et al.*, 1984). Trichloroethylene concentrations in plasma increased two fold, and decreased urinary excretion of a major metabolite of trichloroethylene — trichloroethanol — was observed when ethanol was ingested immediately prior to exposure to trichloroethylene by inhalation (Müller *et al.*, 1975). Drinking of alcoholic beverages inhibits liver metabolism of nitrosamines, such as *N*-nitrosodimethylamine and *N*-nitrosodiethylamine. As a result, nitrosamines are excreted in urine of beer drinkers and volunteers given amines and ethanol (Eisenbrand *et al.*, 1981; Spiegelhalder *et al.*, 1982; Spiegelhalder & Preussmann, 1985).

In chronic alcoholics with normal liver function, xenobiotic metabolism is enhanced in the absence of alcohol. Consumption of 46% of total calories as ethanol for one month by volunteers resulted in a striking increase in the rate of clearance from the blood of meprobamate and pentobarbital (Misra *et al.*, 1971). Similarly, increases in the metabolism of antipyrine (Cushman *et al.*, 1982), tolbutamide (Carulli *et al.*, 1971), warfarin and phenytoin, but not aminopyrine (Iber, 1977), have been described.

When volunteers were given ethanol in the diet in increasing amounts up to 46% of total calories for 16-18 days, electron microscopy of biopsy specimens of the liver revealed a marked increase in the smooth endoplasmic reticulum (Lane & Lieber, 1966). No such change was detected in 17 alcoholics with hepatic steatosis (but not fibrosis; Hakim *et al.*, 1972). These results are probably due to induction of cytochrome P450; for example, hepatic pentobarbital hydroxylase activity, measured in biopsy specimens, was doubled in three nonalcoholic volunteers after 12 days of feeding 42% of total calories as ethanol. No change was detected in the activity of benzo[*a*]pyrene hydroxylase (Rubin & Lieber, 1968).

Alcoholics with normal liver histology had elevated levels of hepatic cytochrome P450 and *in-vitro* activities of monooxygenase, as well as increased clearance of antipyrine *in vivo* (Pelkonen & Sotaniemi, 1982); in contrast, alcoholics with hepatitis or cirrhosis had lower than normal values in all these analyses (Pelkonen & Sotaniemi, 1982; Woodhouse *et al.*, 1983).

It is well accepted that chronic consumption of ethanol enhances the metabolism of many drugs and halogenated hydrocarbons to reactive intermediates, resulting in increased toxicity (Lieber, 1982; Zimmerman, 1986), due probably to induction of P450 IIE1 by ethanol (Coon & Koop, 1987). For example, severe hepatic failure has been reported to develop in chronic alcoholics after ingestion of normally nontoxic doses of acetaminophen (Emby & Fraser, 1977; McClain *et al.*, 1980; Seeff *et al.*, 1986).

(*d*) *Modifying effects of ethanol on intermediary metabolism*

Most of the acute metabolic effects of ethanol that have been observed in experimental animals have also been detected in humans, as reviewed by Lieber (1982). These include elevation of the NADH:NAD redox state (i.e., increases in the lactate:pyruvate and β-hydroxybutyrate:acetoacetate ratios), inhibition of carbohydrate and lipid metabolism and accumulation of hepatic triglycerides (Lieber, 1984a).

It is generally accepted that ethanol metabolism in humans is regulated by the ADH system. This conclusion is supported by the numerous studies in humans which have demonstrated that administration of fructose, which increases rates of NADH reoxidation, elevates rates of ethanol metabolism from 30 to 80%. The absence of elevated alcohol elimination rates in individuals with atypical ADH, who have increased enzyme activity (von Wartburg *et al.*, 1965), further supports the conclusion that the ADH system is regulated predominantly by the NADH:NAD redox state (Thurman *et al.*, 1988).

(*e*) *Major toxic effects*

The clinical features of ethanol intoxication are related to blood ethanol levels: mild intoxication (500-1500 mg/l) is manifested in emotional lability and slight impairment of visual acuity, muscular coordination and reaction time; moderate intoxication (1500-3000 mg/l) results in visual impairment, sensory loss, muscular incoordination, slowed reaction time and slurred speech; severe intoxication (3000-5000 mg/l) is characterized by marked muscular incoordination, blurred or double vision, sometimes stupor and hypothermia, and occasionally hypoglycaemia and convulsions; in coma (>5000 mg/l), there are depressed reflexes, respiratory depression, hypotension and hypothermia. Death may occur from respiratory or circulatory failure or as the result of aspiration of stomach contents in the absence of the gag reflex (Weatherall *et al.*, 1983).

Long-term, high-level alcohol consumption caused toxicity in almost all organ systems of the body (Lieber, 1982).

(i) *Gastrointestinal tract*

Alcoholism commonly affects the mouth, with enlargement of the parotid gland and an increase in salivary secretion in patients with alcoholic liver injury (Dürr *et al.*, 1975; Bode & Menge, 1978). Glossitis and stomatitis are common in alcoholics.

Oesophageal complications that are often diagnosed in alcoholics include oesophagitis, columnar metaplasia (Wienbeck & Berges, 1985) and functional alterations in peristaltic contractions, especially in patients with peripheral neuropathy (Winship *et al.*, 1968).

Ethanol also has acute and chronic effects on gastric secretion and the gastric mucosa. Increased gastric acid secretion occurs as an acute effect (Cooke, 1972). Long-term consumption of alcohol decreases basal and maximal acid output (Chey *et al.*, 1968) and can cause chronic antral gastritis (Parl *et al.*, 1979). Acute mucosal lesions ('haemorrhagic gastritis') are a significant cause of upper gastrointestinal blood loss in alcoholics (Katz *et al.*, 1976).

A number of syndromes or pathological effects of alcoholic beverages in the upper intestine have been attributed to the high alcohol concentrations attained in the upper small intestine, including alterations in intestinal motility (decreased impeding waves in the jejunum; Robles *et al.*, 1974) and impaired transport of, for example, glucose (Thomson & Majumdar, 1981), amino acids (Israel *et al.*, 1969), electrolytes (Mekhjian & May, 1977), thiamine (Wilson & Hoyumpa, 1979), vitamin B12 (Lindenbaum & Lieber, 1969) and folic acid (Halsted *et al.*, 1967).

Since malnutrition impairs the nutrient absorptive function of the gastrointestinal tract, the malnutrition that often accompanies alcoholism may itself contribute to, or exacerbate, the malabsorption seen in alcoholics (Mezey, 1975; Lieber, 1982).

Pyridoxine deficiency occurs in alcoholics, and acetaldehyde has been incriminated in the accelerated destruction of vitamin B6 (Lumeng & Li, 1974). Abnormally low blood levels of vitamin E have been reported in alcoholics (Losowsky & Leonard, 1967). Deficiencies in other vitamins and trace elements have been reviewed (Thomson & Majumdar, 1981).

(ii) *Liver*

Alcoholic liver disease ranges from fatty liver, alcoholic hepatitis and fibrosis to irreversible cirrhosis (for review, see Lieber, 1984b).

Alcoholic hepatitis is characterized by an inflammatory reaction of the liver with necrosis of hepatocytes and may be associated with the occurrence of hyalin bodies (Mallory, 1911; Denk *et al.*, 1975; French & Burbige, 1979; Phillips, 1982; Denk, 1985).

Most studies suggest that intake of more than 120-180 g ethanol per day for more than 15 years is the critical dose-duration factor for the development of cirrhosis (Lelbach, 1975). Some other reports (Péquignot *et al.*, 1978; Tuyns & Péquignot, 1984; Norton *et al.*, 1987) have shown an elevated risk for cirrhosis following even lower daily consumption of ethanol. Risk factors for the development of alcoholic cirrhosis include poor nutrition, genetic susceptibility and female gender (Burnett & Sorrell, 1981; Tuyns & Péquinot, 1984; Norton *et al.*, 1987).

It has been suggested that viral hepatitis B is more common among alcoholics than among corresponding nonalcoholic populations, and an increased prevalence of serological markers of viral hepatitis has been reported in alcoholics (Mills *et al.*, 1979; Pimstone & French, 1984). The extent to which joint exposure to hepatitis B virus and alcohol leads to mutual modification of effects has not been clearly established.

(iii) *Pancreas*

Alcoholic pancreatitis is generally described as both acute and chronic (Sarles & Laugier, 1981). The acute form is associated with considerable mortality (Geokas, 1984). Chronic alcoholic pancreatitis generally develops after eight to ten years of heavy drinking (Strum & Spiro, 1971). Drinking binges (heavy drinking during weekends) often precipitate relapses of pancreatitis in alcoholics; similar excesses by nonalcoholics rarely provoke the disorder (Sarles & Laugier, 1981).

(iv) *Endocrine organs*

Alcohol interacts with the endocrine system, including the hypothalamus, pituitary and gonads. In addition, liver injury may disturb peripheral metabolism of hormones by affecting hepatic blood flow, protein binding, enzymes, cofactors or receptors.

Chronic ethanol abuse increases plasma cortisol levels (Mendelson & Stein, 1966; Mendelson *et al.*, 1971). Ethanol stimulates adrenal medullary secretion of catecholamines; in addition, the peripheral metabolism of the released catecholamines is altered by ethanol (Davis *et al.*, 1967). Alcohol and alcoholic liver injury affect thyroid function; acute administration of ethanol increases the liver:plasma ratio of thyroid hormones (Szilagyi, 1987), a finding that may explain some of the metabolic effects of ethanol.

Blood testosterone concentrations fall reversibly in normal male volunteers within hours of their ingesting sufficient amounts of alcohol to produce hangover (Van Thiel *et al.*, 1983). Chronic intake of alcohol further decreases serum testosterone levels which may lead to testicular atrophy and impotence (Mendelson & Mello, 1974; Gordon *et al.*, 1976; Van Thiel & Lester, 1977; Välimäki *et al.*, 1982; Van Thiel & Gavaler, 1985; Gavaler & Van Thiel, 1987). The finding of simultaneously elevated luteinizing hormone levels, especially in cirrhotics (Välimäki *et al.*, 1982), suggests a primary testicular effect of ethanol.

It is generally accepted that acute ethanol administration has little or no effect on human female hypothalamic-pituitary-gonadal function. On the contrary, chronic ethanol abuse leads to early menopause, lower postmenopausal gonadotropin levels and increased plasma levels of the classic female sex hormones, despite the presence of amenorrhoea (Gavaler

& Van Thiel, 1987). Elevated basal prolactin levels and exaggerated prolactin responses to thyrotropin-releasing hormone have been described in alcoholics (Ylikahri *et al.*, 1980).

(v) *Immune system*

The effects of alcohol on the immune system have been reviewed (Kanagasundaram & Leevy, 1981; Lieber, 1982; MacSween & Anthony, 1985). Studies in patients with alcoholic liver disease have shown decreased immune responsiveness (Berenyi *et al.*, 1974).

(vi) *Heart*

Acute and prolonged ingestion of alcohol has a deleterious effect on left ventricular function (Gould *et al.*, 1971; Regan *et al.*, 1975). The association between heavy drinking and cardiomyopathy is widely recognized (New York Heart Association Criteria Committee, 1964; Wendt *et al.*, 1966; Friedberg, 1971; McDonald *et al.*, 1971; Perloff, 1971; Demakis *et al.*, 1974; Regan *et al.*, 1975).

Protective effects of moderate alcohol consumption with regard to cardiovascular disease are discussed on p. 37.

(*f*) *Effects on reproduction and prenatal toxicity*

Numerous reviews of the reproductive effects and prenatal toxicity of alcohol are available (Jones & Smith, 1975; Warner & Rosett, 1975; Majewski, 1978; Neugut, 1981; Colangelo & Jones, 1982; Streissguth, 1983; Barrison *et al.*, 1985; Gavaler & Van Thiel, 1987). The adverse effects of alcohol in pregnancy have been known since biblical times, and occasional reports were published in the eighteenth and nineteenth centuries about the effects of excessive drinking on pregnancy. Following publication of the term 'fetal alcohol syndrome' by Jones and Smith (1973), contemporary interest in the effects of alcohol in pregnancy increased extensively, and, within eight years, Abel (1981) had published a comprehensive bibliography on the subject containing more than one thousand references.

The 'fetal alcohol syndrome' is characterized by both physical and mental effects. The major physical features are pre- and postnatal growth deficiency with regard to both weight and length, microcephaly, and characteristic facial features, including short palpebral fissures, short upturned nose with hypoplastic philtrum, thinned upper vermilion and retrognathia. The major neurological features are mild to moderate mental retardation, poor coordination, hypotonia, irritability in infancy and hyperactivity in childhood (Clarren & Smith, 1978). The two sexes seem to be equally at risk (Abel, 1979). Not all affected children have all of the features of the syndrome, and difficulty in recognizing the facial features seems to present the major problem in diagnosis. The syndrome was first described in the children of chronic alcoholic women, and much of the subsequent research has been devoted to finding whether the effects are dose-related and whether a threshold exists below which no adverse effect is detectable.

Hanson *et al.* (1978), as part of a large study on drinking, smoking, diet and use of of medicines in 1529 women in Seattle, WA, USA, separated a subgroup of infants born to 70 mothers who drank at least 1 oz (29.6 ml) ethanol per day on average, and these were compared with 93 infants born to mothers drinking <1 oz ethanol per day (five or more drinks per occasion). These 163 infants underwent special examination for features of fetal alcohol syndrome without prior knowledge of the mothers' drinking habits. Fetal alcohol syndrome-type features were diagnosed in 9/70 infants from mothers who consumed 1 oz [≃ 23 g] ethanol per day or more, compared with 2/93 from mothers who consumed less than 1 oz/day ($p = 0.023$). Significantly lower body weight, body length and reduced mental and motor development were found among infants of the mothers who drank more heavily on follow-up of infants of the original cohort at eight months of age (Streissguth *et al.*, 1981).

A prospective study by Olegård *et al.* (1979) in Göteborg, Sweden, in 1977/1978 identified 28 pregnancies in 25 alcoholic women. During the study period, there were about 7600 deliveries in the whole of Göteborg, and the study included antenatal clinics covering about one-third of the population. Five of the pregnancies ended in induced abortions, and two babies died during birth. Of the remaining 21 pregnancy outcomes, seven infants had full fetal alcohol syndrome and seven others partial features of the syndrome.

In a number of other studies, evidence was found for adverse effects of alcohol consumption during pregnancy, but not necessarily typical features of the fetal alcohol syndrome. A prospective study in Boston, MA, USA, by Ouellette *et al.* (1977) on 633 women who had registered for prenatal care at the Boston City Hospital, addressed alcohol intake, smoking, drug use and diet. At publication, 322 babies had been delivered. The abnormality rate, defined as infants with congenital anomalies, growth abnormalities or neurological abnormalities, was 29/42 (71%) in heavy drinkers, 45/128 (36%) in moderate drinkers and 52/150 (35%) in rare drinkers or abstainers ($p < 0.001$). The authors defined heavy drinkers as having an average daily intake of >45 ml [~ 36 g] ethanol per day or more, and abstinent/rare drinkers as less than one drink per month; the remainder were classified as moderate drinkers. There was a marked excess of infants of heavy drinkers who were small for their gestational age or had congenital anomalies or microcephaly. There was no specific pattern of anomalies, such as the fetal alcohol syndrome. [The Working Group noted that this is a high-risk population, among which 35% of all newborns are admitted to intensive care. Also, there was an association between heavy alcohol intake and both smoking and previous use of psychotropic drugs, but these were not corrected for in the analysis.]

A large prospective study in France (Kaminski *et al.*, 1976) was carried out on 9236 women delivered in Paris between 1963 and 1969. Using as the criterion for heavy drinking consumption of 400 ml wine containing 11% or more alcohol [~ 35 g ethanol] (or equivalent in other alcoholic beverages) per day, an excess of stillbirths was reported (2.6 *versus* 1.0%), as well as an excess of babies small for their gestational age (4.8 *versus* 2.5%) and reduced placental weight. The effects of alcohol were still significant ($p \leqslant 0.01$) after adjusting for maternal age, marital state, smoking and previous pregnancy outcomes. Two further studies (Kaminski *et al.*, 1981), one retrospective and the other prospective, did not confirm the increase in stillbirths found in the first study, and none of the three studies showed an increase in congenital malformations associated with alcohol intake.

Sokol *et al.* (1980) reported the results of a study of women from one obstetric hospital in Cleveland, OH, USA, who were classified as alcohol abusers (204), compared with 11 923 in a 'no alcohol group'. Alcohol abuse was associated with reduced birth weight (average reduction, 190 g), a significant increase in congenital anomalies and problems during delivery. Five cases of fetal alcohol syndrome were diagnosed. [The Working Group noted that a number of confounding factors, such as drug abuse and gravidity, were identified but were not controlled for.]

In a later study, the same group of workers (Ernhart *et al.*, 1987) analysed data from 359 mother-infant pairs classified according to alcohol intake, almost all of whom were from lower social classes. The prevalence of the cranio-facial anomalies associated with the fetal alcohol syndrome was related to the amount of maternal drinking during the first trimester of pregnancy. The relationship was most marked at higher levels of consumption (above 3 oz [88.8 ml] ethanol).

A prospective study on 32 019 women attending 13 clinics in California, USA, in 1974-77 was reported by Harlap and Shiono (1980), who studied the relationship between alcohol consumption, smoking and first- and second-trimester abortions. They found a significant increase in the incidence of second-trimester abortions with alcohol intake, giving age-adjusted relative risks of 1.03 (not significant), 1.98 ($p < 0.01$) and 3.53 ($p < 0.01$) for women taking less than one, one to two and three or more drinks [not defined] per day. There was no relationship with the incidence of first-trimester abortions; the effects observed were not explained by age, parity, race, marital status, smoking or the number of previous abortions.

Kline *et al.* (1980) conducted a case-control study on the relationship between alcohol intake and spontaneous abortion. Cases were a consecutive series of spontaneous abortions in three hospitals in Manhattan (NY, USA) between 1974 and 1978. Controls, matched for age and hospital and who had been delivered after 28 weeks' gestation, were selected concurrently, and 657 case-control pairs were included in the analysis. The authors found that 17.0% of cases and only 8.1% of controls reported drinking twice per week or more. The odds ratio, adjusted for three variables (age, interval between last menstrual period and interview and drinking before pregnancy) was 2.6 (95% confidence interval, 1.6-4.2). No significant interaction was found between alcohol intake and several other variables, such as smoking, previous spontaneous abortion, nausea/vomiting, weight, age, race, marijuana use or caffeine use. The effect was dose-related and, for those who drank twice a week or more, each type of beverage was significantly associated with increased risk of abortion. The association for wine and spirits (average intake per occasion, >1 oz [~ 23 g] ethanol) was slightly greater than that for beer (average intake, <1 oz ethanol, except for daily drinkers). The authors concluded that 1 oz ethanol twice per week is about the threshold amount that may produce an abortion.

Marbury *et al.* (1983) reported on a large study on alcohol consumption in 12 440 women from two hospitals in Boston, USA, interviewed at the time of delivery. After controlling for confounding by demographic factors, smoking, parity and obstetric history, alcohol consumption of 14 drinks per week or more was associated only with an increase in abruptio placenta. There was no adverse effect below 14 drinks per week, and no increase in malformations at any intake level.

Full fetal alcohol syndrome is seen only in the children of very heavy drinkers, usually chronic alcoholics. Some of the features of the syndrome are seen, however, at lower doses, and one of the most sensitive effects seems to be reduced birth weight. Little (1977), using multiple linear regression, showed in a study on 263 women that an average intake of 1 oz [~ 23 g] ethanol daily before pregnancy was associated with a decrease in birth weight of 91 g, and the same amount in late pregnancy with a decrease of 160 g. Wright *et al.* (1984) published a review of previous studies, including a detailed analysis of their own study on 1122 pregnancies in the UK, in which they used both the Mantel-Haenszel method and stepwise logistic regression. They found that intake of more than 10 g ethanol per day before or in very early pregnancy doubled the risk of a light (<10th centile) baby. Both of these studies showed an association between alcohol intake and smoking and showed that the effect of smoking on birth weight is independent of, and additive with, the effect of alcohol. Smith *et al.* (1986) showed, in a group of moderate drinkers, that women who stop drinking by mid-pregnancy have a lower risk in terms of both growth and behavioural outcomes than those who continue throughout pregnancy.

Follow-up of children with fetal alcohol syndrome shows that the effects remain severe and permanent, with little or no evidence of catching up either physically or mentally. This observation is independent of whether the child is brought up in his own home or in a foster home, and suggests that the majority of the defects are the result of prenatal exposure to alcohol (Kyllerman *et al.*, 1985; Streissguth *et al.*, 1985).

As well as the facial dysmorphology, growth and mental retardation, a number of other malformations have been observed in association with fetal alcohol syndrome. The most common, occurring in up to 50% of cases, are cardiac malformations, especially atrial and ventricular septal defects (Löser & Majewski, 1977; Dupuis *et al.*, 1978; Sandor *et al.*, 1981), renal defects (DeBeukelaer *et al.*, 1977; Quazi *et al.*, 1979; Havers *et al.*, 1980) and a variety of skeletal defects (Spiegel *et al.*, 1979; Herrmann *et al.*, 1980; Halmesmäki *et al.*, 1985; Pauli & Feldman, 1986). Although mental retardation is a major feature of fetal alcohol syndrome, there have been few reports of brain dysmorphology; however, severe disorders in brain development have been reported (Clarren *et al.*, 1978; Goldstein & Arulanantham, 1978; Peiffer *et al.*, 1979; Wisniewski *et al.*, 1983), suggesting an action at different stages. Other less frequent effects include alteration in palmar creases (Tillner & Majewski, 1978), liver abnormalities (Habbick *et al.*, 1979; Mφller *et al.*, 1979) and eye defects (Strömland, 1981).

Studies of hypothalamic-pituitary hormonal function in children with fetal alcohol syndrome have shown no abnormality, indicating that the deficit in height and weight is not due to lack of growth hormone (Root *et al.*, 1975; Tze *et al.*, 1976; Castells *et al.*, 1981).

(g) *Mutagenicity and chromosomal effects*

Chromosomal aberrations and aneuploid metaphases were found in the peripheral lymphocytes of alcoholics. In 200 alcoholics, de Torok (1972) found a high frequency of metaphases with nonmodal chromosome numbers, particularly in those with alcoholism-related organic brain syndrome, in whom 43.7% of the cells had 45 chromosomes and only 4.4% of the cells had the normal chromosome number of 46. In 100 alcoholics without organic brain syndrome, 23.6% of the cells had 46 chromosomes. In 20 ex-alcoholics who no longer drank, 47.2% of the cells had 46 chromosomes, and, in 60 nonalcoholics, there were

91.6% metaphases with 46 chromosomes. The author stated that a high incidence of structural changes was also observed.

Mitelman and Wadstein (1978), using 72-h cultures, found a significant elevation of the frequencies of hyperploid and hypoploid metaphases and of chromosomal aberrations in cells from ten alcoholics. Significant increases in the incidences of hyperploid and hypoploid metaphases and of metaphases with aberrations were observed using 72-h cultures of cells from 77 alcoholics (Kucheria *et al.*, 1986).

[The Working Group noted that a culture time of three days was used in these studies, which is not ideal since second- and third-division metaphases are present in such cultures. In addition, aneuploidies, especially metaphases with 45 chromosomes, could arise during preparation of the cells.]

In a series of studies with two-day cultures, Obe and his coworkers analysed chromosomal aberrations in lymphocytes of alcoholics (Obe *et al.*, 1977; Obe & Ristow, 1979; Obe *et al.*, 1979, 1980; Obe & Salloch-Vogel, 1985; Obe *et al.*, 1985; Obe, 1986) and found that they had higher frequencies of chromosomal aberrations than nonalcoholics. A comparison of the numbers of exchange-type aberrations per 10^4 metaphases in 379 alcoholics (number of metaphases analysed, 65 952) with historical control values gave the following results: chromatid translocations, 15.62 *versus* 5.13; dicentrics, 19.56 *versus* 8.00; rings, including minutes, 7.88 *versus* 1.77. These results indicate that there are nearly three times more exchange-type aberrations in alcoholics as in nonalcoholics (Obe & Anderson, 1987). In a study of 200 alcoholics, the frequencies of exchange-type aberrations were not correlated with age or sex but were correlated positively with the duration of alcohol dependence; smoking alcoholics had a higher frequency of exchange-type aberrations than nonsmoking alcoholics (Obe *et al.*, 1980). Alcoholics who were not currently drinking alcohol had fewer aberrations than those drinking currently (Obe *et al.*, 1980, 1985).

In a study of peripheral blood lymphocytes from alcohol drinkers and 20 controls, cultured for 48 h, there were more chromosome-type aberrations in those with a daily ethanol consumption of more than 80 ml (Horvat *et al.*, 1983).

Several studies have suggested that alcoholics have higher sister chromatid exchange frequencies in their lymphocytes than nonalcoholics (Butler *et al.*, 1981; Seshadri *et al.*, 1982; Horvat *et al.*, 1983; Hedner *et al.*, 1984; Kucheria *et al.*, 1986). Butler *et al.* (1981) showed that in nine alcoholics who were not currently drinking alcohol there was no elevation in such frequencies. Seshadri *et al.* (1982) reported that sister chromatid exchange frequencies in babies of ten alcoholic mothers who had elevated sister chromatid exchange frequencies were similar to those in babies from nonalcoholic mothers.

[The Working Group noted that in these studies smoking and other confounding factors were frequently not controlled for, which may have influenced the results.]

Activity profiles appear in Appendix 2.

5. EPIDEMIOLOGICAL STUDIES OF CANCER IN HUMANS

As early as 1910, it was observed in Paris, France, that about 80% of patients with cancer of the oesophagus and cardiac region of the stomach were alcoholics, who drank mainly absinthe (Lamy, 1910). In the first half of this century, it was also noted from mortality statistics in various countries that high risks for cancers of the oral cavity, pharynx, oesophagus and larynx occurred among persons employed in the production and distribution of alcoholic beverages (Young & Russell, 1926; Clemmesen, 1941; Kennaway & Kennaway, 1947; Versluys, 1949). Later studies showed that cancers at these sites occur at lower rates of incidence (and mortality) in religious groups that proscribe alcohol intake, such as Seventh-day Adventists (Wynder *et al.*, 1959; Lemon *et al.*, 1964; Phillips *et al.*, 1980), compared with corresponding national populations. Although many aspects of the life style of such populations are particular, differences in drinking (and smoking) habits may contribute to the differences in disease rates. Subsequent to these historical observations and studies of religious groups, analytical studies of the cohort and case-control type have been carried out.

5.1 Measurement of alcohol intake in epidemiological studies

In descriptive studies, discussed below, a very crude level of alcohol intake is typically inferred for a group of individuals, on the basis of characteristics such as treatment for alcoholism. Frequently, even measurements of average alcohol intake in these groups and in the groups with which they are compared are not available.

In case-control and cohort studies involving individual subjects, measurements of alcohol intake are usually obtained by structured interview or questionnaire. The questions asked vary widely among studies, providing markedly different levels of detail about alcohol intake (Room, 1979). In some studies, a single question was asked that provided only a few categories of alcohol consumption. In many studies, separate questions were asked regarding the average frequency (usually in terms of standard units) of drinking beer, wine, spirits and other specific beverages. This information allows a calculation of usual total ethanol intake as well as an estimation of that from the specific beverages. In some studies, further information was collected about alcohol consumption at different ages. In general, details about intraindividual variations, such as 'binge drinking', have not been incorporated in the studies reviewed.

The validity of self-reported alcohol consumption has been reviewed by Midanik (1982). In some populations (Pernanen, 1974), but not necessarily all, self reporting of alcohol intake results in a lower total than that for alcohol sales. However, even if a population as a whole tends to underestimate intake, this may not necessarily be true of participants in epidemiological studies, such as those who volunteer to enrol in a cohort study. Moreover, there is some evidence that underestimation tends to be proportional to consumption, so that the broad ordering of respondents is maintained (Boland & Roizen, 1973).

The reproducibility and validity of the measurements of alcohol consumption used in epidemiological investigations have been examined in several recent studies. Rohan and Potter (1984) interviewed 37 men and 33 women in Australia regarding food and beverage intake twice at a three-year interval; mean intakes were reported almost identically on the two questionnaires, and the correlation between the original report and recalled intake was 0.87 for men and 0.79 for women. In a comparison of intake measured by diet record and a dietary history interview four years later among 79 Dutch men and women, mean alcohol consumption was found to be identical using the two methods, and the correlation among individual subjects was 0.82 (van Leeuwen *et al.*, 1983).

Riboli *et al.* (1986) compared wine intake as assessed by an interviewer-administered questionnaire among 29 Italian adults with consumption reported in a one-week dietary record. The estimate from the questionnaire was about 40% higher than that determined from the diary, and the correlation between the methods was 0.57. In a validation study of a self-administered dietary questionnaire conducted among 173 participants in a large US cohort of women, Willett *et al.* (1987) compared alcohol intake computed from two administrations of a questionnaire at a one-year interval with intake assessed by four one-week diet records collected during the interviewing year. Mean alcohol intake by this group of women was nearly identical whether assessed by either of the two questionnaires or the dietary record: the correlation between the two questionnaires was 0.90, that between the first questionnaire and the diet record, 0.86, and that between the second questionnaire and diet record, 0.90. Furthermore, significant correlations were observed between the questionnaire measure of alcohol intake and plasma high-density lipoprotein-cholesterol levels (which is known to be sensitive to alcohol ingestion), providing qualitative evidence of a physiological response to alcohol intake. It thus appears that alcohol intake can be measured in a reproducible and valid manner by the relatively simple questionnaires employed in many epidemiological studies. Additional characterization of drinking habits, including use of alcohol at different ages and shorter-term patterns of individual variation, may provide useful information and improve the classification of subjects according to long-term alcohol use.

In case-control studies, errors in recall of alcohol intake that are different between cases and controls could distort the relation with cancer risk; it is possible that the occurrence of a grave illness could affect recall. In several studies of dietary recall, it has been noted that current dietary intake has a major influence on the reporting of earlier diet (Jensen *et al.*, 1984). Since alcohol intake may be altered by serious illness or by its treatment, it is possible that studies of prevalent cases of cancer are less reliable than studies of newly diagnosed cases, even if alcohol does not influence prognosis.

5.2 Descriptive studies

Descriptive studies (also referred to as ecological or correlation studies) of the relationship between alcohol consumption and cancer risk entail analysis of the co-variation of population-based measures of those two variables. Variations (known or inferred) in alcohol consumption by time, geographic location and category of person are examined in relation to variations in cancer incidence or mortality rates. Since alcohol consumption tends to be associated with other forms of behaviour that might also influence the risk of developing cancer (especially cigarette smoking and aspects of diet), and for which equivalent measures of exposure are frequently not available, it is not possible in descriptive studies to infer a causal relationship between alcohol consumption and cancer risk. In addition, in descriptive studies, average values of alcohol consumption are attributed to population groups as a whole; depending on the actual distribution of exposures within the population, this can result in considerable misclassification of exposure and consequent errors in estimation of effects.

(*a*) *Geographical and temporal studies*

Geographical and temporal variations in alcohol consumption are usually estimated from systematic records (governmental or commercial) of production and sales, or from changes in the rates of other acknowledged diseases of 'alcohol abuse' (especially alcoholic liver cirrhosis). In some cross-sectional, regional, ecological studies, alcohol consumption in different population subgroups has been estimated by direct survey (e.g., Hinds *et al.*, 1980).

Intrapopulation studies, in which identifiable groups of people with known differences in alcohol consumption (e.g., abstainers, religious groups, ethnic groups) or with known or presumed changes in drinking habits (e.g., migrants) are studied, are also a useful source of descriptive epidemiological data. Again, however, measures of confounding variables are often not available, or, if available, may be difficult to 'control for' in data analysis at the population level.

Descriptive studies have been used most frequently to study alcohol consumption in relation to specific cancers of the upper alimentary tract and larynx. Oesophageal cancers, in particular, have been studied in this way in both developed and developing countries. Many geographic correlation studies have been carried out to examine mortality from alimentary tract cancer in relation to mortality from liver cirrhosis and alcoholism within the departments of France (Lasserre *et al.*, 1967). These studies have consistently shown a strong correlation of oesophageal cancer with the index of alcohol consumption; less strong correlations have been seen for cancers of the mouth, pharynx and stomach. Geographic studies have also been carried out in eastern and southern Africa to examine the substantial local variations in oesophageal cancer mortality in relation to alcohol consumption and to brewing practices (Day *et al.*, 1982). Several international studies have demonstrated a positive correlation between national consumption of beer per head and mortality from cancer of the rectum (Breslow & Enstrom, 1974; Potter *et al.*, 1982).

Time trends in alcohol consumption per head and mortality from selected cancers have been analysed in some countries, predominantly in relation to cancers of the upper alimentary tract and larynx (Tuyns *et al.*, 1977; McMichael, 1979). Positive correlations have been reported consistently for some specific sites. In studies in which simultaneous time trends in several countries have been examined, a role has been suggested for alcohol consumption in the etiology of, for example, cancers of the large bowel (McMichael *et al.*, 1979).

Variations in the male:female ratio of cancer rates in relation to variations in the male:female ratio of mortality from alcoholic liver cirrhosis, or of alcohol consumption as determined by surveys of population samples, have also suggested a role for alcohol consumption in the etiology of cancers of the upper alimentary tract, the larynx, the liver, and, less clearly, the stomach and large bowel (Flamant *et al.*, 1964; Enstrom, 1977; Keller, 1977).

In very few descriptive studies has deliberate attention been paid to the relationship between alcohol consumption and cancers at other possibly relevant sites, such as the breast, pancreas and lung.

(*b*) *Studies of cancer rates in cultural subgroups*

The Mormons (Church of Jesus Christ of Latter-day Saints) expect abstention from alcohol and tobacco by active members; while the Seventh-day Adventists proscribe tobacco smoking, alcohol drinking and meat eating.

Wynder *et al.* (1959) compared the relative frequencies of various cancers in Seventh-day Adventists and in nonmembers recorded in eight US hospitals (83% in California), where Seventh-day Adventists represented approximately 10% of all hospital admissions. There were fewer cancers than expected of the lung (not adenocarcinoma), urinary bladder, uterine cervix, mouth, larynx and oesophagus in the Seventh-day Adventists.

Lemon *et al.* (1964) compared the age- and sex-standardized rates for causes of death of Californian Seventh-day Adventists with those of other Californians in a five-year follow-up of 47 866 members of the Church. A total of 3481 deaths (64.9% of expected for men and 74.1% for women) were reported, and death certificates were obtained for 3451 of them; cancer mortality was 70.6% of the expected value for men and 80.1% for women. The major deficits were in buccal and pharyngeal cancer (3 observed, 16 expected) and lung cancer (19 observed, 50 expected).

Phillips *et al.* (1980) compared cancer mortality among Seventh-day Adventists in California with that of a sample of other Californians who were similar with regard to various demographic and socioeconomic factors. The two cohorts comprised 22 940 Seventh-day Adventists and 112 725 nonmembers, who were followed for 17 (1960-76) and 13 (1960-72) years, respectively, and who had completed the same baseline questionnaire in 1960. Deaths were ascertained by annual follow-up of each study member and by record linkage with the California State death certificate file. Age- and sex-adjusted mortality ratios (Seventh-day Adventists:other Californians and Seventh-day Adventists:US white population for 1960-75) were given for all cancers, for stomach, colorectal, lung, breast and prostatic cancer, and for leukaemias and lymphomas. Significant deficits were detected for all cancers combined, for colorectal cancer, for lung cancer and for other smoking-related cancers.

Jensen (1983) studied 1589 male Copenhagen Temperance Society members in Denmark, 781 of whom were Seventh-day Adventists. Expected numbers of cancer cases were obtained by multiplying sex-, age- and calendar-time-specific incidence rates for the general Copenhagen population by the sex-, age- and time-specific person-years of observation in the several groups. For cancers at all sites, a reduced risk was observed among Seventh-day Adventists (relative risk [RR], 0.7; $p < 0.01$), in contrast to that of members of other temperance societies (RR, 1.1). The author attributed the overall reduction in cancer risk to the deficits of alcohol- and tobacco-related cancers among the Seventh-day Adventists. The risk of cancer of the colon, including cancer of the rectosigmoid junction, was also reduced, whereas the risk for rectal cancer was not significantly different from that of the general population.

A comparison of the cancer incidence rates in Mormons and non-Mormons in Utah, USA, during 1966-70, was carried out by Lyon *et al.* (1976). The study was based on 10 641 cases of cancer in Utah classified according to membership in the Mormon Church. Some beliefs and practices of the Mormon Church include emphasis on family life and education, strict sexual mores, and abstinence from alcohol, tobacco, tea, coffee and nonmedicinal drugs (Lyon *et al.*, 1980). Significantly reduced standardized incidence ratios (SIR) for Mormons:non-Mormons were found for the following cancers: all, 0.9 for men and 0.8 for women; oesophagus, 0.4 ($p < 0.001$) and 0.1 ($p < 0.01$); larynx, 0.4 ($p < 0.001$) and 0.3 ($p = 0.02$); stomach, 0.8 ($p = 0.04$) for men; colon, 0.7 ($p < 0.001$) for women; lung, 0.5 ($p < 0.001$) for men; uterine cervix, invasive, 0.6, *in situ*, 0.4 ($p < 0.001$); and breast, 0.9 ($p = 0.008$) for women. In contrast, male Mormons had slightly but significantly elevated incidences of cancer of the prostate and of the brain and nervous system. The findings were very similar when the analysis was extended to the period 1967-75, thus including 20 379 cases of cancer (Lyon *et al.*, 1980), approximately 90% of which had been histologically confirmed.

Enstrom (1978) examined cancer mortality among male Mormons in California, USA, during 1968-75. The death rate from cancers at combined smoking-related sites was 58% that of the general Californian population, and that from all other cancers, 68%. Most Mormons smoke and drink alcohol about half as much as the general population, being fairly similar in other respects, such as socioeconomic status and urbanization. Active Mormons abstain almost completely from tobacco and alcohol (Enstrom, 1975). In a subsequent report, Enstrom (1980) was able to use Mormon Church records to subdivide the male Mormon population into those who were active members of the Church and those who were not. The deficit in cancer mortality was greater in active than in all male Mormons. For stomach cancer and colon cancer, the age-standardized mortality ratios (SMRs) did not differ noticeably between active and all male Mormons; however, for rectal and lung cancer, the SMRs were much lower in active Mormons (0.4 and 0.2) than in all male Mormons (0.7 and 0.6). [In these studies of Californian Mormons, it is not made clear how well the numerator deaths, as recorded by the state, correspond to the apparent denominator, as provided by the Mormon Church.]

5.3 Analytical studies

(*a*) *General introduction*

The relationship between alcohol intake and cancer at a variety of sites has been assessed in many large cohort studies. With few exceptions, detailed information on type of beverage, amount drunk and on smoking was not available. Tobacco smoking and alcohol drinking are often correlated at the individual level, and tobacco smoke is a cause of cancer at many sites that may also be related to alcohol consumption (IARC, 1986a). However, a major methodological advantage of cohort studies over case-control studies is the lesser probability of selection bias and bias with regard to information on exposure. The most detailed evidence about the relationship between alcohol and cancer at individual sites has come from case-control studies, many of which are described in subsequent sections.

Most of the cohort studies have been of the retrospective (historical) type, comparing cancer incidence or mortality in groups with high alcohol intake (e.g., alcoholics and brewery workers) with that of the general population. The distinction between such cohort studies and descriptive studies is not always clear; several of the investigations of religious groups, described above, could be considered cohort studies but were included with the other studies of these groups for coherence. A few prospective (concurrent) cohort studies in which information on drinking and smoking was available for individual cohort members have been of sufficient size for site-specific risks to be determined.

In a number of cohort studies initiated to study cardiovascular disease, total cancer incidence or mortality has been reported; however, because of the absence of site-specific risk estimates, such studies have not been included.

Since, in some of the cohort studies, the risk of cancer at many different sites was examined, their design is described and commented upon here in order to save unnecessary repetition. Studies in which cancer at only one site was studied are described in the relevant section.

The design of the major retrospective and prospective cohort studies is summarized in Table 45.

(i) *Norwegian Alcoholics Study* (Sundby, 1967)

A total of 1722 men discharged during 1925-39 from the Psychiatric Department of an Oslo hospital with a diagnosis of alcoholism were enrolled in the study and observed until the end of 1962. No information was available on drinking and smoking habits of individual cohort members or of the cohort as a whole, but 408 were considered to be vagrant alcoholics. Evidence of persistent alcoholism was available for about 75% of the vagrants and for 50% of the remaining group. Follow-up was virtually complete, with 1061 deaths. Death certificates were located for 1028 of these, and information on cause of death was available for another 28 persons. The observed numbers of deaths were compared with expected numbers based on causes of deaths for all of Norway (496.9) and for Oslo (629.0).

(ii) *Finnish Alcohol Misusers and Alcoholics Study* (Hakulinen *et al.*, 1974)

Between 1944 and 1959, male 'alcohol misusers' were registered by the Finnish State Alcohol Monopoly on the basis of conviction for drunkenness, sanctions imposed by the municipal social welfare boards, and various breaches against the regulations governing alcohol usage. No information was available on the amount of alcohol consumed by the cohort members, nor on types of beverage or smoking habits. The numbers of incident cases of cancer of the oesophagus, of the liver and of the colon among an estimated 205 000 men born 1881-1932 and alive in 1965-68 were obtained by a manual match between the files of the Finnish Cancer Registry for these years and the files of the Alcohol Misusers Registry. Person-years at risk during the period 1965-68 were estimated from samples, and these formed the basis for computing expected numbers of cases. Lung cancer risk was determined in a similar fashion, but for only one-third of the group in 1968.

A second group of men more than 30 years of age, who in 1967-70 had been listed as chronic alcoholics by the Social Welfare Office of Helsinki, were also studied. The mean annual number of such men was estimated to be 4370. No information was available on type or amount of alcoholic beverages drunk or on tobacco smoking, but the persons in the group of chronic alcoholics were heavy alcohol drinkers, most of whom drank cheap, strong beverages, wines and denatured alcohols. Incident cases of cancer occurring during 1967-70 were identified by record linkage with the Finnish Cancer Registry, and expected numbers were derived on the basis of national incidence rates and computed person-years.

[The Working Group noted that cancer incidence was determined over a brief period (four years) of follow-up. Determination of only a small part of the total experience of each of the underlying source populations of alcohol misusers and chronic alcoholics could introduce bias if the distribution of time since entry into the cohort was limited or skewed and if alcohol-related cancer deaths are distributed unevenly over cohort follow-up time.]

(iii) *UK Alcoholics Study* (Nicholls *et al.*, 1974)

A total of 935 patients who had been discharged from four mental hospitals in or near London, UK, during the years 1953-57, or who had died during the key hospitalization and who had been given a primary or secondary diagnosis implicating abnormal drinking, were followed for 10-15 years. Of the total sample, 70 (7.5%) remained untraced and 233 men (34.4%) and 76 women (29.6%) had died; a total of 112.7 deaths was expected (SMR, 2.7). The SMR for all cancers was 1.7 (37 cases, $p < 0.05$) for men and 1.9 (13 cases, nonsignificant) for women. The study was extended to all of England and Wales 1953-64 by Adelstein and White (1976), who covered a total of 1595 men and 475 women. The SMRs for all causes of deaths were 2.1 for men and 2.8 for women.

Table 45. Main characteristics of cohort studies on the relationship between alcohol and cancers at many sites

Study and reference	Period of enrolment	Population at start (effective population)	Duration of follow-up; no. of deaths; no. of cancers	Completeness of follow-up	Information on		
					Type of beverage	Amount of alcohol	Smoking status
Norwegian Alcoholics (Sundby, 1967)	1925–39	1722 men (1693)	37 years; 1061 deaths; 204 ca deaths	98.3%	–	–	–
Finnish Alcohol Misusers	1944–59	Estimated 205 000 men alive in 1965–68 (born 1881–1932)	Incidence of selected ca sites only; 449 ca cases	–	–	–	–
and Alcoholics (Hakulinen et al. 1974)	1967–70	Mean annual number of men in the registry, 4370	4 years; 81 incident ca cases	–	–	–	–
UK Alcoholics (Nicholls et al., 1974)	1953–57	678 men, 257 women (865)	10–15 years; 309 deaths; 50 ca deaths	92.5%	–	–	–
Massachusetts Alcoholics (Monson & Lyon, 1975)	1930, 1935 or 1940	1139 men, 243 women	41 years; 894 deaths; 105 ca deaths	66%	–	–	–
England and Wales (Adelstein & White, 1976)	1953–64	1595 men 475 women	17 years; 605 men 189 women	–	–	–	–
Dublin Brewery Workers (Dean et al., 1979)	1954–73	– (men)	20 years; 1628 deaths; total no. of ca deaths not stated	–	–[a]	–[a]	–

Table 45 (contd)

Study and reference	Period of enrolment	Population at start (effective population)	Duration of follow-up; no. of deaths; no. of cancers	Completeness of follow-up	Information on		
					Type of beverage	Amount of alcohol	Smoking status
Japanese Prospective (Hirayama, 1979)	1965	122 261 men, 142 857 women (40+ years)	10 years; 27 993 deaths; 7377 ca deaths	–	+	+	+
Danish Brewery Workers (Jensen, 1979, 1980)	1939–63	14 313 men (6 or more months' employment, 14 227)	30 years; 3550 deaths; 951 ca deaths; 1303 incident ca cases	99.4%	–[a]	–[a]	–
US Veterans Alcoholics (Robinette *et al.*, 1979)	1944–45	4401 men	29 years; 1438 deaths; 166 ca deaths	90–98%	–	–	–
Hawaiian Japanese (Blackwelder *et al.*, 1980; Pollack *et al.*, 1984)	1965–68	8006 men (7846)	Av. 14 years; 426 ca deaths (only 5 sites considered)	98%	+	+	+
Kaiser-Permanente (Klatsky *et al.*, 1981)	1964–68	87 926 (8060 men and women)	10 years; 745 deaths; 215 ca deaths	82–92%	–	+	+
Canadian Alcoholics (Schmidt & Popham, 1981)	1951–70	9889 men (9543)	21 years; 1823 deaths; 240 ca deaths	96.5%	–	–[a]	–[a]
Japanese Doctors (Kono *et al.* 1983, 1985, 1986)	1965	6815 (5135 men)	19 years; 1283 deaths;	94%	–	+	+
Framingham (Gordon & Kannel, 1984)	1950–54	5209 (2106 men, 2641 women)	22 years 1167 deaths; 257 ca deaths (only specific sites)	91%	+	+	+

[a]Estimates of type and/or consumption given for the group

(iv) *Massachusetts Alcoholics Study* (Monson & Lyon, 1975)

The study comprised 1382 persons (1139 men and 243 women) admitted to mental hospitals in 1930, 1935 or 1940 with a diagnosis indicative of chronic alcoholism. No information was provided on the amount or type of alcohol consumed by individuals or by the cohort as a whole, or on smoking habits. Death certificates were traced up to 1 January 1971 for 909 members of the cohort (66%), while the vital status of the remainder was unknown. Because of the high percentage of persons lost to follow-up, absolute death rates could not be calculated; instead, the proportional distribution of deaths by cause in the cohort was compared with that of the USA, taking into account age, sex and calendar time. The analysis was restricted to 894 deaths among whites. [The Working Group noted that the high percentage of loss to follow-up seriously limits the usefulness of these data.]

(v) *Dublin Brewery Workers Study* (Dean *et al.*, 1979)

A list of 1628 deaths during the period 1954-73 was provided by a large brewery in Dublin, Ireland. On the basis of death certificates for all but two of these men and of statistics for the population of employees and pensioners in 1957, 1960, 1967 and 1970, RRs for specific causes of death were estimated employing both national and regional rates. The expected number of deaths was 1675.8 (regional rates). It was estimated from previous research that ethanol intake among the brewery workers was 58 g per day, compared with 16-33 g per day for other groups of the Irish population. Beer (stout) was consumed on the premises. No information was available on individual consumption of alcohol or tobacco; smoking was forbidden at the brewery for many years. [The Working Group noted that the cohort at risk was estimated indirectly as 2000-3000 men at any one time during follow-up, and no individual follow-up of cohort members was performed.]

(vi) *Japanese Prospective Study* (Hirayama, 1979)

In 1965, 122 261 men and 142 857 women aged 40 years and over (91-99% of the census population) were interviewed in 29 health centre districts in Japan. The main items studied were diet, smoking, drinking and occupation. A record linkage system with death registrations was established for the annual follow-up. Associations between alcohol and cancer were investigated on the basis of ten-year follow-ups through 1975, when there were 27 993 deaths from all causes (16 515 for men and 11 478 for women) and 7377 from cancer.

(vii) *Danish Brewery Workers Study* (Jensen, 1979, 1980)

A total of 14 313 male members of the Danish Brewery Workers' Union who had been employed for six or more months in a brewery during the period 1939-63 were enrolled in this retrospective cohort study. The brewery workers had the right to consume six bottles (2.1 l) of light pilsener (lager) beer (alcohol content, 3.7 g [~ 78 g ethanol] per 100 ml) on the premises of the brewery per working day; 1063 members of the cohort worked in a mineral-water factory, with no free ration of beer. No information was available on alcohol consumption or smoking habits of individual members of the cohort; but, on the basis of comparisons with alcohol statistics and population surveys, it was estimated that cohort members with employment in a brewery had a four times higher average beer consumption than the general population. Vital status was ascertained for 99.4% of the cohort members.

There were 3550 deaths (SMR, 1.1) in the cohort, and 1303 incident cases of cancer were identified during the period 1943-72 by record linkage with the Danish Cancer Registry. Expected numbers of cancer cases and deaths were computed on the basis of age-, sex-, residence- and time-specific rates. Relationships between use of alcohol and tobacco and cancer of the pharynx, larynx and oesophagus were further explored in a nested case-control study (Adelhardt *et al.*, 1985).

(viii) *US Veterans Alcoholics Study* (Robinette *et al.*, 1979)

A cohort of 4401 US Army service men hospitalized for chronic alcoholism in 1944-45 was drawn as a sample from records of the US Department of Defense and the Veterans' Administration. Of these, 98% were <40 years of age at the time of hospitalization. They were matched for age with an equal number of enlisted men hospitalized for acute nasopharyngitis during the same period. Deaths in these groups were ascertained through the Veterans' Administration Beneficiary Identification and Records Locator Subsystem, and death certificates were obtained to code for cause of death. Follow-up for death was estimated to be 90-98% complete. No information was available on the drinking habits of individual members of the cohort or on average consumption by the cohort members. It was noted that only 7.5% of the chronic alcoholics had been discharged from military service for medical disability, including alcoholism. The mortality experience of the cohort was compared with that of the matched cohort of nasopharyngitis patients, and the mortality of both cohorts was compared with that of US males for selected causes of death. Overall mortality was approximately 80% higher in the alcoholics group than in the nasopharyngitis group (SMR, 1.9).

(ix) *Hawaiian Japanese Study* (Blackwelder *et al.*, 1980; Pollack *et al.*, 1984)

A detailed interview questionnaire on diet, alcohol consumption, smoking history, socioeconomic factors and demographic variables was given to a cohort of 8006 Japanese men included in a study of cancer in Hawaiian Japanese during 1965-68. Because only about 2.5% of the subjects had moved from Oahu, Hawaii, after the initial examination, the authors considered that the surveillance system had allowed identification of virtually all newly diagnosed cancer cases in the cohort. Two kinds of information on alcohol consumption were obtained at interview: usual monthly consumption of wine (including Japanese saké and fortified wines), beer and spirits (including whisky, gin and brandy), and actual intake of each during the 24-h period preceding the interview. Information on usual consumption was converted into ounces of each type of beverage consumed per month and total ounces of ethanol consumed per month. Subsequent cancers occurring up to 31 December 1980 (the average follow-up period was 14 years) were identified from many sources, including the Hawaii Tumor Registry. The relation between alcohol consumption and epithelial cancers of the stomach, colon, lung, rectum and prostate was analysed, controlling for age and cigarette smoking.

(x) *Kaiser-Permanente Study* (Klatsky *et al.*, 1981)

Between July 1964 and August 1968, 87 926 persons responded to a self-administered questionnaire on alcohol intake as part of a multiphasic health examination in Oakland or

San Francisco, California, USA. This corresponded to 48% of the Kaiser Foundation Health Plan members in 1968. Of these, 22.6% reported that they had not drunk alcohol during the preceding year; 8% did not respond satisfactorily. Of 2084 persons who reported taking six or more drinks per day, 2015 were matched to equal numbers of persons who reported taking three to five drinks per day, two or fewer drinks per day, or total abstinence. The overall mortality of persons taking six or more drinks a day was twice that of those taking two or fewer drinks a day. Matching was for sex, race, presence or absence of current cigarette smoking, examination date and age. Altogether, 745 deaths occurred during ten years of follow-up among the 8060 persons in this study. Deaths were ascertained only from the California death index, and it was estimated that 82-92% of all deaths had been identified.

(xi) *Canadian Alcoholics Study* (Schmidt & Popham, 1981)

The cohort consisted of 9889 men (79% middle-class; <1% nonwhite) who had been admitted to the main clinical services for alcoholics in Ontario between 1951 and 1970. No information on individual drinking or smoking habits was available, but investigations of samples of the cohort indicated an average daily consumption of 254 ml [~ 200 g] ethanol and that >92% were still drinking ten years after admission. A total of 94% of cohort members were current smokers, who smoked an average of 28 cigarettes per day. Altogether, 1823 deaths occurred before 1972; 960.9 were expected. Vital status could not be determined for 3.5% of cohort members. Cause-specific mortality was compared with that of the Ontario male population. A further comparison was made with US veterans who smoked 21-39 cigarettes per day, in an indirect attempt to control for the effect of tobacco on the risk of alcohol-related cancers. Results were also reported for 1119 women followed up for 14 years, but only a few cancer deaths were observed (Schmidt & de Lint, 1972).

(xii) *Japanese Doctors Study* (Kono *et al.*, 1983, 1985, 1986)

A survey of smoking and drinking habits was carried out in March and April 1965 on 6815 male physicians in western Japan by means of a self-administered questionnaire. Of these, 5477 provided sufficient identifying information for prospective follow-up; 5135 provided sufficient information on drinking and smoking to classify them as nondrinkers (21%), ex-drinkers (10%), occasional drinkers (31%) and drinkers by daily intake. Similarly, quantitative information on cigarette smoking was available. Follow-up over 19 years revealed 1283 deaths, and was estimated to be 94% complete.

(xiii) *Framingham Study* (Gordon & Kannel, 1984)

Mortality from cancers of the lung, colon, stomach and breast in relation to alcohol consumption was studied in a cohort of 5209 men and women in Framingham, MA, USA. Alcohol consumption, recorded during 1950-54, was examined in relation to cancer mortality over 22 years of follow-up and obtained from 2106 men and 2641 women. [The Working Group noted that cancer is considered in only one table, analysed by a multivariate technique, but the levels of alcohol consumption included in the analysis are not specified.]

(b) *Cancer of the oral cavity and pharynx*

Since nasopharyngeal cancer is rare in most of the countries in which studies have been carried out, it can be assumed that the pharyngeal cancers referred to are predominantly of the oro- and hypopharynx. It is often difficult to determine whether cancers of the oral cavity or pharynx arise in one or other adjacent part classified as different sites in the International Classification of Diseases (ICD) since 1950. For this reason, and because the incidence of tumours at these sites is relatively low, investigators have grouped tumours of the oral cavity and pharynx together in different ways. This may affect the estimates of risk since the strength of the association with alcohol drinking may vary for adjacent parts of the buccal cavity and pharynx.

The risks for oral cavity and pharyngeal cancer in relation to alcohol consumption are summarized in Tables 46-49; whenever the information has been available, the composition of the tumour group has been given.

(i) *Cohort studies* (descriptions of studies of cancers at many sites are given on pp. 158-164)

Increased mortality from cancer of the oral cavity and pharynx has been observed in people with occupations involving high alcohol consumption (Young & Russell, 1926; Registrar General, 1958; Logan, 1982).

The results of the few available cohort studies are summarized in Table 46. Increased relative risks were found in all, notably in the studies of alcoholics carried out in Norway and Finland (Sundby, 1967; Hakulinen *et al.*, 1974), while the RR was only marginally increased among Danish brewery workers (Jensen, 1980).

Alcoholics in Norway, the USA and Canada had RRs for oral cavity and pharyngeal cancer that were two to five times higher than those of the general populations used for comparison (Sundby, 1967; Monson & Lyon, 1975; Robinette *et al.*, 1979; Schmidt & Popham, 1981). No account could be taken of tobacco smoking, which is known to increase the risk for oral cavity and pharyngeal cancer (IARC, 1986a); however, the RR was still increased when mortality from oral cavity and pharyngeal cancer among Canadian alcoholics was compared with that of US veterans who smoked similar numbers of cigarettes per day (3.3-17.7 according to number of cigarettes smoked per day; Schmidt & Popham, 1981). In the Kaiser-Permanente study (Klatsky *et al.*, 1981), the risk for cancer of the oral cavity, pharynx and oesophagus combined was four times higher among consumers of six or more drinks per day than among nondrinkers roughly matched for smoking habits. The RR was only slightly increased (1.4) among Danish brewery workers with an above-average beer consumption (Jensen, 1980). In the Japanese Doctors study, Kono *et al.* (1986) found an increasing risk for cancer of the upper digestive and respiratory tracts with increasing amount of alcohol taken per day, but the data are presented for all of the oral cavity, pharynx, oesophagus and larynx combined. The association remained after stratifying for tobacco consumption.

(ii) *Prevalence study*

Between March 1964 and September 1966, 346 cases (296 male, 47 female, three of

Table 46. Relative risks for oral cavity and pharyngeal cancer in cohort studies

Study and reference	Number of subjects	Relative risk	95% CI	Comments
Oral cavity				
Norwegian Alcoholics (Sundby, 1967)	13 deaths	5.0	[2.6–8.6]	Comparison with Oslo population
Danish Brewery Workers (Jensen, 1980)	18 cases	1.4	0.9–2.3	
Pharynx				
Norwegian Alcoholics (Sundby, 1967)	9 deaths	4.4	[2.1–8.5]	Comparison with Oslo population
Finnish Alcoholics (Hakulinen *et al.*, 1974)	3 cases	5.7	[1.2–16.5]	
Danish Brewery Workers (Jensen, 1980)	12 cases[b]	1.9	1.0–3.4	
Oral cavity and pharynx[c]				
Norwegian Alcoholics (Sundby, 1967)	22 deaths	4.8	[3.0–7.2]	Comparison with Oslo population
Massachusetts Alcoholics (Monson & Lyon, 1975)	13 deaths	3.3	[1.8–5.6]	
US Veterans Alcoholics (Robinette *et al.*, 1979)	14 deaths	2.2	1.1–4.6	90% CI
Danish Brewery Workers (Jensen, 1980)	46 cases	1.3	0.9–1.7	Includes lip
	11 deaths	0.8	0.4–1.5	
Canadian Alcoholics (Schmidt & Popham, 1981)	24 deaths	4.2	[2.7–6.3]	Comparison with Ontario population
		7.2	[5.0–10.7]	Comparison with US veterans
Kaiser-Permanente (Klatsky *et al.*, 1981)	15 deaths[d]	4.0	1.7–7.9	Comparison of consumers of 6+ drinks/day *versus* 0 drinks/day, adjusted for tobacco use
Japanese Doctors (Kono *et al.*, 1986) — Occasional drinkers	3 deaths[e]	[1.0]	–	Crude RR not changed by adjustment for smoking
<2 *go*[f]/day	3 deaths[e]	[1.5]	[0.8–2.4]	
$\geq$2 *go*/day	12 deaths[e]	[8.6]	[6.9–10.6]	

[a] Confidence interval; [ ] when calculated by the Working Group
[b] Excludes nasopharynx
[c] Includes different tumours, depending on study (see text)
[d] Includes oesophagus
[e] Includes oesophagus and larynx
[f] *go* = 27 ml alcohol

unknown sex) of oral and oropharyngeal cancer were diagnosed in Mainpuri District of India (Wahi, 1968). In a study of the prevalence of this cancer in relation to various population characteristics, information was elicited on chewing, smoking and drinking habits and occupation among the oral cancer cases and for a 10% sample of the population. Altogether, 34 997 persons aged 35 years and over were thus interviewed, and period prevalence rates were calculated; those for regular drinkers and nondrinkers were 9.17 and 0.89 per 1000, respectively. The author noted that it was difficult to obtain reliable information about drinking habits in India.

(iii) *Case-control studies*

Cancer of the oral cavity: Data are summarized in Table 47.

In a study of 462 white men with histologically verified squamous-cell carcinoma of the oral cavity and 81 with pharyngeal cancer, Wynder *et al.* (1957a) compared smoking and drinking habits, as well as a number of other risk factors, with those of 207 controls, who did not differ from the cases with regard to age, religion, educational background or hospital status. Information on exposures was obtained by personal interviews carried out in hospitals. The RR increased with increasing number of units (drinks) per day, irrespective of the type of alcoholic beverage. One unit was defined as 8 oz beer [about 9.5 g ethanol], 4 oz wine [about 12 g] or 1 oz whisky [about 9.5 g]. Dose-response relationships remained for both whisky and beer as the predominant drink after adjustment for tobacco smoking. A particularly strong association with alcohol drinking was found for cancers of the floor of the mouth and of the tongue.

In France, Schwartz *et al.* (1962) studied the smoking and drinking habits of 3937 male patients with cancers at various sites and 1807 controls admitted to hospital for traffic and work accidents in Paris and certain other French towns during 1954-58. Controls were matched to patients by age, sex and interviewer. A personal interview elicited information on tobacco smoking, consumption of alcoholic beverages, diet, socioeconomic factors and hereditary factors. In addition, the interviewer sought objective signs of alcoholism. Alcohol intake was measured as the average consumption over the ten years prior to interview. Since patients admitted for accidents are likely to have a higher alcohol consumption than the population giving rise to the cases, alcohol consumption was also compared with that of a second control group consisting of 1196 men with cancers assumed to be unrelated to use of alcohol or tobacco (cancers of the stomach, small intestine, colon, rectum, other digestive system, skin, kidney, prostate, penis, nervous system, endocrine system). No association with alcohol drinking was found for cancer of the lip (49 cases) or for cancer at other sites in the oral cavity after adjustment for tobacco consumption, in comparison with the accident controls. However, alcohol consumption was significantly higher among cases of cancers of the tongue (164 cases; 153 ml [121 g] ethanol/day) and of the oral cavity (144 cases; 138 ml [109 g] ethanol/day), when compared with cancer controls (113 ml [89 g] ethanol/day). [The Working Group noted that RRs could not be calculated from the data presented.]

Vincent and Marchetta (1963) investigated the alcohol and tobacco consumption of 33 men and nine women with cancer of the oral cavity and of 100 male and 50 female controls.

Table 47. Summary of results of case-control studies on oral cavity cancer and alcohol consumption

Place (reference) Site	Subjects (cases, controls)	Alcohol consumption[a]	Relative risk (RR)	95% CI[b]	Comments
USA, New York (Wynder *et al.*, 1957a)	Men	Never	1.0	-	Crude RR calculated
Lip, floor of mouth,	(462, 207)	<1 unit/day	1.2	0.6–2.8	by the Working Group;
gum, buccal mucosa,		1–2 units/day	1.4	0.6–3.1	incidence study
tongue, palate		3–6 units/day	3.1	1.3–7.4	
		>6 units/day	5.2	2.2–12.4	
USA, Buffalo (Vincent & Marchetta, 1963)	Men	Nondrinkers	1.0	-	Crude RR calculated
Tongue[c], floor of mouth,	(33, 100)	<2 oz [47 g]/day	1.7	0.5–5.9	by the Working
palate, gingiva,		>2 oz [47 g]/day	9.7	3.0–31.9	Group
buccal mucosa	Women	Nondrinkers	1.0	-	
	(9, 50)	<2 oz [47 g]/day	5.1	0.9–28.9	
		>2 oz [47 g]/day	41.0	3.4–495.3	
Sri Lanka (Hirayama, 1966)	Men and women	Nondrinkers	1.0	-	RR adjusted for
Lip, floor of mouth,	(76, 228)	Drinkers	1.5	0.9–2.8	chewing, calculated
tongue[c], buccal mucosa					by the Working Group
Puerto Rico (Martinez, 1969)	Men	None	1.0	-	Crude RR calculated
Lip, floor of mouth,	(108, 108)	≤1 unit/day	0.5	0.2–1.5	by the Working Group
tongue, other mouth		2–4 units/day	1.7	0.7–3.9	based on pairs matched
		≥5 units/day	2.8	1.1–7.0	for age and smoking
	Women	None	1.0	-	
	(30, 30)	≥ 1 unit/day	0.8	0.2–3.6	
USA, Buffalo (Bross & Coombs, 1976)	Women	Nondrinkers	1.0	-	RR adjusted for
Mouth, tongue	(145, 1973)	<30 drinks/month	1.3	0.8–2.2	age and smoking,
		≥30 drinks/month	3.4	1.7–6.6	calculated by the Working Group
USA, Buffalo (Graham *et al.*, 1977)	Men	<1 drink/week	1.0	-	Crude RR
Lip, tongue, floor of	(584, 1222)	1–6 drinks/week	1.1	0.8–1.5	
mouth, gum, other mouth		7–13 drinks/week	2.0	1.3–3.0	
		≥14 drinks/week	2.7	1.9–3.7	

Table 47 (contd)

Place (reference) Site	Subjects (cases, controls)	Alcohol consumption[a]	Relative risk (RR)	95% CI[b]	Comments
USA, Multicenter (Williams & Horm, 1977) Lip, tongue	Men (74, 1788)	Nondrinkers	1.0		RR adjusted for age, race and smoking; 95% CI could not be calculated
		≤50 oz-year	1.0		
		≥51 oz-year	1.4	NS	
	Women (20, 3188)	Nondrinkers	1.0		
		≤50 oz-year	0.7		
		≥51 oz-year	9.7	$p < 0.01$	
Gum, mouth	Men (53, 1788)	Nondrinkers	1.0		RR adjusted for age, race and smoking; 95% CI could not be calculated
		≤50 oz-year	2.0	NS	
		≥51 oz-year	3.7	$p < 0.01$	
	Women (25, 3188)	Nondrinkers	1.0		
		≤50 oz-year	1.2	NS	
		≥51 oz-year	1.5	NS	
Canada, British Columbia (Elwood *et al.*, 1984) Tongue, gum, floor of mouth, other	Men and women (133, 133)	<1 oz [24 g]/week	1.0		RR adjusted for smoking and other risk factors; 95% CI could not be calculated
		1-4 oz [24-96 g]/week	1.1		
		5-9 oz [120-216 g]/week	1.4		
		10-20 oz [240-480 g]/week	1.8		
		≥20 oz ≥480 g]/day	4.5		
France, Paris (Brugère *et al.*, 1986) Lip	Men (97, unk.)	0-39 g/day	1.0	-	RR adjusted for smoking; control group from national survey; 95% CI from paper
		40-99 g/day	1.8	0.8-3.9	
		100-159 g/day	4.9	2.1-11.4	
		160+ g/day	10.5	4-27.7	
Tongue, gum, floor of mouth, buccal mucosa	Men (759, unk.)	0-39 g/day	1.0	-	RR adjusted for smoking; control group from national survey; 95% CI from paper
		40-99 g/day	2.7	1.8-4.1	
		100-159 g/day	13.1	8.2-20.8	
		160+ g/day	70.3	42.8-115.4	

[a] g = pure ethanol
[b] Confidence intervals, calculated by the Working Group, when possible, unless otherwise specified; NS, not significant
[c] Anterior two-thirds of the tongue

Controls were selected from the gastrointestinal clinic of the same hospital that gave rise to the cases and were in the same age groups. Crude RRs of 9.7 and 41 (based on three cases, calculated by the Working Group) were seen for men and women who consumed ≥2 oz [47 g] ethanol per day when compared with nondrinkers.

As part of a study of risk factors for oral cancer in Southeast Asia, Hirayama (1966) inquired about drinking, chewing and smoking habits in Sri Lanka. Seventy-six patients with histologically verified oral cavity cancer (54 men, 22 women) and 228 age- and sex-matched controls were interviewed personally about their exposures. There was an association between alcohol drinking and cancer in the whole group (RR, [3.4]; $p < 0.01$) and among nonchewers (RR, [6.2]; $p < 0.05$). [When adjustment was made for tobacco chewing, a RR of 1.5 (95% confidence interval [CI], 0.9-2.8) was found for alcohol drinkers compared with nondrinkers.]

In Puerto Rico, Martinez (1969) studied 153 cases (115 male, 38 female) of squamous-cell carcinoma of the oral cavity and 488 controls (345 male, 144 female) matched for age and sex, as part of a larger investigation including cancers of the oesophagus and pharynx. The study included all cases diagnosed in hospitals and clinics in Puerto Rico during 1966, and three controls for each case, consisting of one patient from the same hospital or clinic at which the case was diagnosed and two neighbourhood controls; the hospital and neighborhood controls were homogeneous for most variables. Information on drinking, smoking and dietary habits was obtained by personal interview. Possible confounding by tobacco use was eliminated by studying a subset of cases and controls also matched on tobacco consumption. The risk for cancer of the oral cavity in men increased with increasing units of alcohol (18 oz beer [~ 21 g ethanol], 8 oz wine [24 g ethanol], 2 oz spirits [19 g ethanol]) taken per day, after taking account of smoking: 0.5 for <1 unit/day; 1.7 for 2.4 units per day; and 2.8 for ≥5 units per day. No association was seen for the small group of women.

Two studies were based on interviews of patients admitted to the Roswell Park Memorial Institute in Buffalo, NY, USA. Bross and Coombs (1976) compared the drinking habits of 145 white women with cancer of the mouth and tongue with those of 1973 controls with non-neoplastic diseases. All information was elicited by personal interview prior to the final diagnosis used for determining the case-control status of the persons. [After adjustment for age and smoking, persons who consumed 30 or more drinks of spirits, bottles of beer or glasses of wine per month had a RR for oral cavity and tongue cancer of 3.4 (95% CI, 1.7-6.6) compared with nondrinkers.] The influence of alcohol was seen in particular among women age 40-64 years at diagnosis. Similar RRs were seen for oral cavity and for tongue cancer separately. Graham *et al.* (1977) compared drinking, smoking and dietary habits and dentition status for 584 white men with histologically confirmed cancer of the oral cavity and 1222 white male controls diagnosed at the same hospital between 1958-65. The crude RR increased with increasing number of drinks taken per week to 2.7 ($p < 0.0001$) in those drinking ≥14 drinks per week. This increase in risk persisted after adjustment for smoking and poor dentition, also identified as risk factors in this study.

The Third National Cancer Survey conducted in the USA in 1967-71 (Cutler *et al.*, 1974) included a patient interview study (Williams & Horm, 1977). A total of 7518 cancer patients were interviewed (57% of those randomly selected for an interview), and the questions included amount and duration of alcohol and tobacco consumption. Quantitative lifetime drinking histories were obtained only for persons who had consumed at least one form of alcohol at least once weekly for at least one year; persons who had never drunk this often were counted as nondrinkers. Drinking and smoking habits of persons with cancers at individual sites known from other studies to be strongly associated with tobacco and alcohol were compared with the habits of persons with cancers at all remaining 'unrelated' sites. These controls consisted of 2102 men and 3464 women. RRs for consumption of wine, beer, spirits and total ethanol were calculated for each related site, adjusted for sex, age and smoking, as compared to other unrelated sites combined. The cut-off point between the two levels of consumption was 51 oz-years, calculated from units/week × number of years of consumption, the unit being glass, can and jigger for the three forms of alcohol used, which were converted to ounces of total ethanol using a standard conversion formula. Lifetime alcohol consumption of 74 men with cancers of the lip and tongue was compared with that of 1788 men with cancers not known to be related to either smoking or drinking. A nonsignificant RR of 1.4 emerged for men with a consumption of ≥51 oz-years ethanol after adjustment for age, race and smoking. Among the 20 women with these cancers, a significantly increased RR of 9.7 was seen for heavy drinkers in comparison with nondrinkers; no elevated risk (RR, 0.7) was seen in those drinking <51 oz-years. Among 53 men with cancer of the gum and mouth, consumers of ≥51 oz-years ethanol had an increased risk (3.7; $p < 0.01$), and the RR increased with increasing lifetime consumption. For 25 women, the RR was not significantly increased (1.2 and 1.5 in those with <51 and with ≥51 oz-years, respectively).

A study of oral cavity, pharyngeal and laryngeal cancers in British Columbia, Canada (Elwood *et al.*, 1984), included 133 cases (83 male, 50 female) of cancer of the oral cavity diagnosed between 1977 and 1980; 133 hospital controls with other cancers were individually matched for age, sex, clinic and time of diagnosis. Patients with diseases presumed by the authors to be unrelated to smoking and alcohol use were included in the control group, which comprised patients with stomach, colorectal and breast cancer. Information on drinking and smoking habits, together with information on social and occupational factors, was obtained by personal interviews. After adjustment for smoking, socioeconomic group, marital status, history of tuberculosis and dental care, a significant increase in trend and risk was observed with increasing amount of alcohol consumed per week. The association with alcohol drinking was stronger than that for smoking.

In France, Brugère *et al.* (1986) reported on systematically recorded information on tobacco use and alcohol consumption for 2540 male cancer patients treated at the Head and Neck Department of the Curie Institute in Paris between 1975 and 1982. Since no control group was available, they compared the alcohol and tobacco consumption of the patients, as recorded on hospital charts, with the consumption of the general population elicited as part of a national survey on health and medical care; for persons in the national survey, the figures were converted to intake in grams of ethanol per day by means of standard measures. A sample of the persons enrolled in the national survey, stratified by age, was used as controls. After adjustment for smoking, the RR for lip cancer among 97 men increased with increasing daily consumption of ethanol, and increasing RRs were also seen among 759 men with cancers of the tongue, gum, floor of mouth and buccal mucosa. [The Working Group noted that information on tobacco and alcohol use was obtained by means of different methods and in different interview situations for cases and controls; the size of the control group is not given.]

Cancer of the pharynx: Six of the studies reviewed above also examined the RR for cancer of the pharynx or epilarynx, when specified, in relation to alcohol intake (Wynder *et al.*, 1957a; Vincent & Marchetta, 1963; Martinez, 1969; Williams & Horm, 1977; Elwood *et al.*, 1984; Brugère *et al.*, 1986). The results of these studies are summarized in Table 48. In all of these investigations, the RR for pharyngeal cancer increased with increasing consumption of alcohol. This increase in risk was also noted in the studies in which the effect of smoking (Martinez, 1969; Williams & Horm, 1977; Brugère *et al.*, 1986), socioeconomic group, marital status, dental care and history of tuberculosis (Elwood *et al.*, 1984) could be taken into account.

A study in Sweden showed that male cases of cancer of the upper hypopharynx (32 patients) and possibly those with cancer of the lower hypopharynx (nine patients) had a higher alcohol intake than 115 controls. No difference was seen for women with regard to cancer of the hypopharynx or cancer of the oral cavity (Wynder *et al.*, 1957b).

Schwartz *et al.* (1962; see description, p. 167) found a higher daily alcohol consumption among 206 cases of hypopharyngeal cancer in France (157 ml/day [~ 124 g ethanol/day]) than among accident controls (126 ml/day [~ 100 g/day]), which was significant after adjustment for tobacco use and after comparison with cancer controls (113 ml/day [~ 89 g/day]). The alcohol consumption of 141 cases of oropharyngeal cancer was significantly higher (144 ml/day [~ 114 g/day]) than that of the cancer controls.

Olsen *et al.* (1985a) studied 32 cases of hypopharyngeal cancer in Denmark (26 male, six female) below the age of 75 years, diagnosed in five treatment centres of the country during the period 1980-82. Controls (1141) were selected at random from the population register and stratified for age, sex and place of residence. Smoking and drinking habits were elicited by self-administered questionnaire. [A nonsignificant RR of 1.8 (95% CI, 0.7-3.3) was calculated for persons who consumed ⩾150 g ethanol per week when compared with persons who consumed less, after adjustment for age, sex and tobacco use.]

Tuyns *et al.* (1988) studied 1147 male cases of hypopharyngeal and laryngeal cancer together with 3057 male population controls in France, Italy, Spain and Switzerland. Detailed information on drinking, smoking and dietary habits was obtained by personal interview. After meticulous reclassification of the site of origin of the cancer, there were 281 cases of hypopharyngeal cancer (piriform sinus, postcricoid area, posterior wall, and hypopharynx unspecified) and 118 cases of epilaryngeal cancer at the junction between the pharynx and larynx (epiglottis, aryepiglottic fold, arytenoid and epilarynx unspecified). The RR increased steeply with daily alcohol consumption, taking account of smoking, age and place of residence.

Cancer of the oral cavity and pharynx combined: In two studies, the risk associated with alcohol drinking has been investigated for cancer of the oral cavity and pharynx together. The results of these studies are summarized in Table 49.

Table 48. Summary of results of case-control studies on pharyngeal cancer and alcohol consumption

Place (reference) Site	Subjects (cases, controls)	Total alcohol consumption[a]	Relative risk (RR)	95% CI[b]	Comments
USA, New York (Wynder & Bross, 1957; Wynder *et al.*, 1957a) Tonsils, pharynx	Men (81, 207)	Never	1.0	-	Crude RR calculated by the Working Group
		<1 unit/day	0.7	0.2–3.6	
		1–2 units/day	1.1	0.2–5.3	
		3–6 units/day	4.4	0.9–21.1	
		>6 units/day	7.7	1.9–31.2	
USA, Buffalo (Vincent & Marchetta, 1963) Piriform sinus, tonsillar fossa and pillar, hypopharynx, posterior third of tongue	Men (33, 100)	Nondrinkers	1.0	-	Crude RR calculated by the Working Group
		<47 g/day	3.8	0.5–28.7	
		>47 g/day	52.5	12.7–217.0	
	Women (7, 50)	Nondrinkers	1.0	-	
		<47 g/day	2.6	0.2–28.5	
		>47 g/day	82.0	14.0–481.2	
Puerto Rico (Martinez, 1969) Naso-, meso- and hypo-pharynx, pharynx, unspecified	Men (39, 39)	None	1.0	-	RR based on pairs matched for age and tobacco use
		≤1 unit/day	4.1	0.6–26.2	
		2–4 units/day	1.4	0.2–9.8	
		>5 units/day	14.7	2.4–89.7	
USA Multicenter (Williams & Horm, 1977) Pharynx	Men (47, 1788)	Nondrinkers	1.0		RR adjusted for smoking, age and race; 95% CI could not be calculated
		≤50 oz-year	1.9		
		≥51 oz-year	6.2	$p < 0.01$	
	Women (18, 3188)	Nondrinkers	1.0		
		<50 oz-year	1.7		
		≥51 oz-year	17	$p < 0.01$	
Denmark (Olsen *et al.*, 1985a) Hypopharynx	Men and women (32, 1141)	<150 g/week	1.0	-	RR adjusted for age, sex and smoking by the Working Group
		≥150 g/week	1.8	0.7–3.3	
France, Paris (Brugère *et al.*, 1986) Oropharynx	Men (634, unk.)	0–39 g/day	1.0	-	RR adjusted for smoking; control group from national survey; 95% CI from paper
		40–99 g/day	2.6	1.6–4.2	
		100–159 g/day	15.2	9.2–25.1	
		160+ g/day	70.3	41.2–120	

Table 48 (contd)

Place (reference) Site	Subjects (cases, controls)	Total alcohol consumption[a]	Relative risk (RR)	95% CI[b]	Comments
Hypopharynx	Men (366, unk.)	0–39 g/day	1.0	-	RR adjusted for smoking; control group from national survey; 95% CI from paper
		40–99 g/day	3.3	1.4–7.9	
		100–159 g/day	28.6	12.5–65.1	
		160+ g/day	143.1	61.9–330.5	
Epilarynx	Men (217, unk.)	0–39 g/day	1.0	-	RR adjusted for smoking; control group from national survey; 95% CI from paper
		40–99 g/day	1.9	0.9–4.8	
		100–159 g/day	18.7	8.1–42.9	
		≥160 g/day	101.4	44–233.9	
Canada, British Columbia (Elwood _et al._, 1984) Oropharynx and hypopharynx, other	Men and women (87, 87)	<24 g/week	1.0		RR adjusted for smoking and other risk factors; 95% CI could not be calculated
		24–120 g/week	3.7		
		120–210 g/week	6.8		
		210–450 g/week	12.2		
		≥450 g/week	12.1		
France, Italy, Spain, Switzerland (Tuyns _et al._, 1988)					
Hypopharynx	Men (281, 3057)	0–20 g/day	1.0	-	RR adjusted for smoking, age and area of residence; 95% CI from paper
		21–40 g/day	1.6	0.7–3.4	
		41–80 g/day	3.2	1.6–6.2	
		81–120 g/day	5.6	2.8–11.2	
		≥121+ g/day	12.5	6.3–25.0	
Epilarynx	Men (118, 3057)	0–20 g/day	1.0	-	RR adjusted for smoking, age and area of residence; 95% CI from paper
		21–40 g/day	0.9	0.3–2.7	
		41–80 g/day	1.5	0.6–3.9	
		81–120 g/day	5.1	2.1–12.4	
		>121 g/day	10.6	4.4–25.8	

[a] g = pure ethanol
[b] Confidence intervals, calculated by the Working Group, when possible, unless otherwise specified

Table 49. Summary of results of case-control studies on oral cavity and pharyngeal cancer combined

Place (reference) Site	Subjects (cases, controls)	Total alcohol consumption[a]	Relative risk (RR)	95% CI[b]	Comments
USA, New York (Keller & Terris, 1965) Tongue, floor of mouth, palate, mesopharynx, hypopharynx, other parts of mouth, multiple sites	Men (134, 134)	Never	1.0	–	RR calculated by Working Group on the basis of pairs matched for smoking
		<9.5 g/day	1.4	0.6–3.0	
		9.5–35 g/day	2.1	0.9–4.8	
		>38g/day	3.7	1.7–7.8	
USA, New York (Feldman *et al.*, 1975; Feldman & Boxer, 1979) Oral cavity, pharynx	Men (96, 182)	None	1.0		RR adjusted for age and tobacco; 95% CI could not be calculated; test for trend significant at $\alpha = 0.005$ level
		<70 g/day	0.6		
		71–138 g/day	2.1		
		>140 g/day	4.5		

[a] g = pure ethanol
[b] Confidence intervals, calculated by the Working Group

In the USA, Keller and Terris (1965) investigated the smoking and drinking histories of 598 male cases of histologically confirmed squamous-cell carcinoma of the oral cavity and pharynx admitted to three Veterans Administration hospitals in New York during the period 1953-63. A similar number of male controls was selected individually as the next admission to the same hospital from persons in the same five-year age group. Information on alcohol and tobacco consumption was abstracted from clinical records based on data that had been elicited routinely by the admitting physicians. The contributions from different alcoholic beverages were summarized as daily intake of ounces of ethanol. After matching for smoking, the RR increased with increasing ethanol consumption in 134 case-control pairs. Rothman (1978) reported that the RR was higher for cancers at various sites in the mouth and mesopharynx than for cancer of the hypopharynx in heavy drinkers (>1.6 oz [>38 g] ethanol/day).

Feldman *et al.* (1975) and Feldman and Boxer (1979) compared the characteristics of a group of 185 male patients with cancers of the head and neck and a control group of 319 patients with other types of cancer admitted to five hospitals in New York City from 1971 to 1973. Only 182 male patients with cancers unrelated to tobacco and alcohol were eventually included in the control group. Information on dietary, smoking and drinking habits during the period five years before diagnosis was obtained by personal interview. The RRs for head and neck cancer were significantly related to alcohol consumption; when the comparison was restricted to the 96 males with cancer of the oral cavity, mesopharynx and hypopharynx, the increasing RR with increasing amount of daily alcohol drinking after adjustment for age and tobacco use became even more pronounced.

(iv) *Risk associated with type of alcoholic beverage*

In retrospective cohort studies of alcoholics, it has generally not been possible to distinguish the effects of different types of beverages. There was, however, a significantly increased risk for cancer of the pharynx (RR, 2.1; 95% CI, 1.0-3.7), but not for cancer of the oral cavity (RR, 1.4; 95% CI, 0.8-2.4), among beer-drinking Danish brewery workers (Jensen, 1979, 1980).

Wynder *et al.* (1957a) examined the dose-response relationships for whisky and beer drinking separately in male cases of oral cavity and pharyngeal cancer. For each type of beverage, an increasing trend was seen with increasing daily alcohol consumption after adjustment for smoking. The RR was highest among whisky drinkers of seven units [~ 65 g ethanol] or more per day, but the RRs for consumers of beer, wine and whisky were not substantially different for 1-6 units of ethanol intake. [The Working Group noted that no adjustment was made for consumption of other beverages.]

Increased RRs, unadjusted for smoking, were also observed by Keller and Terris (1965) for consumers of different types of alcoholic beverages compared with nondrinkers [wine only: RR, 2.5, 95% CI, 1.3-5.1; beer only: 2.6, 1.7-4.0; whisky only: 3.3, 2.1-5.1; mixed drinking: 2.7, 1.9-3.9]. Williams and Horm (1977) found similar patterns of RR controlled for smoking for equivalent lifetime consumption of beer and spirits among male cases of cancers of the lip and tongue, gum and mouth. The RRs for pharyngeal cancer were higher for those who drank wine and beer. The pattern among women was more uneven, possibly due to smaller numbers. [The Working Group noted that no adjustment was made for use of other alcoholic beverages in these two studies.]

(v) *Studies of joint exposure*

Tobacco smoking is causally related to cancer of the oral cavity and pharynx (IARC, 1986a), and alcohol and tobacco consumption are often correlated.

Rothman and Keller (1972) and Rothman (1976) reanalysed the information on consumption of alcohol and tobacco obtained by Keller and Terris (1965) in their study of US veterans. Altogether, 483 cases and 447 controls remained after exclusion of persons for whom there was inadequate information on either smoking or alcohol consumption. When stratifying for smoking, the RR for oral and pharyngeal cancer increased with increasing alcohol consumption at every level of smoking (Table 50). Persons with a daily consumption of ≥1.6 oz [36 g] ethanol had a two- to six-fold increased risk compared with nondrinkers.

Table 50. Relative risks[a] for oral cavity and pharyngeal cancer according to level of exposure to smoking and alcohol[b]

Ethanol/day (g)	Smoking (cigarette equivalents/day)			
	0	<20	20–39	40+
0	1.0	1.6	1.6	3.4
<9.5	1.7	1.9	3.3	3.4
9.5–35	1.9	4.9	4.8	8.2
>37	2.3	4.8	10.0	15.6
Cases/controls	26/85	66/97	248/197	143/68

[a]Risks are expressed relative to a risk of 1.0 for persons who neither smoked nor drank.
[b]From Rothman (1976)

The analysis showed a greater than multiplicative effect between alcohol and tobacco in the development of oral cavity and pharyngeal cancer, and heavy drinkers who were also heavy smokers had a RR of 15.6 when compared with persons who neither smoked nor drank. These results are in agreement with the findings of Wynder *et al.* (1957a), while Graham *et al.* (1977) found an additive effect of smoking and drinking. Elwood *et al.* (1984) could not distinguish statistically between an additive and a multiplicative effect. In the small Danish study of hypopharyngeal cancer (Olsen *et al.*, 1985a), a multiplicative effect was indicated. In the study of Tuyns *et al.* (1988), there was a multiplicative effect of alcohol and tobacco use on the risk of hypopharyngeal/epilaryngeal cancer (Table 51).

(iv) *Effect of alcohol in nonsmokers*

Some investigators have been able to evaluate the risk of oral cavity and pharyngeal cancer associated with alcohol drinking in nonsmokers. Wynder *et al.* (1957a) found no

Table 51. Relative risk for cancer of the hypopharynx/epilarynx according to level of exposure to smoking and alcohol[a]

Ethanol/day (g)	No. of cigarettes/day			
	0–7	8–15	16–25	26+
0–40	1.0	4.7	13.9	4.9
41–80	3.0	14.6	19.5	18.4
81–120	5.5	27.5	48.3	37.6
≥121	14.7	71.6	67.8	135.5
Total no. of cases	32	108	177	92

[a]From Tuyns et al. (1988)

difference in drinking habits among 16 cases of oral cavity and pharyngeal cancer and nine controls who did not smoke. By contrast, a doubling of the RR was seen among nonsmokers (26 cases, 85 controls) who consumed 1.6 oz or more [>37 g ethanol] alcohol per day compared to nondrinkers (Rothman & Keller, 1972; Rothman, 1976). Elwood *et al.* (1984) found a significant positive trend with alcohol intake in nonsmokers when the risk was examined for cancers of the oral cavity, pharynx and extrinsic larynx combined. In the study of Tuyns *et al.* (1988), there were more consumers of 80 g or more of ethanol per day among lifelong nonsmoking cases than among nonsmoking controls. [The Working Group noted that, in these studies, it is usually not possible to distinguish between current nonsmokers and lifelong nonsmokers.]

(c) *Cancer of the larynx*

The various subsites of the larynx must be distinguished from the point of view of degree of potential exposure: the endolarynx is exposed to inhaled agents, while the junctional area between the larynx and the pharynx is exposed to both inhaled and ingested agents. According to the ICD, these borderline areas (i.e., epiglottis free border, posterior surface of suprahyoid portion, junctional region of the three folds, aryepiglottic fold, arytenoid) should be classified partly under 161 (larynx) and partly under 146 and 148 (pharynx). In few studies is it stated whether these anatomical sites are included within the larynx. In some studies, the term 'extrinsic' and 'intrinsic' larynx are used, without specifying the subunits included.

(i) *Cohort studies* (descriptions of studies of cancers at many sites are given on pp. 158-164)

Studies of alcoholics have invariably shown increased risks for laryngeal cancer in comparison with the general population. The results of these studies are summarized in Table 52. It has not been possible to take into account the possible influences of differences

Table 52. Relative risks for laryngeal cancer in cohort studies

Study and reference	Number of subjects	Relative risk	95% CI[a]	Comments
Norwegian Alcoholics (Sundby, 1967)	5 deaths	3.1	[1.0-7.3]	Compared with Oslo inhabitants
Finnish Alcoholics (Hakulinen et al., 1974)	3 cases	1.4	[0.3-4.1]	
Massachusetts Alcoholics (Monson & Lyon, 1975)	6 deaths	3.8	[1.4-8.2]	
US Veterans Alcoholics (Robinette et al., 1979)	11 deaths	1.7	0.7-4.4	90% CI
Danish Brewery Workers (Jensen, 1980)	45 cases[b]	2.0	1.4-2.7	Cohort members drank on average four times more beer than reference population
Canadian Alcoholics (Schmidt & Popham, 1981)	12 deaths	4.3	[1.4-4.9]	Compared with Ontario population
		4.5	[2.3-7.8]	Compared with US veterans

[a]Confidence interval; [ ] when calculated by the Working Group
[b]Includes one case of cancer of the trachea

in smoking habits, which would have been desirable since tobacco smoke causes laryngeal cancer (IARC, 1986a). However, Schmidt and Popham (1981) found a SMR of 4.5 when they compared the number of laryngeal cancer deaths among Canadian alcoholics, who smoked on average 28 cigarettes per day, with that among of US veterans who smoked similar numbers of cigarettes per day. [The Working Group noted that other factors may vary between the two cohorts.] In Danish brewery workers (Jensen, 1980), the SIR for laryngeal (and tracheal) cancer was 3.7 [95% CI, 2.4-5.6] in persons with at least 30 years of employment in beer production, while it was 0.7 [0.04-8.7] in the small group of workers employed in mineral-water production.

These studies corroborate observations from occupational statistics (Young & Russell, 1926; Kennaway & Kennaway, 1947; Versluys, 1949) and clinical studies (Ahlbom, 1937; Jackson & Jackson, 1941; Kirchner & Malkin, 1953) of an association between laryngeal cancer and occupations with easy access to alcoholic beverages and with heavy alcohol drinking.

(ii) *Case-control studies*

The results of case-control studies on laryngeal cancer are summarized in Table 53. As part of a study of patients with cancers of the upper digestive tract and respiratory tract, Wynder *et al.* (1956) compared the smoking and drinking habits of 209 white male laryngeal cancer

Table 53. Summary of results of case-control studies on laryngeal cancer and alcohol consumption

Place (reference)	Subjects (cases, controls)	Alcohol consumption[a]	Relative risk (RR)	95% CI[b]	Comments
USA, New York (Wynder *et al.*, 1956)	Men (209, 209)	Never or <1 unit[c]/day of mainly straight whisky	1.0	-	RR adjusted for smoking, calculated by the Working Group
		1–6 units/day	1.8	0.9–3.2	
		7+ units/day	5.3	2.5–11.2	
		Beer or wine, irrespective of amount consumed	1.8	1.0–2.9	
USA, Buffalo (Vincent & Marchetta, 1963)	Men (23, 100)	<47 g/day	1.0	-	Crude RR calculated by the Working Group
		≥47 g/day	5.9	2.4–14.3	
USA, Multicenter (Wynder *et al.*, 1976)	Men (224, 414)	<1 unit/day [~10 g]	1.0	-	RR adjusted for smoking, calculated by the Working Group
		1–6 units/day [~10–60 g]	1.2	0.8–1.9	
		7+ units/day [>60 g]	2.3	1.5–3.4	
France (Spalajkovic, 1976)	Men[b] (200, 200)	Nondrinkers	1.0	-	Crude RR calculated by the Working Group
		Drinkers	11.2	6.9–18.2	
USA, Multicenter (Williams & Horm, 1977)	Men (99, 1788)	Nondrinkers	1.0	-	RR adjusted for smoking, age and race; 95% CI could not be calculated
		<50 oz-year	2.2	$p < 0.05$	
		≥51 oz-year	2.3	$p < 0.05$	
	Women (11, 3188)	Nondrinkers	1.0	-	95% CI could not be be calculated
		<50 oz-year	0.3	NS	
		≥51 oz-year	0.8	NS	
USA, Washington State (Hinds *et al.*, 1979)	Men (47, 47)	<1 unit[d]/day	1.0	-	Crude RR
		1–2 units/day	2.1	0.7–6.3	
		3–6 units/day	3.8	1.3–10.9	
		>6 units/day	9.0	2.4–34.1	
Canada, Ontario (Burch *et al.*, 1981)	Men (184, 184)	<1.04 oz [24 g]/day	4.4	2.2–8.5	RR adjusted for smoking; 90% CI
		1.04–2.5 oz [24–58 g]/day	3.9	2.1–7.3	
		≥2.6 oz [≥60 g]/day	4.8	2.3–9.9	

Table 53 (contd)

Place (reference)	Subjects (cases, controls)	Alcohol consumption[a]	Relative risk (RR)	95% CI[b]	Comments
Ireland, Dublin (Herity *et al.*, 1981)	Men (59, 200)	Nondrinkers	1.0		Crude RR; 95% CI could not be calculated
		Light drinkers	0.6		
		Heavy drinkers	3.2		
Canada, British Columbia (Elwood *et al.*, 1984)	Men and women (154, 154)	Extrinsic larynx			RR adjusted for smoking, socio-economic group, marital status, dental care and history of tuberculosis; 95% CI could not be calculated
		<1 oz [24 g]/week	1.0		
		1–4 oz [24–96 g]/week	1.7		
		5–9 oz [120–216 g]/week	2.6		
		10–20 oz [240–480 g]/week	5.1		
		>20 oz [>480 g]/week	6.4		
		Intrinsic larynx			
		<1 oz [24 g]/week	1.0		
		1–4 oz [24–96 g]/week	1.1		
		5–9 oz [120–216 g]/week	0.7		
		10–19 oz [240–480 g]/week	2.0		
		≥20 oz [≥480 g]/week	2.2		
Denmark (Olsen *et al.*, 1985b)[e]	Men and women (326, 1134)	0–100 g/week	1.0		RR adjusted for age and tobacco; 95% CI could not be calculated
		101–200 g/week	1.5		
		201–300 g/week	3.2		
		≥301 g/week	4.1		
USA, New Haven, CT (Zagraniski *et al.*, 1986)	Men (87, 153)	Never	1.0	–	RR adjusted for smoking
		Ever	4.2	1.4–12.4	
France, Paris (Brugère *et al.*, 1986)	Men (224, unk.)	Supraglottis			RR adjusted for smoking; control group selected from national survey
		0–39 g/day	1.0	–	
		40–99 g/day	2.6	1.3–5.1	
		100–159 g/day	11.0	5.5–21.7	
		≥160 g/day	42.1	20.5–86.4	
	(242, unk.)	Glottis + subglottis			
		0–39 g/day	1.0	–	
		40–99 g/day	0.8	0.5–1.2	
		100–159 g/day	1.5	0.9–2.6	
		≥160 g/day	6.1	3.4–10.9	

Table 53 (contd)

Place (reference)	Subjects (cases, controls)	Alcohol consumption[a]	Relative risk (RR)	95% CI[b]	Comments
France, Italy, Spain, Switzerland (Tuyns *et al.*, 1988)	(727, 3057)	Endolarynx			
		0–20 g/day	1.0	–	RR adjusted for smoking, age, area of residence
		21–40 g/day	0.9	0.7–1.3	
		41–80 g/day	1.1	0.8–1.5	
		81–120 g/day	1.7	1.2–2.4	
		>121 g/day	2.6	1.8–3.6	

[a] g = pure ethanol
[b] Confidence intervals, calculated by the Working Group, when possible
[c] 1 unit = 8 oz beer [9.5 g pure ethanol], 4 oz wine [12 g] or 1 oz whisky [9.5 g]
[d] 1 unit = 12 oz beer [14.3 g pure ethanol], 4 oz wine [12 g] or 1 oz spirits [9.5 g]
[e] Includes hypopharynx

patients with those of 209 hospital controls matched for age, sex, hospital status and educational and/or religious status. Information was obtained by personal interview without knowledge of the patient's case-control status. The laryngeal cancer patients had a significantly higher alcohol consumption than the control patients. When the comparisons were restricted to the group of patients who smoked 16-34 cigarettes per day, whisky drinkers consuming seven or more units per day had a 9.7-fold increase in risk compared with nondrinkers. After adjustment for smoking, the RR increased with increasing amount of whisky. There was no significant difference in the amounts of alcohol consumed by patients with intrinsic and extrinsic laryngeal cancer. Among 14 female laryngeal cancer cases, alcohol consumption was reported to be similar to that of controls. [The Working Group noted that some of the tumours classified as of the extrinsic larynx might have been of the hypopharynx.]

Schwartz *et al.* (1962; see description, p. 167) found a significantly higher average total ethanol consumption among 249 male laryngeal cancer cases (146 mg/day [115 g/day]) than among 249 accident controls (132 ml/day [104 g/day]); control patients with cancers unrelated to alcohol or tobacco use had an average daily consumption of 113 ml [89 g]. When the comparison was restricted to workers living in the département of Seine, the 63 laryngeal cancer patients had a significantly higher consumption (160 ml [126 g]/day) than the cancer controls (119 ml [94 g]/day) after accounting for differences in age and tobacco consumption.

In a study of patients with cancer of the oral cavity, pharynx or larynx, Vincent and Marchetta (1963) found increased consumption of both alcohol and tobacco among 23 male laryngeal cancer patients as compared with 100 controls selected from the gastrointestinal clinic of the same hospital that gave rise to the cases and in the same age groups. [The Working Group calculated a significant crude RR of 5.9 for consumers of 2 oz [47 g] or more ethanol per day compared with those taking less than 2 oz ethanol per day.]

Wynder *et al.* (1976) also reported RRs for smoking and drinking habits among 224 laryngeal cancer patients from different US hospitals and among 414 controls. Controls were matched to cases by year of interview, hospital status and age at diagnosis. Information on drinking and smoking was obtained by personal interview. There was a significant dose-response relationship for the amount taken per day after adjustment for smoking.

In France, Spalajkovic (1976) compared the alcohol consumption of 200 patients with cancer of the larynx or hypopharynx with that of 200 patients with nonmalignant ear, nose and throat disease. A significant increase in risk was noted for drinkers compared with nondrinkers.

In a study based on the Third National Cancer Survey in the USA (see description, pp. 170-171), significantly increased RRs were noted for alcohol drinking among 99 male laryngeal cancer patients after adjustment for smoking, age and race. No such increase was noted in women (11 cases; Williams & Horm, 1977).

Hinds *et al.* (1979) studied 47 laryngeal cancer cases in Washington State, USA, and 47 neighbourhood controls matched for sex, race and ten-year age group. Exposure information was obtained by interview. The RR for laryngeal cancer increased with increasing alcohol consumption.

In Ontario, Canada, 184 male laryngeal cancer cases were interviewed personally at home on smoking and on alcohol consumption, and on certain occupational exposures, and compared with 184 neighbourhood controls matched for age. Significantly increased RRs were noted for all categories of drinkers compared with nondrinkers. No dose-response relationship was apparent (Burch *et al.*, 1981).

Fifty-nine male laryngeal cancer cases were included in a study of head and neck cancer in Dublin, Ireland (Herity *et al.*, 1981), and their smoking and drinking habits were compared with those of 200 age-matched controls who were at the same hospital with cancers unrelated to smoking or with benign conditions. The RR was 3.2 among drinkers of more than 60 g ethanol per day for ten years, compared with nondrinkers and controlling for tobacco use.

In a study of cancers of the oral cavity, pharynx and larynx in British Columbia, Canada (see description, p. 171), Elwood *et al.* (1984) included 154 cases (130 male, 24 female) of extrinsic and intrinsic laryngeal cancer. Their drinking and smoking habits were compared with those of 374 hospital controls with other cancers. For cancers of the extrinsic and the intrinsic larynx, significant dose-response relationships ($p = 0.001$ and $p = 0.05$, respectively) were observed for alcohol consumption when account was taken of smoking, socioeconomic group, marital status, dental care and history of tuberculosis.

In a case-control study nested within the Danish brewery worker cohort, nonsignificantly increased RRs were associated with moderate and heavy alcohol consumption (Adelhardt *et al.*, 1985). [The Working Group noted the small size of this study.]

In a population-based study which comprised all laryngeal cancer patients below the age of 75 years seen at five departments involved in laryngeal cancer therapy in Denmark between 1980-82, Olsen *et al.* (1985b) investigated 326 patients and 1134 controls. After adjustment for tobacco use, a significant dose-response relationship was seen with total alcohol consumption, measured in grams of ethanol per week.

Zagraniski *et al.* (1986) investigated the drinking habits of 87 white US male laryngeal cancer patients and 153 hospital controls with no prior diagnosis of cancer or respiratory disease. Controls were matched on hospital, year of admission, decade of birth, county of residence, smoking status and type of tobacco used. The case and control groups represented 59% and 48%, respectively, of the originally identified cases and controls. Various measures of alcohol consumption showed an increased RR after adjustment for residual differences in smoking habits between cases and controls.

In France, Brugère *et al.* (1986) (see description, p. 171) investigated 466 men with laryngeal cancer. Increasing RRs with increasing amount of ethanol consumed per day were noted for three different locations in the larynx (supraglottis, glottis, subglottis), and particularly for cancer of the supraglottis.

In the study by Tuyns *et al.* (1988) (see description, p. 172), there were 727 male cases of laryngeal cancer (426 supraglottic, 270 glottic and subglottic and 31 endolarynx not otherwise specified). When their drinking and smoking habits were compared with those of 3057 male population controls, a significantly increasing RR was seen with amount of ethanol drunk daily; the RR for cancer of the endolarynx when comparing consumption of

⩾121 g/day *versus* 0-20 g/day was 2.6 (95% CI, 1.8-3.6). RRs were adjusted for smoking, age and area of residence.

(iii) *Risk associated with type of alcoholic beverages*

Studies have been carried out to investigate whether the ethanol concentrations of different alcoholic beverages entail different RRs for laryngeal cancer. In retrospective cohort studies, it has generally not been possible to distinguish the effects of different types of beverage; however, a significantly increased risk was noted among brewery workers with an above-average beer consumption (Jensen, 1980).

Wynder *et al.* (1956) found the RR to be particularly high for 'heavy' whisky consumers in the USA, but a significant RR [1.7, after adjusting for smoking] was also seen for wine and beer drinking; no difference was found with regard to drinking whisky diluted or undiluted. In a later study in the USA (Wynder *et al.*, 1976), no difference in predominant type of alcoholic beverage was seen between cases and controls, and, in a study based on the Third National Cancer Survey Study, similar RRs were observed with equivalent lifetime consumption of wine, beer and spirits (Williams & Horm, 1977). In Canada, too, the RRs were similar for consumption of comparable amounts of beer and spirits in terms of daily ethanol intake (Burch *et al.*, 1981). In Denmark (Olsen *et al.*, 1985b), the only significantly increased RR was found for drinking beer as the preferred type of alcohol, and the RRs for drinking wine and spirits were not increased. [The Working Group noted that in none of these studies was adjustment made for use of other beverages.]

(iv) *Studies of joint exposure*

An extensive analysis and discussion of the joint effect of alcohol and tobacco is provided by Flanders and Rothman (1982) and by Walter and Iwane (1983), who reanalysed data from the study of Williams and Horm (1977). They restricted the analysis to 87 male cases and 956 male controls with cancers not related to alcohol use, tobacco use or certain occupational exposures; information was also available on age, sex and alcohol and tobacco use. Flanders and Rothman (1982) also reanalysed the data previously reported by Wynder *et al.* (1976), restricting the analysis to 224 male cases and 414 male controls for whom information on both alcohol use and tobacco use was available. The results point to a multiplicative rather than an additive effect, but neither data set is sufficiently extensive to allow a conclusion. Similar limitations apply to two Canadian studies (Burch *et al.*, 1981; Elwood *et al.*, 1984). In the study of Tuyns *et al.* (1988), a multiplicative model provided an adequate description of the data (see Table 54). Other investigators have reported synergism between alcohol and tobacco in the induction of laryngeal cancer (Hinds *et al.*, 1979; Herity *et al.*, 1981, 1982; Olsen *et al.*, 1985b; Zagraniski *et al.*, 1986).

(v) *Effect of alcohol in nonsmokers*[1]

Flanders and Rothman (1982) analysed data from Wynder *et al.* (1976) regarding the drinking habits of nonsmokers and found that there were no drinkers among the five cases

[1]Subsequent to the meeting, the Secretariat became aware of a further study demonstrating an association between laryngeal cancer and alcohol drinking in lifetime nonsmokers (Brownson & Chang, 1987).

Table 54. Relative risks for cancer of the endolarynx, according to level of exposure to smoking and alcohol[a]

Ethanol/day (g)	Cigarettes/day			
	0–7	8–15	16–25	26+
0–40	1.0	6.7	12.7	11.5
41–80	1.7	5.9	12.2	18.5
81–120	2.3	10.7	21.0	23.6
≥121	3.8	12.2	31.6	43.2
Total no. of cases	50	147	357	173

[a]From Tuyns *et al.* (1988)

of laryngeal cancers in nonsmokers. [The Working Group calculated that 1.4 would have been expected on the basis of information for 84 controls.] Burch *et al.* (1981) observed a positive trend in RR with amount of alcohol consumed among lifetime nonsmokers: 7.7 in the highest consumption category (≥2.6 oz [≥60 g] ethanol) compared with nondrinkers. Elwood *et al.* (1984) also found a positive trend with alcohol use in nonsmokers when the risk was examined for cancers of the oral cavity, pharynx and larynx combined. Tuyns *et al.* (1988) found no difference between observed and expected numbers of drinkers among lifelong nonsmokers with cancer of the endolarynx.

(*d*) *Cancer of the oesophagus*

(i) *Cohort studies* (descriptions of studies of cancer at many sites are given on pp. 158-164.)

Almost all of the retrospective cohort studies of persons with an above average intake of alcohol have shown an approximately two-fold increased risk for cancer of the oesophagus compared with rates for the general population (Table 55). In these studies, no information was available on tobacco smoking or other risk factors (e.g., poor diet), which may influence the risk for oesophageal cancer. In the study of Canadian alcoholics (Schmidt & Popham, 1981), the members had an average daily tobacco consumption of 28 cigarettes. The SMR was only marginally affected (2.3) when the observed number of oesophageal cancer deaths was compared with an expected number derived from the death rates for smokers of similar numbers of cigarettes per day in the prospective study of US veterans. [The Working Group noted that it must be assumed that the cohorts studied had rather extreme smoking patterns in order to explain the two-fold increase in risk compared with that of a background population (Axelson, 1978).]

The large Japanese study is the only prospective cohort study in which information is provided on the RR for oesophageal cancer in relation to alcoholic beverage. After

Table 55. Relative risks for oesophageal cancer in cohort studies

Study and reference	Number of subjects	Relative risk	95% CI[a]	Predominant beverage	Comments
Norwegian Alcoholics (Sundby, 1967)	40 deaths	4.1	[2.9–5.6]	Unknown	Compared with Oslo population
Finnish Alcohol Misusers (Hakulinen *et al.*, 1974)	101 cases	1.7	[1.4–2.1]	Unknown	
Finnish Alcoholics (Hakulinen *et al.*, 1974)	4 cases	4.1	[1.4–9.3]	Unknown	
Massachusetts Alcoholics (Monson & Lyon, 1975)	5 deaths	1.9	[0.4–5.5]	Unknown	
Dublin Brewery Workers (Dean *et al.*, 1979)	10 deaths	0.6	[0.3–1.2]	Beer	Based on Dublin rates
Japanese Prospective Study (Hirayama, 1979)	297 deaths	1.1 1.2 1.7 2.0	–	Beer Saké Whisky Shochu	Adjusted for tobacco, age and sex; RRs calculated by the Working Group
US Veterans Alcoholics (Robinette *et al.*, 1979)	13 deaths	2.03	0.9–5.1	Unknown	
DAnish Brewery Workers (Jensen, 1980)	41 cases	2.1	1.5–2.8	Beer	Four times higher beer consumption in cohort than in reference population
Canadian Alcoholics (Schmidt & Popham, 1981)	16 deaths	3.2	[1.8–5.2]	Unknown	Compared with Ontario population
		2.3	[1.3–3.8]		Compared with US veterans

[a]Confidence interval; [ ] when calculated by the Working Group

adjustment for smoking, increased SMRs of 1.7 and 2.0 [calculated by the Working Group] were noted for whisky and *shochu* drinking, respectively (Hirayama, 1979).

(ii) *Case-control studies*

The risk for oesophageal cancer in relation to various total alcohol intakes, the effect of various alcoholic beverages, and interactions with tobacco and nutrition have been quantified in several case-control studies. The results are summarized in Table 56.

Wynder and Bross (1961) studied 150 men with squamous-cell carcinoma of the oesophagus and 150 hospital controls matched for age and sex, primarily with cancer (64%) but excluding smoking-related diseases. Information was obtained by personal interview, in most cases conducted without knowledge of the diagnosis. The oesophageal cancer patients took significantly more drinks per day than the controls, and a dose-response relationship was apparent. A clear dose-response relationship was seen with increasing amounts of whisky and beer consumed daily when the analysis was restricted to smokers of 16-34 cigarettes per day.

Schwartz *et al.* (1962) (see description, p. 167) found that average total alcohol consumption was significantly higher among 362 oesophageal cancer patients (154 ml [122 g] ethanol per day) than among 362 accident controls (136 ml [107 g] ethanol per day) after adjustment for tobacco use. A higher proportion of cases than controls had symptoms of alcoholism. The average difference between cases and cancer controls (113 ml [89 g] ethanol per day) was even higher and remained significant after adjusting for smoking. When the comparison was restricted to workers living in the département of Seine, the 100 oesophageal cancer patients had a significantly higher consumption (157 ml [124 g]/day) than the cancer controls (119 ml [94 g]/day) after accounting for differences in age and tobacco consumption.

In Puerto Rico, Martinez (1969) studied 179 cases (120 male, 59 female) of squamous cell-carcinoma of the oesophagus and 537 controls (360 male, 177 female) matched for age and sex (see description, p. 170). When the independent effect of alcohol consumption was examined by additional matching on tobacco (111 male and 52 female pairs), a clear dose-response relationship was seen in men, even after adjusting for smoking, while no association was apparent in women. [The Working Group noted that only four female cases and four controls consumed two or more units of ethanol/day.]

Two studies of oesophageal cancer in African male cases and hospital controls without cancer in South Africa showed no association with consumption of alcoholic beverages when adjustment was undertaken for smoking habits. Men in Durban had a RR of 0.9 (Bradshaw & Schonland, 1969) and men in Johannesburg a RR of 1.0 (Bradshaw & Schonland, 1974). [RRs were calculated by the Working Group.]

As part of a larger study of various digestive tract cancers, 52 cases of oesophageal cancer in Minnesota, USA, were compared with 1657 hospital controls matched for age, sex, race and hospital to the whole series of digestive tract cancer cases. A significant crude association was found for consumption of beer and spirits but not of wine (Bjelke, 1973).

Table 56. Summary of results of casé-control studies on oesophageal cancer and alcohol consumption

Place (reference)	Subjects (cases, controls)	Alcohol consumption[a]	Relative risk (RR)	95% CI[b]	Comments
USA, New York (Wynder & Bross, 1961)	Men (150, 150)	Never	1.0	-	Crude RR calculated by the Working Group
		<1 unit/day	0.6	0.2-2.5	
		1-2 units/day	1.6	0.4-7.1	
		3-6 units/day	7.1	2.1-26.3	
		7-12 units/day	6.8	1.6-30.4	
		>12 units/day	5.0	1.1-22.6	
		Binges	12.5	1.5-78.4	
Puerto Rico (Martinez, 1969)	Men (111, 111)	None	1.0	-	Crude RR based on pairs matched on smoking, calculated by the Working Group
		<1 unit[c]/day	0.6	0.2-2.0	
		2-4 units/day	2.1	0.8-5.1	
		≥5 units/day	7.7	3.0-20.0	
	Women (52, 52)	None	1.0		
		<1 unit/day	1.9	0.5-6.9	
		≥2 units/day	1.1	0.3-4.6	
South Africa, Durban (Bradshaw & Schonland, 1969, 1974)	Men (98, 341)	Never	1.0		RR adjusted for smoking, calculated by the Working Group
		Ever	0.9	0.4-1.9	
South Africa, Johannesburg (Bradshaw & Schonland, 1974)	Men (196, 1064)	Never	1.0	-	RR adjusted for smoking, calculated by the Working Group; 95% CI from paper
		Ever	1.0	0.6-1.8	
USA, Minnesota (Bjelke, 1973)	Men, women (52, 1657)	Beer <1 time/month	1.0	-	RR adjusted for sex; RR for 6-13 times/months calculated as 2.9 by the Working Group
		1-5 times/month	0.7	0.3-1.9	
		6-13 times/month	2.7	1.2-6.8	
		≥14 times/month	4.4	2.3-8.3	
		Wine <1 time/month	1.0	-	
		1-5 times/month, 6-13 times/month, ≥14 times/month	0.5	0.2-1.2	
		Spirits <1 time/month	1.0	-	RR for 1-5 times/month calculated as 1.7 by the Working Group
		1-5 times per month	1.9	0.9-3.3	
		6-13 times/month	1.6	0.7-4.1	
		≥14 times/month	2.1	1.0-4.3	

Table 56 (contd)

Place (reference)	Subjects (cases, controls)	Alcohol consumption[a]	Relative risk (RR)	95% CI[b]	Comments
Singapore (De Jong et al., 1974)	Men (95, 465)	Never	1.0		Crude RR for samsu (strong liquor) drinking; significant dose-response remains after adjustments; 95% CI could not be calculated
		<daily	2.0		
		Daily	2.9		
USA, Multicenter (Williams & Horm, 1977)	Men (38, 1750)	Nondrinkers	1.0		RR adjusted for age, race and smoking; 95% CI could not be calculated
		<50 oz-year	0.9		
		≥51 oz-year	1.4		
	Women (19, 3169)	Nondrinkers	1.0		
		<50 oz-year	0.9		
		≥51 oz-year	8.1	$p < 0.05$	
France, Brittany (Tuyns et al., 1977)	Men (200, 778)	0-20 g/day	1.0		RR adjusted for smoking; 95% CI could not be calculated
		21-40 g/day	1.2		
		41-60 g/day	3.4		
		61-80 g/day	6.1		
		81-100 g/day	6.6		
		≥101 g/day	18.3		
France, Normandy (Tuyns et al., 1979)	Men (312, 869)	0 g/day	1.0		RR adjusted for smoking calculated by the Working Group; 95% CI could not be calculated
		1-40 g/day	0.8		
		41-80 g/day	2.3		
		≥81 g/day	11.6		
USA, Washington DC (Pottern et al., 1981)	Men (90, 213)	Never drank more than five glasses of alcoholic beverages/week for >1 month	1.0	-	Crude RR; RRs remain high after adjustment for smoking; 95% CI from paper
		1.0-5.9 oz [9.4-55 g]/day	4.0	1.4-12.0	
		6.0-14.9 oz [56-140 g]/day	5.5	2.0-15.0	
		15.0-29.9 oz [141-281 g]/day	7.6	2.7-22.0	
		30.0-80.6 oz [282-757 g]/day	7.5	2.5-22.0	

Table 56 (contd)

Place (reference)	Subjects (cases, controls)	Alcohol consumption[a]	Relative risk (RR)	95% CI[b]	Comments
Uruguay, Montevideo (Vassallo *et al*. 1985)	Men (185, 386)	0–49 ml [39 g]/day	1.0	-	RR adjusted for age and tobacco smoking; 95% CI from paper
		50–99 ml [40–78 g]/day	3.8	2.4–6.2	
		≥100 ml [≥79 g]/day	7.6	4.5–12.8	
Southern Brazil (Victoria *et al*., 1987)	Men, women (171, 342)	Nondrinkers	1.0		*Cachaça* drinking; association persisted after adjustment for confounders; 95% CI could not be calculated
		1–29 g/day	3.5		
		30–89 g/day	6.3		
		90+ g/day	8.2		

[a] g = pure ethanol
[b] Confidence intervals, calculated by the Working Gorup, when possible, unless otherwise indicated
[c] 1 unit = 18 oz beer [21.4 g pure ethanol], 8 oz wine [24 g] or 2 oz spirits [19 g]

De Jong *et al.* (1974) investigated risk factors for oesophageal cancer among Chinese men in Singapore, comparing 95 cases with 465 hospital controls. Significantly elevated RRs were associated with intake of *samsu* (a form of spirits reported by the authors to have an alcohol content equivalent to that of whisky), but not with intake of other spirits. A significant dose-response relationship for *samsu* drinking persisted after adjustment for other identified risk factors, including smoking.

In the study based on the Third National Cancer Survey in the USA (see description, pp. 170-171), Williams and Horm (1977) found nonsignificantly increased RRs among men with oesophageal cancer, but a significant risk (8.1) among women who were classified as heavy drinkers, after controlling for smoking.

Two case-control studies of oesophageal cancer in relation to alcohol and tobacco consumption, as well as to diet, were carried out in a high-incidence area for this cancer in northwestern France (Tuyns, 1970). Aspects of the design of the studies, consumption patterns and selection of control groups have been reported in several papers (Péquignot & Cubeau, 1973; Tuyns & Massé, 1975; Jensen *et al.*, 1978; Tuyns *et al.*, 1983). In the first study, alcohol and tobacco consumption were compared for 200 male cases of oesophageal cancer representative of all cases in the population between 1972 and 1974 and for 778 controls selected randomly from the same population. After adjustment for age and smoking, a clear increase in RR was seen with total amount of alcohol consumed per day, expressed as grams of ethanol derived from different types of alcoholic beverages; adjustment for smoking did not substantially affect the crude risk estimates (Tuyns *et al.*, 1977). In the second study of 743 cases of oesophageal cancer (704 male, 39 female) and 1976 controls chosen at random from the population (923 male, 1053 female) of Normandy, a significantly increased RR (2.7) was observed for any type of alcohol consumption (Tuyns *et al.*, 1982). In a preliminary analysis of information for 312 male cases and 869 hospital-based controls (excluding persons with smoking- and alcohol-related diseases), a clear dose-response relationship was seen (Tuyns *et al.*, 1979). This was sustained by the first detailed report of the full study in which all cases and population controls are compared. The study also showed an association between risk for oesophageal cancer and poor diet, on the basis of an index incorporating citrus fruit, meat and vegetable oils. The risk associated with alcohol intake was independent of poor diet (Tuyns *et al.*, 1987).

Pottern *et al.* (1981) studied black men in Washington DC, USA, who had died from oesophageal cancer in 1975-77. Information was obtained for 120 cases (response rate, 67%) and 250 controls (response rate, 71%) by personal interviews with next-of-kin; about 20% did not provide quantitative information on alcohol intake. Estimates of total ethanol intake were made by combining levels in various beverages. Significantly increased RRs were seen for alcohol drinkers when compared with nondrinkers, and a dose-response relationship emerged. A further analysis of this study (Ziegler, 1986) also showed a relationship with low consumption of various foods and nutrients. The risks associated with alcohol intake and dietary status remained distinct.

All patients admitted to the Oncology Institute of Montevideo, Uruguay, were interviewed with regard to past and current consumption of alcohol, tobacco and *maté* (Vassallo *et al.*, 1985). Between 1979 and 1984, there were 226 cases (185 male, 41 female) of oesophageal cancer, for whom 469 controls (386 male, 83 female) with other neoplastic conditions were selected. There was a significant positive trend with daily intake of spirits in men after adjustment for age and smoking. No data were given for women.

In southern Brazil, 171 histologically confirmed cases of squamous-cell carcinoma of the oesophagus were compared with twice as many individually matched (age, sex, hospital) hospital controls, excluding patients with diseases related to alcohol and tobacco (Victoria *et al.*, 1987). Cases and controls were personally interviewed with regard to consumption of alcohol, tobacco, hot beverages and several foodstuffs. There was an important association with consumption of alcoholic beverages. This was seen in particular for drinking of *cachaça*, a distilled sugar cane spirit which is the most common alcoholic drink in that part of Brazil where it accounts for approximately 80% of alcohol consumption. There were also significant associations with lifetime consumption of beer and wine. The significant association with daily intake and years of drinking *cachaça* persisted after taking account of place of residence, smoking and fruit and meat eating in a logistic regression analysis.

(iii) *Risk associated with type of alcoholic beverage*

In retrospective cohort studies of alcoholics it has generally not been possible to distinguish the effects of different types of beverages; however, in the two studies of brewery workers (Dean *et al.*, 1979; Jensen, 1980), there was evidence that beer was the predominant beverage consumed. The study of Dublin brewery workers showed no increased risk, while the study of Danish brewery workers with high daily beer consumption showed a significant, two-fold risk.

Wynder and Bross (1961) indicated that the RR increased particularly steeply in whisky drinkers, but beer and wine drinkers were also at increased risk for oesophageal cancer. [The Working Group noted that a high RR (6.4) was seen in the category of >6 units of whisky per day, but the average consumption is not given; no adjustment was made for use of other beverages.] In the study of Pottern *et al.* (1981), the RR was highest among consumers of spirits, but the RRs for consumption of beer and wine were compatible with those for spirits. Martinez (1969) found no difference in RR for consumers of commercial rum only, of home-processed rum only or of a mixture of beverages. Tuyns *et al.* (1979) found an indication that oesophageal cancer in Normandy was associated with consumption of all types of alcoholic beverages but noted that the association might be stronger for consumers of distillates of apple cider (approximately 400 g ethanol per l) and of cider itself (approximately 40 g ethanol per l) than for those drinking wine and beer when account was taken of both tobacco and total ethanol intake. In an extended analysis in which cases in Brittany were compared with population controls, beer, cider and wine had the strongest influence on risk, but it could not be ruled out that all types of beverages contributed to the risk in proportion to their alcohol content (Breslow & Day, 1980).

(iv) *Studies of joint exposure*

Tobacco smoking is causally related to oesophageal cancer (IARC, 1986a). Ziegler (1986) found an independent effect of alcohol on oesophageal cancer risk after adjustment for several dietary factors. Similar results were reported from the large case-control study carried out in Normandy (Tuyns *et al.*, 1987), where adjustment for nutrition could not explain the increased risk due to alcohol consumption.

The joint actions of alcohol and tobacco and of alcohol and nutrition have been the subject of several analyses. In their studies in north-western France, Tuyns *et al.* (1977, 1979) found a combined effect of alcohol and tobacco, which they described as multiplicative (Table 57). Similar combined effects of alcohol consumption and nutrition in the causation of oesophageal cancer have been reported; after adjustment for tobacco, a 90-fold increased risk for oesophageal cancer was seen among persons who drank more than 120 g ethanol per day and had a low consumption of citrus fruits, meat and vegetable oils, in comparison with subjects who drank less than 40 g ethanol per day and had a high intake of fresh meat, citrus fruits and vegetable oils (Tuyns *et al.*, 1987).

(v) *Effect of alcohol in nonsmokers*

Tuyns (1983) found that the RR for oesophageal cancer among 39 male and 36 female oesophageal cancer patients who had never smoked increased considerably with increasing alcohol consumption; values were similar in men and women (Table 58).

(*e*) *Cancers of the stomach, colon and rectum*

(i) *Cohort studies* (descriptions of studies of cancers at many sites are given on pp. 158-164).

In general, adjustment for any confounding effects of diet has not been possible in the cohort studies considered below. Dietary factors are thought to be involved in the etiology of stomach cancer and of cancer of the large bowel (colon especially), and dietary habits are likely to vary with alcohol consumption. However, in most of these cohort studies, including the cohorts that were determined retrospectively, information on individual dietary habits was not collected. The studies are summarized in Table 59.

In the study of Norwegian alcoholics (Sundby, 1967), the number of deaths from colon cancer (9) closely matched the expected value (9.4). There was a nonsignificant excess of rectal cancer deaths (SMR, 1.9; 12 cases) and a nonsignificant increase in the risk for death from stomach cancer (SMR, 1.3; 45 cases) when comparison was made with the population of Oslo.

In the Finnish study of alcohol misusers and alcoholics (Hakulinen *et al.*, 1974), the observed number of colon cancer cases (82) within the misusers cohort was fewer than expected (86.6); data for stomach cancer were not reported. For the cohort of chronic alcoholics, the observed numbers of stomach cancers (six) and colon cancers (three) did not clearly differ from those expected (8.0 and 1.6, respectively). Data were not presented for rectal cancer in either cohort.

In the study of UK alcoholics (Adelstein & White, 1976), there were eight deaths from stomach cancer (10.2 expected), nine deaths from cancer of the small intestine and colon (6.8 expected) and four deaths from rectal cancer (4.3 expected).

In the study of alcoholics in Massachusetts (Monson & Lyon, 1975), the proportions of stomach and colorectal cancers were not significantly increased: 15 deaths from stomach

Table 57. Combined effect of alcohol and tobacco on relative risks for cancer of the oesophagus[a]

Ethanol/day (g)	Tobacco consumption/day (g)		
	0-9	10-19	≥20
0-40	1.0	3.4	5.1
41-80	7.3	8.4	12.3
≥81	18.0	19.9	44.4
Total no. of cases	78	58	64

[a]From Tuyns et al. (1977); risks are expressed relative to a risk of 1.0 for persons smoking <10 g/day and drinking ≤40 g/day.

Table 58. Relative risks (RR) for oesophageal cancer in relation to average daily alcohol consumption by nonsmoking males in Normandy, France[a]

Ethanol/day (g)	Males		Females	
	No. of cases	RR	No. of cases	RR
0-40	7	1.0	25	1.0
41-80	15	3.8	8	5.6
81-120	9	10.2	3	11.0
≥121	8	101.0	-	-

[a]From Tuyns (1983)

cancer, seven from colon cancer and four from rectal cancer were observed, whereas 14.6, 11.2 and 5.7 were expected, respectively.

In the Japanese prospective study (Hirayama, 1979), the SMR for death from stomach cancer (1917 deaths) in daily consumers of alcohol as compared with nondrinkers was 1.0 among men. Data are not given for women. Data on alcohol intake in relation to colon cancer (96 deaths) were not tabulated; however, data displayed in a graph indicate that male smokers who drank daily had about a 50% higher risk of intestinal cancer (colon plus small intestine) than smokers who did not drink alcohol; for rectal cancer, no such association was detected. In an earlier report of this study (Hirayama, 1977), the risk for colorectal cancer

Table 59. Relative risks for stomach, colon and rectal cancers in cohort studies

Study and reference	Stomach		Colon		Rectum		Comments
	No. of subjects	Relative risk (95% CI)	No. of subjects	Relative risk (95% CI)	No. of subjects	Relative risk (95% CI)	
Norwegian Alcoholics (Sundby, 1967)	45 deaths	1.3 (0.9–1.7)	9 deaths	1.0 (0.5–1.9)	12 deaths	1.9 2.9	Compared with Oslo population Compared with Norwegian population
Finnish Alcohol Misusers (Hakulinen *et al.*, 1974)	–	–	82 cases	0.95 (0.7–1.1)	–	–	
Finnish Alcoholics (Hakulinen *et al.*, 1974)	6 cases	0.8 (0.3–1.6)	3 cases	1.8 (0.4–5.4)	–	–	
Massachusetts Alcoholics (Monson & Lyon, 1975)	15 deaths	1.0 (0.6–1.7)	7 deaths	0.6 (0.3–1.3)	4 deaths	0.7 (0.2–1.8)	
UK Alcoholics (Adelstein & White, 1976)	8 deaths	0.8 (0.3–1.5)	9 deaths (intestine)	1.3 (0.6–2.5)	4 deaths	0.9 (0.3–2.4)	
Dublin Brewery Workers (Dean *et al.*, 1979)	40 deaths	0.8 (0.6–1.1)	32 deaths	1.3 (0.9–1.9)	32 deaths	1.6 (1.1–2.3)	Compared with Dublin blue-collar workers
US Veterans Alcoholics (Robinette *et al.*, 1979)	9 deaths	1.0 (90% CI, 0.4–2.3)	7 deaths	0.8 (0.3–1.9)	6 deaths	3.3 (0.7–22.4)	
Danish Brewery Workers (Jensen, 1980)	92 cases	0.9 (0.7–1.1)	87 cases	1.1	85 cases	1.0 (0.8–1.3)	Total cohort (brewers and mineral water bottlers)
Canadian Alcoholics (Schmidt & Popham, 1981)	19 deaths	1.0 (0.6–1.6) 1.7 (1.0–2.6)	19 deaths	1.0 (0.6–1.6) 1.0 (intestine) (0.6–1.6)	10 deaths	1.0 (0.5–1.9) 1.1 (0.5–2.0)	Compared with Canadian population Compared with US veterans smoking 21–39 cigarettes/day

was shown to be 1.7 times higher in daily beer drinkers than in nondrinkers. [The Working Group noted that statistical significance was not shown, and separate data were not presented for colon and rectal cancers.]

In the study of alcoholic US veterans (Robinette *et al.*, 1979), the SMR for death from stomach cancer (nine deaths) was 1.0. For colon cancer (seven deaths) and rectal cancer (six deaths), the SMRs were 0.8 and 3.3, respectively.

In the study of Danish brewery workers and mineral-water factory workers (Jensen, 1980), no increase in risk was observed for cancers of the stomach (RR, 0.9; 92 cases), colon and sigmoid (RR, 1.1; 87 cases) or rectum (RR, 1.0; 85 cases). There was no variation in risk for stomach, colon or rectal cancer in relation to duration of employment. [The Working Group noted that this study was designed specifically to examine the relationship between beer drinking and cancer of the large bowel.] The author noted that, if the results of this investigation are taken together with those obtained from the study of the Copenhagen Temperance Society, the risk for rectal cancer can be compared in groups with extreme differences in beer consumption, ranging from the low consumption of (or abstention from) beer in Seventh-day Adventists to the average intake of almost 2.5 l of beer per day for the brewery workers. Since in neither group does the risk for rectal cancer differ from that of the total population, the author concluded that these studies do not indicate a causal association between beer drinking and rectal cancer (Jensen, 1983).

In the study of Dublin brewery workers (Dean *et al.*, 1979), there were 40 deaths from stomach cancer, 32 deaths from cancer of the colon, and 32 from cancer of the rectum. Expected numbers were derived for blue-collar workers in Dublin, in order to control for socioeconomic class; the differences between the observed numbers and those expected for cancers of the stomach (49.2) and colon (24.1) were not significant, but for rectal cancer there was a significant excess of observed (32) to expected (19.7). [The Working Group noted that this study was designed specifically to examine the relationship between beer drinking and cancer of the large bowel.]

In order to to investigate this association further, the relatives of men who had died of rectal cancer were sought and were questioned about the drinking habits of the deceased. For each relative traced, two control relatives were sought from among men who had died of other causes in the same age group, matched for age at death and the year in which they died. It was possible to trace the relatives of 16 of the 32 who had died of cancer of the rectum, of whom 15 drank stout, and 29 of the 64 control relatives, of whom 27 drank stout. The mean alcohol intake of those who had died of cancer of the rectum was reported by the next-of-kin to have been 23.6 pints (13.4 l) of stout per week and 1.8 glasses (0.13 l) of spirits per week. The mean intake for the 29 controls was 16.1 pints (9.1 l) of stout per week and four glasses (0.28 l) of spirits per week. This difference is significant ($p < 0.05$) (Dean *et al.*, 1979). [The Working Group noted the high potential for bias in this comparison because of the low interview rates.]

In the study of Canadian alcoholics (Schmidt & Popham, 1981), the SMR for death from stomach cancer was 0.95 (19 deaths; not significant), that for colon cancer, 1.04 (19 deaths; not significant), and that for rectal cancer, 1.02 (10 deaths; not significant), in comparison with the general male population of Ontario. In comparison with veterans who smoked 21-39 cigarettes daily, the SMRs for cancers of the stomach, intestine and rectum became 1.7, 1.02 and 1.1, respectively. The authors postulate that the nonsignificant excess of stomach cancer deaths was 'probably attributable to a difference in the class composition of the two samples [alcoholics and veterans] rather than to a difference in their drinking habits'.

In the Kaiser-Permanente study (Klatsky *et al.*, 1981), neither stomach cancer (13 deaths) nor colorectal cancer (19 deaths) was associated with level of alcohol consumption.

In the Framingham study (Gordon & Kannel, 1984), there was a strong positive relationship between heavy consumption of alcohol and stomach cancer mortality for people of each sex (five deaths in women, 13 deaths in men). Multivariable analysis of this relationship, controlling for cigarette smoking, systolic blood pressure, age, relative weight and plasma lipoprotein profile, showed significant positive relationships for both women and men. There was no significant relationship between alcohol use and cancer of the colon (17 deaths in men, 19 in women). No data were reported for rectal cancer. [The Working Group noted that the use of standardized logistic regression coefficients precludes quantitative estimates of the relation between alcohol intake and cancer risk.]

In the study of Hawaiian Japanese (Pollack *et al.*, 1984), there were 99 incident cases of stomach cancer, 92 cases of colon cancer, and 62 cases of rectal cancer. There was no evidence of a relationship between alcohol consumption and stomach and colon cancers. After adjusting for age and cigarette smoking, there was a significant trend ($p < 0.001$) for rectal cancer, with increasing incidence rates accompanying successively higher levels of alcohol consumption. [The Working Group calculated the RR for ≥40 oz/month (800 g) in comparison with abstainers to be 2.9.] In order to examine this relationship further, the authors estimated the risk for rectal cancer among subjects who consumed a given amount of each particular type of alcoholic beverage relative to the risk for those who did not consume the beverage at all, controlling for age, smoking and consumption of other types of alcohol. The only category for which the RR for rectal cancer was significantly raised was the highest, consuming 500 oz (15 l) or more of beer per month; the RR for this category was 3.1 ($p < 0.01$). [The Working Group noted that point estimates for lower categories of beer intake are not given but can be derived from a figure presented in the paper as approximately 1.0 for 1-9 oz, 1.5 for 10-99 oz and 1.5 for 100-499 oz per month.]

In the study of Japanese doctors (Kono *et al.*, 1986), age- and smoking-standardized rates for death from stomach cancer (116 deaths) and colorectal cancer (sites combined; 39 deaths) were not clearly related to alcohol consumption category; rates for these cancers were 10-40% higher (not statistically significant) in occasional and daily drinkers than in nondrinkers.

Wu *et al.* (1987) studied a cohort of 11 888 residents of a retirement community in California, USA. Consumption of alcoholic beverages on an average weekday was assessed by a self-administered questionnaire for wine, beer and spirits, and then combined to derive an overall amount of ethanol consumed. Follow-up was carried out by biennial mailed questionnaire and by consulting county death registrations. During 4.5 years of follow-up, 126 incident cases of colorectal cancer occurred. The crude, age-adjusted RRs were 1.5 (95% CI, 1.0-2.4) and 1.9 (1.3-2.9) for those who drank 1-30 ml (0.8-24 g) ethanol/day and those drinking more, respectively, compared with people who did not drink alcohol daily. After multivariable adjustment for smoking, relative weight and physical activity, the RR in men was 2.2 (95% CI, 1.2-3.8). The corresponding analysis for women showed no significant increase in risk. Another analysis of this study, omitting the 20 cases of rectal cancer, gave essentially the same results.

[The Working Group summarized of the results of the retrospective cohort studies of alcoholics and brewery workers, as follows: in eight studies that addressed stomach cancer, 234 cases were observed, with 251 expected; in nine that addressed cancer of the colon (including one on alcohol misusers), 251 cases were observed, with 245 expected; and in seven that addressed rectal cancer, 148 cases were observed, with 129 expected.]

(ii) *Case-control studies*

Stomach cancer (see Table 60): Wynder *et al.* (1963a) conducted a case-control study of stomach cancer and environmental variables, dietary factors, cigarette smoking and alcohol consumption in Iceland, Japan, Slovenia and the USA. A total of 367 male and 154 female cases, and 401 male and 252 female controls (without cancer) were included; all were hospital patients. No clear association was noted between risk for stomach cancer and type of alcohol consumed, although within the US component of the study, beer consumption was more prevalent in both male and female cases than in their controls. [The Working Group noted that, in the absence of quantitative consumption data and control for covariables, interpretation of the data is difficult.]

In a case-control study in New York State, USA, Graham *et al.* (1972) compared 160 men and 68 women with stomach cancer with 228 hospital controls individually matched to cases for sex, age, country of birth and family's ethnic background (as a proxy for socioeconomic status). All patients had originally been hospitalized in 1957-66 and had been interviewed routinely about social, behavioural and dietary traits by trained interviewers who were unaware of the patient's medical status. Usual frequency of consumption of beer, wine, gin, vodka and whisky was assessed, and an index of total alcohol consumption was derived. Comparison of the drinking profiles of cases and controls revealed no difference in overall alcohol intake. [The Working Group noted that it was not possible to estimate RR by level of consumption.]

Haenszel *et al.* (1972) carried out a case-control study of stomach cancer among Japanese in Hawaii. During 1963-69, 220 patients admitted to hospital with stomach cancer (135 men, 85 women) were enrolled for study; 96% of these cases were histologically confirmed. Two hospital controls were selected for each case, matched on sex, age, hospital and date of admission, excluding patients with stomach disorders and other alimentary tract cancers. Study subjects were interviewed about usual past frequency of intake of foods and alcoholic drinks. Saké and beer were the alcoholic drinks for which consumption differed most between cases and controls. The RR in beer drinkers compared with those who did not drink beer was 1.2; the RR for drinking saké was 1.4, confined substantially to those who drank it daily, for whom the RR was 2.2 ($p < 0.05$). [The Working Group noted that, since the data were analysed in a univariate fashion, covariables such as cigarette smoking and major nutrients could not be controlled for.]

Table 60. Summary of results of case-control studies of stomach cancer and alcohol consumption

Place (reference)	Subjects (cases, controls)	Exposure measurement	Results[a]	Comments
UK (Stocks, 1957)	Men (153, 4630)	Frequency of beer consumption	No association	
Iceland, Japan, Slovenia, USA (Wynder _et al_., 1963a)	Men (367, 401) Women (154, 252)	Frequency of alcohol consumption, by type of beverage	Few differences in consumption profile	No quantitative consumption data; no control of covariates
USA, Kansas City (Higginson, 1966)	Men (93, 279)	Open-ended interview about consumption of alcoholic beverages	No difference in overall alcohol consumption profile; prevalence of 'heavy periodical' drinking higher in cases	
USA, Buffalo (Graham _et al_., 1972)	Men (160, 160) Women (68, 68)	Frequency of consumption, by type of beverage	No difference in consumption profile	
Hawaii (Japanese) (Haenszel _et al_., 1972)	Men (135, 270) Women (85, 170)	Frequency of consumption, by type of beverage	Beer: Abstain 1.0 $<$6/month 1.2 [0.7-1.9] $\geq$6/month 1.2 [0.7-2.0] Saké: Abstain 1.0 $<$daily 1.0 [0.6-1.9] $\geq$daily 2.2 [1.1-4.4]	RR not controlled for dietary variables or social class
Norway (Bjelke, 1973)	Men, women (228, 1394)	Frequency of consumption, by type of beverage	No significant difference	RR for high _versus_ low consumers among women gives positive association with beer
USA, Minnesota (Bjelke, 1973)	Men, women (83, 1657)	Frequency of consumption, by type of beverage	No significant difference	

Table 60 (contd)

Place (reference)	Subjects (cases, controls)	Exposure measurement	Results[a]	Comments
USA, Multicenter (Williams & Horm, 1977)	Men (120, 1668) Women (82, 3106)	Frequency and duration of consumption, by type of beverage	Men: no significant association; women: nonsignificant doubling in risk for wine and beer	Controlled for age, race, cigarette smoking
France (Hoey *et al.*, 1981)	Men (40, 168)	Frequency of consumption, by type or amount	<80 g daily, 1.0 ≥80 g daily, 6.9 (3.3–14.3)	No adjustment for socio-economic status
France, Calvados (Tuyns *et al.*, 1982)	Men, women (163, 1976)	Frequency of consumption, by type of beverage	Consumers *versus* nonconsumers: RR, 0.5 (95% CI, 0.2–1.8)	
Greece, Piraeus (Trichopoulos *et al.*, 1985)	Men, women (110, 100)	Frequency and amount of consumption	Nonsignificant positive linear trend in risk Below median, 1.0 Above median, [1.4] [0.8–2.4]	RR calculated by Working Group
Poland, Cracow (Jedrychowski *et al.*, 1986)	Men, women (110, 110)	Usual number of glasses per week, by type of beverage	RR in those drinking vodka before breakfast, 2.1 (1.0–4.2); no other difference	Adjusted for smoking, residence, diet

[a]Relative risk (RR) and 95% confidence interval ([] when calculated by the Working Group), when available

In a study in France (Hoey *et al.*, 1981), 40 newly diagnosed (1978-80) male cases of adenocarcinoma of the stomach were compared with 168 hospital controls. Cases and controls came from the same endoscopy unit, and controls were patients with cancer or polyp of the colon and rectum, hiatal hernia or gallstones. Three-quarters of the cases reported a current wine consumption of one or more litres per day (or an equivalent amount of alcohol from other beverages). The RR for those consuming more than 80 g ethanol daily compared with those consuming less was 6.9. Adjustment for tobacco use (for which an increased RR of 4.8 was found) did not substantially affect the RR observed for alcohol. The authors noted that, although high consumption of wine in France may be related to low social class (as is stomach cancer), social class was not adjusted for in their study.

A case-control study of stomach cancer was conducted by Trichopoulos *et al.* (1985) in Piraeus, Greece. Cases comprised 110 consecutive patients (57 men, 53 women) with histologically confirmed adenocarcinoma of the stomach admitted to two teaching hospitals during 1981-84. Controls comprised 100 orthopaedic patients hospitalized during the same period without cancers or other diseases of the digestive system. All subjects were interviewed by the same interviewer, who recorded the usual frequency of consumption of foods and alcohol before the onset of the present disease/disorder. There was no linear trend of increasing risk with increasing frequency of alcohol consumption. [The Working Group noted, however, that comparison of subjects with consumption above the median (value not given) with those with a consumption below the median yields a RR of 1.4.]

Jedrychowski *et al.* (1986) carried out a case-control study of stomach cancer in relation to diet and alcohol consumption in Cracow, Poland, in 1980-81. Each of an incident series of 110 histologically confirmed cases of adenocarcinoma of the stomach was individually matched by sex and age to a hospital patient without obvious gastrointestinal disease or dietary abnormality, who was interviewed in hospital. Alcohol consumption was recorded as usual number of glasses [volume unspecified] per week of beer, wine and vodka. After adjustment for smoking, residence and diet, the RR for stomach cancer associated with consumption of vodka before breakfast was 2.1, 33 cases reporting this habit; however, there was no overall difference between cases and controls with regard to consumption of beer, wine or spirits (vodka). The authors commented that the observed increase in risk associated with drinking vodka on an empty stomach was biologically plausible. [The Working Group noted that reliance on place of residence as an indicator of social class might have resulted in residual confounding.]

Large-bowel cancer (see Table 61): Wynder and Shigematsu (1967) conducted a case-control study of colorectal cancer, based in a New York hospital, in which 791 cancer cases were compared with two groups of controls matched for age and sex: cancer patients with cancers other than of the alimentary and respiratory tracts and patients with nonneoplastic diseases other than pulmonary arterial disease and chronic respiratory diseases. Information about the amount of alcohol consumed was obtained at interview for 492 cases and 273 controls. Among men, there was no difference in consumption for those with cancers at most subsites in the large bowel, with the exception of patients with rectal cancer in whom there was a significantly higher percentage of heavy drinkers than in the controls. There was no such difference between female cases and controls. There was a significantly higher

Table 61. Summary of results of case-control studies of large-bowel cancer and alcohol consumption

Place (reference)	Subjects (cases, controls)	Exposure measurement	Results[a]	Comments
UK (Stocks, 1957)	Colon and rectum: men (166, 4630)	Frequency of consumption	Beer <daily, 1.0 Beer ≥ daily, 1.4 (0.9-2.1)	RR adjusted for sex and age only, calculated by the Working Group
USA, Kansas City (Higginson, 1966)	Colon and rectum: men (340, 1020)	Open-ended questionnaire about consumption of alcoholic beverages	No difference in alcohol consumption	
USA, New York (Wynder & Shigematsu, 1967)	Colon: men (174, 206) women (114, 67) Rectum: men (140, 206) women (64, 67)	Frequency and pattern of drinking, by type of beverage	Rectal cancer significantly associated with heavy drinking; significantly more beer drinkers among male rectal and colon cancer cases than controls	No adjustment for social and other behavioural factors
Norway (Bjelke, 1973)	Colon: men, women (162, 1394) Rectum: men, women (116, 1394)	Frequency of consumption, by type of beverage	No difference observed	Matching ignored in analysis
USA, Minnesota (Bjelke, 1973)	Colon: men, women (259, 1657) Rectum: men, women (114, 1657)	Frequency of consumption, by type of beverage	Colon: significant positive association with consumption of spirits in men; significantly negative in women Rectum: significant positive association with beer consumption for men and women combined	Matching ignored in analysis
USA, Multicenter (Williams & Horm, 1977)	Colon: men (294, 1329) women (359, 2691) Rectum: men (165, 1329) women (138, 2691)	Frequency and duration of consumption, by type and amount	Colon (men): Total Wine Beer Spirits Abstainers 1.0 1.0 1.0 1.0 <50 oz-yr 1.4 1.1 1.2 1.5 ≥50 oz-yr 1.5* 2.1* 1.7* 1.6* Rectum: RR, 2.0* for high total alcohol intake in women	RR adjusted for age, race, cigarette smoking; *, significant
France, Calvados (Tuyns *et al.*, 1982)	Colon: men, women (142, 1976) Rectum: men, women (198, 1976)	Frequency of consumption, by type of beverage	Colon: 1.4 (0.3-5.7) Rectum: 1.6 (0.5-5.5)	Consumers *versus* abstainers

Table 61 (contd)

Place (reference)	Subjects (cases, controls)	Exposure measurement	Results[a]	Comments
Canada, Toronto (Miller, A.B. *et al.*, 1983)	Colon: men, women (348, 542) Rectum: men, women (194, 335)	Frequency of consumption, by type and amount	No association with colon cancer Rectal cancer: M F Beer: Low 1.0 1.0 Medium 0.7 1.6 High 1.3 1.6	RR adjusted for education, diet, smoking
USA, New York (Kabat *et al.*, 1986)	Rectum: men (130, 336) women (88, 249)	Frequency and duration of consumption, by type of beverage	No association with wine or spirits consumption Beer: M F Abstainers 1.0 1.0 Occasional 1.6 (0.9–2.8) 0.5 (0.3–1.0) 1–7.9 oz [24–190 g]/day 1.3 (0.7–2.4) 0.5 (0.2–1.2) 8–31.9 oz [192–766 g]/day 1.8 (0.9–3.5) 0.7 (0.1–3.2) ≥32 oz [≥768 g]/day 3.5 (1.8–7.0) –	RR, 2.7 (1.3–5.7) for men drinking ≥32 oz [≥768 g]/day, adjusted for religion and education
Australia, Adelaide (Potter & McMichael, 1986)	Colon: men, women (220, 438) Rectum: men, women (199, 396)	Frequency of consumption, by type and amount	Total alcohol: Increased risk (nonsignificant) for colon and rectal cancer in women Spirits: M F Colon cancer 1.0 2.0 Rectal cancer 1.0 1.5	Matched RR (≥12.9 g/day *versus* <0.01 g/day) calculated by Working Group
Australia, Melbourne (Kune *et al.*, 1987a)	Colon and rectum: men, women (715, 727)	Estimated cumulative intake, by type of beverage	Colon: no significant association Rectum: Beer quartiles: M F 1 1.0 1.0 2 1.7* 1.6 3 1.8* 1.6 4 1.9* 2.1	RR adjusted for dietary variables RR changed little when also adjusted for other alcoholic beverages; *, significant

[a] Relative risk (RR); 95% confidence intervals in parentheses

proportion of beer drinkers among male cases of rectal and colon cancer (35% and 31%, respectively), compared with 19% of controls, but there was no difference in other types of alcohol consumed. The authors conclude that 'the excess of heavy drinkers, particularly of beer, among men with rectal cancer appeared to reflect factors such as religious differences, smoking habits and the lower socioeconomic status of that group'. There was no difference in alcohol consumption between the rectal cancer group and the second control group.

Miller, A.B. *et al.* (1983) conducted a case-control study in Toronto, Canada, of 348 patients with colon cancer and 194 with rectal cancer, compared with two series of controls consisting of 542 individually matched neighbourhood and 535 frequency matched hospital controls. Standardized interview information was obtained on usual frequency of food and alcohol consumption. Analysis was done for groups of foods rather than nutrients, and these included alcoholic beverages, in particular beer. There was some evidence of an increased risk for rectal cancer, but not colon cancer, in association with beer intake; nonsignificantly elevated RRs of 1.3 for men and 1.6 for women were found among individuals in the highest consumption tertile. There was no indication of an association between colon or rectal cancer and other types of alcohol consumption.

The association between beer drinking and cancer of the rectum was investigated by Kabat *et al.* (1986) in a case-control study of 130 male and 88 female rectal cancer cases, all histologically confirmed, and 336 males and 249 female controls. The controls consisted of patients with cancers other than of the digestive tract and disease conditions not associated with tobacco use. A maximum of three controls was matched to each case on the basis of age, sex and calendar year of hospital interview. Information on consumption of beer, wine and spirits throughout adulthood (quantity and duration), and on smoking and socio-demographic characteristics was obtained by standardized interview. Beer intake was significantly associated with estimated risk of rectal cancer in men, the RR increasing with consumption. For drinkers of 32 oz or more of beer per day, the RR was 3.5. There was no association with duration of beer drinking. A nonsignificant inverse association with consumption was seen for women; however, only nine cases and 40 controls drank beer more than occasionally. In conditional multiple logistic regression analyses, the RR for beer drinking decreased slightly when controlled for potential confounding variables, and the RR for men drinking $\geq$32 oz/day, when adjusted for religion and education, was 2.7. Consumption of wine or spirits showed no association with rectal cancer.

Potter and McMichael (1986) reported a population-based case-control study of 419 incident cases of large-bowel cancer (220 colon, 199 rectum) and 732 community controls, interviewed regarding diet and alcohol in 1979-81 in Adelaide, Australia. Information regarding food and alcohol intake was obtained using a quantitative frequency questionnaire; the reproducibility of information about alcohol consumption was documented in a study of a subgroup of the study population re-interviewed by that research group in Adelaide (Rohan & Potter, 1984). Analysis by quintile of alcohol consumption showed that total alcohol intake was associated with nonsignificantly increased risks of both colon and rectal cancer in women but not in men. In both men and women, there were increased risks for colon and rectal cancer associated with consumption of spirits. For colon cancer, there was a statistically significant, approximate doubling of risk associated with drinking a glass [volume unspecified] of spirits per day in women, and with drinking two glasses per day in men, relative to abstainers. For rectal cancer, there was a weaker association with consumption of spirits. There was no association between beer consumption and cancer at either site.

As part of a large investigation of colorectal cancer incidence, etiology and survival in Melbourne, Australia, a case-control study was conducted to identify whether diet and alcohol, among other variables, were associated with colorectal cancer (Kune *et al.*, 1987a). The authors compared 715 incident cases of adenocarcinoma of the large bowel with 727 age- and sex-matched community controls. Information about the total lifetime intake of specific alcoholic beverages was obtained by interview, and data were classified by level of consumption of beer, wine, spirits and total alcohol. There was little evidence of an association of any of the alcohol variables with the risk of colon cancer; however, beer was found to be a significant risk factor for rectal cancer in men (RR, 1.0, 1.7, 1.8, 1.9 for four increasing quartiles of consumption), controlling for ten dietary variables and for other categories of alcoholic beverage. This effect was greatest in older men. RRs were similar in women but did not attain significance. Consumption of spirits was associated with a reduced risk of rectal cancer in men. [The Working Group noted that some controls were re-interviewed (Kune *et al.*, 1987b), which seriously limits the interpretation of these findings.]

Stomach and colorectal cancer (see Tables 60 and 61): In an early case-control study by Stocks (1957) in North Wales and Liverpool, UK, trained interviewers obtained histories from hospitalized patients with and without cancer. Within each residential area, the frequency of consumption of alcohol by cancer patients aged 45-74 years was compared with that expected on the basis of sex- and age-specific frequency distributions of the non-cancer patients, who totalled 4630 men and 4900 women 45-74 years old. In men, usable data were available from 153 stomach cancer patients and 166 patients with colorectal cancer; beer drinking was positively associated with intestinal cancer (RR calculated by the Working Group to be 1.4 in those who drank daily or weekly in comparison with those who drank less often) but not with stomach cancer. [The Working Group noted that, because of the very low prevalence of self-reported alcohol consumption in women, no informative comparison could be made.]

A case-control study of 93 male cases of stomach cancer and 279 controls, and of 340 male cases of colorectal cancer and 1020 controls was conducted by Higginson (1966). Cases were patients admitted to seven hospitals in Kansas City, USA, with histologically confirmed cancer; controls were hospital patients with no obvious gastrointestinal disease or recent dietary abnormality, frequency matched with cases for sex, age and race. Alcohol consumption was estimated from interviews conducted in hospital. For both stomach and colorectal cancers, the alcohol consumption profiles of cases and controls were virtually identical. Stomach cancer was associated with 'heavy periodical' (i.e., weekend) drinking, but the numbers involved were small (five cases and three controls).

In Norway, Bjelke (1973) compared 228 stomach cancer cases (147 male, 81 female), 162 colon cancer cases (89 male, 73 female), 116 rectal cancer cases (64 male, 52 female) and 221 unconfirmed cases, with 1394 hospital controls matched for sex, age, hospital and interviewer. Consumption of beer, wine and spirits and other dietary items was assessed by interview in terms of six categories of usual frequency. The prevalence of use of any kind of beverage and the mean frequencies were very similar among cases and controls for cancer at each of the sites, in both men and women. In women, stomach cancer was positively associated with beer consumption, but negatively associated with consumption of spirits. [The Working Group noted that each case series was compared with the whole series of controls without taking the original matching into account.]

In a case-control study carried out in Minnesota, USA, the design of which was very similar to his Norwegian study, Bjelke (1973) compared 83 stomach cancer cases (67 male, 16 female), 259 colon cancer cases (144 male, 115 female) and 144 rectal cancer cases (74 male, 40 female) aged 39-75 years, with 1657 hospital controls matched for age, sex, race and hospital, excluding persons with gastrointestinal diseases and a few other specified conditions. A significant positive association was seen for men and women combined for rectal cancer and beer consumption. For colon cancer and consumption of spirits, the association was significantly positive for men and negative for women.

In a patient interview study (Williams & Horm, 1977) as part of the Third National Cancer Survey (see description, pp. 170-171), 202 stomach cancer cases (120 male, 82 female), 653 colon cancer cases (294 male, 359 female) and 303 rectal cancer cases (165 male, 138 female) were compared with 1209 male and 2609 female controls, who were other cancer cases in the survey. After controlling for age, race and cigarette smoking, the risk for colon cancer among men was significantly increased with high total ethanol consumption (RR, 1.5) and for drinking beer, wine or spirits. The risk for neither rectal nor stomach cancer showed a clear association with alcohol consumption in men. Among women, the risk for rectal cancer was significantly increased (RR, 2.0) with high consumption of total ethanol, while the risks for colon and stomach cancers showed no statistically significant increase. There was a moderate association between stomach cancer in women and consumption of wine and beer (but not spirits).

Tuyns *et al.* (1982) conducted a population-based case-control study in which 163 stomach cancer cases, 142 colon cancer cases and 198 rectal cancer cases were identified and interviewed prospectively, during 1975-80, in Calvados, France. A total of 1976 population controls were interviewed during 1973-80, comprising a random sample of all people aged over 20 years in the source population. A standard interview questionnaire was used, which was developed for French patterns of alcohol consumption and administered by specially trained dieticians. There were nonsignificantly increased RRs for colon cancer (1.4; 95% CI, 0.3-5.7) and rectal cancer (1.6; 0.5-5.5) in alcohol consumers *versus* abstainers, and a nonsignificantly decreased RR for stomach cancer (0.5; 0.2-1.8).

(*f*) *Cancer of the liver*

(i) *Cohort studies* (descriptions of studies of cancers at many sites are given on pp. 158-164)

In most of the cohort studies on liver cancer, summarized in Table 62, it is probable that several cases classified as having primary liver cancer in fact had metastatic liver cancer,

Table 62. Relative risks for liver cancer in cohort studies

Study and reference	No. of subjects	Relative risk[a]	Comments
Norwegian Alcoholics (Sundby, 1967)	6 deaths	2	Compared with Norwegian population
Finnish			
Alcohol Misusers	66 cases	1.5*	
Alcoholics (Hakulinen *et al.*, 1974)	2 cases	2.5	
Massachussetts Alcoholics (Monson & Lyon, 1975)	4 deaths	1	
UK Alcoholics (Adelstein & White, 1976)	5 deaths	5.8* in males	
Dublin Brewery Workers (Dean *et al.*, 1979)	7 deaths	1.3	
US Veterans Alcoholics (Robinette *et al.*, 1979)	2 deaths	>1	
Danish Brewery Workers (Jensen, 1980)	29 cases	1.5*	
Canadian Alcoholics (Schmidt & Popham, 1981)	4 deaths	2	
Japanese Prospective Study (Hirayama, 1981)	-	1.3* nonsmokers, 0.9 <200 000 cig., 1.3 200 000–400 000 cig., 1.2 >400 000 cig., 1.5	Daily drinkers; RRs calculated by the Working Group
Japanese Doctors (Kono *et al.*, 1986)	51 deaths	ex-drinkers, 1.4 (0.4–4.8) occasional drinkers, 1.5 (0.6–3.8) daily drinkers <2 *go*, 2.0 (0.8–5.1) daily drinkers >2 *go*, 2.7 (1.0–6.8)	RR adjusted for age and smoking
Japan (Shibata *et al.*, 1986)	21 deaths	7.5* for *shochu* drinkers	Fishing area - RR not adjusted for smoking

[a]*, significant; ;95% confidence interval in parentheses

because of difficulties in diagnosis. Furthermore, it is clear that, in some of these studies, cases of primary liver cancer were grouped with other cancers. Both practices would tend to affect (probably underestimate) the strength of the association between alcohol consumption and risk for primary liver cancer.

In the prospective Japanese study (Hirayama, 1975, 1978, 1981), the most recent (Hirayama, 1981) age-adjusted rate ratio for primary liver cancer between daily drinkers and nondrinkers was calculated by the Working Group to be 1.3, which is significantly different from the null value of 1.0. [The Working Group noted that data on hepatitis B virus serology were not available.]

In the study of Japanese doctors (Kono *et al.*, 1983, 1985, 1986), the numbers of deaths (and age-adjusted death rates per 10 000 per year) are given for primary liver cancer (ICD-8 155, 197.8) as follows: seven deaths (3.6) among nondrinkers, four (4.9) among ex-drinkers, 14 (5.7) among occasional drinkers, 13 (7.1) among daily drinkers of less than 2 *go* (1 *go* = 180 ml saké = 22 g ethanol) and 13 (9.0) among daily drinkers of more than 2 *go*. Excluding ex-drinkers, and using logistic regression to control for age and tobacco smoking, the partial regression coefficient for alcohol intake is 0.317 (standard error, 0.125). The Working Group calculated that this corresponds to a statistically significant RR for primary liver cancer of 1.4 for an increase in alcohol consumption of 1 *go* per day. In categorical assessments, the RR (and 95% CI) for primary liver cancer, with nondrinkers as referents, were 1.4 (0.4-4.8) for ex-drinkers, 1.5 (0.6-3.8) for occasional drinkers, 2.0 (0.8-5.1) for daily drinkers of less than 2 *go*, and 2.7 (1.0-6.8) for daily drinkers of more than 2 *go*. [The Working Group noted that data on hepatitis B virus serology are not available, and that no information is given about the actual proportion of cases with primary liver cancer in the rubric 197.8, unspecified liver cancer.]

In the study of Hawaiian Japanese (Blackwelder *et al.*, 1980), seven deaths were due to primary liver cancer and 16 to cirrhosis of the liver. The mean ethanol consumption in the seven individuals with primary liver cancer had been 12.0 ml [9.5 g]/day, compared to 36.8 ml [29 g]/day among individuals who had died from cirrhosis of the liver, and to 13.6 ml [11 g]/day in living members of the cohort. All values were ascertained at the initial baseline examination and were not age-standardized.

Another cohort study in which role of alcohol and tobacco in the etiology of primary liver cancer was explored in the general Japanese population was recently reported (Shibata *et al.*, 1986). The study was based on follow-up of 639 men in a farming area and 677 men in a fishing area, in the context of a longitudinal study to evaluate risk factors for coronary heart disease. There was no effect of saké drinking in either the farming or the fishing area nor any effect of drinking *shochu* (a distilled alcoholic beverage made in Japan, containing about 25% alcohol) in the farming area. However, in the fishing area, the observed (18) to expected (2.4) ratio among *shochu* drinkers was 7.5 ($p < 0.001$), with an apparent but nonsignificant dose-trend. [The Working Group noted that the association is not confounded by tobacco smoking, but the lack of data concerning hepatitis B virus, the absence of a similar association with *shochu* in the other study area, and the small overall study size make interpretation of these findings difficult.]

In several studies of cohorts of persons with high alcohol intake, the observed number of deaths from primary liver cancer has been compared with the number expected on the basis of the age-, sex- and calendar-time-specific mortality from this cancer in a reference population. In the study of Norwegian alcoholics (Sundby, 1967), six deaths were observed, with 3.1 expected in Norway. In the Canadian study of Schmidt and de Lint (1972) on alcoholics, no death from primary liver cancer was observed. [The Working Group estimated that approximately two would have been expected on the basis of expected figures in studies of similar size and background rates.] In this study, a high excess of deaths due to cirrhosis of the liver was observed (56 among men and 12 among women, with 4.9 and 0.5 expected), but the authors of the study consider it unlikely that deaths due to primary liver cancer had been misdiagnosed as due to cirrhosis, since most deaths occurred in large hospitals and autopsies were performed on 55% of those who died from cirrhosis.

In a five-year mortality study in one company in the USA of 922 alcoholics and an equal number of nonalcoholics, individually matched by age, sex, payroll, class and geographic location, no death from primary liver cancer was observed (Pell & D'Alonzo, 1973). [The Working Group estimated that approximately one would have been expected.] An excess of deaths due to cirrhosis of the liver was found among alcoholics (11 deaths due to cirrhosis, compared to none among nonalcoholics).

In the study of UK alcoholics (Nicholls *et al.*, 1974; Adelstein & White, 1976), there were five deaths from liver cancer (including extrahepatic bile ducts) among men, while 0.9 would have been expected, giving a significant SMR of 5.8. In the study of Finnish alcohol misusers and alcoholics (Hakulinen *et al.*, 1974), there were 66 cases of primary liver cancer in the misusers cohort and two in the alcoholics cohort, with 44.3 and 0.8 expected, respectively; the first comparison gave a significant result. In the study of Massachussets alcoholics, Monson and Lyon (1975) found four deaths from primary liver cancer (including biliary passages), with 4.2 expected. In the cohort study of male Dublin brewery workers (Dean *et al.*, 1979), there were seven deaths from primary liver cancer with 5.5 expected from Dublin death rates. In the cohort study of male Danish brewery workers (Jensen, 1980), there were 29 incident cases of primary liver cancer with 19.2 expected; this result was significant. In the study of alcoholic US veterans (Robinette *et al.*, 1979), there were two deaths in a category that included primary liver cancer (as well as other rare cancers in ICD-8 rubrics 152, 156, 158 and 159), whereas no such death was observed in a comparison age-matched group. In the cohort study of male alcoholics in Canada (Schmidt & Popham, 1981), four deaths from primary liver cancer (ICD-8, 155, 156) were observed with 2.0 expected.

[The Working Group noted that, taken together, the results of these ten cohort studies on alcoholics generate 125 observed cases of liver cancer *versus* 83.3 expected. The ratio, based on the three most reliable studies, is 1.5 (1.2-1.9). The ratio based on the total numbers of observed and expected cases in all the cohorts is 1.5 (1.3-1.8). Both are significant at the 1% level.]

(ii) *Case control studies*

The results of case-control studies of primary liver cancer are summarized in Table 63.

Table 63. Summary of results of case-control studies of primary liver cancer and alcohol consumption

Place (reference)	Subjects (cases, controls)	Exposure measurement	Results[a]
France, Paris (Schwartz *et al.*, 1962)	Men (61, 61)	Average daily ethanol intake	High but equal ethanol consumption among cases and controls
USA, Multicenter (Williams & Horm, 1977)	Men (18, 1770) Women (10, 3178)	Three categories of wine, beer, spirits or total	Suggestive positive but not significant association Men / Women Nondrinkers 1.0 / 1.0 Moderate drinkers 0.5 / 5.1 Heavier drinkers 2.8 / -
Switzerland, Geneva (Infante *et al.*, 1980b)	Men (31, 207) Women (4, 226)	Main daily and life-long ethanol consumption	Ethanol consumption among cases twice as high as that among controls
Philippines (Bulatao-Jayme *et al.*, 1982)	Men (74, 74) Women (16, 16)	Categorization into 'heavy' (38.4 g) and 'light' (9.8 g) drinkers using mean ethanol intake per day of all subjects	Light aflatoxin, light alcohol: 1.0 Light aflatoxin, heavy alcohol: 3.9* Heavy aflatoxin, light alcohol: 17.5* Heavy aflatoxin, heavy alcohol: 35.0*
Hong Kong (Lam *et al.*, 1982)	Men (95, 95) Women (12, 12)	'Alcohol consumption', details not given	No significant positive association
USA, New Jersey (Stemhagen *et al.*, 1983)	Men (178, 356) Women (87, 174)	Categorization into nondrinker, light, moderate, medium-heavy and heavy drinker	In both sexes, statistically significant linear trends with increasing ethanol consumption Men / Women Nondrinkers 1.0 / 1.0 Light 1.0 (0.5-2.1) / 1.7 (0.7-4.2) Moderate 1.2 (0.5-2.7) / 2.2 (0.9-5.7) Medium 2.5 (1.0-6.5) / 3.7 (0.2-93.6) Heavy 2.0 (0.8-5.1) / 5.6 (0.8-38.6)

Table 63 (contd)

Place (reference)	Subjects (cases, controls)	Exposure measurement	Results[a]
USA, Los Angeles County (Yu *et al.*, 1983)	Men (50, 50) Women (28, 28)	Three categories of ethanol intake: low, moderate, high	0–9 g/day, 1.0 10–79 g/day, 0.9 (0.4–1.9) ≥80 g/day, 4.2 (1.3–13.8)
Sweden (Hardell *et al.*, 1984)	Hepatocellular carcinoma: men (83, 166) Cholangiocarcinoma: men (15, 30)	Categorization into nondrinkers, light consumers of spirits (≤4 bottles/year), moderate consumers (>1 bottle/month–<1 bottle/week), heavy consumers (>1 bottle/week) (1 bottle = 370 ml spirits)	Alcohol: 0–79 g/day / ≥80 g/day Non-/ex-smokers: 1.0 / ∞ ≤1 pack/day: 1.4 (0.6–3.4) / 0.8 (0.1–4.6) >1 pack/day: 1.8 (0.7–5.0) / 14.0 (1.7–113.9) Nondrinkers, 1.0 Light drinkers, 2.1 (0.9–5.1) Moderate drinkers, 2.9 (1.0–8.7) Heavy drinkers, 4.3 (1.8–10.8)
USA, five states (Austin *et al.*, 1986)	Men (60, 110) Women (26, 51)	Categorization into no use, infrequent use, occasional use, regular use (at least once/day)	Statistically significant dose-dependent association with frequency of alcohol intake Nondrinkers 1.0 Infrequent drinkers 1.4 Occasional drinkers 2.3 Regular drinkers 2.6
Greece, Athens (Trichopoulos *et al.*, 1987)	Men (173, 400)	Total daily ethanol consumption in grams	No association for ethanol consumption with or without underlying cirrhosis; for liver cancer with cirrhosis, 'heavy' ethanol consumption (>70 g/day), adjusted RR, 1.2

[a]Relative risk; 95% confidence intervals in parentheses; *, significant

In a large case-control study of all cancers in Paris, Schwartz *et al.* (1957, 1962; see description, p. 167) grouped 61 male cases of primary liver cancer, pancreatic cancer and cancers of the peritoneum, and compared them with matched hospital controls. The proportion of alcoholics and the mean alcohol intake were almost identical in the two groups.

In a study conducted within the Third National Cancer Survey (Williams & Horm, 1977; see description, pp. 170-171), there were 18 cases of primary liver cancer in men and ten among women. Men in the higher time-weighted alcohol consumption category had a RR for primary liver cancer of 2.8, after adjustment for smoking, but there was no elevation of risk among men in the moderate consumption category (RR, 0.5). There were no women in the higher alcohol consumption category; among those in the moderate consumption category, the tobacco-adjusted RR for primary liver cancer was 5.1. None of these associations was significant.

In a case-control study in Geneva, with 31 male and four female cases of histologically confirmed primary liver cancer and 207 and 226 population controls (among whom the participation rate was 70%), Infante *et al.* (1980a,b) found substantially higher age-standardized alcohol consumption among the cases than among the controls (47 g ethanol in men; 12 g in women). The differences in alcohol consumption were not related to the small differences in tobacco smoking between cases and controls. Alcohol consumption was not higher among primary liver cancer cases with cirrhosis (72 g in men, 23 g in women) than among those without cirrhosis (101 g in men). [The Working Group noted that information concerning hepatitis B virus serology was not available.]

In a case-control study of 90 histologically confirmed cases of primary liver cancer (74 male, 16 female) and 90 age- and sex-matched hospital controls with normal liver function tests in the Philippines, Bulatao-Jayme *et al.* (1982) investigated the role of alcohol and aflatoxin intake in the etiology of primary liver cancer. Intake of alcohol and of aflatoxin (see IARC, 1976b, 1987a) were ascertained using dietary questionnaires and on the basis of aflatoxin contamination of various foods and the ethanol content of alcoholic beverages. In comparison with 'light aflatoxin-light alcohol' consumers (referent group), the RRs were 3.9 among 'light aflatoxin-heavy alcohol' consumers, 17.5 among 'heavy aflatoxin-light alcohol' consumers and 35.0 among 'heavy aflatoxin-heavy alcohol' consumers. [The Working Group noted that the lack of data concerning hepatitis B virus serology in this study, and the probable correlation between prevalence of hepatitis B surface antigen carrier state and both alcohol and aflatoxin intake hinder interpretation of the results.]

In a study of 107 cases (95 male, 12 female; 106 histologically confirmed) and 107 controls matched for sex, age and hospital in Hong Kong, Lam *et al.* (1982) found that serum hepatitis B surface antigen carrier state and tobacco smoking were independent risk factors for primary hepatocellular carcinoma. While no data were reported, the authors stated that neither alcohol intake nor aflatoxin contamination of foods was significantly related.

Stemhagen *et al.* (1983) studied 265 cases (178 male, 87 female) of histologically confirmed primary liver cancer (216 hepatocellular carcinoma) and 530 controls (356 male, 174 female) matched for age, sex and county of residence in New Jersey, USA, by interviews mostly (96%) with next-of-kin; dead cases were matched through death certificates with dead controls. There were statistically significant linear trends with increasing alcohol consumption up to RRs of 2.0 and 5.6 among heavily drinking men and women, respectively. Drinking habits were also studied by type of alcohol consumed, but the numbers were small, and the only remarkable finding was a strong association among women between exclusive beer drinking (RR, 10.6; 95% CI, 2.6-42.9) and primary liver cancer. No association was found between primary liver cancer and tobacco smoking, probably because most of the controls had tobacco-related diseases, notably ischaemic heart disease. [The Working Group noted that data concerning hepatitis B virus serology were not available.]

Yu *et al.* (1983) studied 78 cases (50 male, 28 female) of hepatocellular cancer identified through the Los Angeles County Cancer Surveillance Program and 78 age-, sex- and race-matched neighbourhood controls in California, USA, and found a statistically significant association with high ethanol consumption: the RR (and 95% CI) for intake of 10-79 g/day was 0.9 (0.4-1.9) and that for ≥80 g/day was 4.2 (1.3-13.8). [The Working Group noted that information concerning hepatitis B virus serology was not available.]

In a study in Sweden (Hardell *et al.*, 1984), 83 male deaths from histologically confirmed hepatocellular carcinoma and 15 from histologically confirmed intrahepatic cholangiocellular carcinoma, identified through the Swedish Cancer Registry, were each matched with two deceased population controls drawn from the National Population Register; relatives were asked to complete written questionnaires. A statistically significant, dose-dependent association of consumption of spirits was found with hepatocellular carcinoma and a suggestive association with intrahepatic cholangiocarcinoma. Only 34% of the hepatocellular carcinoma cases were reported to have cirrhosis. [The Working Group noted that data on hepatitis B virus serology were not available.]

In a study in five states in the USA on 86 cases (60 male, 26 female) of hepatocellular carcinoma (80 histologically confirmed), diagnosed in any of 12 hospitals, and 161 (110 male, 51 female) age-, sex- and race-matched controls, excluding those with tobacco-related diseases and primary liver diseases, Austin *et al.* (1986) found that chronic hepatitis B virus infection was strongly related to hepatocellular carcinoma and that there was also a moderately strong, dose-dependent association between alcohol consumption and risk for liver cancer, adjusted for age and hepatitis B virus status.

Trichopoulos *et al.* (1987) studied 194 cases (173 male, 21 female) of hepatocellular carcinoma (113 histologically confirmed) admitted to three major hospitals in Athens, Greece, and 456 (400 male, 56 female) hospital controls with diagnoses other than cancer or liver disease. A strong, highly significant association was seen between hepatocellular carcinoma and both serum hepatitis B surface antigen carrier status and tobacco consumption, but there was no association (with or without underlying cirrhosis which was, in most cases, hepatitis B virus-related) with ethanol consumption after adjustment for age, sex, carrier status and tobacco smoking.

(iii) *Studies of joint exposure*

Hirayama (1981) found an interaction between tobacco smoking and alcohol drinking in the causation of primary liver cancer. The rate ratios, calculated by the Working Group, between daily drinkers and other males were 0.9 among nonsmokers, 1.3 among cumulative smokers of up to 200 000 cigarettes, 1.2 among cumulative smokers of 200 000-400 000 cigarettes, and 1.5 among cumulative smokers of more than 400 000 cigarettes. [The Working Group noted that details which would allow alternative statistical calculations to be made are not given.] Yu *et al.* (1983) found a stronger association with alcohol drinking among heavy cigarette smokers than among those who smoked less. Heavy smokers (>1 pack/day) who were also heavy drinkers (>80 g ethanol/day) had a RR of 14.0 (1.7-113.9), while the RR for all heavy drinkers was 4.2. Austin *et al.* (1986) found no interactive effect of tobacco and alcohol consumption and risk for hepatocellular carcinoma.

Interactive effects between ethanol and hepatitis B virus in the causation of primary liver cancer have been postulated by several authors on the basis of relatively small or inadequately controlled clinical, pathological or clinicopathological studies. Support for this notion was recently provided by a case-control study (Oshima *et al.*, 1984) on liver cancer, performed within a cohort of 8646 male voluntary blood donors who were found to be hepatitis B surface antigen-positive during examination at the Red Cross Blood Center in Osaka, Japan, during the period 1972-75 and were followed through 31 December 1980, for an average period of 6.2 years. Twenty cases of primary liver cancer were found (3.03 expected; RR, 6.6). For these 20 cases of liver cancer and 40 age-matched controls selected from healthy hepatitis B virus carriers, detailed information on tobacco smoking and alcohol drinking was obtained. Drinking habits were classified into three categories: heavy (not less than 3 *go* of saké or other alcoholic beverages, equivalent to 80 ml [63 g] ethanol/day), moderate and none or light (less than 1 *go* of saké or the equivalent of 27 ml [21 g] ethanol/day). A strong, dose-dependent, significant, positive association (RR, up to 8.0; 95% CI, 1.3-49.5) between alcohol drinking and primary liver cancer was observed, which was apparently not confounded by tobacco smoking (also positively related to the occurrence of primary liver cancer).

Possible interactions between ethanol and aflatoxins in the etiology of liver cancer have been investigated in two studies; a more than additive effect was reported by Bulatao-Jayme *et al.* (1982), whereas no effect of either ethanol or aflatoxin was found by Lam *et al.* (1982).

(g) *Cancer of the pancreas*

(i) *Cohort studies* (descriptions of studies of cancer at many sites are given on pp. 158-164)

In none of the nine cohorts with high alcohol intake (see Table 64) was there a significantly elevated number of pancreatic cancers (Sundby, 1967; Schmidt & de Lint, 1972; Hakulinen *et al.*, 1974; Adelstein & White, 1976; Dean *et al.*, 1979; Monson & Lyon, 1979; Robinette *et al.*, 1979; Jensen, 1980; Schmidt & Popham, 1981). In only four studies was the observed number of cases greater than five: seven in a follow-up of the study of Adelstein and White (1976; Nicholls *et al.*, 1974), 17 in the study of Dean *et al.* (1979), 44 in the study of Jensen (1980) and 11 in that of Schmidt and Popham (1981).

Table 64. Relative risks (RR) for pancreatic cancer in cohort studies

Study and reference	No. of subjects	RR	Comments
Norwegian Alcoholics (Sundby, 1967)	5 deaths	1.6	Compared with Norwegian population
		0.9	Compared with Oslo population
Canadian Alcoholics (Schmidt & de Lint, 1972)	1 death		
Finnish Alcoholics (Hakulinen *et al.*, 1974)	4 cases	1.8	
Massachusetts Alcoholics (Monson & Lyon, 1975)	3 deaths	0.6	
UK Alcoholics (Adelstein & White, 1976)	7 deaths	1.5	
Dublin Brewery Workers (Dean *et al.*, 1979)	17 deaths	1.2	Compared with Dublin population
		1.5	Compared with Irish population
US Veterans Alcoholics (Robinette *et al.*, 1979)	4 deaths	0.9	
Danish Brewery Workers (Jensen, 1980)	44 cases	1.1	
Canadian Alcoholics (Schmidt & Popham, 1981)	11 deaths	1.2	Compared with Ontario population
		1.1	Compared with US veterans
		0.8	Compared with US veterans with similar smoking habits

In the Japanese prospective study, the SMR for pancreatic cancer among men who consumed alcoholic beverages daily compared with those who did not was 1.1 after eight years (Hirayama, 1975), 0.9 after nine years (Hirayama, 1978) and 0.8 after 16 years (Hirayama, 1985). Furthermore, there was no evidence for an interaction between alcohol intake and tobacco smoking in the causation of pancreatic cancer (Hirayama, 1979).

In the Kaiser-Permanente study (Klatsky *et al.*, 1981), the numbers of pancreatic cancer deaths (and ten-year cumulated mortality per 1000 persons) were two (1.0) among nondrinkers, five (2.5) among light drinkers (two or fewer drinks/day); three (1.5) among moderate drinkers (three to five drinks/day); and six (3.0) among heavy drinkers (six or more drinks/day). The association appears to be positive but it is not statistically significant and does not show a clear dose-dependent pattern. Although subjects were matched for smoking habits, some residual confounding by duration and intensity of smoking could not be excluded.

Heuch *et al.* (1983) reported a cohort of 16 713 subjects, comprising a random sample of Norwegian males (48%), brothers of Norwegians who had emigrated to the USA (20%), and spouses and siblings (males and females) of individuals interviewed in a case-control study of gastrointestinal cancer (32%). For only 4995 men was information on both alcohol drinking and tobacco smoking or chewing available; among these, 18 histologically verified cases of pancreatic cancer occurred. Among 'frequent current users' of alcohol (drinking of beer or spirits at least 14 times per month), five histologically verified cases of cancer of the pancreas were observed, whereas the tobacco-adjusted expected number was 1.7. Among nondrinkers, the observed and expected numbers were three and 7.6, whereas in the intermediate category of moderate alcohol drinkers the corresponding figures were ten and 8.7. The authors interpreted their findings as strongly supportive of a causal role for alcohol ($p = 0.001$ for trend). [However, the authors' estimate of a RR of 10.8 between frequent and nonusers, which the Working Group was unable to reproduce, is based on only 18 cases and has a lower 95% confidence limit of 2.2 (Velema *et al.*, 1986). The Working Group noted that this fact, together with the apparent high nonparticipation rate of heavy drinkers during the formative phase of the cohort, and the conflicting evidence derived from histologically confirmed and nonconfirmed pancreatic cancer cases (among the latter, the association with alcohol intake appears to be negative), make a causal interpretation of the findings difficult.]

In the study of Japanese doctors (Kono *et al.*, 1983, 1986), deaths (and age-adjusted death rates) from pancreatic cancer (per 10 000 persons per year) were three (1.7) among nondrinkers, two (2.4) among ex-drinkers, five (2.1) among occasional drinkers, one (0.5) among daily drinkers of less than 2 *go* and three (2.4) among daily drinkers of more than 2 *go*. Excluding ex-drinkers, and using logistic regression to control for age and smoking, gives a partial regression coefficient for alcohol intake corresponding to a SMR of 1.0, implying that alcohol drinking does not increase the risk for pancreatic cancer.

In the study of Hawaiian Japanese (Blackwelder *et al.*, 1980), 13 deaths from pancreatic cancer were identified within eight years of the initial examination. The mean ethanol consumption in these 13 individuals was 13.7 ml (11 g)/day compared to 13.6 ml (11 g)/day in living members of the cohort.

Furthermore, in the five-year mortality study of 922 alcoholics and an equal number of nonalcoholics, individually matched by age, sex, payroll, class and geographical location in a US company, there were two deaths from pancreatic cancer among alcoholics and none among nonalcoholics (Pell & D'Alonzo, 1973).

[The Working Group noted that the observed number of deaths due to pancreatic cancer in all the cohort studies on alcoholics combined was 98, with ~ 84.4 expected. The pooled SMR (and 95% CI) is thus 1.2 (0.9-1.4).]

(ii) *Case-control studies*

The results of case-control studies of pancreatic cancer are summarized in Table 65.

Table 65. Summary of results of case-control studies of pancreatic cancer and alcohol intake

Place (reference)	Subjects (cases, controls)	Exposure measurement	Results[a]
Japan (Ishii *et al*., 1968, 1973)	Men, women (475, 122 261)	Categories of alcohol intake	RR, ~1.5 for drinkers *versus* nondrinkers
USA, three cities (Wynder *et al*., 1973a)	Men (100, 200) Women (42, 107)	Categorization into nondrinkers, occasional drinkers, regular drinkers	RR [1.3 (0.8–2.0)] for drinkers *versus* nondrinkers
USA, Multicenter (Williams & Horm, 1977)	Men (901, 1770) Women (85, 3178)	Three categories of wine, beer, spirits and total alcohol	RR (heavier *versus* nondrinkers) men, 1.3 women, 0.6
Switzerland, Geneva (Raymond *et al*., 1987)	Men, women (88, 336)	Mean weekly consumption of red wine and beer	90% CI red wine <1270 ml/week 1.0 (0.5–1.9) ≥1270 ml/week 0.9 (0.4–1.7) beer <900 ml/week 0.7 (0.3–1.3) ≥900 ml/week 2.9 (1.3–6.3)
USA (Lin & Kessler, 1981)	Men (57, 57) Women (37, 37)	No clear definition	Patients drank more wine than controls (16.5% *versus* 8.3%), $p < 0.05$ for ≥2 glasses/day
USA, Boston and Rhode Island (MacMahon *et al*., 1981)	Men (218, 307) Women (149, 337)	Categorization into nondrinkers, occasional drinkers, regular drinkers	Men / Women nondrinkers 1.0 / 1.0 occasional 1.3 (0.7–2.6) / 0.8 (0.5–1.3) regular 1.3 (0.6–2.6) / 0.5 (0.3–1.1)
Greece, Athens (Manousos *et al*., 1981)	Men (32, 172) Women (18, 34)	Regular drinkers of >10 g ethanol daily	RR 0.7 (0.3–1.3) for regular drinkers *versus* others
USA, California (Haines *et al*., 1982)	Men (56, 112) Women (60, 120)	Categorization into alcohol intake < once a day, regular daily consumption, patients with alcohol-related problems	No association

Table 65 (contd)

Place (reference)	Subjects (cases, controls)	Exposure measurement	Results[a]
USA, several states (Wynder *et al.*, 1983)	Men (153, 5469) Women (122, 2525)	Daily alcohol intake	RR for drinkers of >5 oz daily *versus* nondrinkers men, 1.6 (0.9–2.6) women, 0.9 (0.3–2.1)
France, Marseilles (Durbec *et al.*, 1983)	Men (37, 100) Women (32, 99)	Daily ethanol intake in grams	RR for median drinkers (~40 g/day) *versus* nondrinkers, [2.4 (1.2–4.3)]
Japan, Tokyo (Kodama & Mori, 1983a,b)	Men (59, 72) Women (25, 29)	Habitual daily consumption	RR for habitual drinkers *versus* others, [0.6 (0.3–1.2)]
USA, Baltimore (Gold *et al.*, 1985)	Men (94, 188) Women (103, 206)	Categorization into nondrinkers, drinkers (any amount or frequency)	No or inverse association
USA, Los Angeles County (Mack *et al.*, 1986)	Men (282, 282) Women (208, 208)	Daily ethanol intake in grams; total and from various sources	Alcohol (g/day) <40 0.7 (0.5–1.1) 40–79 0.8 (0.5–1.3) >79 1.2 (0.7–2.2)
Sweden, Stockholm and Uppsala (Norell *et al.*, 1986)	Men (55, 110) Women (44, 88)	Daily ethanol consumption in grams	Alcohol (g/day) / *vs* hospital controls / *vs* population controls 0–1 1.0 1.0 2–9 0.5 (0.3–0.9) 0.7 (0.5–1.2) ≥10 0.5 (0.3–1.0) 0.6 (0.3–1.1) (90% CI)

[a]Relative risk (RR) with 95% confidence intervals, except where noted; [ ] when calculated by the Working Group

On the basis of a clinical series of 83 patients with cancer of the pancreas in New Orleans, USA, and a comparison series of 100 patients assembled independently and subsequently, Burch and Ansari (1968) speculated that chronic alcoholism may substantially increase the risk for pancreatic cancer. [The Working Group noted that this clinical study was not conducted as, and does not have the methodological characteristics of, a case-control investigation.]

In a large case-control study of all cancers in Paris, Schwartz *et al.* (1957, 1962; see description, p. 167) grouped 61 male cases of pancreatic cancer, primary liver cancer and cancers of the peritoneum and compared them with matched hospital controls. The proportion of alcoholics and the mean alcohol intake were almost identical in the two groups.

Using as background data the results from a large population survey of 122 261 adults in 29 health districts in Japan, Ishii *et al.* (1968) analysed information gathered by questionnaire from 475 patients with pancreatic cancer, hospitalized in 100 collaborating institutions. They reported an increased RR (~ 1.5) for drinkers of alcoholic beverages. [The Working Group noted that the statistical significance of the finding was not given and that differences in tobacco smoking between cases and controls were not accounted for in the analysis.]

In a case-control study in three US cities, Wynder *et al.* (1973a,b) compared 100 men and 42 women with adenocarcinoma of the pancreas with 200 men and 107 women with diseases not related to tobacco use. They found a slight, nonsignificant, dose-unrelated association between alcohol consumption and risk for pancreatic cancer [RR, 1.3].

There were 224 cases of pancreatic cancer in the study of Williams and Horm (1977; for description, see pp. 170-171), but total ethanol consumption could be assessed for only 91 male and 85 female cases. Among men, the data indicate an overall slight, nonsignificant positive association between ethanol consumption and pancreatic cancer risk after adjustment for age, sex, race, education and smoking (RR, 1.3). Among women there was no association with ethanol consumption (RR, 0.6).

In a study in Geneva, Switzerland, the age-standardized mean daily ethanol consumption of histologically confirmed cases of pancreatic cancer from Geneva University Hospital was 46 g for men and 13 g for women; the corresponding consumption figures among population controls (among whom participation was 70%) were 47 g for men and 12 g for women; the differences are nonsignificant [RR for drinkers *versus* nondrinkers, ~ 1] (Voirol *et al.*, 1980). In a later analysis of the same data and a few additional cases, Raymond *et al.* (1987) observed, however, a significantly increased risk among beer drinkers (RR, 2.9). [The Working Group noted that there was no *a priori* hypothesis with regard to beer and that several comparisons, including one of individual beverages, had been undertaken.]

Lin and Kessler (1981) carried out a case-control study on 109 patients with histologically confirmed pancreatic cancer from collaborating hospitals in five metropolitan areas of the USA; 15 of the cases were islet-cell tumours. Controls were patients without cancer matched 1:1 with the patients for sex, age, race and marital status. The patients tended to drink more wine (16.5% *versus* 8.3%; $p < 0.05$ for two or more glasses/day) than the controls. [The Working Group noted that patients with tobacco- and alcohol-related diseases were not excluded from the controls and that no information was given on how alcohol consumption was analysed.]

In a study on 367 patients (218 men, 149 women) with histologically verified cancer of the pancreas from 11 hospitals in Massachusetts and Rhode Island, USA, and 644 controls with diseases unrelated to use of tobacco or alcohol, MacMahon *et al.* (1981) found no evidence of an association between alcohol intake and pancreatic cancer risk; the overall age- and sex-adjusted RR for regular drinkers was calculated by the Working Group to be 0.9 when adjusted for tobacco (95% CI, 0.6-1.3), with no evidence of increased risk at any level of consumption or with any type of alcoholic beverage.

In a study on 50 patients (32 men, 18 women) with histologically verified cancer of the pancreas from five hospitals in Athens, Greece, and 206 hospital controls (172 men, 34 women) with diagnoses other than cancer or disease of the liver or pancreas, Manousos *et al.* (1981) found a statistically significant association between pancreatic cancer and cigarette smoking but no association with regular drinking of alcoholic beverages (>10 g ethanol daily). The RR, adjusted for age, sex and tobacco use, was 0.7 for regular drinkers in comparison with nondrinkers.

In a study in California, USA, based on review of the medical records of 116 histologically confirmed cases of pancreatic cancer (56 male, 60 female) from two medical centres, two controls, matched for sex, age, race, hospital and year of admission, were matched for every cancer case: one control with malignant disease, the other with nonmalignant disease (Haines *et al.*, 1982). No association was found between alcohol intake and risk for pancreatic cancer.

In a US study on 275 histologically confirmed incident cases of primary pancreatic cancer (153 male, 122 female) from 17 hospitals and 7994 hospital controls (5469 male, 2525 female) with diseases unrelated to tobacco and stratified for age and smoking, Wynder *et al.* (1983) found slight, dose-unrelated, nonsignificant associations between alcohol intake and pancreatic cancer. Heavy drinkers (≥15 oz [~120 g] ethanol/day) had tobacco-adjusted RRs of 1.6 among men and 0.9 among women, when compared to nondrinkers.

In a study of 69 histologically verified cases of adenocarcinoma of the pancreas (37 male, 32 female) from three gastroenterology departments in Marseilles, France, and 199 controls (100 male, 99 female) matched for sex, age and neighbourhood, without gastrointestinal diseases, Durbec *et al.* (1983) found, in a logistic conditional regression model, a positive association between total alcohol intake (particularly wine of high alcohol content) and pancreatic cancer risk [RR for drinkers *versus* nondrinkers, 2.4]. The RR was reduced after controlling for fat and carbohydrate intake, and there were unexpected negative associations with duration of alcohol consumption; there was no increased risk with regular drinking of aperitives and spirits. [The Working Group noted that these findings, the lack of association with tobacco smoking, and the unspecified participation rate among the potential controls make interpretation of the results difficult.]

In a study on 84 primary pancreatic carcinoma cases (59 male, 25 female) confirmed at autopsy and 113 randomly selected autopsy controls (72 male, 29 female) in Tokyo, Japan,

Kodama and Mori (1983a,b) found no evidence for an increase in pancreatic cancer risk among regular drinkers of saké or other alcoholic beverages, on the basis of information derived from clinical records. The Working Group calculated a RR of 0.6 among habitual drinkers, not adjusted for smoking.

Gold *et al.* (1985) matched 94 male and 103 female cases of histologically confirmed pancreatic cancer from 16 hospitals in Baltimore, MD, USA, using an age-, race- and sex-matched case-control design, with both a hospital control series and a random-digit-dialling population control series. Proxy interviews were undertaken for 75% of the cases; controls were interviewed directly. No association was found between alcohol intake and cancer of the pancreas. The RR in comparison with the hospital controls was calculated by the Working Group to be 1.1 (0.7-1.7) and that in comparison with population controls to be 0.6. The inverse association was more evident among wine drinkers: the RR was calculated by the Working Group to be 0.9 (0.5-1.4) in comparison with hospital controls and 0.5 (0.3-0.8) with population controls.

In a population-based case-control study in Los Angeles, USA (Mack *et al.*, 1986), 282 male and 208 female cases of histologically confirmed pancreatic cancer in persons less than 65 years of age were identified from a cancer registry and compared with 282 male and 208 female matched neighbourhood controls. Information about alcohol intake was obtained by proxy interview for most cases and by personal interview for most controls. A nonsignificant inverse association was found between cancer of the pancreas and alcohol intake from any source; the inverse association was more pronounced for table wine consumption. The estimated RRs (*versus* nondrinkers) were 0.7 (0.5-1.1) for consumers of less than 40 g ethanol daily, 0.8 (0.5-1.3) for consumers of 40-79 g ethanol daily and 1.2 (0.7-2.2) for consumers of more than 79 g ethanol daily (not controlled for tobacco). No interaction between alcohol intake and smoking was evident.

A population-based case-control study in Sweden involved 55 male and 44 female cases of histologically confirmed cancer of the pancreas compared with an age- and sex-matched control series of hospital patients with inguinal hernia and another from the general population (Norell *et al.*, 1986). Inverse associations were noted in both comparisons, with RRs for frequent *versus* infrequent alcohol use of 0.5 (*versus* hospital controls) and 0.7 (*versus* population controls). The latter RR was calculated by the Working Group.

(*h*) *Cancer of the breast*

(i) *Cohort studies*

Four cohort studies in general populations have been published in which the association between alcohol intake and breast cancer has been examined (see Table 66).

Hiatt and Bawol (1984) followed 88 477 female members of the Kaiser Foundation health care plan in California (USA) who were more than 15 years of age at enrolment and had completed a questionnaire on the use of alcoholic beverages. Between 1960 and 1972, 1169 incident cases of breast cancer occurred; multivariate analysis was done on 694 cases over 30 years of age. After controlling for age, race, education, smoking, body mass index, cholesterol level and reproductive factors (all of which made only small differences), the

Table 66. Relative risks for breast cancer in cohort studies

Reference	Population	No. of cases	Alcohol consumption	Relative risk	95% confidence interval	Comment
Hiatt & Bawol (1984)	88 477 US health-plan members (1960–72); follow-up until 1977, aged >15 years	694	0 drinks/day	1.0		Controlled for race, education, smoking, body mass index, cholesterol, reproductive factors; no data on specific beverages
			<3 drinks/day	1.0		
			≥3 drinks/day	1.4	[1.0–1.7][a]	
Hiatt *et al.* (1987)	69 000 US health-plan members; five years of follow-up (1979–84)	303	Nondrinkers	1.0		Controlled for age, race, body mass index, smoking; effect not limited to any specific bevereage. RR highest among white and Hispanic and postmenopausal women
			Past drinkers	2.2	1.2–3.9	
			1–2 drinks/day	1.5	1.0–2.3	
			3–5 drinks/day	1.5	0.8–2.8	
			≥6 drinks/day	3.3	1.2–9.3	
Schatzkin *et al.* (1987)	USA, First National Health and Nutrition Examination Survey (1971–75); 7188 women 25–74 years of age; median follow-up, 10 years	121	No drinks in last year	1.0		Controlled for education, body mass index, dietary fat, reproductive factors; no data on specific beverage use; highest RR among youngest and thinnest women
			>0.1–1.2 g/day	1.4	0.8–2.5	
			1.3–4.9 g/day	1.6	0.9–3.1	
			≥5 g/day	2.0	1.1–3.7	
Willett *et al.* (1987)	USA, 89 538 registered nurses aged 34–59 years followed up for 4 years	601	0 g/day	1.0		Significantly increased RR independently for 5+ g/day of beer, 1.4 (1.1–1.8), liquor, 1.4 (1.1–1.7), but not wine, 1.1 (0.9–1.4). RR highest among thinner women and those without other risk factors for breast cancer (2.5; 1.5–4.2)
			<1.5 g/day	1.0	0.8–1.3	
			1.5–4.9 g/day	0.9	0.7–1.2	
			5.0–14.9 g/day	1.3	1.0–1.6	
			≥15 g/day	1.6	1.3–2.0	

[a] Calculated by the Working Group

SIRs were 1.0 for fewer than three drinks [not further specified] per day and 1.4 for three or more drinks per day. [The Working Group noted that, because of the way in which the question on alcohol use was asked, the authors were not able to divide the group consuming fewer than three drinks per day more finely, or to examine the effects of specific beverages.]

Hiatt *et al.* (1987) presented preliminary data in an abstract[1] on a separate cohort of 69 000 US women belonging to the same health care plan. During five years of follow-up (1979-84), 303 incident cases of breast cancer occurred. After controlling for age, race, body mass index and cigarette smoking, the SIRs were 1.5 for those consuming one to two drinks of any alcoholic beverage per day, 1.5 for those consuming three to five drinks per day, and 3.3 for those consuming six or more drinks per day. RRs were strongest among white and Hispanic and among postmenopausal women.

Schatzkin *et al.* (1987) analysed data from the first US National Health and Nutrition Examination Survey. At enrolment, 7188 women 25-74 years of age examined during 1971-75 were available for analysis. During a median of ten years of follow-up, 121 incident cases of breast cancer were diagnosed. After controlling for the effects of education, body mass index, dietary fat (based on a single 24-h recall) and reproductive factors, the adjusted RRs were similar or slightly higher than the crude relationships. When compared with women reporting no alcohol use during the previous year, the SIRs were 1.4 for women reporting an intake of $<$0.1-1.2 g ethanol per day, 1.6 for 1.3-4.9 g per day and 2.0 for $\geqslant$5 g per day. No data were available on the use of specific beverages. The highest SIRs were seen among the youngest and thinnest women.

Willett *et al.* (1987) examined the risk for breast cancer in relation to alcohol intake among members of the US Nurses' Health Study cohort. The alcohol intake of 89 538 registered nurses aged 34-59 years was assessed by questionnaire in 1980. The evaluation was validated by comparison with intake measured by a detailed day-by-day recording of all foods and beverages taken by a subgroup of 173 participants (see p. 154). In this study, comprehensive data on other dietary factors, including dietary fat, protein, fibre and vitamin A were also collected. During a follow-up of four years, 601 incident cases of breast cancer were ascertained. In comparison with women reporting no alcohol intake during the year prior to the baseline questionnaire, the RRs controlled for reproductive factors were 1.0 for $<$1.5 g ethanol per day, 0.9 for 1.5-4.9 g/day, 1.3 for 5.0-14.9 g/day and 1.6 for $\geqslant$15 g/day (Mantel extension χ for linear trend, 4.2; $p < 0.0001$). Controlling for nutritional factors as well as for family history of breast cancer and reproductive variables had no influence on the association of alcohol with risk for breast cancer. When the use of $\geqslant$5 g ethanol per day from specific alcoholic beverages was examined, controlling for the use of other alcoholic beverages simultaneously in a multivariate model, significant associations were found for beer (RR, 1.4) and spirits (1.4), but not for wine (1.1). For the latter, the CI includes the estimates for the other beverages, indicating that an association with wine is still quite plausible. The association with breast cancer risk was strongest among the women who were 45-54 years old and thinner. The relationship between alcohol intake and breast

[1]Subsequent to the meeting, this study was published in full (Hiatt *et al.*, 1988).

cancer tended to be somewhat stronger among current and past smokers than among those who had never smoked; however, this difference in RR was not significant. A particularly strong association was observed among those consuming 15 g or more ethanol per day and who had no other risk factor for breast cancer (RR, 2.5). Information on earlier alcohol intake was not collected; however, no elevation in risk for breast cancer was seen among women who were currently nondrinkers and reported that their alcohol intake had greatly decreased during the previous ten years. The authors noted that differential detection of breast cancer among alcohol users was unlikely to explain the positive associations because the percentage of cases with metastases in one or more lymph nodes was similar among the users and nonusers of alcohol.

(Descriptions of studies of cancers at many sites are given on pp. 158-164).

In the Framingham Heart Study (Gordon & Kannel, 1984), 28 deaths from breast cancer were ascertained. A small, nonsignificant, negative logistic regression coefficient was noted for alcohol intake. [The Working Group noted the small number of cases and the limited analysis.]

In the Kaiser-Permanente Study (Klatsky *et al.*, 1981), a total of 11 deaths from breast cancer was found; no relationship with alcohol consumption was detected. [The Working Group noted that the number of cases was too small to examine the relationship with alcohol intake.]

Adelstein and White (1976) identified 475 women in the UK Alcoholics Study and ascertained deaths for a period of up to 21 years. Ten deaths due to breast cancer occurred compared with an expected number of 4.9, yielding a SMR of 2.0. No control for confounding effects was possible.

A few breast cancer deaths were reported in the other cohort studies on alcoholics: Schmidt and deLint (1972), two cases; Monson and Lyon (1975), three cases (4.1 expected).

(ii) *Case-control studies*

Case-control studies of alcohol and breast cancer are summarized in Table 67.

In the study by Williams and Horm (1977; see description, pp. 170-171), 1167 breast cancer cases were reported, 1118 with known smoking and drinking habits. Data on other risk factors for breast cancer were not available. Overall, for women consuming less than 51 oz [<1200 g ethanol]-years, the RR was 1.3 ($p < 0.05$), and that for women consuming 51 or more oz-years was 1.6 ($p < 0.01$). For women consuming less than 51 and 51 or more oz-years of specific beverages, the RRs were 1.7 ($p < 0.01$) and 1.1 for wine, 1.2 and 1.4 for beer, and 1.4 ($p < 0.01$) and 1.4 ($p < 0.05$) for spirits. [The Working Group noted that the relationships with specific beverages were not controlled for the use of other alcoholic beverages, with which they tend to be highly correlated.]

Rosenberg *et al.* (1982) utilized data from a large drug-surveillance programme conducted in Canada, Israel and the USA to examine the relationship between alcohol intake and breast cancer risk. They identified 1152 incident cases (30-69 years old) and compared their alcohol use with that of two control series: 519 women with endometrial or ovarian cancer and 2702 women hospitalized for nonmalignant diseases. Drinkers of each

Table 67. Summary of results of case-control studies of breast cancer and alcohol intake

Place (reference)	Subjects (cases, controls)	Alcohol consumption[a]	Relative risk (RR)[b] (95% confidence interval)					Comments
			None	Total	Wine	Beer	Spirits	
USA, Multicenter (Williams & Horm, 1977)	1118, 3178	<50 oz [1200 g]-year	1.0	1.3*	1.7*	1.2	1.4*	Controlled for smoking, age, race
		≥51 oz [1200 g]-year	1.0	1.6*	1.1	1.4	1.4*	
			None	Total	Wine	Beer	Spirits	
Canada, Israel, USA (Rosenberg et al., 1982)	1152, 519 endometrial or ovarian cancer	<4 days/week	1.0	1.5 (1.1-2.1)	1.8*	2.0*	1.2	Control for educational level and reproductive factors had minimal effect on RR
		≥4 days/week		2.0 (1.3-2.0)	2.3	2.2	2.1*	
		Ex-drinker		1.3 (0.7-2.3)				
	1152, 2702 nonmalignant disorders	<4 days/week	1.0	1.9 (1.5-2.4)	2.2*	1.2	1.1	
		≥4 days/week		2.5 (1.9-3.4)	1.9*	2.1*	2.5*	
		Ex-drinker		1.6 (1.1-2.4)				
USA, Roswell Park, NY (Byers & Funch, 1982)	1314, 770	0 drinks/months (never)	1.0					No relation with beer, wine, spirits
		0 drinks/month (ex)	0.6					
		<3 drinks/month	1.1					
		3-8 drinks/month	1.0					
		9-25 drinks/month	1.1					
		≥26 drinks/month	1.1					
USA (Paganini-Hill & Ross 1983)	239, 239	Never drink	1.0					No relation with beer, wine, spirits
		≤1 drink/day	1.0					
		≥2 drinks/day	1.0					
USA (Begg et al., 1983)	997, 730	0 drinks/week	1.0					Adjusted for age and smoking
		1-7 drinks/week	0.9 (0.8-1.1)					
		>7 drinks/week	1.4 (0.9-2.0)					

Table 67 (contd)

Place (reference)	Subjects (cases, controls)	Alcohol consumption[a]	Relative risk (RR)[b] (95% confidence interval)	Comments
USA (Webster, L.A. *et al.*, 1983)	1226, 1279	0 g/week	1.0	Alcohol questions not clearly directed to period before diagnosis; no effect of beer, wine, spirits
		<50 g/week	0.9 (0.7–1.2)	
		50–149 g/week	0.9 (0.7–1.2)	
		150–199 g/week	1.1 (0.7–1.7)	
		200–249 g/week	1.1 (0.7–1.9)	
		250–299 g/week	1.0 (0.5–1.7)	
		≥300 g/week	1.1 (0.6–1.8)	
France (Lê *et al.*, 1984)	1010, 1950	Alcohol with meals	None 1.0; Total 1.5*; Cider 1.5; Beer 2.4*; Wine 1.4*	Matched for all characteristics; unknown participation rates; control for reproductive factors and dairy products did not affect risk
			Total alcohol	
	500, 945	0 g/week	1.0	
		1–79 g/week	1.0 (0.7–1.4)	
		80–159 g/week	1.4 (1.0–2.0)	
		160–239 g/week	1.5 (1.0–2.1)	
		≥240 g/week	1.2 (0.7–2.0)	
Northern Italy (Talamini *et al.*, 1984)	368, 373	Ever *versus* never	2.5 (1.7–3.7)	High participation rates, controlled for education, occupation and reproductive factors
		Wine: no use	1.0	
		<0.5 l [~50 g 100% ethanol]/day	2.4 (1.6–3.5)	
		≥0.5 l/day	16.7 (3.1–89.7)	
Milan, Italy (La Vecchia *et al.*, 1985)	437, 437	0 drinks/day	1.0	High participation rates, adjusted for reproductive factors, social class and years of education and limited dietary variables. Effect strongest among 40–49-years old
		≤3 drinks/day	1.3 (0.9–1.8)	
		>3 drinks/day	2.1 (1.1–4.0)	
		wine:		
		0 drink/day	1.0	
		≤3 drinks/day	1.2 (0.9–1.6)	
		>3 drinks/day	2.2 (1.1–4.7)	
		beer: any use	1.3 (0.8–2.1)	
		spirits: any use	1.4 (0.9–2.2)	

Table 67 (contd)

Place (reference)	Subjects (cases, controls)	Alcohol consumption[a]	Relative risk (RR)[b] (95% confidence interval)	Comments
USA, North Carolina (O'Connell *et al.*, 1987)	276, 1519	<1 drink/week ≥1 drink/wee	1.0 1.5 (1.0–2.1) premonopausal women, 1.9 (1.1–3.3) postmenopausal women, 1.2 (0.7–2.0)	Adjusted for race, oestrogen use, oral contraceptive use, cigarette smoking; no specific data on beverages
USA (Harvey *et al.*, 1987)	1524, 1896	Never 0.1–13 g/week 14–91 g/week 92–182 g/wee >183 g/week	1.0 1.1 (0.9–1.3) 1.1 (0.9–1.3) 1.3 (1.0–1.7) 1.7 (1.2–2.4)	Controlled for income, education and reproductive factors; effect almost entirely attributable to alcohol before age 30; independent effects of beer and spirits
Greece (Katsouyanni *et al.* 1986)	120, 120	Alcohol intake	Nonsignificant inverse trend	Low power; alcohol consumption levels not provided
Chile (Medina *et al.*, 1983)	76, 76	None Occasional Moderate Not specified	1.0 0.8 (0.4–1.8) 2.8 (0.7–10.9) 1.9 (0.5–6.7)	No adjustment for potential confounders

[a] g = 100% ethanol
[b] *, significant

specific beverage were asked whether they consumed that beverage on fewer than four or on more than four days per week. Using the cancer series as a control group, women drinking on fewer than four days per week experienced a RR of 1.5 compared with nondrinkers; the corresponding RR for those drinking four or more drinks per day was 2.0. With the nonmalignant series as the control group, the RR was 1.9 for fewer than four days per week and 2.5 for four or more days per week. Control for years of education and reproductive variables in multiple logistic regression analysis did not alter the relationship of alcohol use with breast cancer appreciably. When examined by specific beverage type, similar RRs were observed for beer, wine and spirits. [The Working Group noted that these were not controlled for correlated use.]

Byers and Funch (1982), responding in a letter to the report of Rosenberg *et al.*, provided data from a large case-control study conducted in Roswell Park Memorial Hospital in the USA during 1957-65. The drinking habits of 1314 incident cases of breast cancer (30-69 years old) were compared with those of 770 patients with nonneoplastic conditions who attended the same institution. These investigators found no relationship between breast cancer risk and alcohol use at any level, nor with consumption of beer, wine or spirits. The authors noted that their subjects had been raised in a rural area during the Prohibition era, which may have resulted in the observed low level of alcohol consumption.

Paganini-Hill and Ross (1983), also in a letter responding to the report of Rosenberg *et al.*, described the relationship between alcohol intake and breast cancer in a US retirement community in California. These authors identified 239 prevalent cases and compared their current alcohol intake with that of 239 matched community controls of similar social class. No elevation in risk was found for those consuming one or more drinks per day, and no association was found with either wine, beer or spirits. A subsample of 25 cases reported that they had not reduced their alcohol intake after the diagnosis of cancer.

In another letter following the report of Rosenberg *et al.*, Begg *et al.* (1983) compared the alcohol use among 997 breast cancer cases ascertained as part of the US Eastern Cooperative Oncology Group with that among 730 patients with other malignancies not thought to be related to alcohol use. After adjustment for age and smoking, the RRs were 0.9 for one to seven drinks per week and 1.4 for seven or more drinks per week (not significant).

Webster, L.A. *et al.* (1983) examined the relation between alcohol use and breast cancer in a large, multicentred US case-control study based on tumour registries that was primarily designed to address the effect of steroid hormone use on risk for this disease. Cases consisted of 1226 women, 20-54 years old, who were compared with 1279 controls identified by random digit telephone dialling. The response rates for interview were 82% for cases and 85% for those identified as potential controls. [The Working Group noted that the number of controls who were not contacted at all is never known when using the random-digit dialling procedure.] Women were first asked whether they had consumed any alcoholic beverage during the preceding five years. Those responding positively were then asked about their usual consumption of beer, wine and spirits. The authors noted that both the cases and controls reported intakes that were higher than those noted in national surveys. No relationship between alcohol use and breast cancer risk was observed; even for use of more than 300 g ethanol per week, the RR was only 1.1. No association with beer, wine or spirits was seen. [The Working Group noted that, since the cases were identified through tumour registries and were thus interviewed several months after diagnosis, it is possible that they had reduced their intake due to their disease and that this was reflected in their responses to questions about current intake; the questions on the amount of alcohol consumed were not specifically directed to the period before the diagnosis of breast cancer.]

In a study in France, Lê *et al.* (1984, 1986) reported on the association of alcohol use with breast cancer risk among patients attending 66 private surgical clinics. A simple measure of alcohol intake (whether or not it was usually consumed with meals) was available for the entire group of 1010 incident cases and 1950 clinical controls. A positive relationship with breast cancer risk was observed (RR, 1.5; $p = 0.0001$); controlling for the effects of reproductive factors and a limited set of dietary questions (mainly on consumption of dairy products) did not appreciably alter this finding (RR, 1.9; 1.4-2.6). Additional detailed questions on alcohol use were subsequently posed to the remaining 500 cases and 945 control women.The RRs were 1.0 for 1-79 g ethanol/week, 1.4 for 80-159 g/week, 1.5 for 160-239 g/week and 1.2 for 240 or more g/week. In this population, most alcohol was taken in the form of wine. A significant elevation in risk was also associated with beer consumption; no significant association was found for alcohol in the form of cider, but the use of this beverage was relatively low.

Talamini *et al.* (1984) conducted a case-control study in a northern Italian population that included information on the use of wine, the primary form of alcohol consumed in that area. They identified 368 cases (27-79 years old); controls consisted of 373 women hospitalized with acute conditions. Participation rates were 98% for both cases and controls. Multivariate analyses were used to control for the effects of education, occupation and reproductive variables; these analyses did not appreciably alter the crude relationships. In comparison with nondrinkers, the RR for use of <0.5 l of wine per day [~ 50 g ethanol] was 2.4, and for use of ≥0.5 l of wine per day, the RR was 16.7.

In another study from northern Italy, La Vecchia *et al.* (1985) obtained information on the number of drinks of specific alcoholic beverages per day from 437 incident cases of breast cancer (26-74 years old) and 437 patients hospitalized with acute conditions. Analyses were conducted adjusting for social class, years of education and reproductive variables. For women consuming three or fewer drinks per day, the RR was 1.3, and for those drinking more than three drinks per day it was 2.1. For consumption of more than three drinks of wine per day, the RR was 2.2. The effect was strongest for women 40-49 years old: RR of 3.5 for more than three drinks/day.

In a study from North Carolina, USA, O'Connell *et al.* (1987) studied alcohol intake among 276 incident cases and 1519 community controls. Analyses were adjusted for race, oestrogen use, oral contraceptive use and cigarette smoking. For women consuming one or more drinks of any alcoholic beverage per week compared with those consuming none or less than one drink per week, the RR was 1.5. No data on specific beverages were available. In this study, the effect of alcohol was limited to premenopausal women, among whom the RR was 1.9, as compared with 1.2 among postmenopausal women.

Harvey *et al.* (1987) conducted a nested case-control study within a population of participants in a national US cancer screening programme. A total of 1524 incident cases of breast cancer were identified in white women that had been diagnosed at least three years after entry into the screening programme. A total of 1896 control subjects were identified from among participants who did not develop cancer. In comparison with women who had never drunk alcohol, the RR was 1.1 for drinking 0.1-13 g ethanol per week, 1.1 for 14-91 g/week, 1.3 for 92-182 g/week and 1.7 for ≥183 g/week. Controlling for education, income and reproductive factors did not appreciably affect the RRs. Independent associations were observed for consumption of ≥92 g/week beer (RR, 1.7) and spirits (2.1) but not for wine (0.8). The authors noted that the lack of effect of wine may have been due to the small number of wine drinkers. The influence of alcohol use at different ages was examined in this study; the positive association with breast cancer was entirely attributable to alcohol use before the age of 30. For women who consumed >92 g ethanol per week before age 30, the risk for breast cancer was elevated whether or not they drank at later ages. However, the number of women who drank before age 30 and later stopped was small (15 cases), so that the distinction between those who continued and those who stopped is unstable. For alcohol consumption at less than 30 years of age, the association with risk for breast cancer did not vary by age at diagnosis, suggesting that a latent period effect was not present.

[The Working Group noted that in the studies of O'Connell *et al.* (1987) and Harvey *et al.* (1987) hospital or clinic controls were not used. Thus, the possibly lower alcohol consumption of hospital controls relative to members of the community at large (Anon., 1985b) is an unlikely explanation for the positive associations found between breast cancer and alcohol use.]

In a small case-control study in Greece of 120 cases and 120 orthopaedic patients as controls, Katsouyanni *et al.* (1986) observed a nonsignificant inverse relationship between alcohol intake and risk for breast cancer. [The Working Group noted that alcohol intake was not a focus of this study and few details are provided; levels of alcohol intake were not described.]

Medina *et al.* (1983) reported a small, hospital-based case-control study of breast cancer in Chile. Controls were patients hospitalized for cholecystectomy and matched by age with cases; 76 pairs were interviewed. In comparison with nondrinkers, moderate alcohol users (not defined) experienced a nonsignificant elevation in risk for breast cancer (RR, 2.8).

(iii) *Risk associated with type of alcoholic beverage*

In ten of the studies, data were collected on intake of specific alcoholic beverages. Wine intake was significantly associated with breast cancer in five studies (Williams & Horm, 1977; Rosenberg *et al.*, 1982; Lê *et al.*, 1984; Talamini *et al.*, 1984; La Vecchia *et al.*, 1985); beer intake was significantly associated with increased risk in four (Rosenberg *et al.*, 1982; Lê *et al.*, 1984; Harvey *et al.*, 1987; Willett *et al.*, 1987); and intake of spirits was significantly associated with increased risk in four (Williams & Horm, 1977; Rosenberg *et al.*, 1982; Harvey *et al.*, 1987; Willett *et al.*, 1987). Byers and Funch (1982), Paganini-Hill and Ross (1983) and Webster, L.A. *et al.* (1983) found no association with consumption of beer, wine or spirits.

The examination of the effects of specific beverages is complicated by the tendency among women, at least in some populations, to drink more than one type of alcoholic beverage. The effects of specific beverages are thus best studied using multivariate analyses in which the use of each beverage is controlled for use of the others. Only in the studies of Harvey *et al.* (1987) and Willett *et al.* (1987) was this form of analysis used; both showed significant independent effects of beer and spirits but not of wine. Although the effect of wine appears to be less than that of beer or spirits, the CI for wine drinking included the estimate for the other two beverages, precluding a firm conclusion about the effect of wine.

(iv) *Studies of joint exposure*

In most reports, data have not been included on the effects of joint exposures, and in those in which they were, the subgroups analysed differed. Age and menopausal status have been examined most commonly in connection with alcohol use, and, because of their high correlation, these variables are not distinguished for this purpose. Of the six studies that examined this association (La Vecchia *et al.*, 1985; Harvey *et al.*, 1987; Hiatt *et al.*, 1987; O'Connell *et al.*, 1987; Schatzkin *et al.*, 1987; Willett *et al.*, 1987), four found a higher RR among younger or premenopausal women, one showed no evidence for an interaction (Harvey *et al.*, 1987), and one found a higher RR among postmenopausal women (Hiatt *et al.*, 1987). The only other suggestion of an interaction, which has been observed in more than one study, is the observation of a higher RR among thin women (Schatzkin *et al.*, 1987; Willett *et al.*, 1987). Expressing alcohol intake in dose per kilogram of body mass did not appreciably alter the relation of alcohol intake with risk for breast cancer in the latter study. The RRs tend to be somewhat higher among women with no other risk factor for breast cancer; as noted previously, the RR was 2.5 for ⩾15 g ethanol per day among women with no other risk factor compared with the RR of 1.5 among other women (Willett *et al.*, 1987).

(*i*) *Cancer of the lung*

(i) *Cohort studies* (descriptions of studies of cancers at many sites are given on pp. 158-164)

Data from cohort studies on alcohol consumption and lung cancer are summarized in Tables 68 and 69.

In the study of Norwegian alcoholics (Sundby, 1967), 19 lung cancer deaths were observed with 13.2 expected on the basis of mortality figres for Oslo. No information on tobacco use was available, but the SMR for bronchitis was 2.3 when compared with Norwegian rates. In the study of Pell and D'Alonzo (1973), described on p. 210, five cases of lung cancer were observed in alcoholics and two in controls.

In the study of US veterans (Robinette *et al.*, 1979), mortality from lung cancer in alcoholics was no different from that in nasopharyngitis controls (64 and 66 deaths, respectively). Mortality from respiratory diseases as a whole, however, was significantly higher than in white US men (SMR, 1.36; $p < 0.01$). [The Working Group noted that smoking was not controlled for.]

Table 68. Relative risks (RR) for lung cancer in cohort studies without individual control of tobacco use

Study and reference	No. of subjects	RR[a]	Comments
Norwegian Alcoholics (Sundby, 1967)	19 deaths	3.5* 1.4	Compared with Norwegian population Compared with Öslo population
USA (Pell & D'Alonzo, 1973)	5 deaths	2.5	Two deaths among one-to-one matched controls
US Veterans Alcoholics (Robinette *et al.*, 1979)	64 deaths	1.1 (90% confidence interval, 0.8-1.4)	
Finnish Alcohol Misusers (Hakulinen *et al.*, 1974)	200 cases	2*	Expectancy (99.2) computed from whole population rates, but observed drawn from only the first third of the cohort in alphabetical order
Finnish Alcoholics (Hakulinen *et al.*, 1974)	33 cases	1.6*	
Massachusetts Alcoholics (Monson & Lyon, 1975)	19 deaths	1.3	
UK Alcoholics (Adelstein & White, 1976)	44 deaths	Men: 1.0 Women: 3.2*	
Dublin Brewery Workers (Dean *et al.*, 1979)	98 deaths	1.1 (0.9 if socio-economic status adjusted for)	Smoking was forbidden at the brewery for many years; according to relatives, 26 of 45 deceased smoked 23 cigarettes per day on average
Japanese Prospective Study (Hirayama, 1979)	611 deaths	Drinking / Smoking / RR Daily / Daily / 5.5 Occasionally / Daily / 4.7 No / Daily / 5.4 Not daily / No / 1.0	Actual numbers not stated

Table 68 (contd)

Study and reference	No. of subjects	RR[a]	Comments
Danish Brewery Workers (Jensen, 1980)	287 cases 280 deaths	1.2	Excess of the same order as for mineral-water bottlers (who did not have the right to free beer, data not shown) and as excess expected among persons of low socioeconomic class in Denmark
Canadian Alcoholics (Schmidt & Popham, 1981)	89 deaths	1.7, compared with Ontario population 1.0, compared with US veterans who smoked 21–29 cigarettes/day	Only 2% of cohort were lifetime nonsmokers, 94% were current smokers and 88% smoked >20 cigarettes/day

[a]*, significant

Table 69. Relative risks (RR) for lung cancer in cohort studies with quantitative information on consumption and individual control for tobacco use

Study and reference	Results			Comments
Kaiser Permanente (Klatsky *et al.*, 1981)	Usual no. of drinks/day in the last year	No. of lung cancer deaths and % mortality	RR	Among nonsmokers, the proportion of ex-smokers increases significantly with alcohol consumption, as well as the proportion of heavy smokers in the category of presently smoking. Furthermore, heavy drinkers include a 'slightly larger fraction who had smoked for over 20 years and of persons who inhaled' [data not shown]. Residual confounding highly probable
	0 (and ex-drinkers)	15 0.75%	1.0	
	≤2	7 0.35%	0.5	
	3–5	16 0.79%	1.1	
	≥6	24 1.19%	1.6*	
Norway (Kvåle *et al.*, 1983)	Vit. A index	No.	RR	RR for highest *versus* low current alcohol intake by vitamin A index, adjusted for age, smoking, geographical region, urban/rural residence and socio-economic status. Paper focuses on vitamin A and not on alcohol; a table refers to 65 histologically verified cases, but the overall incidence was 168
	Low	25	3.7	
	Medium	21	1.4	
	High	19	0.2	
	Total	65	1.3	
Framingham Study (Gordon & Kannel, 1984)	On the basis of 42 male and 9 female lung cancer deaths, a positive association (among males only) with level of alcohol consumption disappears after controlling for cigarettes/day, age, blood pressure, relative weight and lipoproteins			Ex-drinkers are grouped with nondrinkers; paper focuses on overall mortality and the categorization of alcohol consumption for studying cancer is not reported.

Table 69 (contd)

Study and reference	Results				Comments
Hawaiian-Japanese (Pollack *et al.*, 1984)	Usual monthly alcohol consumption (oz/month)	Age- and tobacco-adjusted incidence	RR		Alcohol used: 10% wine, 3.7% beer, 38% whisky. Crude data not shown, so importance of tobacco confounding and likelihood of residual confounding cannot be assessed. Incidence per 100 000 person-years, based on 89 incident cases confirmed by histological study
	None	70.1	1.00		
	<5	47.5	0.68		
	5–14	91.3	1.30		
	15–39	120.2	1.72		
	$\geq$40	130.5	1.86		
Japanese Doctors (Kono *et al.*, 1986)	Drinking habit	No. of deaths	Age-adjusted death rate	Age- and tobacco-adjusted RR	Apparent dose-effect relationship among consumers cannot be explained by residual tobacco confounding since there is no tobacco confounding.
	Never	24	11.5	1	
	Ex-drinker	5	5.4	0.6 (0.2–1.5)	
	Occasional	12	4.9	0.4* (0.2–0.8)	
	<43 mg/day	17	9.2	0.8 (0.4–1.4)	
	$\geq$43 mg/day	16	12.4	0.9 (0.5–1.7)	

In the Finnish study of alcoholics and alcohol misusers study (Hakulinen *et al.*, 1974), 200 cases of lung cancer were detected in alcohol misusers while 99 were expected (SIR, 2.0); 33 cases were observed among chronic alcoholics with 20.2 expected (SIR, 1.6). [The Working Group noted that, if the high RRs for alcohol misusers were due to confounding by tobacco, there would have been extreme differences in the smoking habits of the misusers and the control population; a lower SIR was seen for the alcoholics, who certainly drank more heavily than the misusers.]

In the study of Massachusetts alcoholics (Monson & Lyon, 1975), the proportionate cancer mortality ratio for lung cancer was 1.3, based on 19 lung cancer deaths. [The Working Group noted that there was no adjustment for smoking.]

In the UK follow-up study of alcoholics (Adelstein & White, 1976), a significant excess of lung cancer deaths was observed in women (8 *versus* 2.5 expected) but not in men (36 *versus* 35.3). [The Working Group noted that information on tobacco use was not available.]

In the study of Dublin brewery workers (Dean *et al.*, 1979), the SMR for lung cancer, adjusted for socioeconomic level, was 0.9.

In the Japanese prospective study (Hirayama, 1979), an analysis of the effect of drinking alcoholic beverages (none, occasionally, daily) in daily smokers was based on 611 deaths from lung cancer among men. The SMRs (compared with men who did not smoke or drink daily) were 5.4, 4.7 and 5.5, respectively, indicating no variation in relation to alcohol drinking. In a further analysis of 1324 lung cancer deaths observed in 16 years of follow-up of 122 261 males (Hirayama, 1985), the SMR associated with alcohol consumption [not otherwise defined], adjusted for tobacco, was 1.6. [The Working Group noted that the levels of exposure to alcohol and tobacco were not defined.]

In the study of Danish brewery workers (Jensen, 1980), both the SMR and SIR for lung cancer were 1.2 (95% CI, 1.0-1.3). The excess was of the same order among beer production workers (SIR, 1.1) and mineral-water bottlers (SIR, 1.3), was independent of duration of employment, and corresponded with expected social class differences. No data on smoking were provided, but the SMR for bronchitis was less than 1, indicating that smoking rates were not higher than in the general population.

In the study of Canadian alcoholics (Schmidt & Popham, 1981), the SMR for lung cancer was 1.7 ($p < 0.01$) in comparison with the population of Ontario; however, in comparison with the stratum of US veterans who most closely resembled the alcoholics in their smoking habits (21-39 cigarettes per day), the SMR for lung cancer was 1.0.

In the Kaiser-Permanente study (Klatsky *et al.*, 1981), cumulative mortality from lung cancer over ten years' follow-up was 0.7% (15 deaths) in persons consuming no drinks per day, 0.4% (7 deaths) in those consuming two or fewer, 0.8% (16 deaths) in those taking three to five, and 1.2% (24 deaths) in those taking six or more drinks per day. The authors noted that, although the groups were matched for smoking status, the group of heavy drinkers included more individuals who smoked heavily and the group of nondrinkers more individuals who had never smoked. [The Working Group noted that, although there was a significant difference between the two lowest consumption groups and the highest, the reported residual confounding by tobacco makes interpretation difficult.]

In a prospective cohort study on the effects of dietary vitamin A on lung cancer (Kvåle *et al.*, 1983) in Norway, in which 13 785 men and 2928 women were followed for 11.5 years, 168 incident cases of lung cancer were diagnosed. Alcohol use was analysed in a subset of the cohort in which the relevant information on consumption of alcohol, tobacco and vitamin A was available. The relative odds ratios estimated for the highest of three levels of alcohol consumption [groups not defined] *versus* the lowest were 3.7, 1.4, 0.2 and 1.3 for low, medium and high vitamin A index groups and for the whole group, respectively. The figures were based on 65 cases and were adjusted for age, cigarette smoking (never, ex-, current smokers of 1-19 and ≥20 cigarettes/day), region and urban/rural residence and socio-economic group.

In the Framingham study (Gordon & Kannel, 1984), 42 deaths from lung cancer deaths were observed in men. There was a nonsignificant association between lung cancer and alcohol consumption; but even this disappeared in logistic regression analysis, standardized for number of cigarettes per day, systolic blood pressure, age, relative weight and plasma lipoprotein levels. Only nine deaths from lung cancer were observed among women.

In the study of Hawaiian Japanese (Pollack *et al.*, 1984), with 89 incident cases of lung cancer, age- and smoking-adjusted incidence rates of lung cancer showed a significantly positive trend with total alcohol consumption. The SIRs compared with abstainers were 2.2 for those drinking at least 1.5 l of wine/month and 2.6 for those who drank at least 1.5 l of whisky/month; these were significantly elevated. Tobacco was controlled for by classifying smoking habits as never, former and current smokers; the results were the same when the subjects were classified into nonsmokers and current smokers, further subdivided according to the amount smoked (data not shown). The authors could not exclude the possibility that the apparent association between lung cancer and alcohol consumption was due to residual confounding by tobacco.

In the study of Japanese doctors (Kono *et al.*, 1986), there were 74 deaths from lung cancer. Nondrinkers had the highest SMR for lung cancer; among the drinkers, the SMRs rose with increasing alcohol consumption and were 0.6 for ex-drinkers, 0.4 for occasional drinkers, 0.8 for drinkers of <2 *go* [43 g ethanol] per day and 0.9 for drinkers of >2 *go* per day. Confounding by tobacco was controlled for by classifying smoking habits into five categories (non-, ex- and current smoker consuming 1-9, 10-19, 20+ cigarettes/day). [The Working Group considered that the observed dose-response effect among current drinkers is unlikely to reflect residual confounding by smoking, since adjustment for smoking had little effect on the estimates of alcohol-related RR.]

Three of the cohort studies described above (Klatsky *et al.*, 1981; Pollack *et al.*, 1984; Kono *et al.*, 1986) provide some information on the smoking-adjusted risk for lung cancer at various levels of alcohol consumption. There was a consistent pattern of decreased risk at low levels of alcohol consumption compared to non-/never drinkers and, among consumers, an increasing trend in risk with increasing level of consumption. In general, within each study, differences in risk associated with different levels of consumption are not statistically significant. Overall, the apparent increase in risk with increasing level of consumption is most likely to be attributable to residual confounding.

(ii) *Case-control studies*

Data from case-control studies on the association between alcohol consumption and lung cancer incidence are summarized in Table 70.

In a study on cancer incidence in North Wales and Liverpool, UK, in relation to habits and environment (Stocks, 1957; for description, see p. 206), the association of beer drinking with risk for lung cancer was studied by interviewing 485 male lung cancer patients aged 45-74 years, or their family members, and 4630 controls matched for age and area of residence. Of the cases, 328 were daily or weekly beer drinkers, while 273.0 would have been expected; the association was limited to those who smoked fewer than 100 cigarettes per week. [The Working Group noted that confounding could not be excluded.]

In a large case-control study in Paris, France (Schwartz *et al.*, 1962; for description, see p. 167), a significant difference was seen in the alcohol consumption of 1159 cases with bronchial cancer and that of 1196 controls with tobacco-unrelated cancers; this almost disappeared, however, after adjustment for smoking.

In a hospital-based case-control study in Durban, South Africa (Bradshaw & Schonland, 1969), 45 lung cancer patients and 341 controls without malignant disease were interviewed with regard to their alcohol consumption (use of Bantu beer, European spirits or local concoctions). A significantly greater number of cases than controls were consumers of local concoctions (53.3 *versus* 24.9%). [The Working Group noted that no adjustment was made for smoking habits or for age.]

Keller (1977) compared the relative frequency of lung cancer among patients discharged from the US complex of veterans' hospitals with cirrhosis and any cancer (286 men) with the relative frequency among patients without cirrhosis and any cancer (374 men). The frequency was not increased over that in patients without cirrhosis, even when cancers of the mouth, pharynx and digestive organs were excluded.

In the patient interview study of Williams and Horm (1977; for description, see pp. 170-171), an association was seen between the level of wine, beer, spirits or total ethanol consumption and lung cancer in both men and women. This association disappeared completely, however, when the analysis was performed on a subgroup for which the data allowed controlling for smoking (568 male and 155 female cases).

In a case-control study in Dublin, Ireland (Herity *et al.*, 1982), the alcohol consumption of 68 lung cancer patients was compared with that of a control group used in a previous study (Herity *et al.*, 1981) that examined the association between alcohol consumption and cancer of the larynx (see description, p. 184). The odds ratio of those with heavy alcohol consumption (in excess of 90 g ethanol per day for ten years) compared to non- and light drinkers was 2.1. The risk was greatly reduced, however, when alcohol intake was considered in the context of tobacco smoking (fewer than 20 cigarettes/day, 20 or more cigarettes/day). The authors concluded that the results were attributable almost entirely to confounding.

Table 70. Summary of results of case-control studies of lung cancer and alcohol intake

Place (reference)	Subjects (cases, controls)	Alcohol consumption	Results[a]					Comments
France, Paris (Schwartz et al., 1962)	Men (1159, 1196)	Mean alcohol consumption based on wine, cider, beer and spirits consumed over the last ten years	Highly significant difference (135 ml/day versus 113; χ^2, 42.5) decreases dramatically when cigarettes/day controlled for (χ^2, 5.8)					Authors considered that, with further adjustments, the significance of the association would disappear.
South Africa, Durban (Bradshaw & Schonland, 1969)	Men (45, 341)	User/nonuser of beer/European spirits or concoctions	More cases than controls were users of local concoctions					No individual control for tobacco use
USA, Multicenter (Williams & Horm, 1977)	Men (737, 2102)			Men		Women		RR for drinkers versus nondrinkers
	Men, adjusted for smoking (568, 2102)			Age-adj.	Age- & tobacco-adj.	Age-adj.	Age- & tobacco-adj.	
	Women (194, 3464)		Wine <50 oz-yr	0.9	0.6	0.9	0.7	
	Women, adjusted for smoking (155, 3464)		≥51 oz-yr	1.4	1.1	1.8	1.1	
			Beer <50 oz-yr	1.3	1.2	1.6	0.8	
			≥51 oz-yr	1.7*	1.1	2.3*	1.1	
			Spirits <50 oz-yr	1.2	0.9	1.7*	1.2	
			≥51 oz-yr	1.6*	1.1	1.3	0.6	
			Ethanol <50 oz-yr	1.2	0.9	1.5	1.1	
			≥51 oz-yr	1.6*	1.0	1.5	0.7	
Ireland, Dublin (Herity et al., 1981)	Men (59, 152)	Median lifetime exposure (90 g ethanol/day)		Alcohol				Tobacco-specific and crude RR for alcohol consumption. Risk of drinking above median is explained almost totally by association of heavy drinking with heavy smoking. The residual effect among light [1.5] and among heavy [1.2] smokers seems compatible with residual confounding.
			Smoking	None and light		Heavy		
			None and light	1.0		1.5 (0.4-5.2)		
			Heavy	10.6 (4.6-24.1)		12.4 (5.4-28.4)		
			All	1.0		2.1 (1.1-3.8)		

[a]*, significant

(j) *Cancer of the urinary bladder*

(i) *Cohort studies* (descriptions of studies of cancers at many sites are given on pp. 158-164)

Cohort studies on mortality according to alcohol consumption which mention bladder cancer deaths are summarized in Table 71. In the prospective Japanese study (Hirayama, 1979), analysis of 77 deaths from bladder cancer in men showed no significant difference in the SMRs for daily drinkers and nondrinkers among daily smokers. In the study of Danish brewery workers (Jensen, 1980), the risk for bladder cancer was not elevated. In two small studies (Pell & D'Alonzo, 1973; Robinette *et al.*, 1979), the numbers of observed and expected cases of bladder cancer were one and 0 and none and 3, respectively.

Table 71. Relative risks (RR) for bladder cancer in cohort studies

Study and reference	No. of subjects	Results and comments
USA, one company (Pell & D'Alonzo, 1973)	1 death	None among one-to-one matched controls not known to be alcoholic
Finnish Alcoholics (Hakulinen *et al.*, 1974)	5 cases	3.2 expected; RR, 1.6 (urinary organs)
Massachussets Alcoholics (Monson & Lyon, 1975)	4 deaths	3.9 expected; RR, 1.0 (bladder and other urinary organs)
Japanese Prospective Study (Hirayama, 1979)	77 deaths	Drinking / Smoking / RR: daily / daily / 1.4 occasionally / daily / 1.6 no / daily / 1.4 no / no / 1.0 No. of subjects and significance not stated
US Veterans Alcoholics (Robinette *et al.*, 1979)	0	Three expected
Danish Brewery Workers (Jensen, 1980)	75 cases	86.7 expected; RR, 0.9 (95% confidence interval, 0.7-1.1)

In four further cohort studies, no distinction was made between deaths from cancer of the bladder and other parts of the urinary tract and death from other genitourinary cancers. In the study of Hawaiian Japanese (Blackwelder *et al.*, 1980), ten subjects who had died from prostatic or urinary tract cancer had had a higher unadjusted mean ethanol consumption (26.7 ml (21 g) per day) than survivors (13.6 ml (11 g) per day). A further follow-up of the same cohort showed no excess of prostatic or urinary bladder cancer

(Pollack *et al.*, 1984), but the data were not adjusted for age or tobacco use. In the Kaiser-Permanente study (Klatsky *et al.*, 1981), the distribution of 22 deaths from genitourinary cancer (ICD-8 180-189) among nondrinkers and drinkers of one to two, three to five and six or more drinks per day suggested no association. In the study of chronic alcoholics in Helsinki (Hakulinen *et al.*, 1974), five incident cases of cancers of urinary organs except prostate were observed, with 3.2 expected. In the study of Massachussets alcoholics (Monson & Lyon, 1975), four cases of cancer of the bladder and other urinary organs were observed; 3.9 were expected.

(ii) *Case-control studies*

Data from studies in which the association between alcohol consumption and bladder cancer risk was considered are shown in Table 72.

In the hospital-based case-control study in Paris, France (Schwartz *et al.*, 1957, 1962; see description, p. 167), the average daily ethanol consumption of the 214 cases (113 ml (89 g) per day) was not different from that of the accident controls (120 ml (95 g) per day) or of the cancer controls (113 ml (89 g)/day).

In a hospital-based case-control study in New York, USA (Wynder *et al.*, 1963b) of 200 male bladder cancer patients and an equal number of age-matched hospital controls (excluding patients with respiratory or upper gastrointestinal cancer or myocardial infarction), no association was detected between bladder cancer and the number of drinks consumed per day. [The Working Group noted that smoking was not controlled for.]

Dunham *et al.* (1968) interviewed 493 patients with bladder cancer (98.8% histologically confirmed) and 527 controls (mostly patients with diseases other than of the urinary tract and other than cancer) in New Orleans, USA, about factors that might have influenced their diseases (e.g., use of alcoholic beverages). No consistently positive or negative correlation with the use of alcoholic beverages was detected. [The Working Group noted the incomplete reporting of the results, and the lack of statistical evaluation and adjustment for smoking.]

In a case-control study in Canada (Morgan & Jain, 1974), 74 female and 155 male incident cases of histologically verified transitional-cell carcinoma of the bladder were compared with individually age- and sex-matched controls with benign prostatic hypertrophy (158 men) or stress incontinence (73 women). Alcohol use and smoking habits were analysed by a postal questionnaire comprising a seven-day diary of all fluid intake. Alcohol intake (ever/never) was not significantly related to cancer incidence when stratification by smoking habits (ever/never) was performed. A crude odds ratio of 1.2 fell to 1.1 after adjustment for tobacco use and sex, as calculated by the Working Group.

In the patient interview study of Williams and Horm (1977; see description pp. 170-171), no association was detected between consumption of beer, wine or spirits or total ethanol consumption and bladder cancer. The analysis was based on 229 male and 77 female cases not controlled for smoking, and 206 and 73 cases controlled for smoking. After controlling for tobacco use, the association becomes negative, especially among women. A nonsignificant positive trend with high-level beer consumption in men disappears when tobacco use is taken into account.

Table 72. Summary of results of case-control studies of bladder cancer and alcohol intake

Place (reference)	Subjects (cases, controls)	Alcohol consumption	Results[a]	Comments
USA, New York (Wynder et al., 1963b)	Men (200, 200)	No. of drinks		Crude RR and 95% CI calculated by the Working Group
		<1/month	1.0	
		1/month–6/week	1.1 (0.6–2.0)	
		1–2/day	0.9 (0.5–1.7)	
		3–6/day	1.2 (0.6–2.4)	
		7–12/day	2.1 (0.8–5.6)	
		12+	0.7 (0.2–2.7)	
		Sporadic binges	0.8 (0.3–2.4)	
USA, New Orleans (Dunham et al., 1968)	Men, women (493, 527)	Present or past occasional, light, moderate or heavy drinking		Data not shown; no consistently positive or negative association
Canada, Toronto (Morgan & Jain, 1974)	Men, women (229, 231)	Users versus non-users	1.2 (0.8–1.7) 1.1 (0.7–1.6) after adjustment for tobacco use (yes/no) and sex	Crude RR and 95% CI calculated by the Working Group
USA, Multicenter (Williams & Horm, 1977)	Men (229, 2102) Men, smoking controlled for (206, 1788) Women (77, 3464) Women, smoking controlled for (73, 3188)	Two cumulative lifetime drinking categories versus non-drinkers (at least one serving at least once a week for one year)	A nonsignificant positive trend with high-level beer consumption in men (RR, 1.4) disappears when tobacco is taken into account (RR, 1.1)	
Denmark (Mommsen et al., 1982)	Men (165, 165)	Users versus non-users	2.5 (1.0–6.3) 1.6 after adjustment for smoking (yes/no) and other variables	Crude RR

Table 72 (contd)

Place (reference)	Subjects (cases, controls)	Alcohol consumption	Results[a]		Comments
USA, ten areas (Thomas *et al*., 1983)	Men, women (2982, 3313)	Servings/week	Men	Women	Adjusted RR
		0	1.0	1.0	
		<3	0.9	0.8	
		4–6	0.9	0.9	
		7–13	1.0	0.8	
		14–17	0.9	1.0	
		28–41	1.1	0.9	
		≥42	1.0	0.7	
Federal Republic of Germany (Claude *et al*., 1986)	Men (340, 340) Women (91, 91)	Beer (l/day)	Men	Women	No evidence of effect among nonsmokers
		0.1–0.5	1.2	1.4	
		0.6–1.0	2.1*		
		>1	2.8*		
		Wine (l/day)			
		0.1–0.3	1.0	1.9	
		>0.3	0.8		
		Spirits (l/week)			
		0.1–0.5	1.5	1.2	
		>0.5	2.7*		
USA, Missouri (Brownson *et al*., 1987)	Men (846, 2536)	Never	1.0		Adjusted RR
		Ex	0.9 (0.5–1.5)		
		Current <2 drinks/day	1.2 (0.9–1.5)		
		Current ≥2 drinks/day	0.8 (0.6–1.1)		

[a]Relative risk (RR) and 95% confidence interval (CI); *, significant

In a population-based case-control study in Denmark (Mommsen *et al.*, 1982), 165 incident male cases of bladder cancer (91.5% invasive bladder cancer) and an equal number of age-, sex-and geographical area-adjusted controls were interviewed by telephone. Alcohol consumption was related to cancer incidence (crude odds ratio, 2.5; not significant). In a multivariate logistic analysis, the effect of alcohol after adjustment for cigarette smoking (yes/no), prostatic symptoms and occupation was reduced to 1.6.

In a population-based case-control study in ten areas of the USA (Thomas *et al.*, 1983), 2982 incident cases of histologically confirmed bladder cancer and 3313 general population controls were interviewed. Cases were 73% of eligible incident cases from cancer registries; controls were 82% of those identified through random selection from census fields and through random-digit telephone dialing. Alcohol consumption was estimated separately for beer, wine and spirits as the number of servings (a can, bottle or draught of beer, a 118-ml glass of wine or a 44-ml jigger of spirits) consumed during a typical week in the previous winter. After adjustment for potential confounding factors (age, sex, race, geographical location, cigarette smoking status, hazardous occupational exposure), no association between total ethanol consumption (odds ratio, 0.7-1.1) or consumption of wine, beer or spirits (odds ratio, 0.6-1.2) and bladder cancer was detected.

In a case-control study in northern Federal Republic of Germany (Claude *et al.*, 1986), 340 male and 91 female patients with histologically proven tumours of the lower urinary tract and the same number of age- and sex-matched hospital or local controls with no tumour, mainly from urological departments, were interviewed directly about consumption of different alcoholic beverages. After adjustment for smoking (lifetime cifarette consumption), beer drinkers had an overall increased RR and a clear dose-response relationship with daily intake. Drinkers of spirits also had an elevated odds ratio [1.9], while no association was found with drinking of wine. No increased risk was seen for nonsmokers who drank beer and spirits. In a multiple regression analysis, after adjustment for high-risk occupation, the risk for consumption of beer and spirits was substantially reduced and was no longer significant after adjustment for daily fluid intake. [The Working Group noted that beer and spirits were included in fluid intake and the adjustment may thus have erroneously biased the estimate of RR towards 1.]

In a case-control study based on patients registered by the Missouri Cancer Registry (Brownson *et al.*, 1987), 823 histologically verified incident cases of bladder cancer in white men were compared with 2469 cases of cancer unrelated to tobacco use (three controls per case, frequency-matched by age groups; 40% prostatic cancer and 33.5% cancers of the digestive organs and peritoneum). [The Working Group noted that the distribution of cases and controls by alcohol consumption, on which the RRs were computed, included a larger number of subjects than stated in the description of sources: 846 cases and 2536 controls with known alcohol use plus 216 cases and 596 controls with unknown alcohol use.] Information on alcohol and tobacco consumption and main occupation is systematically reported to the Registry by Missouri hospitals using a standardized protocol. No association with alcohol consumption was found, whether controlling for tobacco use and age or not. The age- and tobacco-adjusted RRs for ex-drinkers and for current drinkers (*versus* nondrinkers) were 0.9 and 1.1, respectively. Exclusion of cases of colon and rectal cancers from among the controls did not change the results.

(*k*) *Cancers at other sites*

(i) *Soft tissue*

Data on malignant tumours of soft tissue (ICD 171) are provided in the study of Danish brewery workers (based on eight observed incident cases), which shows a RR of 1.2 [95% CI, 0.52-2.36] for the whole cohort (Jensen, 1980; see pp. 162-163), and in the study of Williams and Horm (1977; see pp. 170-171), based on 45 male and 39 female cases, which shows no association.

(ii) *Skin*

In the study of Danish brewery workers (Jensen, 1980; see pp. 162-163), 77 cases of epithelial skin cancer (ICD 173) were observed with 101.9 expected (SIR, 0.8; 95% CI, 0.6-0.9). In the same study, 15 cases of melanoma were observed (SIR, 1.3; 95% CI, 0.7-2.1). In the study of chronic alcoholics in Helsinki (Hakulinen *et al.*, 1974; see p. 159), five cases of skin cancer (including basal-cell carcinoma) were observed with 6.6 expected.

In the case-control study in France (Schwartz *et al.*, 1962; see p. 167), the average ethanol consumption (129 ml (112 g)/day) of 154 patients with skin cancer (not otherwise specified) was very close to that of accident controls (139 ml; 110 g) and of cancer controls (113 ml; 89 g).

The interview study of Williams and Horm (1977; see pp. 170-171) suggested an association of melanoma with moderate alcohol consumption in men but not in women and not for higher consumption levels. The analysis was based on 40 male and 59 female cases of melanoma.

(iii) *Ovary*

The association between ovarian cancer and alcohol consumption has been considered in four case-control studies.

A study of 92 cases of ovarian malignancies and 92 cases of benign ovarian tumours in the USA, matched for age, residence and date of surgery, showed no significant difference between alcohol users and nonusers (West, 1966). [The Working Group noted that the actual figures are not given.]

The patient interview study of the Third National Cancer Survey (Williams & Horm, 1977; see description pp. 170-171), based on 180 cases and 3367 controls with cancers unrelated to tobacco use, provides a nonsignificant RR of 0.9 (not controlled for smoking) for both drinkers of 1-50 and 51 or more oz-years of ethanol, with reference to nondrinkers. For 153 cases of ovarian cancer in which smoking was controlled, the RRs were even lower.

A hospital-based case-control study at the Roswell Park Memorial Institute, USA, of 274 epithelial carcinomas of the ovary in white women aged 30-79 years and of 1034 controls (excluding cancer, gastrointestinal and endocrine disease) showed no association with alcohol consumption for women over 49 years of age (RR, 0.8-1.1). There was, however, a nonsignificant decreasing trend with increasing consumption (RR, 0.84 for one to eight drinks/week and 0.56 for nine or more) for women 30-49 years old (Byers *et al.*, 1983).

In the USA, a population-based case-control study of ovarian cancer in women under 55 years of age based on 433 incident cases (71% of total incidence) and 2915 controls (83% of potential controls selected through random-digit telephone dialing) showed a significantly lower risk (0.5; 93% CI 0.2-0.9) for 'heavy' users (250 g ethanol per week or more), especially among younger women. The estimates were adjusted for age, smoking, education, reproductive factors and oral contraceptive use (Gwinn *et al.*, 1986).

(iv) *Other organs of the female genital tract*

In the study of Canadian alcoholics (Schmidt & de Lint, 1972; see p. 164), five deaths from cancer of the uterus (not otherwise specified) were observed, with 1.4 expected. In the study of UK alcoholics (Adelstein & White, 1976; see p. 159), four deaths from cervical cancer were observed, with 0.9 expected.

The study of Williams and Horm (1977; see description pp. 170-171) showed no evidence of an association for cancers of the cervix, uterine corpus and vulva (based on 249, 345 and 30 cases, respectively, adjusted for age, race and tobacco use). The estimated RRs for both cervical and uterine corpus cancers were slightly lower than 1.0.

A study of 257 pairs of cervical cancer patients and controls (23-86 years old) in Lesotho, South Africa, showed a three-fold elevated risk among women who consumed indigenous alcohol and a two-fold risk for women who drank European alcoholic beverages after adjustment for tobacco use and other beverages (Martin & Hill, 1984).

[The Working Group noted that no adjustment for social and sexual variables was attempted in these studies.]

(v) *Prostate*

In the study of Norwegian alcoholics (Sundby, 1967; see pp. 158-159), 16 deaths from prostatic cancer were observed while 11.4 were expected on the basis of mortality in Oslo. Three deaths from prostatic cancer were observed in the follow-up of 922 alcoholics employed by a US company and none among matched controls (Pell & D'Alonzo, 1973; see p. 210). One case of prostatic cancer, with 2.8 expected, was observed among chronic alcoholics in Helsinki (Hakulinen *et al.*, 1974; see p. 159), and three cases, with 2.4 expected, were observed in the study of UK alcoholics (Adelstein & White, 1976; see p. 159).

In the Japanese prospective study (Hirayama, 1979; see p. 162), 63 deaths from prostatic cancer were reported; the SMR for daily drinking and daily smoking, as compared with nonsmokers and men who did not drink daily was 1.0 and 0.90 for daily smoking only. [The Working Group noted that the actual figures were not given.]

In the study of alcoholic US veterans (Robinette *et al.*, 1979; see p. 163), two deaths from prostatic cancer were observed, corresponding to a SMR of 0.55 (90% CI, 0.07-2.93). In the cohort of Danish brewery workers (Jensen, 1980; see pp. 162-163), 80 incident cases of prostatic cancer were observed, with 81.1 expected (SIR, 1.0; 95% CI, 0.8-1.2) in the total cohort. In the study of Canadian alcoholics, 11 deaths were seen; the SMR was 1.09 with reference to the Ontario population, and 1.43 with reference to US veterans who smoked 21-39 cigarettes/day (Schmidt & Popham, 1981).

The study of Hawaiian Japanese (Pollack *et al.*, 1984; see p. 163) provides age- and smoking-adjusted incidence rates according to amount of ethanol consumed, based on 84 incident cases of prostatic cancer. These suggest no evidence of a trend with increasing consumption.

In the case-control study of alcohol and cancer in France (Schwartz *et al.*, 1962; see description p. 167), the average consumption of 139 patients with prostatic cancer (110 ml (87 g) ethanol/day) was similar to that of controls (113 ml (89 g)).

A hospital-based case-control study in New York City of 217 patients with clinical cancer of the prostate and 200 controls with no known disease of the prostate showed no difference in alcohol consumption between the two groups (77% and 81%, respectively, were alcohol drinkers). Alcohol consumption was categorized into 1-2, 3-6, 7 or more units/day or binge, where a unit is 1 oz spirits, 4 oz wine or 8 oz beer (Wynder *et al.*, 1971).

In the study of Keller (1977; see p. 239), the age-adjusted relative frequency of prostatic cancer was slightly lower among cirrhotics. [The Working Group noted that when cases of cancer of the upper respiratory and digestive organs were excluded from the controls, the proportion of prostatic cancer among cirrhotics was slightly higher (16.7%) than among noncirrhotics (13.7%).]

In the study of Williams and Horm (1977; see pp. 170-171), of 531 cases of prostatic cancer and 1656 controls with cancer not related to tobacco use, the age- and race-adjusted odds ratios for consuming 1-50 and ≥51 oz-years of ethanol were, respectively, 0.78 and 0.84. Controlling for tobacco (465 cases and 1323 controls) did not change the estimates (odds ratios, 0.78 and 0.87).

(vi) *Testis*

Cohort studies provide no evidence that alcohol drinking in adult life affects testicular cancer incidence. The study of Danish brewery workers (Jenson, 1980; see pp. 162-163) shows a RR of 0.7 (95% CI, 0.4-1.1), based on 15 observed incident cases. In the study of alcoholic US veterans (Robinette *et al.*, 1979; see p. 163), no death from testicular cancer was observed, but there were two in the one-to-one matched comparison group.

In the hospital-based case-control study in Paris (Schwartz *et al.*, 1962; see p. 167), the average ethanol consumption reported by 37 patients with testicular cancer (112 ml (88 g)/day) was very close to that reported by the cancer control group (113 ml (89 g)) and lower than that of the accident controls (139 ml (110 g)).

In a case-control study of prenatal and perinatal factors for testicular cancer (Brown *et al.*, 1986), the alcohol consumption of the mothers of 202 cases was compared with that of 206 cases of other cancers as controls. Mothers were interviewed, and 20.3% reported consuming one to 14 drinks of alcoholic beverages per week, with a median of one drink. The crude RR (1.6; 95% CI, 1.0-2.7) for maternal alcohol consumption was confounded by smoking. No clear dose-response relationship was seen: the RR was 2.3 (1.0-5.2) for more than one drink per week and 1.1 (0.6-2.2) for one drink per week. The association was no longer significant when smoking and birth weight were taken into account in multivariate analyses.

(vii) *Kidney*

Two deaths from kidney cancer were observed in alcoholics and one in matched nonalcoholics in the cohort study of US company (Pell & D'Alonzo, 1973; see p. 210). One death from cancer of the 'kidney, ureter or other' was observed in the study of alcoholic US veterans, and four were seen in the comparison group (Robinette *et al.*, 1979; see p. 163).

In the Japanese prospective study (Hirayama, 1979; see p. 162), the SMR for kidney cancer was 1.4 for daily drinking and daily smoking and 1.4 for daily smokers only, compared with subjects who did not smoke and did not drink daily. [The Working Group noted that the actual number of cases was not given.]

In the study of Danish brewery workers (Jensen, 1980; see pp. 162-163), the RR for kidney cancer was 1.0 (95% CI, 0.7-1.4), based on 38 incident cases in the total cohort.

In the study of Schwartz *et al.* (1962; see p. 167), the average ethanol consumption of 69 kidney cancer cases (108 ml (85 g)/day) was similar to that of cancer controls (113 ml (89 g)). Accident controls consumed an average of 126 ml (99 g)/day .

The study of Williams and Horm (1977; see pp. 170-171) showed no association with alcohol consumption in either the 73 male or 53 female cases.

(viii) *Brain*

No death from brain cancer was seen in alcoholics but one in nonalcoholic controls in the study of Pell and D'Alonzo (1973; see p. 210). Among chronic alcoholics in Helsinki (Hakulinen *et al.*, 1974; see p. 159), two cases of cancer of the nervous system were observed when 1.9 were expected. The Japanese prospective study (Hirayama, 1979; see p. 162) suggested no effect of alcohol on brain cancer mortality: SMR, 1.2 for daily smoking and daily drinking, 1.5 for daily smoking and occasional drinking and 1.1 for daily smoking only.

A significant excess of brain tumours (five observed deaths against none in matched control patients with nasopharyngitis) was observed in the study of alcoholics among US veterans (Robinette *et al.*, 1979; see p. 163).

Among Danish brewery workers (Jensen, 1980; see pp. 162-163), the RR for brain and nervous system cancers, based on 37 incident cases, was 1.1 (95% CI, 0.8-1.5).

The study of Williams and Horm (1977; see pp. 170-171) compared 75 male and 61 female cases of cancer of the nervous system with cases of cancer unrelated to tobacco use. A significant negative association for the highest category of total ethanol consumption (RR, 0.4) was observed for men only.

(ix) *Thyroid cancer*

In the study of chronic alcoholics in Helsinki (Hakulinen *et al.*, 1974; see p. 159), one case of thyroid cancer was observed with 0.4 expected.

Among men in the study of Williams and Horm (1977; see pp. 170-171), there was a positive trend, with RRs of 1.1 and 1.7 for the two categories of total ethanol consumption when not controlled for smoking (based on five and nine cases, respectively). Among women, the corresponding figures were 1.6 (based on 18 cases) and 0.6 (based on two cases). The analysis comprised 30 men and 86 women with thyroid tumours.

(x) *Lymphatic and haematopoietic system*

One case of lymphoma and one of leukaemia were observed in the study of chronic alcoholics in Helsinki (Hakulinen *et al.*, 1974; see p. 159), with 1.7 and 1.2 expected, respectively.

The study of Williams and Horm (1977; see pp. 170-171) suggested that subjects with low alcohol consumption may have a lower risk of lymphosarcomas or Hodgkin's disease and a higher risk for leukaemias with respect to nondrinkers; the differences were not statistically significant, however, and there was no difference for subjects in the highest consumption category.

The study of alcoholic US veterans showed a SMR of 0.9 (based on 13 observed deaths) for lymphatic and haematopoietic cancers and a SMR of 0.5 (based on three observed cases) for leukaemia (Robinette *et al.*, 1979; see p. 163).

In the Hawaiian Japanese prospective study (Blackwelder *et al.*, 1980; see p. 163), 13 subjects died from cancer of the lymphatic and haematopoietic tissues in eight years. Their mean ethanol consumption (43.9 ml (35 g)/day) was higher than that of survivors (13.6 ml (11 g)/day). These figures are not, however, adjusted for age.

The study of Danish brewery workers (Jensen, 1980; see pp. 162-163) showed a SIR of 1.0 (based on 68 observed incident cases; 95% CI, 0.8-1.3) for lymphatic and haematopoietic cancers in the total cohort.

In the study of Keller (1977; see p. 239), the age-adjusted relative frequency of cancers of lymphatic and haematopoietic tissues was lower among cirrhotics both before and after exclusion of patients with alcohol-related cancers from among the controls.

6. SUMMARY OF DATA REPORTED AND EVALUATION

6.1 Chemical composition, consumption and trends

Alcoholic beverages are produced from raw materials by fermentation. The predominant types of commercially produced alcoholic beverages are beer, wine and spirits. The main components of all alcoholic beverages are ethanol and water; beers also contain substantial amounts of carbohydrates. Many compounds that have been identified as common to all alcoholic beverages are present in different quantities depending on the beverage. Some components and occasional contaminants include known and suspected carcinogens. Beers and wines also contain vitamins and other nutrients which are usually absent from distilled spirits. Despite the differences in concentration, the average intake of ethanol per drink is approximately constant across beverage types.

Alcoholic beverages, both home-made and commercially produced, have long been consumed in most parts of the world. Recorded consumption tends to be higher in societies with populations of European origin and lower in Muslim societies. In most of the developed countries, a majority of adults consume alcoholic beverages at least occasionally.

Since 1950, consumption per head has increased substantially in most parts of the world, although since the mid-1970s a reduction in the rate of increase and, in some countries, a decline in consumption have occurred. Drinking patterns — overall level of alcohol consumption, choice of alcoholic beverages, differences by sex and age and temporal variations — differ among and within societies.

6.2 Experimental carcinogenicity data

Ethanol and some alcoholic beverages were tested for carcinogenicity in five studies in mice by oral administration. Ethanol was also tested in one experiment by transplacental exposure or exposure *via* mother's milk. Due to severe limitations in experimental design or conduct, these studies could not be used for an evaluation of carcinogenicity.

Two studies involved oral administration of ethanol and of one alcoholic beverage to rats. One study was inadequate for evaluation, and in the other no difference in the incidence of tumours was found.

In seven studies, ethanol or an alcoholic beverage was administered to rats as a control in studies of combined effects with a known carcinogen. In one of these, involving male animals only, ethanol administered in water as the drinking fluid significantly increased the incidences of hepatocellular carcinomas and of tumours of the pituitary gland, of the adrenal gland and of pancreatic islet cells, but neither isocaloric nor isonutrient diets were used. All of these studies, however, suffered from various limitations and could not be used for evaluation.

Ethanol and certain alcoholic beverages were administered to hamsters by oral administration in four studies, three of which were designed to ascertain combined effects with known carcinogens. All of these studies suffered from various limitations and could not be evaluated. One study in mice involving application of ethanol or residues of alcoholic beverages to the skin could also not be evaluated.

In experiments in which various carcinogens were administered orally with ethanol as a vehicle, ethanol enhanced the incidence of nasal cavity tumours induced in mice by *N*-nitrosodimethylamine and enhanced the incidences of oesophageal/forestomach tumours and lung tumours induced in mice by *N*-nitrosodiethylamine or *N*-nitrosodi-*n*-propylamine.

In further studies, various carcinogens were administered by different routes simultaneously with ethanol in water as the drinking fluid or in liquid diets. Ethanol enhanced the incidence of benign tumours of the nasal cavity induced in rats by *N'*-nitrosonornicotine given in a liquid diet, and enhanced the incidences of nasal cavity and tracheal tumours and of neoplastic nodules of the liver induced in hamsters by *N*-nitrosopyrrolidine given by intraperitoneal injection. Administration of ethanol in the drinking-water enhanced the incidences of hepatocellular carcinomas and of liver angiosarcomas induced in rats by inhalation of vinyl chloride.

In a number of other experiments, ethanol had no modifying effect on the overall incidence of tumours in mice, rats or hamsters given *N*-nitrosomethylbenzylamine, *N*-nitrosobis(2-oxopropyl)amine, *N*-methyl-*N'*-nitro-*N*-nitrosoguanidine, 7,12-dimethyl-benz[*a*]anthracene or 1,2-dimethylhydrazine by various routes of administration.

There is *sufficient evidence* for the carcinogenicity of acetaldehyde (the major metabolite of ethanol) in experimental animals.

6.3 Human carcinogenicity data

Cancers of the oral cavity and pharynx

In six retrospective cohort studies of persons with an intake of alcoholic beverages higher than that of the reference population and including alcoholics and brewery workers, the risk for cancers of the oral cavity and pharynx (effectively excluding the nasopharynx) has been examined. In five studies of alcoholics, the relative risk was significantly increased by between two and five fold.

In two prospective cohort studies, the risk for cancers of the oral cavity, pharynx, larynx and oesophagus combined and for cancers of the oral cavity, pharynx and oesophagus combined increased with the daily number of drinks.

Case-control studies have been performed of cancers of the oral cavity (11 studies), pharynx (ten studies), and oral cavity and pharynx combined (two studies). In all but two of the studies, the risk increased significantly with increasing level of consumption of alcoholic beverages; in two studies, nonsignificant increases were observed. These results persisted after adjustment for tobacco smoking. The risk increased with daily intake of alcoholic beverages at any level of tobacco smoking in six studies in which this was examined, and the risk for cancer increased with amount drunk by nonsmokers in three out of four studies in which this aspect was examined.

Epidemiological studies clearly indicate that drinking of alcoholic beverages is causally related to cancers of the oral cavity and pharynx (excluding the nasopharynx). There is no indication that the effect is dependent on type of beverage.

Cancer of the larynx

Data on laryngeal cancer were provided by six retrospective cohort studies — five of alcoholics and one of brewery workers. The risk for laryngeal cancer was significantly increased by two to five fold in four of the studies.

Fourteen case-control studies in North America and Europe all showed that the relative risk increased with level of intake of alcoholic beverages. Three large studies indicated that the risk associated with intake of alcoholic beverages was stronger for cancer at sites at the junction between the larynx and pharynx than for cancer of the endolarynx. These results persisted after adjustment for tobacco smoking. In nine of the studies in which this was examined, it was reported that the association with drinking of alcoholic beverages was seen at any level of smoking. Three studies have been carried out on small groups of lifetime nonsmokers; the relative risk increased with amount of drinking in one, but no difference was seen in the proportion of drinkers and nondrinkers in the two others.

Epidemiological studies clearly indicate that drinking of alcoholic beverages is causally related to laryngeal cancer. There is no indication that the effect is dependent on type of beverage.

Cancer of the oesophagus

Seven of eight retrospective cohort studies of alcoholics and brewery workers showed two- to four-fold increased risks of cancer of the oesophagus, although this was nonsignificant in two. Of 13 case-control studies, 11 showed significantly increased relative risks with level of intake of alcoholic beverages. The increased risk persisted after adjustment for tobacco smoking and was seen at all levels of tobacco smoking in the two studies in which this was examined. The risk increased with intake of alcoholic beverages in a small number of persons who had never smoked in the only study in which this aspect was examined.

Epidemiological studies clearly indicate that drinking of alcoholic beverages is causally related to cancer of the oesophagus. There is no indication that the effect is dependent on type of beverage.

Cancer of the stomach

In three of 13 cohort studies, stomach cancer risk was increased in association with consumption of alcoholic beverages, but in only one was this statistically significant. Summation of observed and expected numbers of cases of stomach cancer in the eight retrospective cohorts of persons with above-average consumption of alcoholic beverages indicates a slight deficit in risk.

Data have been reported from 12 case-control studies on the relationship between drinking of alcoholic beverages and stomach cancer. In two studies, the risk for stomach cancer was positively and significantly associated with consumption of alcoholic beverages. In another study, a significant increase in risk was found with one specific drinking practice. One study reported a nonsignificant reduction in the risk for stomach cancer associated with drinking of alcoholic beverages.

In most epidemiological studies of alcoholic beverages and stomach cancer, including all nine retrospective cohort studies, there was no adjustment for any possible confounding effect of diet.

In view of the overall lack of excess risk for stomach cancer in the cohort studies, the inconsistent results of the case-control studies, and the inadequate control for dietary and socioeconomic factors, there is little in the aggregate data to suggest a causal role for drinking of alcoholic beverages in stomach cancer.

Cancer of the large bowel

Two of 13 cohort studies of colon cancer showed an increase in risk, while another showed a nonsignificantly decreased risk associated with raised consumption of alcoholic beverages. Summation of observed and expected numbers of cases of colon cancer in the nine retrospective cohorts of persons with above-average consumption of alcoholic beverages indicates no overall shift in the risk.

For rectal cancer, the risk was increased in association with drinking of alcoholic beverages in four of nine cohort studies. In two of these four studies, a significant increase was seen in relation to beer consumption, including one study in which there was evidence of a dose-response relationship up to a three-fold increase in risk. In the two others, nonsignificant, two- to three-fold increases in the risk for rectal cancer in alcoholics were reported. Summation of observed and expected numbers of cases of rectal cancer in the seven retrospective cohorts of persons with above-average consumption of alcoholic beverages indicates a slight (15%) excess of cases.

Of the four cohort studies in which data were reported on colon and rectal cancers combined, one showed a significant, two-fold increase, while two others showed a nonsignificant increase in risk with raised consumption of alcoholic beverages.

In four of eight case-control studies of colon cancer, a significant positive relationship was evident with drinking of specific beverages: with beer consumption in two studies, and with spirits consumption in three studies.

In six of nine case-control studies of rectal cancer, a significant positive relationship with drinking of alcoholic beverages was reported. In three studies, beer consumption was significantly associated with rectal cancer in men only; in one study, this association was significant for men and women combined. Of the other two studies with significant positive results, one showed an association with consumption of spirits, the other with total ethanol consumption. A case-control analysis within one of the studies of brewery workers showed a positive relationship between drinking of stout and rectal cancer risk.

In most epidemiological studies of consumption of alcoholic beverages and large-bowel cancer, including all nine retrospective cohort studies, there was no adjustment for any possible confounding effect of diet.

In view of the inconsistent findings from epidemiological studies and the probability of uncontrolled confounding by dietary factors, no conclusion can be drawn about the role of consumption of alcoholic beverages in the causation of colon cancer.

Overall, some of the epidemiological studies provide suggestive but inconclusive data for a causal role of drinking of alcoholic beverages, most often beer consumption, in rectal cancer.

Cancer of the liver

Of four cohort studies of the general population, two showed a significantly increased risk for liver cancer among drinkers of alcoholic beverages, whereas in a third study an increased risk was found only among a subgroup of drinkers in one of the two populations studied. Three of ten cohort studies of persons with high intake of alcoholic beverages showed a significant association between consumption of alcoholic beverages and liver cancer, whereas in five other studies the association was positive but nonsignificant. Summation of observed and expected numbers of cases of liver cancer in these ten studies on special cohorts indicates a significant 50% increase in risk.

Six of ten case-control studies showed significant associations at the two- to three-fold level between consumption of alcoholic beverages and primary liver cancer.

A particularly strong association between consumption of alcoholic beverages and primary liver cancer was demonstrated in a cohort study of hepatitis B surface antigen-positive volunteer blood donors. The results of one case-control and one cohort study suggest that the risk for liver cancer is particularly high among people who both drink alcoholic beverages and smoke cigarettes.

Potential confounding due to hepatitis B virus, tobacco smoking and aflatoxin was not explored in all the studies; whenever it was, it did not alter the findings qualitatively. The available results, taken together, indicate that drinking of alcoholic beverages is causally related to liver cancer.

Cancer of the pancreas

Of five cohort studies of the general population, only one showed a significantly increased incidence of cancer of the pancreas among regular drinkers of alcoholic beverages; of ten cohort studies of persons with high intake, none showed a significant association between consumption of alcoholic beverages and pancreatic cancer risk. Of 14 case-control studies, only one has indicated an increased pancreatic cancer risk among regular drinkers of alcoholic beverages. Taken together, the results of these 29 studies suggest that consumption of alcoholic beverages is unlikely to be causally related to cancer of the pancreas.

Cancer of the breast

A significant positive association between intake of alcoholic beverages and breast cancer incidence was seen in each of four large prospective studies and in seven of 13 case-control studies. Nonsignificant positive associations of similar magnitude were observed in two of the case-control studies, in which there were relatively few persons. A dose-response relationship, generally with up to 1.5- to two-fold risks, has been observed. The consistency of this positive association makes it unlikely that the relationship is due to chance or methodological bias. There is no indication that the association is dependent on type of beverage.

Confounding due to currently recognized risk factors for breast cancer was controlled for in most studies; in no instance did adjustment for these factors appreciably alter the estimated risk. In view of the modest elevations in relative risks observed, the possibility of confounding by an unrecognized factor cannot be ruled out entirely, especially since much of the etiology of breast cancer remains unexplained. In order that such a factor be sufficient to explain the observed associations with the drinking of alcoholic beverages, however, it would have to be much more strongly associated with the occurrence of breast cancer than the known common risk indicators and, also, highly correlated with consumption of alcoholic beverages.

The modest elevation in relative risk that has been observed is potentially important because of the high incidence of breast cancer in many countries. Although the available data indicate a positive association between drinking of alcoholic beverages and breast cancer in women, a firm conclusion about a causal relationship cannot be made at present.

Cancer of the lung

Fifteen cohort studies of alcoholics, of persons with higher than average consumption of alcoholic beverages and of the general population have yielded inconsistent results on an association between drinking of alcoholic beverages and the risk for lung cancer. Smoking was taken into account in only five of these studies. In five case-control studies, there was no association between risk for lung cancer and consumption of alcoholic beverages. In view of the lack of excess risk in case-control studies and the inconsistent results of cohort studies, there is no indication that drinking of alcoholic beverages has a causal role in lung cancer.

Cancers at other sites

Overall, studies on cancers of the urinary bladder, kidney, ovary, prostate and lymphatic and haematopoietic system show no association with consumption of alcoholic beverages. The sparsity of the observations on cancers of the skin, corpus and cervix uteri, vulva, testis, brain, thyroid and soft tissues precludes an evaluation.

6.4 Other relevant data

Toxic effects and metabolism

The concentrations of ethanol attained in humans in the upper gastrointestinal tract after consumption of alcoholic beverages can cause local irritation. Long-term, excessive drinking of alcoholic beverages can also cause fatty liver, alcoholic hepatitis, cell necrosis, fibrosis and cirrhosis in the liver.

In humans and experimental animals, ethanol metabolism generates acetaldehyde, predominantly in the liver, and low concentrations of acetaldehyde are found in the blood. In alcoholics, the rate of ethanol oxidation is enhanced, resulting in increased levels of acetaldehyde in the liver and blood. In some ethnic groups, the absence of a specific form of aldehyde dehydrogenase leads to elevated acetaldehyde concentrations in tissues and blood after ingestion of alcohol.

An acute effect of ethanol is inhibition of the metabolism of xenobiotics in humans and experimental systems. In rodents, administration of nitrosamines together with ethanol results in increased DNA alkylation in some extrahepatic tissues such as oesophagus and kidney. Long-term ingestion of ethanol by humans and experimental animals increases levels of cytochrome P450 in the liver, resulting in enhanced metabolism of a wide variety of xenobiotics.

Alterations in hormonal status have been described after either acute or chronic ingestion of ethanol in some studies in humans and experimental animals.

Effects on reproduction

In humans, ethanol is a developmental toxin, and various effects have been associated with ethanol intake. Excessive consumption of alcoholic beverages during pregnancy is associated with the development of a syndrome of physical and mental manifestations in the offspring — the fetal alcohol syndrome; it may also cause defects in the central nervous system, heart, kidney and limbs. Moderate consumption can be associated with reduced birth weight and behavioural deficits, but effects generally have not been observed with an intake of about one drink per day.

Ethanol at high blood levels affects the structure of the reproductive organs and causes significant reductions in fetal body weight, increased resorptions and teratogenic effects in a number of species. Behavioural development of mice and rats was affected by exposure to ethanol *in utero* in some, but not all, studies; exposure *in utero* or during lactation reduced postnatal growth.

Ethanol crosses the placenta in a variety of species, and both ethanol and acetaldehyde have been found in fetal tissues after dosage of pregnant rodents with ethanol. Both ethanol and acetaldehyde can cause embryonal developmental abnormalities *in vitro*.

Genetic and related effects

Increased frequencies of chromosomal aberrations, sister chromatid exchanges and aneuploidies were found in the peripheral lymphocytes of alcoholics.

In rodents exposed *in vivo*, ethanol induced dominant lethal mutations in mice and rats and aneuploidy in germ cells of mice, but did not induce chromosomal aberrations in rats or Chinese hamsters. It induced sister chromatid exchanges in mice and rats but not in Chinese hamsters. It did not induce micronuclei in mice, but conflicting results were obtained in rats. It induced sister chromatid exchanges in mouse embryos exposed *in vivo* and, in one study, chromosomal aberrations in rat embryos exposed *in vivo*.

In most studies of human cells *in vitro*, ethanol did not induce chromosomal aberrations in the absence of an exogenous metabolic system or sister chromatid exchanges in the presence or absence of an exogenous metabolic system. In limited studies, ethanol gave positive results in tests for morphological cell transformation in mouse C3H 10T1/2 cells but not in Syrian hamster embryo cells. In rodent cells *in vitro*, sister chromatid exchanges were induced in the presence, but generally not in the absence, of an exogenous metabolic system. Neither micronuclei nor chromosomal aberrations were induced in the absence of an exogenous metabolic system. Ethanol did not induce DNA damage or mutation in rodent cells *in vitro*. It did not induce mutation or recombination in *Drosophila*.

In plant roots, ethanol induced chromosomal aberrations and sister chromatid exchanges and, in one study, micronuclei in tetrads. In fungi, it induced mutations and nondisjunction; in single studies, it induced mitotic crossing-over but not gene conversion. Ethanol did not induce mutation or DNA damage in bacteria.

Ethanol-free extracts of some alcoholic beverages induced sister chromatid exchanges in human cells *in vitro* and mutation in bacteria.

6.5 Evaluation[1]

There is *inadequate evidence* for the carcinogenicity of ethanol and of alcoholic beverages in experimental animals.

There is *sufficient evidence* for the carcinogenicity of alcoholic beverages in humans.

---

[1]For definition of the italicized terms, see Preamble pp. 27-30.

The occurrence of malignant tumours of the oral cavity, pharynx, larynx, oesophagus and liver is causally related to the consumption of alcoholic beverages.

Alcoholic beverages *are carcinogenic to humans* (Group 1).

ETHANOL

Nonmammalian systems													Mammalian systems																											
Proka-ryotes		Lower eukaryotes				Plants			Insects				*In vitro*																*In vivo*											
													Animal cells								Human cells								Animals							Humans				
D	G	D	R	G	A	D	G	C	R	G	C	A	D	G	S	M	C	A	T	I	D	G	S	M	C	A	T	I	D	G	S	M	C	DL	A	D	S	M	C	A
–	–		?	+	+			+	–[1]	–			–[1]	–[1]	+	–[1]	–[1]		?	+[1]			–	–[1]	–						+	?	–	+	+		+		+	+

A, aneuploidy; C, chromosomal aberrations; D, DNA damage; DL, dominant lethal mutation; G, gene mutation; I, inhibition of intercellular communication; M, micronuclei; R, mitotic recombination and gene conversion; S, sister chromatid exchange; T, cell transformation

7. REFERENCES

Abel, E.L. (1978) Effect of ethanol on pregnant rats and their offspring. *Psychopharmacology*, *57*, 5-11

Abel, E.L. (1979) Sex ratio in fetal alcohol syndrome. *Lancet*, *ii*, 105

Abel, E.L. (1980) Fetal alcohol syndrome: behavioral teratology. *Psychol. Bull.*, *87*, 29-50

Abel, E.L. (1981) *Fetal Alcohol Syndrome*, Vol. 1, Boca Raton, FL, CRC Press

Abel, E.L. (1985a) Prenatal effects of alcohol on growth: a brief overview. *Fed. Proc.*, *44*, 2318-2322

Abel, E.L. (1985b) Alcohol enhancement of marijuana-induced fetotoxicity. *Teratology*, *31*, 35-40

Abel, E.L. & Dintcheff, B.A. (1978) Effects of prenatal alcohol exposure on growth and development in rats. *J. Pharmacol. exp. Ther.*, *207*, 916-921

Abel, E.L. & Dintcheff, B.A. (1986) Saccharin preference in animals prenatally exposed to alcohol: no evidence of altered sexual dimorphism. *Neurobehav. Toxicol. Teratol.*, *8*, 521-523

Abel, E.L. & Greizerstein, H.B. (1979) Ethanol-induced prenatal growth deficiency: changes in fetal body composition. *J. Pharmacol. exp. Ther.*, *211*, 668-671

Abernethy, D.J., Frazelle, J.H. & Boreiko, C.J. (1982) Effects of ethanol, acetaldehyde and acetic acid in the C3H/10T1/2 C18 cell transformation system (Abstract No. Bf-1). *Environ. Mutagenesis*, *4*, 331

Adam, L. & Postel, W. (1987) Gas chromatographic analysis of ethyl carbamate (urethane) in spirits (Ger.). *Branntweinwirtschaft*, *March*, 66-68

Addiction Research Foundation (1985) *Statistics On Alcohol and Drug Use in Canada and Other Countries*, Vol. 1, *Statistics on Alcohol Use*, Toronto, pp. 214-218

Adelhardt, M., Jensen, O.M. & Hansen, H.S. (1985) Cancer of the larynx, pharynx, and oesophagus in relation to alcohol and tobacco consumption among Danish brewery workers. *Dan. med. Bull.*, *32*, 119-123

Adelstein, A. & White, G. (1976) Alcoholism and mortality. *Popul. Trends*, *6*, 7-13

Agarwal, D.P. & Goedde, H.W. (1986) *Ethanol oxidation: ethnic variations in metabolism and response*. In: Kalow, W. *et al.*, eds, *Ethnic Differences in Reactions to Drugs and Xenobiotics* (*Progress in Clinical & Biological Research Series, Vol. 214*), New York, Alan R. Liss, pp. 99-112

Agarwal, D.P., Harada, S. & Goedde, H.W. (1981) Racial differences in biological sensitivity to ethanol: the role of alcohol dehydrogenase and aldehyde dehydrogenase isozymes. *Alcohol. clin. exp. Res.*, *5*, 12-16

Aguilar, M.V., Martinez, M.C. & Masoud, T.A. (1987) Arsenic content in some Spanish wines. Influence of the wine-making technique on arsenic content in musts and wines. *Z. Lebensmittel-untersuch. Forsch.*, *185*, 185-187

Ahlbom, H.E. (1937) Predisposition factors to squamous-cell carcinoma of the mouth, throat and oesophagus. Statistical study on material in the Radiumhemmet Hospital, Stockholm (Ger.). *Acta radiol.*, *18*, 163-185

Alfonso, M., Parafita, M.A., Mancebo, M.J. & Marcó, J. (1985) Further evidence for effects of ethanol on gonadotrophins and prolactin secretion in female rats. *Gen. Pharmacol.*, *16*, 43-47

Alvarez, M.R., Cimino, L.E., Jr, Cory, M.J. & Gordon, R.E. (1980a) Ethanol induction of sister chromatid exchanges in human cells *in vitro*. *Cytogenet. Cell Genet.*, *27*, 66-69

Alvarez, M.R., Cimino, L.E., Jr & Pusateri, T.J. (1980b) Induction of sister chromatid exchanges in mouse fetuses resulting from maternal alcohol consumption during pregnancy. *Cytogenet. Cell Genet.*, *28*, 173-180

Amacher, D.E., Paillet, S.C., Turner, G.N., Ray, V.A. & Salsburg, D.S. (1980) Point mutations at the thymidine kinase locus in L5178Y mouse lymphoma cells. II. Test validation and interpretation. *Mutat. Res.*, *72*, 447-474

Amerine, M.A., Berg, H.W. & Cruess, W.V. (1972) *The Technology of Wine Making*, 3rd ed., Westport, CT, Avi Publishing Co.

Anderson, L.M., Harrington, G.W., Pylypiw, H.M., Jr, Hagiwara, A. & Magee, P.N. (1986) Tissue levels and biological effects of *N*-nitrosodimethylamine in mice during chronic low or high dose exposure with or without ethanol. *Drug Metab. Disposition*, *14*, 733-739

Anderson, R.A., Jr (1982) *The possible role of paternal alcohol consumption in the etiology of the fetal alcohol syndrome*. In: Abel, E.L., ed., *Fetal Alcohol Syndrome*, Vol. 3, *Animal Studies*, Boca Raton, FL, CRC Press, pp. 83-112

Anderson, R.A., Jr, Willis, B.R. & Oswald, C. (1985) Spontaneous recovery from ethanol-induced male infertility. *Alcohol*, *2*, 479-484

Anon. (1966) *Encyclopaedia Britannica*, Chicago, IL, William Benton

Anon. (1980) *Farm Chemicals Handbook*, Willoughby, OH, Meister Publishing, p. D279

Anon. (1985a) The facts about 'alcohol equivalence'. *Brew. Dig.*, *November*, 22-26

Anon. (1985b) Does alcohol cause breast cancer? *Lancet*, *i*, 1311-1312

Anon. (1987) Yellow 6 labeling for alcoholic beverages proposed. *Food chem. News*, *7 September*, 37

Arimoto, S., Nakano, N., Ohara, Y., Tanaka, K. & Hayatsu, H. (1982) A solvent effect on the mutagenicity of tryptophan-pyrolysate mutagens in the *Salmonella*/mammalian microsome assay. *Mutat. Res.*, *102*, 105-112

Athanasiou, K. & Bartsocas, C.S. (1980) The effect of pine resin on chromosome breakage and sister-chromatid exchanges in human peripheral lymphocytes. *Mutat. Res.*, *79*, 79-80

Austin, H., Delzell, E., Grufferman, S., Levine, R., Morrison, A.S., Stolley, P.D. & Cole, P. (1986) A case-control study of hepatocellular carcinoma and the hepatitis B virus, cigarette smoking, and alcohol consumption. *Cancer Res.*, *46*, 962-966

Axelson, O. (1978) Aspects on confounding in occupational health epidemiology. *Scand. J. Work Environ. Health*, *4*, 98-102

Badr, F.M. & Badr, R.S. (1975) Induction of dominant lethal mutation in male mice by ethyl alcohol. *Nature*, *253*, 134-136

Badr, F.M. & Hussain, F. (1977) Action of ethanol and its metabolite acetaldehyde in human lymphocytes. In vivo and in vitro study (Abstract). *Genetics*, *86*, S2-S3

Badr, F.M., Badr, R.S., Asker, R.L. & Hussain, F.H. (1977) *Evaluation of the mutagenic effects of ethyl alcohol by different techniques*. In: Gross, M.M., ed., *Alcohol Intoxication and Withdrawal*, IIIa, *Biological Aspects of Ethanol*, New York, Plenum Press, pp. 25-46

Bakken, A.M., Farstad, M. & Berge, R. (1979) The formation of alkyl palmitate by rat liver microsomes. *FEBS Lett.*, *99*, 47-50

Balboni, C. (1963) *Alcohol in relation to dietary patterns.* In: Lucia, S.P., ed., *Alcohol and Civilization*, New York, McGraw-Hill, pp. 61-74

Baldwin, S. & Andreasen, A.A. (1974) Congener development in bourbon whisky matured at various proofs for twelve years. *J. Assoc. off. anal. Chem.*, *57*, 940-950

Baldwin, S., Black, R.A., Andreasen, A.A. & Adams, S.L. (1967) Aromatic congener formation in maturation of alcoholic distillates. *J. agric. Food Chem.*, *15*, 381-385

Bandas, E.L. (1982) Study of the role of metabolites and impurities in the mutagenic action of ethanol on yeast mitochondria. *Genetika*, *18*, 1056-1061

Bandas, E.L. & Zakharov, I.A. (1980) Induction of *rho*⁻ mutations in yeast *Saccharomyces cerevisiae* by ethanol. *Mutat. Res.*, *71*, 193-199

Bandion, F., Valenta, M. & Kain, W. (1976) Contribution to an evaluation of benzaldehyde contents in stone fruit fine brandies and stone fruit liquors (Ger.). *Mitt. Rebe Wein Obstbau Früchteverwent. Klosterneuburg*, *26*, 131-138

Banduhn, N. & Obe, G. (1985) Mutagenicity of methyl 2-benzimidazolecarbamate, diethylstilbestrol and estradiol: structural chromosomal aberrations, sister-chromatid exchanges, C-mitoses, polyploidies and micronuclei. *Mutat. Res.*, *156*, 199-218

Bannigan, J. & Burke, P. (1982) Ethanol teratogenicity in mice: a light microscopic study. *Teratology*, *26*, 247-254

Barale, R., Rusciano, D., Stretti, G., Zucconi, D., Monaco, M., Mosesso, P. & Principe, P. (1983) The induction of forward gene mutation and gene conversion in yeasts by treatment with cyclophosphamide *in vitro* and *in vivo*. *Mutat. Res.*, *111*, 295-312

Baraona, E. (1985) *Ethanol and lipid metabolism.* In: Seitz, H.K. & Kommerell, B., eds, *Alcohol Related Diseases in Gastroenterology*, Berlin (West), Springer, pp. 65-95

Baraona, E., Pirola, R.C. & Lieber, C.S. (1974) Small intestinal damage and changes in cell population produced by ethanol ingestion in the rat. *Gastroenterology*, *66*, 226-234

Baraona, E., Leo, M.A., Borowsky, S.A. & Lieber, C.S. (1975) Alcoholic hepatomegaly: accumulation of protein in the liver. *Science*, *190*, 794-795

Baraona, E., Leo, M.A., Borowsky, S.A. & Lieber, C.S. (1977) Pathogenesis of alcohol-induced accumulation of protein in the liver. *J. clin. Invest.*, *60*, 546-554

Baraona, E., Pikkarainen, P., Salaspuro, M., Finkelman, F. & Lieber, C.S. (1980) Acute effects of ethanol on hepatic protein synthesis and secretion in the rat. *Gastroenterology*, *79*, 104-111

Baraona, E., Matsuda, Y., Pikkarainen, P., Finkelman, F. & Lieber, C.S. (1981a) *Effect of ethanol on hepatic protein secretion and microtubules. Possible mediation by acetaldehyde.* In: Galanter, M. ed., *Currents in Alcoholism*, Vol. VIII, New York, Grune & Stratton, pp. 421-434

Baraona, E., Guerra, M. & Lieber, C.S. (1981b) Cytogenetic damage of bone marrow cells produced by chronic alcohol consumption. *Life Sci.*, *29*, 1797-1802

Baraona, E., Finkelman, F. & Lieber, C.S. (1984) Reevaluation of the effects of alcohol consumption on rat liver microtubules: effects of feeding status. *Res. Commun. chem. Pathol. Pharmacol.*, *44*, 265-278

Baraona, E., DiPadova, C. & Lieber, C.S. (1985) Transport of acetaldehyde in red blood cells from liver to other tissues (Abstract No. 405). *Hepatology*, *5*, 1048

Baraona, E., Julkunen, R., Tannenbaum, L. & Lieber, C.S. (1986) Role of intestinal bacterial overgrowth in ethanol production and metabolism in rats. *Gastroenterology*, *90*, 103-110

Barauskaite, S.V. (1985) *Carcinogenic effect of ethyl alcohol* (Abstract) (Russ.). In: *Proceedings of a Conference on Current Developments of Drugs Synthesis and Research, 27-28 June, Kaunas (Lithuania), USSR*, p. 159

Barilyak, I.R. & Kozachuk, S.Y. (1983) Embryotoxic and mutagenic activity of ethanol and acetaldehyde after intra-amniotic injection (Russ.). *Tsitol. Genet.*, *17*, 57-60

Barlow, O.W., Beams, A.J. & Goldblatt, H. (1936) Studies of the pharmacology of ethyl alcohol. I. A comparative study of the pharmacologic effects of grain and synthetic ethyl alcohols. II. A correlation of the local irritant, anesthetic and toxic effects of three potable whiskeys with their alcohol content. *J. Pharmacol. exp. Ther.*, *56*, 117-146

Barrison, I.G., Waterson, E.J. & Murray-Lyon, I.M. (1985) Adverse effects of alcohol in pregnancy. *Br. J. Addict.*, *80*, 11-22

Barron, S. & Riley, E.P. (1985) Pup-induced maternal behavior in adult and juvenile rats exposed to alcohol prenatally. *Alcohol. clin. exp. Res.*, *9*, 360-365

Barron, S., Riley, E.P. & Smotherman, W.P. (1986) The effect of prenatal alcohol exposure on umbilical cord length in fetal rats. *Alcohol. clin. exp. Res.*, *10*, 493-495

Bartsch, W., Sponer, G., Dietmann, K. & Fuchs, G. (1976) Acute toxicity of various solvents in the mouse and rat. *Arzneimittelforschung*, *26*, 1581-1583

Bassir, O. & Maduagwu, E.N. (1978) Occurrence of nitrate, nitrite, dimethylamine, and dimethylnitrosamine in some fermented Nigerian beverages. *J. agric. Food Chem.*, *26*, 200-203

Baumes, R., Cordonnier, R., Nitz, S. & Drawert, F. (1986) Identification and determination of volatile constituents in wines from different vine cultivars. *J. Sci. Food Agric.*, *37*, 927-943

Beaud, P. & Ramuz, A. (1978) General composition of morello cherry brandies: comparison with kirsch (Fr.). *Trav. Chim. aliment. Hyg.*, *69*, 536-543

Begg, C.B., Walker, A.M., Wessen, B. & Zelen, M. (1983) Alcohol consumption and breast cancer. *Lancet*, *i*, 293-294

Berenyi, M.R., Straus, B. & Cruz, D. (1974) In vitro and in vivo studies of cellular immunity in alcoholic cirrhosis. *Am. J. dig. Dis.*, *19*, 199-205

Bernhard, C.G. & Goldberg, L. (1935) Absorption and oxidation of alcohol in alcoholics (Ger.). *Acta med. scand.*, *86*, 152-215

Bernstein, L. & Khan, A. (1973) Rapid spectrophotometric determination of oxalate in beer and wort. *Am. Soc. brew. Chem. Proc.*, 20-23

Best, C.H., Hartroft, W.S., Lucas, C.C. & Ridout, J.H. (1949) Liver damage produced by feeding alcohol or sugar and its prevention by choline. *Br. med. J.*, *ii*, 1001-1006

Bhalla, V.K., Chen, C.J.H. & Gnanaprakasam, M.S. (1979) Effects of in vivo administration of human chorionic gonadotropin and ethanol on the process of testicular receptor depletion and replenishment. *Life Sci.*, *24*, 1315-1324

Biles, B. & Emerson, T.R. (1968) Determination of fibres in beer. *Nature*, *219*, 93-94

Bird, R.P., Draper, H.H. & Basrur, P.K. (1982) Effect of malonaldehyde and acetaldehyde on cultured mammalian cells: production of micronuclei and chromosomal aberrations. *Mutat. Res.*, *101*, 237-246

Bjelke, E. (1973) *Epidemiologic Studies of Cancer of the Stomach, Colon, and Rectum: With Special Emphasis on the Role of Diet*, Thesis, University of Minnesota

Blackwelder, W.C., Yano, K., Rhoads, G.G., Kagan, A., Gordon, T. & Palesch, Y. (1980) Alcohol and mortality: the Honolulu Heart Study. *Am. J. Cancer*, *68*, 164-169

Blakley, P.M. & Scott, W.J., Jr (1984a) Determination of the proximate teratogen of the mouse fetal alcohol syndrome. 2. Pharmacokinetics of the placental transfer of ethanol and acetaldehyde. *Toxicol. appl. Pharmacol.*, *72*, 364-371

Blakley, P.M. & Scott, W.J., Jr (1984b) Determination of the proximate teratogen of the mouse fetal alcohol syndrome. 1. Teratogenicity of ethanol and acetaldehyde. *Toxicol. appl. Pharmacol.*, *72*, 355-363

Blevins, R.D. & Shelton, M.S. (1983) Response of *Salmonella typhimurium* mutants to 3D9-THC and in conjunction with known mutagens. *J. environ. Sci. Health*, *A18*, 413-443

Blevins, R.D. & Taylor, D.E. (1982) Mutagenicity screening of twenty-five cosmetic ingredients with the *Salmonella*/microsome test. *J. environ. Sci. Health*, *A17*, 217-239

Bleyman, M.A. & Thurman, R.G. (1979) Comparison of acute and chronic ethanol administration on rates of ethanol elimination in the rat *in vivo*. *Biochem. Pharmacol.*, *28*, 2027-2030

Bo, W.J., Krueger, W.A., Rudeen, P.K. & Symmes, S.K. (1982) Ethanol-induced alterations in the morphology and function of the rat ovary. *Anat. Rec.*, *202*, 255-260

Bode, C., Goebell, H. & Stähler, M. (1970) Alteration of alcohol-dehydrogenase activity in rat liver following protein deficiency and ethanol (Ger.). *Z. ges. exp. Med.*, *152*, 111-124

Bode, J.C. & Menge, H. (1978) Gastrointestinal tract and alcohol (Ger.). *Internist*, *19*, 116-122

Boeck, D. & Kieninger, H. (1979) Nucleic bases and nucleosides in several beers (Ger.). *Brauwissenschaft*, *32*, 160-166

Boggan, W.O., Randall, C.M., DeBeukelaer, M. & Smith, R. (1979) Renal anomalies in mice prenatally exposed to ethanol. *Res. Commun. chem. Pathol. Pharmacol.*, *23*, 127-142

Böhlke, J.U., Singh, S. & Goedde, H.W. (1983) Cytogenetic effects of acetaldehyde in lymphocytes of Germans and Japanese: SCE, clastogenic activity, and cell cycle delay. *Hum. Genet.*, *63*, 285-289

Bokkenheuser, V.D., Winter, J., Mosenthal, A.C., Mosbach, E.H., McSherry, C.K., Ayengar, N.K.N., Andrews, A.W., Lebherz, W.B., III, Pienta, R.J. & Wallenstein, S. (1983) Fecal steroid 21-dehydroxylase, a potential marker for colorectal cancer. *Am. J. Gastroenterol.*, *78*, 469-475

Boland, B. & Roizen, R. (1973) Sales slips and survey responses: new data on the reliability of survey consumption measures. *Drinking Drug Pract. Surv.*, *8*, 5-10

Bond, N.W. (1986) Prenatal alcohol exposure and offspring hyperactivity: effects of *para*-chlorophenylalanine and methysergide. *Neurobehav. Toxicol. Teratol.*, *8*, 667-673

Bosin, T.R., Krogh, S. & Mais, D. (1986) Identification and quantification of 1,2,3,4-tetrahydro-β-carboline-3-carboxylic acid and 1-methyl-1,2,3,4-tetrahydro-β-carboline-3-carboxylic acid in beer and wine. *J. agric. Food Chem.*, *34*, 843-847

Bosron, W.F., Li, T.-K. & Vallee, B.L. (1980) New molecular forms of human liver alcohol dehydrogenase: isolation and characterization of ADH Indianapolis. *Proc. natl Acad. Sci. USA*, *77*, 5784-5788

Boveris, A., Oshino, N. & Chance, B. (1972) The cellular production of hydrogen peroxide. *Biochem. J.*, *128*, 617-630

Bradshaw, E. & Schonland, M. (1969) Oesophageal and lung cancers in Natal African males in relation to certain socio-economic factors. An analysis of 484 interviews. *Br. J. Cancer*, *23*, 275-284

Bradshaw, E. & Schonland, M. (1974) Smoking, drinking, and oesophageal cancer in African males of Johannesburg, South Africa. *Br. J. Cancer*, *30*, 157-163

Brander, C.F., Kepner, R.E. & Webb, A.D. (1980) Identification of some volatile compounds of wine of *Vitis vinifera* cultivar Pinot noir. *Am. J. Enol. Vitic.*, *31*, 69-75

Braun, R., Schöneich, J., Weissflog, L. & Dedek, W. (1982) Activity of organophosphorus insecticides in bacterial tests for mutagenicity and DNA repair — direct alkylation vs. metabolic activation and breakdown. I. Butonate, vinylbutonate, trichlorfon, dichlorvos, demethyl dichlorvos and demethyl vinylbutonate. *Chem.-biol. Interactions*, *39*, 339-350

Breslow, N.E. & Day, N. (1980) *Statistical Methods in Cancer Research*, Vol. I, *The Analysis of Case-control Studies* (*IARC Scientific Publications No. 32*), Lyon, International Agency for Research on Cancer, pp. 227-233

Breslow, N.E. & Enstrom, J.E. (1974) Geographic correlations between cancer mortality rates and alcohol-tobacco consumption in the United States. *J. natl Cancer Inst.*, *53*, 631-639

Brodie, B.B., Butler, W.M., Jr, Horning, M.G., Maickel, R.P. & Maling, M.H. (1961) Alcohol-induced triglyceride deposition in liver through derangement of fat transport. *Am. J. clin. Nutr.*, *9*, 432-435

Broitman, S.A., Gottlieb, L.S. & Vitale, J.J. (1976) Augmentation of ethanol absorption by mono- and disaccharides. *Gastroenterology*, *70*, 1101-1107

Bross, I.D.J. & Coombs, J. (1976) Early onset of oral cancer among women who drink and smoke. *Oncology*, *33*, 136-139

Brown, L.M., Pottern, L.M. & Hoover, R.N. (1986) Prenatal and perinatal risk factors for testicular cancer. *Cancer Res.*, *46*, 4812-4816

Brown, N.A., Goulding, E.H. & Fabro, S. (1979) Ethanol embryotoxicity: direct effects on mammalian embryos *in vitro*. *Science*, *206*, 573-575

Brownson, R.C. & Chang, J.C. (1987) Exposure to alcohol and tobacco and the risk of laryngeal cancer. *Arch. environ. Health*, *42*, 192-196

Brownson, R.C., Chang, J.C. & Davis, J.R. (1987) Occupation, smoking, and alcohol in the epidemiology of bladder cancer. *Am. J. publ. Health*, *77*, 1298-1300

Brugère, J., Guenel, P., Leclerc, A. & Rodriguez, J. (1986) Differential effects of tobacco and alcohol in cancer of the larynx, pharynx, and mouth. *Cancer*, *57*, 391-395

Brusick, D.J., Jagannath, D.R., Myhr, B., Sernaw, R. & Chappel, C.I. (1988) Genetic toxicology evaluation of commercial beers. II. Mutagenic activity of commercial beer products in *Salmonella typhimurium* strains TA-98, TA-100 and TA-102. *Mutat. Res.* (in press)

Bruun, K. (1985) *Formulating comprehensive national alcohol policies.* In: Grant, M., ed., *Alcohol Policies* (*WHO Regional Publications, European Series No. 18*), Copenhagen, World Health Organization, pp. 137-142

Bruun, K., Edwards, G., Lumio, M., Mäkelä, K., Pan, L., Popham, R.E., Room, R., Schmidt, W., Skog, O.-J., Sulkunen, P. & Österberg, E. (1975) *Alcohol Control Policies in Public Health Perspective*, Vol. 25, Helsinki, The Finnish Foundation for Alcohol Studies, pp. 34-91

Bücher, T. & Klingenberg, M. (1958) Pathway of hydrogen in living organisms (Ger.). *Angew. Chem.*, *70*, 552-570

Buday, A.Z., Belleau, G. & Van Gheluwe, G. (1972) Quantitative determination of nucleic acid derivatives by reflectance measurements. *Am. Soc. brew. Chem. Proc.*, 56-60

Bulatao-Jayme, J., Almero, E.M., Castro Ma, C.A., Jardeleza Ma, T.R. & Salamat, L.A. (1982) A case-control dietary study of primary liver cancer risk from aflatoxin exposure. *Int. J. Epidemiol.*, *11*, 112-119

Bull, P., Yanez, L. & Nervi, F. (1987) Mutagenic substances in red and white wine in Chile, a high risk area for gastric cancer. *Mutat. Res.*, *187*, 113-117

Burch, G.E. & Ansari, A. (1968) Chronic alcoholism and carcinoma of the pancreas. A correlative hypothesis. *Arch. intern. Med.*, *122*, 273-275

Burch, J.D., Howe, G.R., Miller, A.B. & Semenciw, R. (1981) Tobacco, alcohol, asbestos, and nickel in the etiology of cancer of the larynx: a case-control study. *J. natl Cancer Inst.*, *67*, 1219-1224

Burnett, D.A. & Sorrell, M.F. (1981) Alcoholic cirrhosis. *Clin. Gastroenterol.*, *10*, 443-455

Burnett, K.G. & Felder, M.R. (1980) Ethanol metabolism in *Peromyscus* genetically deficient in alcohol dehydrogenase. *Biochem. Pharmacol.*, *29*, 125-130

Burns, E.M., Kruckeberg, T.W., Kanak, M.F. & Stibler, H. (1986) Ethanol exposure during brain ontogeny: some long-term effects. *Neurobehav. Toxicol. Teratol.*, *8*, 383-389

Butler, M.G., Sanger, W.G. & Veomett, G.E. (1981) Increased frequency of sister-chromatid exchanges in alcoholics. *Mutat. Res.*, *85*, 71-76

Byers, T. & Funch, D.P. (1982) Alcohol and breast cancer. *Lancet*, *i*, 799-800

Byers, T., Marshall, J., Graham, S., Mettlin, C. & Swansom, M. (1983) A case-control study of dietary and nondietary factors in ovarian cancer. *J. natl Cancer Inst.*, *71*, 681-686

Cabeça-Silva, C., Madeira-Lopes, A. & van Uden, N. (1982) Temperature relations of ethanol-enhanced petite mutation in *Saccharomyces cerevisiae*: mitochondria as targets of thermal death. *FEMS Microbiol. Lett.*, *15*, 149-151

Cabras, P., Meloni, M. & Pirisi, F.M. (1987) *Pesticide fate from vine to wine.* In: Ware, G.W., ed., *Reviews of Environmental Contamination and Toxicology*, Vol. 99, New York, Springer, pp. 83-117

Cadotte, M., Allard, S. & Verdy, M. (1973) Lack of effect of ethanol *in vitro* on human chromosomes. *Ann. Génét.*, *16*, 55-56

Caetano, R., Suzman, R.M., Rosen, D.H. & Voorhees-Rosen, D.J. (1983) The Shetland Islands: longitudinal changes in alcohol consumption in a changing environment. *Br. J. Addict.*, *78*, 21-36

Carroll, R.B. (1970) Analysis of alcoholic beverages by gas-liquid chromatography. *Q. J. Stud. Alcohol*, *5* (Suppl.), 6-19

Carter, E.A. & Isselbacher, K.J. (1971) The metabolism of ethanol to carbon dioxide by stomach and small intestinal slices. *Proc. Soc. exp. Biol. Med.*, *138*, 817-819

Carulli, N., Manenti, F., Gallo, M. & Salvioli, G.F. (1971) Alcohol-drugs interaction in man: alcohol and tolbutamide. *Eur. J. clin. Invest.*, *1*, 421-424

Casazza, J.P. & Veech, R.L. (1985) The production of 1,2-propanediol in ethanol treated rats. *Biochem. biophys. Res. Commun.*, *129*, 426-430

Castells, S., Mark, E., Abaci, F. & Schwartz, E. (1981) Growth retardation in fetal alcohol syndrome. Unresponsiveness to growth-promoting hormones. *Dev. Pharmacol. Ther.*, *3*, 232-241

Castonguay, A., Rivenson, A., Trushin, N., Reinhardt, J., Spathopoulos, S., Weiss, C.J., Reiss, B. & Hecht, S.S. (1984) Effects of chronic ethanol consumption on the metabolism and carcinogenicity of *N'*-nitrosonornicotine in F344 rats. *Cancer Res.*, *44*, 2285-2290

Cederbaum, A.I. & Dicker, E. (1983) Inhibition of microsomal oxidation of alcohols and of hydroxyl-radical scavenging agents by the iron-chelating agent desferrioxamine. *Biochem. J.*, *210*, 107-113

Cederbaum, A.I., Dicker, E., Lieber, C.S. & Rubin, E. (1978) Ethanol oxidation by isolated hepatocytes from ethanol-treated and control rats; factors contributing to the metabolic adaptation after chronic ethanol consumption. *Biochem. Pharmacol.*, *27*, 7-15

Charalambous, G., Bruckner, K.J., Hardwick, W.A. & Linnebach, A. (1974) Separation, identification and determination of beer flavor compounds by high pressure liquid chromatography — Part II. *Tech. Q. Master Brew. Assoc. Am.*, *11*, 150-154

Chaubey, R.C., Kavi, B.R., Chauhan, P.S. & Sundaram, K. (1977) Evaluation of the effect of ethanol on the frequency of micronuclei in the bone marrow of Swiss mice. *Mutat. Res.*, *43*, 441-444

Chauhan, P.S., Aravindakshan, M., Kumar, N.S. & Sundaram, K. (1980) Failure of ethanol to induce dominant lethal mutations in Wistar male rats. *Mutat. Res.*, *79*, 263-275

Checiu, M. & Sandor, S. (1982) The effect of chronic oral alcoholization upon late fetal development in mice. *Morphol. Embryol.*, *28*, 15-19

Checiu, M. & Sandor, S. (1986) The effect of ethanol upon early development in mice and rats. IX. Late effect of acute preimplantation intoxication in mice. *Morphol. Embryol.*, *32*, 5-11

Chen, E.C.-H. & Van Gheluwe, G. (1979) Analysis of histamine in beer. *J. Am. Soc. brew. Chem.*, *37*, 91-95

Chen, J.J. & Smith, E.R. (1979) Effects of perinatal alcohol on sexual differentiation and open-field behavior in rats. *Horm. Behav.*, *13*, 219-231

Chen, T.-H., Kavanagh, T.J., Chang, C.C. & Trosko, J.E. (1984) Inhibition of metabolic cooperation in Chinese hamster V79 cells by various organic solvents and simple compounds. *Cell Biol. Toxicol.*, *1*, 155-171

Chernoff, G.F. (1977) The fetal alcohol syndrome in mice: an animal model. *Teratology*, *15*, 223-229

Chernoff, G.F. (1979) Introduction: a teratologist's view of the fetal alcohol syndrome. *Curr. Alcohol.*, *7*, 7-13

Chernoff, G.F. (1980) The fetal alcohol syndrome in mice: maternal variables. *Teratology*, *22*, 71-75

Cherrington, E.H., ed. (1924) *Standard Encyclopedia of the Alcohol Problem*, Vol. 2, Westerville, OH, American Issue Publishing, pp. 580-597

Chey, W.Y., Kusakcioglu, O., Dinoso, V. & Lorber, S.H. (1968) Gastric secretion in patients with chronic pancreatitis and in chronic alcoholics. *Arch. intern. Med.*, *122*, 399-403

Cheynier, V. & Rigaud, J. (1986) HPLC separation and characterization of flavonols in the skins of *Vitis vinifera* var. Cinsault. *Am. J. Enol. Vitic.*, *37*, 248-252

Christoph, N., Schmitt, A. & Hildenbrand, K. (1986) Study of the formation and behaviour of urethane during distillation in the manufacture of spirits (Ger.). *Alkohol-Ind.*, *15*, 347-354

Cicero, T.H. & Badger, T.M. (1977) Effects of alcohol on the hypothalamic-pituitary-gonadal axis in the male rat. *J. Pharmacol. exp. Ther.*, *201*, 427-433

Cicero, T.J., Meyer, E.R. & Bell, R.D. (1979) Effects of ethanol on the hypothalamic-pituitary-luteinizing hormone axis and testicular steroidogenesis. *J. Pharmacol. exp. Ther.*, *208*, 210-215

Clarren, S.K. & Smith, D.W. (1978) The fetal alcohol syndrome. *New Engl. J. Med.*, *298*, 1063-1067

Clarren, S.K., Alvord, E.C., Jr, Sumi, S.M., Streissguth, A.P. & Smith, D.W. (1978) Brain malformations related to prenatal exposure to alcohol. *J. Pediatr.*, *92*, 64-67

Clarren, S.K., Bowden, D.M. & Astley, S.J. (1987a) Pregnancy outcomes after weekly oral administration of ethanol during gestation in the pig-tailed macaque (*Macaca nemestrina*). *Teratology*, *35*, 345-354

Clarren, S.K., Bowden, D.M. & Astley, S.J. (1987b) Teratogenesis from once per week oral ingestion of ethanol in a non-human primate (Abstract No. 53). *Teratology*, *35*, 66A

Claude, J., Kunze, E., Frentzel-Beyme, R., Paczkowski, K., Schneider, J. & Schubert, H. (1986) Life-style and occupational risk factors in cancer of the lower urinary tract. *Am. J. Epidemiol.*, *124*, 578-589

Clemmesen, J. (1941) *Cancer and Occupation in Denmark, 1935-1939*, Copenhagen, Nyt Nordisk Forlag

Colangelo, W. & Jones, D.G. (1982) The fetal alcohol syndrome: a review and assessment of the syndrome and its neurological sequelae. *Prog. Neurobiol.*, *19*, 271-314

Collis, C.H., Cook, P.J., Foreman, J.K. & Palframan, J.F. (1971) A search for nitrosamines in East African spirit samples from areas of varying oesophageal cancer frequency. *Gut*, *12*, 1015-1018

Connor, C.L. & Chaikoff, I.L. (1938) Production of cirrhosis in fatty livers with alcohol. *Proc. Soc. exp. Biol. Med.*, *32*, 356-359

Cooke, A.R. (1972) Ethanol and gastric function. *Gastroenterology*, *62*, 501-502

Coon, M.J. & Koop, D.R. (1987) Alcohol-inducible cytochrome P-450 (P-450$_{ALC}$). *Arch. Toxicol.*, *60*, 16-21

Cortés, F., Mateos, S. & Escalza, P. (1986) Cytotoxic and genotoxic effects of ethanol and acetaldehyde in root-meristem cells of *Allium cepa*. *Mutat. Res.*, *171*, 139-143

Cotruvo, J.A., Simmon, V.A. & Spanggord, R.J. (1977) Investigation of mutagenic effects of products of ozonation reactions in water. *Ann. N.Y. Acad. Sci.*, *298*, 124-140

Crecelius, E.A. (1977) Arsenite and arsenate levels in wine. *Bull. environ. Contam. Toxicol.*, *18*, 227-230

Creus, A., Xamena, N. & Marcos, R. (1983) Positive response of diethylstilbestrol in the sex-linked recessive lethal assay in *Drosophila* after larval feeding. *Mutat. Res.*, *122*, 309-313

Crone, C. (1965) The permeability of brain capillaries to non-electrolytes. *Acta physiol. scand.*, *64*, 407-417

Crow, K.E., Cornell, N.W. & Veech, R.L. (1977) The rate of ethanol metabolism in isolated rat hepatocytes. *Alcohol. clin. exp. Res.*, *1*, 43-50

Cunningham, H.M. & Pontefract, R. (1971) Asbestos fibres in beverages and drinking water. *Nature*, *232*, 332-333

Cushman, P., Barboriak, J.J., Liao, A. & Hoffman, N.E. (1982) Association between plasma high density lipoprotein cholesterol and antipyrine metabolism in alcoholics. *Life Sci.*, *30*, 1721-1724

Cutler, S.J., Scotto, J., Devesa, S.S. & Connelly, R.R. (1974) Third National Cancer Survey — an overview of available information. *J. natl Cancer Inst.*, *53*, 1565-1575

Czajka, M.R., Tucci, S.M. & Kaye, G.I. (1980) Sister chromatid exchange frequency in mouse embryo chromosomes after in utero ethanol exposure. *Toxicol. Lett.*, *6*, 257-261

Daft, P.A., Johnston, M.C. & Sulik, K.K. (1986) Abnormal heart and great vessel development following acute ethanol exposure in mice. *Teratology*, *33*, 93-104

Daniel, A. & Roane, D. (1987) Aneuploidy is not induced by ethanol during spermatogenesis in the Chinese hamster. *Cytogenet. Cell Genet.*, *44*, 43-48

Darroudi, F. & Natarajan, A.T. (1987) Induction of chromosomal aberrations and sister chromatid exchanges in CHO cells by mutagenic metabolites activated by plant microsomal extracts. *Biol. Zbl.*, *106*, 169-174

David, R.M. & Nerland, D.E. (1983) Induction of mouse liver glutathione *S*-transferase by ethanol. *Biochem. Pharmacol.*, *32*, 2809-2811

Davis, V.E., Brown, H., Huff, J.A. & Cashaw, J.L. (1967) Ethanol-induced alterations of norepinephrine metabolism in man. *J. Lab. clin. Med.*, *69*, 787-799

Day, N.E., Muñoz, N. & Ghadirian, P. (1982) *Epidemiology of esophageal cancer: a review.* In: Correa, P. & Haenszel, W., eds, *Epidemiology of Cancer of the Digestive Tract*, The Hague, Martinus Nijhoff, pp. 21-57

Dean, G., MacLennan, R., McLoughlin, H. & Shelley, E. (1979) Causes of death of blue-collar workers at a Dublin brewery, 1954-73. *Br. J. Cancer*, *40*, 581-589

DeBeukelaer, M.M., Randall, C.L. & Stroud, D.R. (1977) Renal anomalies in the fetal alcohol syndrome. *J. Pediatr.*, *91*, 759-760

De Flora, S., Zanacchi, P., Camoirano, A., Bennicelli, C. & Badolati, G.S. (1984a) Genotoxic activity and potency of 135 compounds in the Ames reversion test and in a bacterial DNA-repair test. *Mutat. Res.*, *133*, 161-198

De Flora, S., Camoirano, A., Zanacchi, P. & Bennicelli, C. (1984b) Mutagenicity testing with TA97 and TA102 of 30 DNA-damaging compounds, negative with other *Salmonella* strains. *Mutat. Res.*, *134*, 159-165

De Jong, U.W., Breslow, N., Goh Ewe Hong, J., Sridharan, M. & Shanmugaratnam, K. (1974) Aetiological factors in oesophageal cancer in Singapore Chinese. *Int. J. Cancer*, *13*, 291-303

Demakis, J.G., Proskey, A., Rahimtoola, S.H., Jamil, M., Sutton, G.C., Rosen, K.M., Gunnar, R.M. & Tobin, J.R., Jr (1974) The natural course of alcoholic cardiomyopathy. *Ann. intern. Med.*, *80*, 293-297

Denk, H. (1985) *Ethanol Mallory bodies and the microtubular system.* In: Seitz, H.K. & Kommerell, B., eds, *Alcohol Related Diseases in Gastroenterology*, Berlin (West), Springer, pp. 154-171

Denk, H., Gschnait, F. & Wolff, K. (1975) Hepatocellular hyalin (Mallory bodies) in long term griseofulvin-treated mice: a new experimental model for the study of hyalin formation. *Lab. Invest.*, *32*, 773-776

Desser, H. & Bandion, F. (1985) Evaluation of the changes in concentrations of biogenic amines in wines after certain treatments and during the storage of bottled wine (Ger.). *Mitt. Hoeheren Bundeslehr-Versuchsanst. Wein-Obstbau Klosterneuburg*, *35*, 16-19

Dexter, J.D., Tumbleson, M.E., Decker, J.D. & Middleton, C.C. (1980) Fetal alcohol syndrome in Sinclair (S-1) miniature swine. *Alcohol. clin. exp. Res.*, *4*, 146-151

Di Luzio, N.R. & Hartman, A.D. (1967) Role of lipid peroxidation in the pathogenesis of the ethanol-induced fatty liver. *Fed. Proc.*, *26*, 1436-1442

Ding, X., Koop, D.R., Crump, B.L. & Coon, M.J. (1986) Immunochemical identification of cytochrome P-450 isozyme 3a (P-450_{ALC}) in rabbit nasal and kidney microsomes and evidence for differential induction by alcohol. *Mol. Pharmacol.*, *30*, 370-378

Dioguardi, N., Idéo, G., Del Ninno, E. & de Franchis, R. (1970) Induction of liver UDPGT by ethanol. *Lancet*, *i*, 1063

DiStefano, R. (1983) Identification of ethyl esters of 2-hydroxyglutaric acid and 2-hydroxyglutaric acid γ-lactone in wines (Ital.). *Vitis*, *22*, 220-224

Dölle, W. (1969) Cobalt-induced heart disease in chronic beer drinkers (Ger.). *Internist*, *10*, 29-30

Drawert, F. & Barton, H. (1973) Critical contribution to the analysis of aflatoxins in wine (Ger.). *Wein Wiss.*, *56*, 1247-1250

Drawert, F. & Barton, H. (1974) Detection of aflatoxin in wine (Ger.). *Z. Lebensmitteluntersuch. Forsch.*, *154*, 223-224

Drawert, F., Leupold, G. & Lessing, V. (1975) *Group separation and gas chromatographic analysis of beer constituents* (Ger.). In: *Proceedings of the 15th European Brewery Convention Congress, Nice*, pp. 791-802

Drawert, F., Leupold, G. & Lessing, V. (1976) Quantitative gas chromatographic determination of organic acids, neutral substances (carbohydrates) and amino acids in wort and beer (Ger.). *Brauwissenschaft*, *29*, 345-353

Driver, H.E. & McLean, A.E.M. (1986) Dose-response relationships for initiation of rat liver tumours by diethylnitrosamine and promotion by phenobarbitone or alcohol. *Food chem. Toxicol.*, *24*, 241-245

Dunham, L.J., Rabson, A.S., Stewart, H.L., Frank, A.S. & Young, J.L. (1968) Rates, interview, and pathology study of cancer of the urinary bladder in New Orleans, Louisiana. *J. natl Cancer Inst.*, *41*, 683-709

Dupuis, C., Dehaene, P., Deroubaix-Tella, P., Blanc-Garin, A.P., Rey, C. & Carpentier-Courault, C. (1978) Cardiopathies of children born to alcoholic mothers (Fr.). *Arch. Mal. Coeur*, *71*, 565-572

Durbec, J.P., Chevillotte, G., Bidart, J.M., Berthezene, P. & Sarles, H. (1983) Diet, alcohol, tobacco and risk of cancer of the pancreas: a case-control study. *Br. J. Cancer*, *47*, 463-470

Dürr, H.K., Bode, J.C., Gieseking, R., Haase, R., von Arnim, I. & Beckmann, B. (1975) Changes in exocrine function of the parotid gland and pancreas of patients with liver cirrhosis and chronic alcoholism (Ger.). *Verh. Dtsch. Ges. inn. Med.*, *81*, 1322-1324

de Duve, C. & Baudhuin, P. (1966) Peroxisomes (microbodies and related particles). *Physiol. Rev.*, *46*, 323-357

Eastwood, G.L. & Kirchner, J.P. (1974) Changes of the fine structure of mouse gastric epithelium produced by ethanol and urea. *Gastroenterology*, *67*, 71-84

Edwards, G., Chandler, J. & Hensman, C. (1972) Drinking in a London suburb: I. Correlates of normal drinking. *Q. J. Stud. Alcohol, Suppl. 6*, 69-93

Edwards, G., Gross, M.M., Keller, M., Moser, J. & Room, R., eds (1977) *Alcohol-related Disabilities* (*WHO Offset Publication No. 32*), Geneva, World Health Organization

Edwards, J.A. & Price Evans, D.A. (1967) Ethanol metabolism in subjects possessing typical and atypical liver alcohol dehydrogenase. *Clin. Pharmacol. Ther.*, *8*, 824-829

Edwards, T.L., Singleton, V.L. & Boulton, R. (1985) Formation of ethyl esters of tartaric acid during wine aging: chemical and sensory effects. *Am. J. Enol. Vitic.*, *36*, 118-124

Eisenbrand, G., Spiegelhalder, B. & Preussmann, R. (1981) *Analysis of human biological specimens for nitrosamine contents*. In: Bruce, W.R., Correa, P., Lipkin, M., Tannenbaum, S.R. & Wilkins, T.D., eds, *Gastrointestinal Cancer: Endogenous Factors* (*Banbury Report 7*), Cold Spring Harbor, NY, CSH Press, pp. 275-283

Elliott, C.R., Prasad, J.S., Husby, A.D., Ellingson, R.J., Holtzman, J.L. & Crankshaw, D.L. (1985) Effects of chronic ethanol consumption on male Syrian hamster hepatic microsomal mixed-function oxidases. *Alcohol*, *2*, 17-22

Ellis, F.W., Pick, J.R. & Sawyer, M. (1977) Effects of ethanol administration during pregnancy on fetal development in beagle dogs (Abstract No. 76). *Fed. Proc.*, *36*, 285

Elwood, J.M., Pearson, J.C.G., Skippen, D.H. & Jackson, S.M. (1984) Alcohol, smoking, social and occupational factors in the aetiology of cancer of the oral cavity, pharynx and larynx. *Int. J. Cancer*, *34*, 603-612

Elzay, R.P. (1966) Local effect of alcohol in combination with DMBA on hamster cheek pouch. *J. dent. Res.*, *45*, 1788-1795

Elzay, R.P. (1969) Effect of alcohol and cigarette smoke as promoting agents in hamster pouch carcinogenesis. *J. dent. Res.*, *48*, 1200-1205

Emby, D.J. & Fraser, B.N. (1977) Hepatotoxicity of paracetamol enhanced by ingestion of alcohol. Report of two cases. *S. Afr. med. J.*, *51*, 208-209

Enstrom, J.E. (1975) Cancer mortality among Mormons. *Cancer*, *36*, 825-841

Enstrom, J.E. (1977) Colorectal cancer and beer drinking. *Br. J. Cancer*, *35*, 674-683

Enstrom, J.E. (1978) Cancer and total mortality among active Mormons. *Cancer*, *42*, 1943-1951

Enstrom, J.E. (1980) Cancer mortality among Mormons in California during 1968-75. *J. natl Cancer Inst.*, *65*, 1073-1082

Eriksson, C.J.P. & Deitrich, R.A. (1983) *Metabolic mechanisms in tolerance and physical dependence on alcohol.* In: Kissin, B. & Begleiter, H., eds, *The Pathogenesis of Alcoholism: Biological Factors*, New York, Plenum Press, pp. 253-283

Ernhart, C.B., Sokol, R.J., Martier, S., Moron, P., Nadler, D., Ager, J.W. & Wolf, A. (1987) Alcohol teratogenicity in the human: a detailed assessment of specificity, critical period, and threshold. *Am. J. Obstet. Gynecol.*, *156*, 33-39

Eschnauer, H. (1967) Trace elements in wine (Ger.). *Z. Lebensmitteluntersuch. Forsch.*, *134*, 13-17

Eschnauer, H. (1982) Trace elements in must and wine: primary and secondary contents. *Am. J. Enol. Vitic.*, *33*, 226-230

Espinet, C. & Argilés, J.M. (1984) Ethanol and acetaldehyde concentrations in the rat foeto-maternal system after an acute ethanol administration given to the mother. *Arch. int. Physiol. Biochim.*, *92*, 339-344

Estival, A., Clemente, F. & Ribet, A. (1981) Ethanol metabolism by the rat pancreas. *Toxicol. appl. Pharmacol.*, *61*, 155-165

Etiévant, P.X. (1981) Volatile phenol determination in wine. *J. agric. Food Chem.*, *29*, 65-67

Farinati, F., Zhou, Z., Bellah, J., Lieber, C.S. & Garro, A.J. (1985) Effect of chronic ethanol consumption on activation of nitrosopyrrolidine to a mutagen by rat upper alimentary tract, lung, and hepatic tissue. *Drug Metab. Disposition*, *13*, 210-214

Fazakas-Todea, I., Checiu, M. & Sandor, S. (1985) The effect of ethanol upon early development in mice and rats. VIII. The effect of chronic consumption of some beverages upon preimplantation development in rats. *Morphol. Embryol.*, *31*, 249-256

Feinman, L., Baraona, E., Matsuzaki, S., Korsten, M. & Lieber, C.S. (1978) Concentration dependence of ethanol metabolism *in vivo* in rats and man. *Alcohol. clin. exp. Res.*, *2*, 381-385

Feldman, J.G. & Boxer, P. (1979) Relationship of drinking to head and neck cancer. *Prev. Med.*, *8*, 507-519

Feldman, J.G., Hazan, M., Nagarajan, M. & Kissin, B. (1975) A case-control investigation of alcohol, tobacco, and diet in head and neck cancer. *Prev. Med.*, *4*, 444-463

Fernandez, K., Caul, W.F., Boyd, J.E., Henderson, G.I. & Michaelis, R.C. (1983) Malformations and growth of rat fetuses exposed to brief periods of alcohol *in utero*. *Teratog. Carcinog. Mutagenesis*, *3*, 457-460

Fillmore, K. & Caetano, R. (1982) *Epidemiology of alcohol abuse and alcoholism in occupations.* In: *Occupational Alcoholism: A Review of Research Issues* (*National Institute on Alcohol Abuse and Alcoholism Research Monograph No. 8; DHHS Publication No. (ADM) 82-1184*), Washington DC, US Government Printing Office, pp. 21-88

Finnish Foundation for Alcohol Studies (1977) *International Statistics on Alcoholic Beverages, Production, Trade and Consumption 1950-1972*, Forssa, Aurasen Kirjapaino, pp. 209-222

Fisher, S.E., Inselman, L.S., Duffy, L., Atkinson, M., Spencer, H. & Chang, B. (1985) Ethanol and fetal nutrition: effect of chronic ethanol exposure on rat placental growth and membrane-associated folic acid receptor binding activity. *J. pediatr. Gastroenterol. Nutr.*, *4*, 645-649

Fisher, S.E., Duffy, L. & Atkinson, M. (1986) Selective fetal malnutrition: effect of acute and chronic ethanol exposure upon rat placental Na,K-ATPase activity. *Alcohol. clin. exp. Res.*, *10*, 150-153

Flamant, R., Lasserre, O., Lazar, P., Leguerinais, J., Denoix, P. & Schwartz, D. (1964) Differences in sex ratio according to cancer site and possible relationship with use of tobacco and alcohol. Review of 65,000 cases. *J. natl Cancer Inst.*, *32*, 1309-1316

Flanders, W.D. & Rothman, K.J. (1982) Interaction of alcohol and tobacco in laryngeal cancer. *Am. J. Epidemiol.*, *115*, 371-379

Food and Agriculture Organization (1979) *Perspective on Mycotoxins* (*FAO Food and Nutrition Paper 13*), Rome, pp. 64-65

Forney, R.B., Hughes, F.W., Richards, A.B. & Gates, P.W. (1963) Toxicity and depressant action of ethanol and hexobarbital after pretreatment with asparagine. *Toxicol. appl. Pharmacol.*, *5*, 790-793

Forsander, O.A. (1970) Influence of ethanol on the redox state of the liver. *Q. J. Stud. Alcohol*, *31*, 550-570

Forsander, O.A., Räihä, N., Salaspuro, M. & Mäenpää, P. (1965) Influence of ethanol on the liver metabolism of fed and starved rats. *Biochem. J.*, *94*, 259-265

Fournet, B. & Montreuil, J. (1975) Identification and quantification of organic acids in various French beers (Fr.). *Cah. Nutr. Diét.*, *10*, 69-71

Freedman, A. & Shklar, G. (1978) Alcohol and hamster buccal pouch carcinogenesis. *Oral Surg.*, *46*, 794-805

French, S.W. & Burbige, E.J. (1979) *Alcoholic hepatitis: clinical, morphologic, pathogenic and therapeutic aspects.* In: Popper, H. & Shaffner, F., eds, *Progress in Liver Diseases*, Vol. VI, New York, Grune & Stratton, pp. 557-579

Frey, W.A. & Vallee, B.L. (1980) Digitalis metabolism and human liver alcohol dehydrogenase. *Proc. natl Acad. Sci. USA*, *77*, 924-927

Friedberg, C.K. (1971) Symposium: cardiomyopathy. Introduction. *Circulation*, *44*, 935-941

Friedman, L.A. & Kimball, A.W. (1986) Coronary heart disease mortality and alcohol consumption in Framingham. *Am. J. Epidemiol.*, *124*, 481-489

Fukui, M. & Wakasugi, C. (1972) Liver alcohol dehydrogenase in a Japanese population. *Jpn. J. legal Med.*, *26*, 46-51

Gabrial, G.N., Schrager, T.F. & Newberne, P.M. (1982) Zinc deficiency, alcohol, and a retinoid: association with esophageal cancer in rats. *J. natl Cancer Inst.*, *68*, 785-789

Gallup, G., Jr, Shriber, J., III & McMurray, C. (1985) *Alcohol Use and Abuse in America* (*Gallup Report No. 242*), Princeton, NJ, Gallup Poll, p. 68

Garcia Heras, J., Herrera, J., Lovell, M., Coco, I. & Coco, R. (1982) Induction of sister chromatid exchanges in mouse kidney fibroblasts by medroxyprogesterone acetate. *Medicina*, *42*, 255-258

Garro, A.J., Seitz, H.K. & Lieber, C.S. (1981) Enhancement of dimethylnitrosamine metabolism and activation to a mutagen following chronic ethanol consumption. *Cancer Res.*, *41*, 120-124

Gascon-Barré, M. (1982) Interrelationships between vitamin D_3 and 25-hydroxyvitamin D_3 during chronic ethanol administration in the rat. *Metabolism*, *31*, 67-72

Gascon-Barré, M. & Joly, J.-G. (1981) The biliary excretion of [^{3}H]-25-hydroxyvitamin D_3 following chronic ethanol administration in the rat. *Life Sci.*, *28*, 279-286

Gavaler, J.S. & Van Thiel, D.H. (1987) Reproductive consequences of alcohol abuse: males and females compared and contrasted. *Mutat. Res.*, *186*, 269-277

Geokas, M.C. (1984) Ethanol and the pancreas. *Med. Clin. N.A.*, *68*, 57-75

Gibel, W. (1967) Experimental studies on syncarcinogenesis in oesophageal carcinoma (Ger.). *Arch. Geschwulstforsch.*, *30*, 181-189

Giknis, M.L.A. & Damjanov, I. (1983) The transplacental effects of ethanol and metronidazole in Swiss Webster mice. *Toxicol. Lett.*, *19*, 37-42

Giknis, M.L.A., Damjanov, I. & Rubin, E. (1980) The differential transplacental effects of ethanol in four mouse strains. *Neurobehav. Toxicol.*, *2*, 235-237

Glinsukon, T., Taycharpipranai, S. & Toskulkao, C. (1978) Aflatoxin B_1 hepatotoxicity in rats pretreated with ethanol. *Experientia*, *34*, 869-870

Goad, P.T., Hill, D.E., Slikker, W., Jr, Kimmel, C.A. & Gaylor, D.W. (1984) The role of maternal diet in the developmental toxicology of ethanol. *Toxicol. appl. Pharmacol.*, *73*, 256-267

Gold, E.B., Gordis, L., Diener, M.D., Seltser, R., Boitnott, J.K., Bynum, T.E. & Hutcheon, D.F. (1985) Diet and other risk factors for cancer of the pancreas. *Cancer*, *55*, 460-467

Goldstein, G. & Arulanantham, K. (1978) Neural tube defect and renal anomalies in a child with fetal alcohol syndrome. *J. Pediatr.*, *93*, 636-637

Golimowski, J., Valenta, P. & Nürnberg, H.W. (1979a) Toxic trace metals in food. I. A new voltammetric procedure for toxic trace metal control of wines. *Z. Lebensmitteluntersuch. Forsch.*, *168*, 353-359

Golimowski, J., Valenta, P., Stoeppler, M. & Nürnberg, H.W. (1979b) Trace metals in food. II. A comparative study of the levels of toxic trace metals in wine by differential pulse anodic stripping voltammetry and electrothermal atomic absorption spectrometry. *Z. Lebensmitteluntersuch. Forsch.*, *168*, 439-443

Gordon, B.H.J., Baraona, E., Miyakawa, H., Finkelman, F. & Lieber, C.S. (1985) Exaggerated acetaldehyde response after ethanol administration during pregnancy and lactation in rats. *Alcohol. clin. exp. Res.*, *9*, 17-22

Gordon, G.G., Altman, K., Southren, A.L., Rubin, E. & Lieber, C.S. (1976) The effect of alcohol (ethanol) administration on sex-hormone metabolism in normal men. *New Engl. J. Med.*, *295*, 793-797

Gordon, T. & Kannel, W.B. (1984) Drinking and mortality: the Framingham study. *Am. J. Epidemiol.*, *120*, 97-107

Gould, L., Zahir, M., DeMartino, A. & Gomprecht, R.F. (1971) Cardiac effects of a cocktail. *J. Am. med. Assoc.*, *218*, 1799-1802

Graf, U., Würgler, F.E., Katz, A.J., Frei, H., Juon, H., Hall, C.B. & Kale, P.G. (1984) Somatic mutation and recombination test in *Drosophila melanogaster*. *Environ. Mutagenesis*, *6*, 153-188

Graham, S., Schotz, W. & Martino, P. (1972) Alimentary factors in the epidemiology of gastric cancer. *Cancer*, *30*, 927-938

Graham, S., Dayal, H., Rohrer, T., Swanson, M., Sultz, H., Shedd, D. & Fischman, S. (1977) Dentition, diet, tobacco and alcohol in the epidemiology of oral cancer. *J. natl Cancer Inst.*, *59*, 1611-1618

Granerus, G., Svensson, S.-E. & Wetterqvist, H. (1969) Histamine in alcoholic drinks. *Lancet*, *i*, 1320

Grant, M. (1985) *Establishing priorities for action*. In: Grant, M., ed., *Alcohol Policies* (*WHO Regional Publications, European Series No. 18*), Copenhagen, World Health Organization, pp. 1-8

Greenfield, N.J., Pietruszko, R., Lin, G. & Lester, D. (1976) The effect of ethanol ingestion on the aldehyde dehydrogenases of rat liver. *Biochim. biophys. Acta*, *428*, 627-632

Greenwald, E.K., Martz, R.C., Harris, B., Brown, D.J., Forney, R.B. & Hughes, F.W. (1968) Ethyl alcohol toxicity in the bat (*Myotis lucifugus*). *Toxicol. appl. Pharmacol.*, *13*, 358-362

Griciute, L. (1981) *Influence of ethyl alcohol on experimental carcinogenesis* (Russ.) (Abstract). In: *Proceedings of the 5th Conference of the Oncologists of Estonian SSR, Latvian SSR and Lithuanian SSR, 26-28 October, Tallin, USSR*, p. 170

Griciute, L., Castegnaro, M. & Béréziat, J.-C. (1981) Influence of ethyl alcohol on carcinogenesis with *N*-nitrosodimethylamine. *Cancer Lett.*, *13*, 345-352

Griciute, L., Castegnaro, M. & Béréziat, J.-C. (1982) *Influence of ethyl alcohol on the carcinogenic activity of* N-*nitrosodi*-n-*propylamine*. In: Bartsch, H., Castegnaro, M., O'Neill, I.K. & Okada, M., eds, N-*Nitroso Compounds: Occurrence and Biological Effects* (*IARC Scientific Publications No. 41*), Lyon, International Agency for Research on Cancer, pp. 643-648

Griciute, L., Castegnaro, M. & Béréziat, J.-C. (1984) *Influence of ethyl alcohol on carcinogenesis induced with* N-*nitrosodiethylamine*. In: Börzsönyi, M., Day, N.E., Lapis, K. & Yamasaki, H., eds, *Models, Mechanisms and Etiology of Tumour Promotion* (*IARC Scientific Publications No. 56*), Lyon, International Agency for Research on Cancer, pp. 413-417

Griciute, L., Castegnaro, M., Béréziat, J.-C. & Cabral, J.R.P. (1986) Influence of ethyl alcohol on the carcinogenic activity of *N'*-nitrosonornicotine. *Cancer Lett.*, *31*, 267-275

Griciute, L., Castegnaro, M. & Béréziat, J.C. (1987) *Influence of ethyl alcohol on carcinogenesis induced by volatile* N-*nitrosamines detected in alcoholic beverages*. In: Bartsch, H., O'Neill, I.K. & Schulte-Hermann, R., eds, *Relevance of* N-*Nitroso Compounds to Human Cancer: Exposures and Mechanisms* (*IARC Scientific Publications No. 84*), Lyon, International Agency for Research on Cancer, pp. 264-265

Grigor, M.R. & Bell, I.C., Jr (1973) Synthesis of fatty acid esters of short-chain alcohol: an acyltransferase in rat liver microsomes. *Biochim. biophys. Acta*, *306*, 26-30

Grunnet, N. (1973) Oxidation of acetaldehyde by rat-liver mitochondria in relation to ethanol oxidation and the transport of reducing equivalents across the mitochondrial membrane. *Eur. J. Biochem.*, *35*, 236-243

Gualandi, G. & Bellincampi, D. (1981) Induced gene mutation and mitotic non-disjunction in *A. nidulans*. *Toxicol. Lett.*, *9*, 389-394

Guerri, C. & Sanchis, R. (1986) Alcohol and acetaldehyde in rat's milk following ethanol administration. *Life Sci.*, *38*, 1543-1556

Guymon, J.F. & Crowell, E.A. (1972) GC-separated brandy components derived from French and American oaks. *Am. J. Enol. Vitic.*, *23*, 114-120

Gwinn, M.L., Webster, L.A., Lee, N.C., Layde, P.M. & Rubin, G.L. (1986) Alcohol consumption and ovarian cancer risk. *Am. J. Epidemiol., 123*, 759-766

Habbick, B.F., Zaleski, W.A., Casey, R. & Murphy, F. (1979) Liver abnormalities in three patients with fetal alcohol syndrome. *Lancet, i*, 580-581

Habs, M. & Schmähl, D. (1981) Inhibition of the hepatocarcinogenic activity of diethylnitrosamine (DENA) by ethanol in rats. *Hepato-gastroenterology, 28*, 242-244

Haenszel, W., Kurihara, M., Segi, M. & Lee, R.K.C. (1972) Stomach cancer among Japanese in Hawaii. *J. natl Cancer Inst., 49*, 969-988

Haggard, H.W. & Jellinek, E.M. (1942) *Alcohol Explored*, Garden City, NY, Doubleday, Doran & Co., pp. 189-195

Hahn, H.K.J. & Burch, R.E. (1983) Impaired ethanol metabolism with advancing age. *Alcohol. clin. exp. Res., 7*, 299-301

Haines, A.P., Moss, A.R., Whittemore, A. & Quivey, J. (1982) A case-control study of pancreatic carcinoma. *J. Cancer Res. clin. Oncol., 103*, 93-97

Hajjar, J.-J., Murphy, D., Tomicic, T. & Scheig, R. (1981) Effect of amino acids and dipeptides on ethanol absorption across the rat intestine. *Pharmacology, 23*, 177-184

Hakim, J., Feldmann, G., Troube, H., Boucherot, J. & Boivin, P. (1972) Comparative study of bilirubin and *para*-nitrophenol glucuronyl transferase activities. II. Effect of chronic alcohol intoxication in man (Fr.). *Pathol. Biol., 20*, 277-285

Hakulinen, T., Lehtimäki, L., Lehtonen, M. & Teppo, L. (1974) Cancer morbidity among two male cohorts with increased alcohol consumption in Finland. *J. natl Cancer Inst., 52*, 1711-1714

Halkka, O. & Eriksson, K. (1977) *The effects of chronic ethanol consumption on goniomitosis in the rat*. In: Gross, M.M., ed., *Alcohol Intoxication and Withdrawal*, IIIa, *Biological Aspects of Ethanol*, New York, Plenum Press, pp. 1-6

Halmesmäki, E., Raivio, K. & Ylikorkala, O. (1985) A possible association between maternal drinking and fetal clubfoot. *New Engl. J. Med., 312*, 790

Halsted, C.H., Griggs, R.C. & Harris, J.W. (1967) The effect of alcoholism on the absorption of folic acid (H^3-PGA) evaluated by plasma levels and urine excretion. *J. Lab. clin. Med., 69*, 116-131

Halsted, C.H., Robles, E.A. & Mezey, E. (1973) Distribution of ethanol in the human gastrointestinal tract. *Am. J. clin. Nutr., 26*, 831-834

Hamada, H., Toshimitsu, N., Kojima, M. & Morita, T. (1985) Effects of ethanol on the induction of respiration-deficient mutants in yeast by metal ions. *Chem. pharm. Bull., 33*, 3507-3509

Hamilton, S.R., Hyland, J., McAvinchey, D., Chaudhry, Y., Hartka, L., Kim, H.T., Cichon, P., Floyd, J., Turjman, N., Kessie, G., Nair, P.P. & Dick, J. (1987a) Effects of chronic dietary beer and ethanol consumption on experimental colonic carcinogenesis by azoxymethane in rats. *Cancer Res., 47*, 1551-1559

Hamilton, S.R., Sohn, O.S. & Fiala, E.S. (1987b) Effects of timing and quantity of chronic dietary ethanol consumption on azoxymethane-induced colonic carcinogenesis and azoxymethane metabolism in Fischer 344 rats. *Cancer Res., 47*, 4305-4311

Handa, R.J., McGivern, R.F., Noble, E.S. & Gorski, R.A. (1985) Exposure to alcohol *in utero* alters the adult patterns of luteinizing hormone secretion in male and female rats. *Life Sci., 37*, 1683-1690

Handler, J.A. & Thurman, R.G. (1987) Rates of H_2O_2 generation from peroxisomal β-oxidation are sufficient to account for fatty acid-stimulated ethanol metabolism in perfused rat liver. *Alcohol*, *4*, 131-134

Hanson, J.W., Streissguth, A.P. & Smith, D.W. (1978) The effects of moderate alcohol consumption during pregnancy on fetal growth and morphogenesis. *J. Pediatr.*, *92*, 457-460

Hardell, L., Bengtsson, N.O., Jonsson, U., Eriksson, S. & Larsson, L.G. (1984) Aetiological aspects on primary liver cancer with special regard to alcohol, organic solvents and acute intermittent porphyria — an epidemiological investigation. *Br. J. Cancer*, *50*, 389-397

Harger, R.N. & Hulpieu, H.R. (1956) *The pharmacology of alcohol.* In: Thompson, G.N., ed., *Alcoholism*, Springfield, IL, Charles C. Thomas, pp. 103-232

Harger, R.N., Hulpieu, H.R. & Lamb, E.B. (1937) The speed with which various parts of the body reach equilibrium in the storage of ethyl alcohol. *J. biol. Chem.*, *120*, 689-704

Harlap, S. & Shiono, P.H. (1980) Alcohol, smoking, and incidence of spontaneous abortions in the first and second trimester. *Lancet*, *ii*, 173-176

Harrison, B. (1971) *Drink and the Victorians. The Temperance Question in England 1815-1872*, Pittsburgh, University of Pittsburgh Press, p. 132

Harsanyi, Z., Granek, I.A. & Mackenzie, D.W.R. (1977) Genetic damage induced by ethyl alcohol in *Aspergillus nidulans*. *Mutat. Res.*, *48*, 51-74

Harvey, E.B., Schairer, C., Brinton, L.A., Hoover, R.N. & Fraumeni, J.F., Jr (1987) Alcohol consumption and breast cancer. *J. natl Cancer Inst.*, *78*, 657-661

Hashimoto, S. & Recknagel, R.O. (1968) No chemical evidence of hepatic lipid peroxidation in acute ethanol toxicity. *Exp. mol. Pathol.*, *8*, 225-242

Hasumura, Y., Teschke, R. & Lieber, C.S. (1974) Increased carbon tetrachloride hepatotoxicity, and its mechanism, after chronic ethanol consumption. *Gastroenterology*, *66*, 415-422

Havers, W., Majewski, F., Olbing, H. & Eikenberg, H.-U. (1980) Anomalies of the kidneys and genitourinary tract in alcohol embryopathy. *J. Urol.*, *124*, 108-110

Hawkins, R.D. & Kalant, H. (1972) The metabolism of ethanol and its metabolic effects. *Pharmacol. Rev.*, *24*, 67-157

He, S.-M. & Lambert, B.O. (1985) Induction and persistence of SCE-inducing damage in human lymphocytes exposed to vinyl acetate and actaldehyde in vitro. *Mutat. Res.*, *158*, 201-208

Hedner, K., Wadstein, J. & Mitelman, F. (1984) Increased sister chromatid exchange frequency in chronic alcohol users. *Hereditas*, *101*, 265-266

ter Heide, R. (1984) *Instrumental analysis of alcoholic beverages.* In: Nykänen, L. & Lehtonen, P., eds, *Flavour Research of Alcoholic Beverages* (*Foundation for Biotechnical and Industrial Fermentation Research 3*), Helsinki, pp. 149-165

ter Heide, R. (1986) *The flavour of distilled beverages.* In: Morton, I.D. & MacLeod, A.J., eds, *Food Flavours*, Part B, *The Flavour of Beverages*, Amsterdam, Elsevier, pp. 239-336

ter Heide, R., de Valois, P.J., Visser, J., Jaegers, P.P. & Timmer, R. (1978) *Concentration and identification of trace constituents in alcoholic beverages.* In: Charalambous, G., ed., *Analysis of Foods and Beverages. Headspace Techniques*, New York, Academic Press, pp. 249-281

ter Heide, R., Schaap, H., Wobben, H.J., de Valois, P.J. & Timmer, R. (1981) *Flavor constituents in rum.* In: Charalambous, G. & Inglett, G., eds, *The Quality of Foods and Beverages*, Vol. 1, *Chemistry and Technology*, New York, Academic Press, pp. 183-200

Henderson, G.I., Turner, D., Patwardhan, R.V., Lumeng, L., Hoyumpa, A.M. & Schenker, S. (1981) Inhibition of placental valine uptake after acute and chronic maternal ethanol consumption. *J. Pharmacol. exp. Ther.*, *216*, 465-472

Henefer, E.P. (1966) Ethanol, 30 per cent, and hamster pouch carcinogenesis. *J. dent. Res.*, *45*, 838-844

Herity, B., Moriarty, M., Bourke, G.J. & Daly, L. (1981) A case-control study of head and neck cancer in the Republic of Ireland. *Br. J. Cancer*, *43*, 177-182

Herity, B., Moriarty, M., Daly, L., Dunn, J. & Bourke, G.J. (1982) The role of tobacco and alcohol in the aetiology of lung and larynx cancer. *Br. J. Cancer*, *46*, 961-964

Herrmann, J., Pallister, P.D. & Opitz, J.M. (1980) Tetraectrodactyly and other skeletal manifestations in the fetal alcohol syndrome. *Eur. J. Pediatr.*, *133*, 221-226

Hétu, C., Yelle, L. & Joly, J.-G. (1982) Influence of ethanol on hepatic glutathione content and on the activity of glutathione S-transferases and epoxide hydrase in the rat. *Drug Metab. Disposition*, *10*, 246-250

Heuch, I., Kvåle, G., Jacobsen, B.K. & Bjelke, E. (1983) Use of alcohol, tobacco and coffee, and risk of pancreatic cancer. *Br. J. Cancer*, *48*, 637-643

Heymann, H., Noble, A.C. & Boulton, R.B. (1986) Analysis of methoxypyrazines in wines. 1. Development of a quantitative procedure. *J. agric. Food Chem.*, *34*, 268-271

Hiaring, P.E. (1986) J. Lohr: pioneer in reverse osmosis. *Wines Vines*, *67*, 34-36

Hiatt, R.A. & Bawol, R.D. (1984) Alcoholic beverage consumption and breast cancer incidence. *Am. J. Epidemiol.*, *120*, 676-683

Hiatt, R., Klatsky, A. & Armstrong, M.A. (1987) Heavy alcohol consumption may increase the risk of breast cancer (Abstract No. 3305). *Fed. Proc.*, *46*, 883

Hiatt, R.A., Klatsky, A.L. & Armstrong, M.A. (1988) Alcohol consumption and the risk of breast cancer in a prepaid health plan. *Cancer Res.*, *48*, 2284-2287

Higginson, J. (1966) Etiological factors in gastrointestinal cancer in man. *J. natl Cancer Inst.*, *37*, 527-545

Hill, A. & Wolff, S. (1983) Sister chromatid exchanges and cell division delays induced by diethylstilbestrol, estradiol, and estriol in human lymphocytes. *Cancer Res.*, *43*, 4114-4118

Hill, D.E., Slikker, W., Jr, Goad, P.T., Bailey, J.R., Sziszak, T.J. & Hendrickx, A.G. (1983) Maternal, fetal, and neonatal elimination of ethanol in nonhuman primates. *Dev. Pharmacol. Ther.*, *6*, 259-268

Hinds, M.W., Thomas, D.B. & O'Reilly, H.P. (1979) Asbestos, dental X-rays, tobacco, and alcohol in the epidemiology of laryngeal cancer. *Cancer*, *44*, 1114-1120

Hinds, M.W., Kolonel, L.N., Lee, J. & Hirohata, T. (1980) Associations between cancer incidence and alcohol cigarette consumption among five ethnic groups in Hawaii. *Br. J. Cancer*, *41*, 929-940

Hiramatsu, R. & Furutani, F. (1978) Persistences of sprayed malathion and trichlorfon in grape berries and grape products (Jpn.). *Yamaguchi-ken Nogyo Shikenjo Kenkyu Hokoku*, *30*, 37-44 [*Chem. Abstr.*, *89*, 192446g]

Hirayama, T. (1966) An epidemiological study of oral and pharyngeal cancer in Central and South-east Asia. *Bull. World Health Org.*, *34*, 41-69

Hirayama, T. (1975) *Prospective studies on cancer epidemiology based on census population in Japan.* In: Bucalossi, P., Veronesi, U. & Cascinelli, N., eds, *Proceedings of the XIth International Cancer Congress, Florence 1974*, Vol. 3, *Cancer Epidemiology, Environmental Factors*, Amsterdam, Excerpta Medica, pp. 26-35

Hirayama, T. (1977) *Changing patterns of cancer in Japan with special reference to the decrease in stomach cancer mortality.* In: Hiatt, H.H., Watson, J.D. & Winsten, J.A., eds, *Origins of Human Cancer*, Book A, *Incidence of Cancer in Humans*, Cold Spring Harbor, NY, CSH Press, pp. 55-75

Hirayama, T. (1978) *Prospective studies on cancer epidemiology based on census population in Japan.* In: Nieburgs, H.E., ed., *Prevention and Detection of Cancer*, Vol. 1, *Etiology*, New York, Marcel Dekker, pp. 1139-1148

Hirayama, T. (1979) Diet and cancer. *Nutr. Cancer, 1*, 67-81

Hirayama, T. (1981) *A large-scale cohort study on the relationship between diet and selected cancers of digestive organs.* In: Bruce, W.R., Correa, P., Lipkin, M., Tannenbaum, S.R. & Wilkins, T.D., eds, *Gastrointestinal Cancer: Endogenous Factors* (*Banbury Report 7*), Cold Spring Harbor, NY, CSH Press, pp. 409-429

Hirayama, T. (1985) *A cohort study on cancer in Japan.* In: Blot, W.J., Hirayama, T. & Hoel, D.G., eds, *Statistical Methods for Cancer Epidemiology*, Hiroshima, Radiation Effects Research Foundation, pp. 73-91

Ho, B.T., Fritchie, G.E., Idänpään-Heikkilä, J.E. & McIsaac, W.M. (1972) Placental transfer and tissue distribution of ethanol-1-^{14}C. A radioautographic study in monkeys and hamsters. *Q. J. Stud. Alcohol, 33*, 485-493

Hoeft, H. & Obe, G. (1983) SCE-inducing congeners in alcoholic beverages. *Mutat. Res., 121*, 247-251

Hoerner, M., Behrens, U.J., Worner, T. & Lieber, C.S. (1986) Humoral immune response to acetaldehyde adducts in alcoholic patients. *Res. Commun. chem. Pathol. Pharmacol., 54*, 3-12

Hoey, J., Montvernay, C. & Lambert, R. (1981) Wine and tobacco: risk factors for gastric cancer in France. *Am. J. Epidemiol., 113*, 668-674

Hohorst, H.J., Kreutz, F.H. & Bücher, T. (1959) On the metabolite concentration of the liver of the rat (Ger.). *Biochem. Z., 332*, 18-46

Holmberg, B., Kronevi, T. & Ekner, A. (1986) *Subchronic Toxicity Investigation of Ethyl Alcohol: A Test for Lowest Effective Dose (LED) to be Used in a Long-Term Bioassay for Carcinogenicity* (*Arbete och Hälsa Vetenskaplig Skriftserie 14*), Solna, Arbetarskyddsstyrelsen

Holtzman, J.L., Gebhard, R.L., Eckfeldt, J.H., Mottonen, L.R., Finley, D.K. & Eshelman, F.N. (1985) The effects of several weeks of ethanol consumption on ethanol kinetics in normal men and women. *Clin. Pharmacol. Ther., 38*, 157-163

Hood, R.D., Lary, J.M. & Blacklock, J.B. (1979) Lack of prenatal effects of maternal ethanol consumption in CD-1 mice. *Toxicol. Lett., 4*, 79-82

Hoofdproduktschap voor Akkerbouwprodukten (Central Commodity Board for Arable Products) (1984) *Alcohol. Biomedical and Social Aspects of the Use of Alcoholic Beverages* (Dutch), Amsterdam

Horak, W., Fuchs, H. & Bäcker, P. (1974a) Analysis of rum (Part I) (Ger.). *Alkohol-Ind., 87*, 217-218

Horak, W., Fuchs, H. & Bäcker, P. (1974b) Analysis of rum (Part II) (Ger.). *Alkohol-Ind., 87*, 245-249

Horgan, M.M., Sparrow, M.D. & Brazeau, R., eds (1986) *Alcohol Beverage Taxation and Control Policies*, 6th ed., Ottawa, Brewers Association of Canada

Horie, A., Kohchi, S. & Kuratsune, M. (1965) Carcinogenesis in the esophagus. II. Experimental production of esophageal cancer by administration of ethanolic solution of carcinogens. *Gann*, *56*, 429-441

Horiguchi, T., Suzuki, K., Comas-Urrutia, A.C., Mueller-Heubach, E., Boyer-Milic, A.M., Baratz, R.A., Morishima, H.O., James, L.S. & Adamsons, K. (1971) Effect of ethanol upon uterine activity and fetal acid-base state of the rhesus monkey. *Am. J. Obstet. Gynecol.*, *109*, 910-917

Horn, R.S. & Manthei, R.W. (1965) Ethanol metabolism in chronic protein deficiency. *J. Pharmacol. exp. Ther.*, *147*, 385-390

Horton, A.A. (1971) Induction of aldehyde dehydrogenase in a mitochondrial fraction. *Biochim. biophys. Acta*, *253*, 514-517

Horvat, D., Rozgaj, R., Račić, J., Mimica, M., Čorović, N. & Pavičević, L. (1983) Chromosome damages in chronic alcohol consumers. *Coll. Antropol.*, *7*, 71-77

Howarth, A.E. & Pihl, E. (1985) High-fat diet promotes and causes distal shift of experimental rat colonic cancer — beer and alcohol do not. *Nutr. Cancer*, *6*, 229-235

Hulpieu, H.R. & Cole, V.V. (1946) Potentiation of the depressant action of alcohol by adrenalin. *Q. J. Stud. Alcohol*, *7*, 89-97

Hunt, P.A. (1987) Ethanol-induced aneuploidy in male germ cells of the mouse. *Cytogenet. Cell Genet.*, *44*, 7-10

IARC (1974) *IARC Monographs on the Evaluation of Carcinogenic Risk of Chemicals to Man*, Vol. 7, *Some Antithyroid and Related Substances, Nitrofurans and Industrial Chemicals*, Lyon

IARC (1975) *IARC Monographs on the Evaluation of Carcinogenic Risk of Chemicals to Man*, Vol. 8, *Some Aromatic Azo Compounds*, Lyon, pp. 257-266

IARC (1976a) *IARC Monographs on the Evaluation of Carcinogenic Risk of Chemicals to Man*, Vol. 12, Some Carbamates, Thiocarbamates and Carbazides, Lyon

IARC (1976b) *IARC Monographs on the Evaluation of Carcinogenic Risk of Chemicals to Man*, Vol. 10, Some Naturally Occurring Substances, Lyon

IARC (1976c) *IARC Monographs on the Evaluation of Carcinogenic Risk of Chemicals to Man*, Vol. 11, *Cadmium, Nickel, Some Epoxides, Miscellaneous Industrial Chemicals and General Considerations on Volatile Anaesthetics*, Lyon

IARC (1977a) *IARC Monographs on the Evaluation of Carcinogenic Risk of Chemicals to Man*, Vol. 14, *Asbestos*, Lyon

IARC (1977b) *IARC Monographs on the Evaluation of the Carcinogenic Risk of Chemicals to Man*, Vol. 15, *Some Fumigants, the Herbicides 2,4-D and 2,4,5-T, Chlorinated Dibenzodioxins and Miscellaneous Industrial Chemicals*, Lyon

IARC (1978) *IARC Monographs on the Evaluation of the Carcinogenic Risk of Chemicals to Humans*, Vol. 17, *Some* N-*Nitroso Compounds*, Lyon

IARC (1979a) *IARC Monographs on the Evaluation of the Carcinogenic Risk of Chemicals to Humans*, Vol. 19, *Some Monomers, Plastics and Synthetic Elastomers, and Acrolein*, Lyon

IARC (1979b) *IARC Monographs on the Evaluation of the Carcinogenic Risk of Chemicals to Humans*, Vol. 20, *Some Halogenated Hydrocarbons*, Lyon

IARC (1980) *IARC Monographs on the Evaluation of the Carcinogenic Risk of Chemicals to Humans*, Vol. 23, *Some Metals and Metallic Compounds*, Lyon

IARC (1982a) *IARC Monographs on the Evaluation of the Carcinogenic Risk of Chemicals to Humans*, Vol. 29, *Some Industrial Chemicals and Dyestuffs*, Lyon

IARC (1982b) *IARC Monographs on the Evaluation of the Carcinogenic Risk of Chemicals to Humans*, Vol. 27, *Some Aromatic Amines, Anthraquinones and Nitroso Compounds, and Inorganic Fluorides Used in Drinking-water and Dental Preparations*, Lyon

IARC (1983a) *IARC Monographs on the Evaluation of the Carcinogenic Risk of Chemicals to Humans*, Vol. 31, *Some Food Additives, Feed Additives and Naturally Occurring Substances*, Lyon

IARC (1983b) *IARC Monographs on the Evaluation of the Carcinogenic Risk of Chemicals to Humans*, Vol. 30, *Miscellaneous Pesticides*, Lyon

IARC (1983c) *IARC Monographs on the Evaluation of the Carcinogenic Risk of Chemicals to Humans*, Vol. 32, *Polynuclear Aromatic Compounds*, Part 1, *Environmental and Experimental Data*, Lyon

IARC (1985) *IARC Monographs on the Evaluation of the Carcinogenic Risk of Chemicals to Humans*, Vol. 36, *Allyl Compounds, Aldehydes, Epoxides and Peroxides*, Lyon

IARC (1986a) *IARC Monographs on the Evaluation of the Carcinogenic Risk of Chemicals to Humans*, Vol. 38, *Tobacco Smoking*, Lyon

IARC (1986b) *IARC Monographs on the Evaluation of the Carcinogenic Risk of Chemicals to Humans*, Vol. 39, *Some Chemicals Used in Plastics and Elastomers*, Lyon

IARC (1986c) *IARC Monographs on the Evaluation of the Carcinogenic Risk of Chemicals to Humans*, Vol. 40, *Some Naturally Occurring and Synthetic Food Components, Furocoumarins and Ultraviolet Radiation*, Lyon

IARC (1987a) *IARC Monographs on the Evaluation of Carcinogenic Risks to Humans*, Suppl. 7, *Overall Evaluations of Carcinogenicity: An Updating of* IARC Monographs *Volumes 1 to 42*, Lyon

IARC (1987b) *IARC Monographs on the Evaluation of Carcinogenic Risks to Humans*, Suppl. 6, *Genetic and Related Effects: An Updating of Selected* IARC Monographs *from Volumes 1 to 42*, Lyon

Iber, F.L. (1977) Drug metabolism in heavy consumers of ethyl alcohol. *Clin. Pharmacol. Ther.*, *22*, 735-742

Idéo, G., de Franchis, R., del Ninno, E. & Dioguardi, N. (1971) Ethanol increases liver uridine-diphosphate-glucuronyltransferase. *Experientia*, *27*, 24-25

Igali, S. & Gazso, L. (1980) Mutagenic effect of alcohol and acetaldehyde on *Escherichia coli* (Abstract). *Mutat. Res.*, 209-210

Ihemelandu, E.C. (1984) Effect of maternal alcohol consumption on pre-and post-natal muscle development of mice. *Growth*, *48*, 35-43

Ijiri, I. (1974) Studies on the relationship between the concentrations of blood acetaldehyde and urinary catecholamine and the symptoms after drinking alcohol (Jpn.). *Jpn. J. Stud. Alcohol*, *9*, 35-59

Ikawa, M., Impraim, C.C., Wang, G. & Yoshida, A. (1983) Isolation and characterization of aldehyde dehydrogenase isozymes from usual and atypical human livers. *J. biol. Chem.*, *258*, 6282-6287

Infante, F., Voirol, M., Brahime-Reteno, O., Raymond, L., Hollenweger, V. & Loizeau, E. (1980a) Alcohol, tobacco and diet in relation to cancers of the liver and cirrhosis: preliminary results (Fr.). *Schweiz. med. Wochenschr.*, *110*, 875-876

Infante, F., Voirol, M., Raymond, L., Hollenweger, V., Conti, M.C. & Loizeau, E. (1980b) *Alcohol, tobacco and nutriments consumption in liver cancer and cirrhosis patients in Geneva.* In: *Alcohol and the Gastrointestinal Tract* (*Les Colloques de l'INSERM 95*), Paris, Institut National de Science et de la Recherche Médicale, pp. 53-58

Inoue, K., Fukunaga, M. & Yamasawa, K. (1980) Correlation between human erythrocyte aldehyde dehydrogenase activity and sensitivity to alcohol. *Pharmacol. Biochem. Behav.*, *13*, 295-297

Interesse, F.S., Lamparelli, F. & Alloggio, V. (1984) Mineral contents of some southern Italian wines. 1. Determination of B, Al, Si, Ti, V, Cr, Mn, Fe, Ni, Cu, Zn, Mo, Sn, Pb by inductively coupled plasma atomic emission spectrometry (ICP-AES). *Z. Lebensmitteluntersuch. Forsch.*, *178*, 272-278

Iseri, O.A., Lieber, C.S. & Gottlieb, L.S. (1966) The ultrastructure of fatty liver induced by prolonged ethanol ingestion. *Am. J. Pathol.*, *48*, 535-555

Ishii, K., Nakámura, K., Ozaki, H., Yamada, N. & Takeuchi, T. (1968) Epidemiology of pancreatic cancer (Jpn.). *Jpn. J. clin. Med.*, *26*, 1839-1842

Ishii, K., Takeuchi, T. & Hirayama, T. (1973) Chronic calcifying pancreatitis and pancreatic carcinoma in Japan. *Digestion*, *9*, 429-437

Israel, Y., Valenzuela, J.E., Salazar, I. & Ugarte, G. (1969) Alcohol and amino acid transport in the human small intestine. *J. Nutr.*, *98*, 222-224

Israel, Y., Videla, L. & Bernstein, J. (1975) Liver hypermetabolic state after chronic alcohol consumption: hormonal interrelations and pathogenic implications. *Fed. Proc.*, *34*, 2052-2059

Jackson, C. & Jackson, C.L. (1941) Cancer of the larynx. Its increasing incidence. *Arch. Otolaryngol.*, *33*, 45-65

Jackson, M. (1982) *The World Guide to Beer*, London, New Burlington Books

Jacobsen, E. (1952) The metabolism of ethyl alcohol. *Pharmacol. Rev.*, *4*, 107-135

James, D.A. & Smith, D.M. (1982) Analysis of results from a collaborative study of the dominant lethal assay. *Mutat. Res.*, *97*, 303-314

Jansson, T. (1982) The frequency of sister chromatid exchanges in human lymphocytes treated with ethanol and acetaldehyde. *Hereditas*, *97*, 301-303

Jedrychowski, W., Wahrendorf, J., Popiela, T. & Rachtan, J. (1986) A case-control study of dietary factors and stomach cancer risk in Poland. *Int. J. Cancer*, *37*, 837-842

Jellinek, E.M. (1954) *International experience with the problem of alcoholism.* In: *Proceedings of a Meeting of Expert Committees on Mental Health and Alcohol, 27 Sept-2 Oct 1954, Geneva, Switzerland* (*WHO/MENT/587; WHO/APD/ALC/12*), Geneva, World Health Organization, pp. 1-28

Jenkins, W.J. & Peters, T.J. (1980) Selectively reduced hepatic acetaldehyde dehydrogenase in alcoholics. *Lancet*, *i*, 628-629

Jenkins, W.J., Cakebread, K. & Palmer, K.R. (1984) Effect of alcohol consumption on hepatic aldehyde dehydrogenase activity in alcoholic patients. *Lancet*, *i*, 1048-1049

Jensen, O.M. (1979) Cancer morbidity and causes of death among Danish brewery workers. *Int. J. Cancer*, *23*, 454-463

Jensen, O.M. (1980) *Cancer Morbidity and Causes of Death Among Danish Brewery Workers*, Lyon, International Agency for Research on Cancer

Jensen, O.M. (1983) Cancer risk among Danish male Seventh-day Adventists and other temperance society members. *J. natl Cancer Inst.*, *70*, 1011-1014

Jensen, O.M., Tuyns, A.J. & Péquignot, G. (1978) Usefulness of population controls in retrospective studies of alcohol consumption. Experience from a case-control study of esophageal cancer in Ille-et-Vilaine, France. *Q. J. Stud. Alcohol*, *39*, 175-182

Jensen, O.M., Wahrendorf, J., Rosenqvist, A. & Geser, A. (1984) The reliability of questionnaire-derived historical dietary information and temporal stability of food habits in individuals. *Am. J. Epidemiol.*, *120*, 281-290

Johansson, I. & Ingelman-Sundberg, M. (1985) Carbon tetrachloride-induced lipid peroxidation dependent on an ethanol-inducible form of rabbit liver microsomal cytochrome P-450. *FEBS Lett.*, *183*, 265-269

Johnson, H. (1985) *The World Atlas of Wine*, 3rd ed., London, Mitchell Beazley International

Joly, J.-G., Ishii, H., Teschke, R., Hasumura, Y. & Lieber, C.S. (1973) Effect of chronic ethanol feeding on the activities and submicrosomal distribution of reduced nicotinamide adenine dinucleotide phosphate-cytochrome P-450 reductase and the demethylases for aminopyrine and ethylmorphine. *Biochem. Pharmacol.*, *22*, 1532-1535

Jones, K.L. & Smith, D.W. (1973) Recognition of the fetal alcohol syndrome in early infancy. *Lancet*, *ii*, 999-1001

Jones, K.L. & Smith, D.W. (1975) The fetal alcohol syndrome. *Teratology*, *12*, 1-10

Jones, W.L. & Stewart, D.B. (1984) Effects of orally-administered ethanol on mammary gland morphology and functional efficiency in lactating rats. *Exp. Pathol.*, *25*, 205-213

Jounela-Eriksson, P. & Lehtonen, M. (1981) *Phenols in the aroma of distilled beverages*. In: Charalambous, G. & Inglett, G., eds, *The Quality of Foods and Beverages*, Vol. 1, *Chemistry and Technology*, New York, Academic Press, pp. 167-181

Jouret, C. & Puech, J.L. (1975) The importance of lignin in the maturing of rum (Fr.). *Ann. Technol. agric.*, *24*, 325-333

Kabat, G.C., Howson, C.P. & Wynder, E.L. (1986) Beer consumption and rectal cancer. *Int. J. Epidemiol.*, *15*, 494-501

Käfer, E. (1984) Disruptive effects of ethyl alcohol on mitotic chromosome segregation in diploid and haploid strains of *Aspergillus nidulans*. *Mutat. Res.*, *135*, 53-75

Kahn, A.J. (1968) Effect of ethanol exposure during embryogenesis and the neonatal period on the incidence of hepatoma in C3H male mice. *Growth*, *32*, 311-316

Kahn, J.H. & Conner, H.A. (1972) Rapid gas-liquid chromatographic determination of phenethyl alcohol in alcoholic distillates. *J. Assoc. off. anal. Chem.*, *55*, 1155-1158

Kahn, J.H., LaRoe, E.G. & Conner, H.A. (1968) Whiskey composition: identification of components by single-pass gas chromatography-mass spectrometry. *J. Food Sci.*, *33*, 395-400

Kalant, H. (1971) *Absorption, diffusion, distribution, and elimination of ethanol: effects on biological membranes*. In: Kissin, K. & Begleiter, H., eds, *The Biology of Alcoholism*, Vol. 1, *Biochemistry*, New York, Plenum Press, pp. 1-62

Kaminski, M., Rumeau-Rouquette, C. & Schwartz, D. (1976) Alcohol consumption among pregnant women and pregnancy outcome (Fr.). *Rev. Epidémiol. Santé publique*, *24*, 27-40

Kaminski, M., Franc, M., Lebouvier, M., du Mazaubrun, C. & Rumeau-Rouquette, C. (1981) Moderate alcohol use and pregnancy outcome. *Neurobehav. Toxicol. Teratol.*, *3*, 173-181

Kanagasundaram, N. & Leevy, C.M. (1981) *Ethanol, immune reactions and the digestive system*. In: Leevy, C.M., ed., *Clinics in Gastroenterology*, Vol. 10, *Alcohol in the GI Tract*, London, W.B. Saunders, pp. 295-306

Kater, R.M.H., Carulli, N. & Iber, F.L. (1969) Differences in the rate of ethanol metabolism in recently drinking alcoholic and nondrinking subjects. *Am. J. clin. Nutr.*, *22*, 1608-1617

Katsouyanni, K., Trichopoulos, D., Boyle, P., Xirouchaki, E., Trichopoulou, A., Lisseos, B., Vasilaros, S. & MacMahon, B. (1986) Diet and breast cancer: a case-control study in Greece. *Int. J. Cancer*, *38*, 815-820

Katz, D., Pitchumoni, C.S., Thomas, E. & Antonelle, M. (1976) The endoscopic diagnosis of upper-gastrointestinal hemorrhage. Changing concepts of etiology and management. *Dig. Dis.*, *21*, 182-189

Kaufman, M.H. (1983) Ethanol-induced chromosomal abnormalities at conception. *Nature*, *302*, 258-260

Kaufman, M.H. & Bain, I.M. (1984a) Influence of ethanol on chromosome segregation during the first and second meiotic divisions in the mouse egg. *J. exp. Zool.*, *230*, 315-320

Kaufman, M.H. & Bain, I.M. (1984b) The development potential of ethanol-induced monosomic and trisomic conceptuses in the mouse. *J. exp. Zool.*, *231*, 149-155

Keiding, S., Christensen, N.J., Damgaard, S.E., Dejgård, A., Iversen, H.L., Jacobsen, A., Johansen, S., Lundquist, F., Rubinstein, E. & Winkler, K. (1983) Ethanol metabolism in heavy drinkers after massive and moderate alcohol intake. *Biochem. Pharmacol.*, *32*, 3097-3102

Keilin, D. & Hartree, E.F. (1936) Coupled oxidation of alcohol. *Proc. R. Soc. Med. (Lond.)*, *119*, 141-159

Keilin, D. & Hartree, E.F. (1945) Properties of catalase. Catalysis of coupled oxidation of alcohols. *Biochem. J.*, *39*, 293-301

Keller, A.Z. (1977) Alcohol, tobacco and age factors in the relative frequency of cancer among males with and without liver cirrhosis. *Am. J. Epidemiol.*, *106*, 194-202

Keller, A.Z. & Terris, M. (1965) The association of alcohol and tobacco with cancer of the mouth and pharynx. *Am. J. publ. Health*, *55*, 1578-1585

Kennaway, E.L. & Kennaway, N.M. (1947) A further study of the incidence of cancer of the lung and larynx. *Br. J. Cancer*, *1*, 260-298

Keppen, L.D., Pysher, T. & Rennert, O.M. (1985) Zinc deficiency acts as a co-teratogen with alcohol in fetal alcohol syndrome. *Pediatr. Res.*, *19*, 944-947

Kesäniemi, Y.A. & Sippel, H.W. (1975) Placental and foetal metabolism of acetaldehyde in rat. I. Contents of ethanol and acetaldehyde in placenta and foetus of the pregnant rat during ethanol oxidation. *Acta pharmacol. toxicol.*, *37*, 43-48

Ketcham, A.S., Wexler, H. & Mantel, N. (1963) Effects of alcohol in mouse neoplasia. *Cancer Res.*, *23*, 667-670

Khanna, J.M. & Israel, Y. (1980) *Ethanol metabolism*. In: Javitt, N.B., ed., *International Review of Physiology*, I, *Liver and Biliary Tract Physiology*, Vol. 21, Baltimore, MD, University Park Press, pp. 275-315

Kieffer, J.D. & Ketchel, M.M. (1970) Blockade of ovulation in the rat by ethanol. *Acta endocrinol.*, *65*, 117-124

Kieninger, H., Hums, N. & Tavera, M. (1976) Separation and quantitative determination of purines and pyrimidines in wort and beer. Part 1 (Ger.). *Brauwissenschaft*, *29*, 71-75

Kiessling, K.H. (1962) The occurrence of acetaldehyde in various parts of the rat brain after alcohol injection, and its effect on the pyruvate oxidation. *Exp. Cell Res.*, *27*, 367-368

Kikugawa, K., Kato, T. & Hayatsu, H. (1985) Screening of mutagenicity of processed foods by the use of blue cotton (Jpn.). *J. Food Hyg. Soc. (Jpn)*, *26*, 432-436

Kimura, E.T., Ebert, D.M. & Dodge, P.W. (1971) Acute toxicity and limits of solvent residue for sixteen organic solvents. *Toxicol. appl. Pharmacol.*, *19*, 699-704

Kirchner, J.A. & Malkin, J.S. (1953) Cancer of the larynx. Thirty-year survey at New Haven Hospital. *Arch. Otolaryngol.*, *58*, 19-30

Klassen, R.W. & Persaud, T.V.N. (1976) Experimental studies on the influence of male alcoholism on pregnancy and progeny. *Exp. Pathol.*, *12*, 38-45

Klassen, R.W. & Persaud, T.V.N. (1978) Influence of alcohol on the reproductive system of the male rat. *Int. J. Fertil.*, *23*, 176-184

Klatsky, A.L., Friedman, G.D. & Siegelaub, A.B. (1981) Alcohol and mortality: a ten-year Kaiser-Permanente experience. *Ann. intern. Méd.*, *95*, 139-145

Klein, D. (1981) Nitrosamines in beers and whiskies (Fr.). *Méd. Nutr.*, *17*, 293-300, 303

Kline, J., Shrout, P., Stein, Z., Susser, M. & Warburton, D. (1980) Drinking during pregnancy and spontaneous abortion. *Lancet*, *ii*, 176-180

Knupfer, G. & Room, R. (1964) Age, sex and social class as factors in amount of drinking in a metropolitan community. *Soc. Probl.*, *12*, 224-240

Kodama, T. & Mori, W. (1983a) Morphological behavior of carcinoma of the pancreas. 1. Histological classification and electron microscopical observation. *Acta pathol. jpn.*, *33*, 467-481

Kodama, T. & Mori, W. (1983b) Morphological lesions of the pancreatic ducts. Significance of pyloric gland metaplasia in carcinogenesis of exocrine and endocrine pancreas. *Acta pathol. jpn.*, *33*, 645-660

Kohila, T., Eriksson, K. & Halkka, O. (1976) Goniomitosis in rats subjected to ethanol. *Med. Biol.*, *54*, 150-151

Koike, K., Hashimoto, N., Kitami, H. & Okada, K. (1972) Flash exchange gas chromatography of volatile amines in beer. *Rep. Res. Lab. Kirin Brew.*, *15*, 25-29

Koivula, T. & Lindros, K.O. (1975) Effects of long-term ethanol treatment on aldehyde and alcohol dehydrogenase activities in rat liver. *Biochem. Pharmacol.*, *24*, 1937-1942

Königstein, M., Larisch, M. & Obe, G. (1984) Mutagenicity of antiepileptic drugs. I. Carbamazepine and some of its metabolites. *Mutat. Res.*, *139*, 83-86

Konishi, N., Kitahori, Y., Shimoyama, T., Takahashi, M. & Hiasa, Y. (1986) Effects of sodium chloride and alcohol on experimental esophageal carcinogenesis induced by *N*-nitrosopiperidine in rats. *Jpn. J. Cancer Res. (Gann)*, *77*, 446-451

Kono, S., Ikeda, M., Ogata, M., Tokudome, S., Nishizumi, M. & Kuratsune, M. (1983) The relationship between alcohol and mortality among Japanese physicians. *Int. J. Epidemiol.*, *12*, 437-441

Kono, S., Ikeda, M., Tokudome, S., Yoshimura, T., Nishizumi, M. & Kuratsune, M. (1985) Alcohol and cancer in male Japanese physicians. *J. Cancer Res. clin. Oncol.*, *109*, 82-85

Kono, S., Ikeda, M., Tokudome, S., Nishizumi, M. & Kuratsune, M. (1986) Alcohol and mortality: a cohort study of male Japanese physicians. *Int. J. Epidemiol.*, *15*, 527-532

Koop, D.R. & Casazza, J.P. (1985) Identification of ethanol-inducible P-450 isozyme 3a as the acetone and acetol monooxygenase of rabbit microsomes. *J. biol. Chem.*, *260*, 13607-13612

Koop, D.R., Morgan, E.T., Tarr, G.E. & Coon, M.J. (1982) Purification and characterization of a unique isozyme of cytochrome P-450 from liver microsomes of ethanol-treated rabbits. *J. biol. Chem.*, *257*, 8472-8480

Kopun, M. & Propping, P. (1977) The kinetics of ethanol absorption and elimination in twins and supplementary repetitive experiments in singleton subjects. *Eur. J. clin. Pharmacol.*, *11*, 337-344

Korsten, M.A., Matsuzaki, S., Feinman, L. & Lieber, C.S. (1975) High blood acetaldehyde levels after ethanol administration. Difference between alcoholic and nonalcoholic subjects. *New Engl. J. Med.*, *292*, 386-389

Korte, A. & Obe, G. (1981) Influence of chronic ethanol uptake and acute acetaldehyde treatment on the chromosomes of bone-marrow cells and peripheral lymphocytes of Chinese hamsters. *Mutat. Res.*, *88*, 389-395

Korte, A., Slacik-Erben, R. & Obe, G. (1979) The influence of ethanol treatment on cytogenetic effects in bone marrow cells of Chinese hamsters by cyclophosphamide, aflatoxin B_1 and patulin. *Toxicology*, *12*, 53-61

Korte, A., Wagner, H.M. & Obe, G. (1981) Simultaneous exposure of Chinese hamsters to ethanol and cigarette smoke: cytogenetic aspects. *Toxicology*, *20*, 237-246

Kortteinen, T. (1986) Utilization of agricultural produce in the production of alcohol — world trends 1961-1983. *Contemp. Drug Probl.*, *12*, 679-706

Kozachuk, S.Y. & Barilyak, I.R. (1982) Ultrastructure and histochemical characteristics of embryonic hepatocytes under the action of ethanol (Russ.). *Tsitol. Genet.*, *16*, 59-68

Krebs, C. (1928) Experimental alcoholic tumours in white mice (Ger.). *Z. Immunol.-Forsch. exp. Ther.*, *59*, 203-218

Krebs, H.A., Freedland, R.A., Hems, R. & Stubbs, M. (1969) Inhibition of hepatic gluconeogenesis by ethanol. *Biochem. J.*, *112*, 117-124

Krikun, G. & Cederbaum, A.I. (1984) Stereochemical studies on the cytochrome P-450 and hydroxyl radical dependent pathways of 2-butanol oxidation by microsomes from chow-fed, phenobarbital-treated, and ethanol-treated rats. *Biochemistry*, *23*, 5489-5494

Krogh, P., Hald, B., Gjertsen, P. & Myken, F. (1974) Fate of ochratoxin A and citrinin during malting and brewing experiments. *Appl. Microbiol.*, *28*, 31-34

Kronick, J.B. (1976) Teratogenic effects of ethyl alcohol administered to pregnant mice. *Am. J. Obstet. Gynecol.*, *124*, 676-680

Krueger, W.A., Bo, W.J. & Rudeen, P.K. (1982) Female reproduction during chronic ethanol consumption in rats. *Pharmacol. Biochem. Behav.*, *17*, 629-631

Kucheria, K., Taneja, N. & Mohan, D. (1986) Chromosomal aberrations and sister chromatid exchanges in chronic male alcoholics. *Indian J. med. Res.*, *83*, 417-421

Kune, S., Kune, G.A. & Watson, L.F. (1987a) Case-control study of alcoholic beverages as etiological factors: the Melbourne Colorectal Cancer Study. *Nutr. Cancer*, *9*, 43-56

Kune, S., Kune, G.A. & Watson, L.F. (1987b) Observation on the reliability and validity of the design and diet history method in the Melbourne Colorectal Cancer Study. *Nutr. Cancer*, *9*, 5-20

Kuratsune, M., Kohchi, S., Horie, A. & Nishizumi, M. (1971) Test of alcoholic beverages and ethanol solutions for carcinogenicity and tumor-promoting activity. *Gann*, *62*, 395-405

Kuwano, A. & Kajii, T. (1987) Synergistic effect of aphidicolin and ethanol on the induction of common fragile sites. *Hum. Genet.*, *75*, 75-78

Kvåle, G., Bjelke, E. & Gart, J.J. (1983) Dietary habits and lung cancer risk. *Int. J. Cancer*, *31*, 397-405

Kvelland, I. (1983) The mutagenic effect in bacteriophage T4D of a hair dye, 1,4-diaminoanthraquinone, and of two solvents, dimethylsulfoxide and ethanol. *Hereditas*, *99*, 209-213

Kyllerman, M., Aronson, M., Sabel, K.-G., Karlberg, E., Sandin, B. & Olegård, R. (1985) Children of alcoholic mothers. Growth and motor performance compared to matched controls. *Acta paediatr. scand.*, *74*, 20-26

Lafond, J.S., Fouron, J-.C., Bard, H. & Ducharme, G. (1985) Effects of maternal alcohol intoxication on fetal circulation and myocardial function: an experimental study in the ovine fetus. *J. Pediatr.*, *107*, 947-950

Lam, K.C., Yu, M.C., Leung, J.W.C. & Henderson, B.E. (1982) Hepatitis B virus and cigarette smoking: risk factors for hepatocellular carcinoma in Hong Kong. *Cancer Res.*, *42*, 5246-5248

Lambert, B., Chen, Y., He, S.M. & Sten, M. (1985) DNA cross-links in human leucocytes treated with vinyl acetate and acetaldehyde in vitro. *Mutat. Res.*, *146*, 301-303

Lamboeuf, Y., de Saint Blanquat, G. & Derache, R. (1981) Mucosal alcohol dehydrogenase- and aldehyde dehydrogenase-mediated ethanol oxidation in the digestive tract of the rat. *Biochem. Pharmacol.*, *30*, 542-545

Lamy, L. (1910) Statistical clinical study of 134 cases of cancer of the oesophagus and cardia (Fr.). *Arch. Mal. Appar. digest.*, *4*, 451-475

Lane, B.P. & Lieber, C.S. (1966) Ultrastructural alterations in human hepatocytes following ingestion of ethanol with adequate diets. *Am. J. Pathol.*, *49*, 593-603

Lange, L.G. (1982) Nonoxidative ethanol metabolism: formation of fatty acid ethyl esters by cholesterol esterase. *Proc. natl Acad. Sci. USA*, *79*, 3954-3957

Laposata, E.A. & Lange, L.G. (1986) Presence of nonoxidative ethanol metabolism in human organs commonly damaged by ethanol abuse. *Science*, *231*, 497-499

Laser, H. (1955) Peroxidatic activity of catalase. *Biochem. J.*, *61*, 122-127

Lasker, J.M., Ardies, C.M., Bloswick, B.P. & Lieber, C.S. (1986a) Immunochemical evidence for an ethanol-inducible form of liver microsomal cytochrome P-450 in rodents and primates (Abstract No. 1077). *Fed. Proc.*, *45*, 1665

Lasker, J.M., Bloswick, B.P., Ardies, C.M. & Lieber, C.S. (1986b) Evidence for an ethanol-inducible form of liver microsomal cytochrome P-450 in humans (Abstract No. 13). *Hepatology*, *6*, 1108

Lasker, J.M., Raucy, J., Kubota, S., Bloswick, B.P., Black, M. & Lieber, C.S. (1987) Purification and characterization of human liver cytochrome P-450-ALC. *Biochem. biophys. Res. Commun.*, *148*, 232-238

Lasne, C., Gu, Z.W., Venegas, W. & Chouroulinkov, I. (1984) The in vitro micronucleus assay for detection of cytogenetic effects induced by mutagen-carcinogens: comparison with the in vitro sister-chromatid exchange assay. *Mutat. Res.*, *130*, 273-282

Lasserre, O., Flamant, R., Lellouch, J. & Schwartz, D. (1967) Alcohol and cancer (Study of geographical pathology in French departments) (Fr.). *Bull. INSERM*, *22*, 53-60

Lau, V.K. & Lindsay, R.C. (1972) Quantification of monocarbonyl compounds in staling beer. *Tech. Q. Master Brew. Assoc. Am.*, *9*, XVII-XVIII

La Vecchia, C., Decarli, A., Franceschi, S., Pampallona, S. & Tognoni, G. (1985) Alcohol consumption and the risk of breast cancer in women. *J. natl Cancer Inst.*, *75*, 61-65

Lê, M.G., Hill, C., Kramar, A. & Flamant, R. (1984) Alcohol beverage consumption and breast cancer in a French case-control study. *Am. J. Epidemiol.*, *120*, 350-357

Lê, M.G., Moulton, L.H., Hill, C. & Kramar, A. (1986) Consumption of dairy produce and alcohol in a case-control study of breast cancer. *J. natl Cancer Inst.*, *77*, 633-636

Lebsack, M.E., Gordon, E.R. & Lieber, C.S. (1981) The effect of chronic ethanol consumption on aldehyde dehydrogenase activity in the baboon. *Biochem. Pharmacol.*, *30*, 2273-2277

Lee, J.S.K. & Fong, L.Y.Y. (1979) Mutagenicity of Chinese alcoholic spirits. *Food Cosmet. Toxicol.*, *17*, 575-578

Lee, M. (1985) Potentiation of chemically induced cleft palate by ethanol ingestion during gestation in the mouse. *Teratog. Carcinog. Mutagenesis*, *5*, 433-440

Lee, M. & Leichter, J. (1983) Skeletal development in fetuses of rats consuming alcohol during gestation. *Growth*, *47*, 254-262

van Leeuwen, F.E., de Vet, H.C.W., Hayes, R.B., van Staveren, W.A., West, C.E. & Hautvast, J.G.A.J. (1983) An assessment of the relative validity of retrospective interviewing for measuring dietary intake. *Am. J. Epidemiol.*, *118*, 752-758

Lehtonen, M. (1973) Detection of aflatoxins in wines. *Chem. mikrobiol. Technol. Lebensm.*, *2*, 161-164

Lehtonen, M. (1983) High performance liquid chromatography determination of nonvolatile phenolic compounds in matured distilled alcoholic beverages. *J. Assoc. off. anal. Chem.*, *66*, 71-78

Lehtonen, M. & Suomalainen, H. (1979) The analytical profile of some whisky brand. *Process Biochem.*, *14*, 5-6,8-9,26

Lehtonen, P. (1984) *Liquid chromatographic determination of phenolic aldehydes from distilled alcoholic beverages.* In: Nykänen, L. & Lehtonen, P., eds, *Flavour Research of Alcoholic Beverages*, Vol. 3, *Instrumental and Sensory Analysis*, Helsinki, Foundation for Biotechnical and Industrial Fermentation Research, pp. 121-130

Lehtonen, P. (1986) Isolation and HPLC determination of amines in wine. *Z. Lebensmitteluntersuch. Forsch.*, *183*, 177-181

Leichter, J. & Lee, M. (1979) Effect of maternal ethanol administration on physical growth of the offspring in rats. *Growth*, *43*, 288-297

Lelbach, W.K. (1975) Cirrhosis in the alcoholic and its relation to the volume of alcohol abuse. *Ann. N.Y. Acad. Sci.*, *252*, 85-105

Leloir, L.F. & Muñoz, J.M. (1938) Ethyl alcohol metabolism in animal tissues. *Biochem. J.*, *32*, 299-307

Lemon, F.R., Walden, R.T. & Woods, R.W. (1964) Cancer of the lung and mouth in Seventh-day Adventists. Preliminary report on a population study. *Cancer*, *17*, 486-497

Lemperle, E., Kerner, E. & Heizmann, R. (1975) Study of aflatoxin content of wines (Ger.). *Wein Wiss.*, *30*, 82-86

Leo, M.A. & Lieber, C.S. (1983) Hepatic fibrosis after long-term administration of ethanol and moderate vitamin A supplementation in the rat. *Hepatology*, *3*, 1-11

Leo, M.A., Lowe, N. & Lieber, C.S. (1987) Potentiation of ethanol-induced hepatic vitamin A depletion by phenobarbital and butylated hydroxytoluene. *J. Nutr.*, *117*, 70-76

Leppänen, O. & Ronkainen, P. (1982) A sensitive method for the determination of nitrosamines in alcoholic beverages. *Chromatographia*, *16*, 219-223

Leppänen, O., Ronkainen, P., Koivisto, T. & Denslow, J. (1979) A semi-automatic method for the gas chromatographic determination of vicinal diketones in alcoholic beverages. *J. Inst. Brew.*, *85*, 278-281

Lester, D. & Keokosky, W.Z. (1967) Alcohol metabolism in the horse. *Life Sci.*, *6*, 2313-2319

Li, T.-K. & Magnes, L.J. (1975) Identification of a distinctive molecular form of alcohol dehydrogenase in human livers with high activity. *Biochem. biophys. Res. Commun.*, *63*, 202-208

Li, T.-K., Bosron, W.F., Dafeldecker, W.P., Lange, L.G. & Vallee, B.L. (1977) Isolation of II-alcohol dehydrogenase of human liver: is it a determinant of alcoholism? *Proc. natl Acad. Sci. USA*, *74*, 4378-4381

Liddle, P.A.P. & Bossard, A. (1984) *The analysis of anethole and anethole-flavoured beverages by gas chromatography*. In: Nykänen, L. & Lehtonen, P., eds, *Flavour Research of Alcoholic Beverages*, Vol. 3, *Instrumental and Sensory Analysis*, Helsinki, Foundation for Biotechnical and Industrial Fermentation Research, pp. 99-109

Liddle, P.A.P. & Bossard, A. (1985) *Volatile naturally-occurring restricted compounds derived from flavourings, and their determination in foods and beverages*. In: Adda, J., ed., *Progress in Food Flavour Research*, Amsterdam, Elsevier, pp. 467-476

Lieber, C.S. (1970) New pathway of ethanol metabolism in the liver. *Gastroenterology*, *59*, 930-937

Lieber, C.S. (1982) *Medical Disorders of Alcoholism, Pathogenesis and Treatment*, Philadelphia, PA, W.B. Saunders

Lieber, C.S. (1983) *Ethanol metabolism and toxicity*. In: Hodgson, E., Bend, J.R. & Philpot, R.M., eds, *Reviews in Biochemical Toxicology*, Vol. 5, New York, Elsevier, pp. 267-311

Lieber, C.S. (1984a) *Metabolism and metabolic effects of alcohol*. In: Geokas, M.C., ed, *The Medical Clinics of North America*, Vol. 68, *Symposium on Ethyl Alcohol and Disease*, Philadelphia, W.B. Saunders, pp. 3-31

Lieber, C.S. (1984b) Alcohol and the liver: 1984 update. *Hepatology*, *4*, 1243-1260

Lieber, C.S. (1985a) *Ethanol metabolism and pathophysiology of alcoholic liver disease*. In: Seitz, H.K. & Kommerell, B., eds, *Alcohol Related Diseases in Gastroenterology*, Berlin (West), Springer, pp. 19-47

Lieber, C.S. (1985b) Alcohol and the liver: metabolism of ethanol, metabolic effects and pathogenesis of injury. *Acta med. scand., Suppl. 703*, 11-55

Lieber, C.S. & Davidson, C.S. (1962) Some metabolic effects of ethyl alcohol. *Am. J. Med.*, *33*, 319-327

Lieber, C.S. & DeCarli, L.M. (1968) Ethanol oxidation by hepatic microsomes: adaptive increase after ethanol feeding. *Science*, *162*, 917-918

Lieber, C.S. & DeCarli, L.M. (1970) Hepatic microsomal ethanol-oxidizing system: in vitro characteristics and adaptive properties *in vivo*. *J. biol. Chem.*, *245*, 2505-2512

Lieber, C.S. & DeCarli, L.M. (1972) The role of the hepatic microsomal ethanol oxidizing system (MEOS) for ethanol metabolism *in vivo*. *J. Pharmacol. exp. Ther.*, *181*, 279-287

Lieber, C.S. & DeCarli, L.M. (1974) An experimental model of alcohol feeding and liver injury in the baboon. *J. med. Primatol.*, *3*, 153-163

Lieber, C.S. & Schmid, R. (1961) The effect of ethanol on fatty acid metabolism: stimulation of hepatic fatty acid synthesis *in vitro*. *J. clin. Invest.*, *40*, 394-399

Lieber, C.S., Jones, D.P., Mendelson, J. & DeCarli, L.M. (1963) Fatty liver, hyperlipemia and hyperuricemia produced by prolonged alcohol consumption, despite adequate dietary intake. *Trans. Assoc. Am. Phys.*, *76*, 289-300

Lieber, C.S., DeCarli, L.M. & Rubin, E. (1975) Sequential production of fatty liver, hepatitis, and cirrhosis in sub-human primates fed ethanol with adequate diets. *Proc. natl Acad. Sci. USA*, *72*, 437-441

Lieber, C.S., Leo, M.A., Mak, K.M., DeCarli, L.M. & Sato, S. (1985) Choline fails to prevent liver fibrosis in ethanol-fed baboons but causes toxicity. *Hepatology*, *5*, 561-572

Lieber, C.S., Baraona, E., Leo, M.A. & Garro, A. (1987) Metabolism and metabolic effects of ethanol, including interaction with drugs, carcinogens and nutrition. *Mutat. Res.*, *186*, 201-234

Lieberman, F.L. (1963) The effect of liver disease on the rate of ethanol metabolism in man. *Gastroenterology*, *44*, 261-266

Liebich, H.M., König, W.A. & Bayer, E. (1970) Analysis of the flavor of rum by gas-liquid chromatography and mass spectrometry. *J. chromatogr. Sci.*, *8*, 527-533

Lin, J.-Y. & Tai, M.-W. (1980) Mutagenicity of Chinese wine treated with nitrite. *Food Cosmet. Toxicol.*, *18*, 241-243

Lin, R.S. & Kessler, I.I. (1981) A multifactorial model for pancreatic cancer in man. Epidemiologic evidence. *J. Am. med. Assoc.*, *245*, 147-152

Lindenbaum, J. & Lieber, C.S. (1969) Alcohol-induced malabsorption of vitamin B12 in man. *Nature*, *224*, 806

Lindros, K.O. (1978) Acetaldehyde — its metabolism and role in the actions of alcohol. *Res. Adv. Alcohol Drug Probl.*, *4*, 111-176

Lindros, K.O., Oshino, N., Parrilla, R. & Williamson, J.R. (1974) Characteristics of ethanol and acetaldehyde oxidation on flavin and pyridine nucleotide fluorescence changes in perfused rat liver. *J. biol. Chem.*, *249*, 7956-7963

Lindros, K.O., Stowell, A., Pikkarainen, P. & Salaspuro, M. (1980) Elevated blood acetaldehyde in alcoholics with accelerated ethanol elimination. *Pharmacol. Biochem. Behav.*, *13* (Suppl. 1), 119-124

Lindros, K.O., Stowell, L., Väänänen, H., Sipponen, P., Lamminsivu, U., Pikkarainen, P. & Salaspuro, M. (1983) Uninterrupted prolonged ethanol oxidation as a main pathogenetic factor of alcoholic liver damage: evidence from a new liquid diet animal model. *Liver*, *3*, 79-91

Little, R.E. (1977) Moderate alcohol use during pregnancy and decreased infant birth weight. *Am. J. publ. Health*, *67*, 1154-1156

Litvinov, N.N., Voronin, V.M. & Kazatchkov, V.I. (1986a) Evaluation of carcinogenicity of nitrosodimethylamine used in combination with benzene, cadmium, boron or ethanol (Russ.). *Vopr. Onkol.*, *32*, 80-84

Litvinov, N.N., Voronin, V.M. & Kazatchkov, V.I. (1986b) Studies of carcinogenesis modifying properties of aniline, carbon tetrachloride, benzene and ethanol (Russ.). *Eksp. Onkol.*, *8*, 21-23

Lochry, E.A., Randall, C.L., Goldsmith, A.A. & Sutker, P.B. (1982) Effects of acute alcohol exposure during selected days of gestation in C3H mice. *Neurobehav. Toxicol. Teratol.*, *4*, 15-19

Logan, W.P.D. (1982) *Cancer Mortality by Occupation and Social Class, 1851-1971* (*IARC Scientific Publications No. 36*), Lyon, International Agency for Research on Cancer, p. 240

Lolli, G., Serianni, E., Golder, G.M. & Luzzatto-Fegiz, P. (1958) *Alcohol in Italian Culture*, Glencoe, IL, The Free Press, pp. 52-62

Loquet, C., Toussaint, G. & LeTalaer, J.Y. (1980) *Detection of mutagens in various alcoholic beverages, particularly in apple brandy, a product of western France*. In: Holmstedt, B., Lauwerys, R., Mercier, M. & Roberfroid, M., eds, *Mechanisms of Toxicity and Hazard Evaluation*, Amsterdam, Elsevier, pp. 287-290

Loquet, C., Toussaint, G. & LeTalaer, J.Y. (1981) Studies on mutagenic constituents of apple brandy and various alcoholic beverages collected in western France, a high incidence area of oesophageal cancer. *Mutat. Res.*, *88*, 155-164

Lord, T. (1979) *The World Guide to Spirits*, London, Quarto Publishing

Löser, H. & Majewski, F. (1977) Type and frequency of cardiac defects in embryofetal alcohol syndrome. Report of 16 cases. *Br. Heart J.*, *39*, 1374-1379

Losowsky, M.S. & Leonard, P.J. (1967) Evidence of vitamin E deficiency in patients with malabsorption or alcoholism and the effects of therapy. *Gut*, *8*, 539-543

Lumeng, L. & Crabb, D.W. (1984) Rate-determining factors for ethanol metabolism in fasted and castrated male rats. *Biochem. Pharmacol.*, *33*, 2623-2628

Lumeng, L. & Li, T.-K. (1974) Vitamin B_6 metabolism in chronic alcohol abuse. *J. clin. Invest.*, *53*, 693-704

Lyon, J.L., Klauber, M.R., Gardner, J.W. & Smart, C.R. (1976) Cancer incidence in Mormons and non-Mormons in Utah, 1966-1970. *New Engl. J. Med.*, *294*, 129-133

Lyon, J.L., Gardner, J.W. & West, D.W. (1980) Cancer incidence in Mormons and non-Mormons in Utah during 1967-75. *J. natl Cancer Inst.*, *65*, 1055-1061

Ma, T.-H., Harris, M.M., Van Anderson, A., Ahmed, I., Mohammad, K., Bare, J.L. & Lin, G. (1984) Tradescantia-micronucleus (Trad-MCN) tests on 140 health-related agents. *Mutat. Res.*, *138*, 157-167

MacAndrew, C. & Edgerton, R.B. (1969) *Drunken Comportment — A Social Explanation*, Chicago, IL, Aldine Publications

Macdonald, C.M. (1973) The effects of ethanol on hepatic lipid peroxidation and on the activities of glutathione reductase and peroxidase. *FEBS Lett.*, *35*, 227-230

Macdonald, C.M., Dow, J. & Moore, M.R. (1977) A possible protective role for sulphydryl compounds in acute alcoholic liver injury. *Biochem. Pharmacol.*, *26*, 1529-1531

Mack, T.M., Yu, M.C., Hanisch, R. & Henderson, B.E. (1986) Pancreas cancer and smoking, beverage consumption, and past medical history. *J. natl Cancer Inst.*, *76*, 49-60

MacMahon, B., Yen, S., Trichopoulos, D., Warren, K. & Nardi, G. (1981) Coffee and cancer of the pancreas. *New Engl. J. Med.*, *304*, 630-633

MacSween, R.N.M. & Anthony, R.S. (1985) *Immune mechanisms in alcoholic liver disease*. In: Hall, P., ed., *Alcoholic Liver Disease*, London, Edward Arnolds, pp. 69-89

Magrinat, G., Dolan, J.P., Biddy, R.L., Miller, L.D. & Korol, B. (1973) Ethanol and methanol metabolites in alcohol withdrawal. *Nature*, *244*, 234-235

Majchrowicz, E. & Mendelson, J.H. (1970) Blood concentrations of acetaldehyde and ethanol in chronic alcoholics. *Science*, *168*, 1100-1102

Majewski, F. (1978) On the damaging effect of alcohol on offspring (Ger.). *Nervenarzt*, *49*, 410-416

Mak, K.M., Leo, M.A. & Lieber, C.S. (1984) Ethanol potentiates squamous metaplasia of the rat trachea caused by vitamin A deficiency. *Trans. Assoc. Am. Phys.*, *97*, 210-221

Mak, K.M., Leo, M.A. & Lieber, C.S. (1987) Effect of ethanol and vitamin A deficiency on epithelial cell proliferation and structure in the rat esophagus. *Gastroenterology, 93*, 362-370

Mäkelä, K., Room, R., Single, E., Sulkunen, P., Walsh, B., Bunce, R., Cahannes, M., Cameron, T., Giesbrecht, N., de Lint, J., Mäkinen, H., Morgan, P., Mosher, J., Moskalewicz, J., Müller, R., Österberg, E., Wald, I. & Walsh, D. (1981) *Alcohol, Society and the State: 1. A Comparative Study of Alcohol Control*, Toronto, Addiction Research Foundation

Mallory, F.B. (1911) Cirrhosis of the liver. Five different types of lesions from which it may arise. *Bull. Johns Hopkins Hosp., 22*, 69-75

Mallov, S. & Bloch, J.L. (1956) Role of hypophysis and adrenals in fatty infiltration of liver resulting from acute ethanol intoxication. *Am. J. Physiol., 184*, 29-34

Mandard, A.M., Marnay, J., Hélie, H., Tuyns, A.J. & Le Talaer, J.Y. (1981) No effect of ethanol or apple brandy on the upper digestive tract and oesophagus of the Wistar rat. Part of a project to assess etiological factors of cancer of the oesophagus in the west of France (Fr.). *Bull. Cancer, 68*, 49-58

Mändl, B., Wullinger, F., Wagner, D., Binder, W., Schneider, K., Schlosser, A. & Piendl, A. (1971a) Comparison of different aged beers (Ger.). *Brauwelt, 111*, 732-735

Mändl, B., Wullinger, F., Wagner, D., Binder, W., Schneider, K., Schlosser, A. & Piendl, A. (1971b) Comparison of some European beers (Ger.). *Brauwelt, 111*, 1502-1506, 1508-1509, 1511

Mändl, B., Wullinger, F., Wagner, D., Geiger, E., Holzmann, A., Schneider, K. & Piendl, A. (1973) Composition of some American beers (Ger.). *Brauwelt, 113*, 1727, 1729

Mändl, B., Wullinger, F., Becker, H., Wagner, D., Jost, P., Geiger, E., Voss, H., Holzmann, A., Schneider, K. & Piendl, A. (1975) Composition of beers from Cologne (Ger.). *Brauwelt, 115*, 881-883, 886-888

Mändl, B., Wullinger, F. & Wagner, D. (1979) Purines in beer (Ger.). *Brauwissenschaft, 32*, 221-226

Mankes, R.F., LeFevre, R., Benitz, K.-F., Rosenblum, I., Bates, H., Walker, A.I.T., Abraham, R. & Rockwood, W. (1982) Paternal effects of ethanol in the Long-Evans rat. *J. Toxicol. environ. Health, 10*, 871-878

Mankes, R.F., Hoffman, T., LeFevre, R., Bates, H. & Abraham, R. (1983) Acute embryopathic effects of ethanol in the Long-Evans rat. *J. Toxicol. environ. Health, 11*, 583-590

Mann, L.I., Bhakthavathsalan, A., Liu, M. & Makowski, P. (1975) Placental transport of alcohol and its effects on maternal and fetal acid-base balance. *Am. J. Obstet. Gynecol., 122*, 837-844

Manousos, O., Papadimitriou, C., Trichopoulos, D., Polychronopoulou, A., Koutselinis, A. & Zavitsanos, X. (1981) Epidemiologic characteristics and trace elements in pancreatic cancer in Greece. *Cancer Detect. Prev., 4*, 439-442

Marbury, M.C., Linn, S., Monson, R., Schoenbaum, S., Stubblefield, P.G. & Ryan, K.J. (1983) The association of alcohol consumption with outcome of pregnancy. *Am. J. publ. Health, 73*, 1165-1168

Marché, M., Joseph, E., Goizet, A. & Audebert, J. (1975) Theoretical study on cognac, its composition and its natural ageing in oak barrels. III. Principal components of oak wood and substances presumed to be present in spirits (Fr.). *Rev. fr. Oenol., 57*, 13-18

Marjanen, L.A. (1973) Comparison of aldehyde dehydrogenases from cytosol and mitochondria of rat liver. *Biochim. biophys. Acta, 327*, 238-246

Marmot, M.G. (1984) Alcohol and coronary heart disease. *Int. J. Epidemiol., 13*, 160-167

Marnett, L.J., Hurd, H.K., Hollstein, M.C., Levein, D.E., Esterbauer, H. & Ames, B.N. (1985) Naturally occurring carbonyl compunds are mutagens in Salmonella tester strain TA104. *Mutat. Res.*, *148*, 25-34

Marniemi, J., Aitio, A. & Vainio, H. (1975) Ethanol induced alteration of microsomal membrane bound enzymes of rat liver *in vitro*. *Acta pharmacol. toxicol.*, *37*, 222-232

Marshall, M., ed. (1979) *Beliefs, Behaviors and Alcoholic Beverages: A Cross-Cultural Survey*, Ann Arbor, MI, University of Michigan Press, pp. 1-11

Marshall, M., ed. (1982) *Through a Glass Darkly: Beer and Modernization in Papua New Guinea* (*Monograph 18*), Boroko, Papua New Guinea, Institute of Applied Social and Economic Research

Martin, P.M.D. & Hill, G.B. (1984) Cervical cancer in relation to tobacco and alcohol consumption in Lesotho, southern Africa. *Cancer Detect. Prev.*, *7*, 109-115

Martinez, F., Happa, J. & Arias, F. (1985) Biochemical and morphologic effects of ethanol on fetuses from normally ovulating and superovulated mice. *Am. J. Obstet. Gynecol.*, *151*, 428-433

Martinez, I. (1969) Factors associated with cancer of the esophagus, mouth, and pharynx in Puerto Rico. *J. natl Cancer Inst.*, *42*, 1069-1094

Massey, R.C., Crews, C. & McWeeny, D.J. (1982) Method for high-performance liquid chromatographic measurement of *N*-nitrosamines in food and beverages. *J. Chromatogr.*, *241*, 423-427

Matsuda, Y., Baraona, E., Salaspuro, M. & Lieber, C.S. (1979) Effects of ethanol on liver microtubules and Golgi apparatus. Possible role in altered hepatic secretion of plasma proteins. *Lab. Invest.*, *41*, 455-463

Matthewson, K., Al Mardini, H., Bartlett, K. & Record, C.O. (1986) Impaired acetaldehyde metabolism in patients with non-alcoholic liver disorders. *Gut*, *27*, 756-764

Mayer, K. & Pause, G. (1973) Non-volatile biogenic amines in wine (Ger.). *Mitt. Geb. Lebensm. Hyg.*, *64*, 171-179

Mayevsky, A., Bar-Sagie, D. & Bartoov, B. (1983) Sperm cell motility as a new experimental model for toxicological studies. *Arch. Toxicol.*, *Suppl. 6*, 295-299

McCann, J., Choi, E., Yamasaki, E. & Ames, B.N. (1975) Detection of carcinogens as mutagens in the *Salmonella*/microsome test: assay of 300 chemicals, *Proc. natl Acad. Sci. USA*, *72*, 5135-5139

McClain, C.J., Kromhout, J.P., Peterson, F.J. & Holtzman, J.L. (1980) Potentiation of acetaminophen hepatotoxicity by alcohol. *J. Am. med. Assoc.*, *244*, 251-253

McCoy, G.D. (1980) Differential effects of ethanol and other inducers of drug metabolism on the two forms of hamster liver microsomal aniline hydroxylase. *Biochem. Pharmacol.*, *29*, 685-688

McCoy, G.D., Chen, C.-H.B., Hecht, S.S. & McCoy, E.C. (1979) Enhanced metabolism and mutagenesis of nitrosopyrrolidine in liver fractions isolated from chronic ethanol-consuming hamsters. *Cancer Res.*, *39*, 793-796

McCoy, G.D., Hecht, S.S., Katayama, S. & Wynder, E.L. (1981) Differential effect of chronic ethanol consumption on the carcinogenicity of *N*-nitrosopyrrolidine and *N'*-nitrosonornicotine in male Syrian golden hamsters. *Cancer Res.*, *41*, 2849-2854

McCoy, G.D., Hecht, S.S. & Furuya, K. (1986) The effect of chronic ethanol consumption on the tumorigenicity of *N*-nitrosopyrrolidine in male Syrian golden hamsters. *Cancer Lett.*, *33*, 151-159

McDonald, C.D., Burch, G.E. & Walsh, J.J. (1971) Alcoholic cardiomyopathy managed with prolonged bed rest. *Ann. intern. Med.*, *74*, 681-691

McGivern, R.F., Clancy, A.N., Hill, M.A. & Noble, E.P. (1984) Prenatal alcohol exposure alters adult expression of sexually dimorphic behavior in the rat. *Science*, *224*, 896-898

McGlashan, N.D., Walters, C.L. & McLean, A.E.M. (1968) Nitrosamines in African alcoholic spirits and oesophageal cancer. *Lancet*, *ii*, 1017

McGlashan, N.D., Patterson, R.L.S. & Williams, A.A. (1970) N-Nitrosamines and grain-based spirits. *Lancet*, *ii*, 1138

McLain, D.E. & Roe, D.A. (1984) Fetal alcohol syndrome in the ferret (*Mustela putorius*). *Teratology*, *30*, 203-210

McMichael, A.J. (1979) Laryngeal cancer and alcohol consumption in Australia. *Med. J. Austr.*, *1*, 131-134

McMichael, A.J., Potter, J.D. & Hetzel, B.S. (1979) Time trends in colo-rectal cancer mortality in relation to food and alcohol consumption: United States, United Kingdom, Australia and New Zealand. *Int. J. Epidemiol.*, *8*, 295-303

McWeeny, D.J. & Bates, M.L. (1980) Discrimination between synthetic and natural ethyl alcohol in spirits and fortified wines. *J. Food Technol.*, *15*, 407-412

Medina, E., Pascual, J.P., Medina, K.A.M. & Medina, R. (1983) Factors associated with occurrence of breast cancer in women in Chile: study of cases and controls (Sp.). *Rev. med. Chile*, *111*, 1279-1286

Mekhjian, H.S. & May, E.S. (1977) Acute and chronic effects of ethanol on fluid transport in the human small intestine. *Gastroenterology*, *72*, 1280-1286

Mello, N.K., Bree, M.P., Mendelson, J.H. & Ellingboe, J. (1983) Alcohol self-administration disrupts reproductive function in female macaque monkeys. *Science*, *221*, 677-679

Mendelson, J.H. & Mello, N.K. (1974) *Alcohol, aggression and androgens*. In: Frazier, S.H., ed., *Aggression*, Baltimore, MD, Williams & Wilkins, pp. 225-247

Mendelson, J.H. & Stein, S. (1966) Serum cortisol levels in alcoholic and nonalcoholic subjects during experimentally induced ethanol intoxication. *Psychosom. Med.*, *28*, 616-626

Mendelson, J.H., Ogata, M. & Mello, N.K. (1971) Adrenal function and alcoholism. I. Serum cortisol. *Psychosom. Med.*, *33*, 145-157

Mendenhall, C.L. & Chedid, A. (1980) Peliosis hepatis. Its relationship to chronic alcoholism, aflatoxin B_1, and carcinogenesis in male Holtzman rats. *Dig. Dis. Sci.*, *25*, 587-592

Mesley, R.J., Lisle, D.B., Richards, C.P. & Wardleworth, D.F. (1975) The analytical identification of rum. *Ann. Technol. agric.*, *24*, 361-370

Meyer, L.S. & Riley, E.P. (1986) Social play in juvenile rats prenatally exposed to alcohol. *Teratology*, *34*, 1-7

Mezey, E. (1975) Intestinal function in chronic alcoholism. *Ann. N.Y. Acad. Sci.*, *252*, 215-227

Mezey, E. (1976) Ethanol metabolism and ethanol-drug interactions. *Biochem. Pharmacol.*, *25*, 869-875

Mezey, E. (1985) *Effect of ethanol on intestinal morphology, metabolism, and function*. In: Seitz, H.K. & Kommerell, B., eds, *Alcohol Related Diseases in Gastroenterology*, Berlin (West), Springer, pp. 342-360

Mezey, E., Potter, J.J., Harmon, S.M. & Tsitouras, P.D. (1980) Effects of castration and testosterone administration on rat liver alcohol dehydrogenase activity. *Biochem. Pharmacol.*, *29*, 3175-3180

Mezey, E., Potter, J.J., French, S.W., Tamura, T. & Halsted, C.H. (1983) Effect of chronic ethanol feeding on hepatic collagen in the monkey. *Hepatology*, *3*, 41-44

Michaelis, A., Ramshorn, K. & Rieger, R. (1959) Ethanol — radiomimetic agent in *Vicia fabia* L. (Ger.). *Naturwissenschaften*, *46*, 381-382

Midanik, L. (1982) The validity of self-reported alcohol consumption and alcohol problems: a literature review. *Br. J. Addict.*, *77*, 357-382

Mildau, G., Preuss, A., Frank, W. & Heering, W. (1987) Ethyl carbamate (urethane) in alcoholic beverages: improved analysis and light-dependent formation (Ger.). *Dtsch. Lebensm.-Rundsch.*, *83*, 69-74

Miller, A.B., Howe, G.R., Jain, M., Craib, K.J.P. & Harrison, L. (1983) Food items and food groups as risk factors in a case-control study of diet and colo-rectal cancer. *Int. J. Cancer*, *32*, 155-161

Miller, M.W. (1986) Effects of alcohol on the generation and migration of cerebral cortical neurons. *Science*, *233*, 1308-1311

Miller, S.I., Del Villano, B.C., Flynn, A. & Krumhansl, M. (1983) Interaction of alcohol and zinc in fetal dysmorphogenesis. *Pharmacol. Biochem. Behav.*, *18*, 311-315

Miller, W.R. & Hester, R.K. (1986) Inpatient alcoholism treatment. Who benefits? *Am. Psychol.*, *41*, 794-805

Mills, P.R., Pennington, T.H., Kay, P., MacSween, R.N.M. & Watkinson, G. (1979) Hepatitis B_S antibody in alcoholic cirrhosis. *J. clin. Pathol.*, *32*, 778-782

Milon, H., Morin, Y. & Bonenfant, J.-L. (1968) Epidemic of cardiomyopathy in beer drinkers (Fr.). *Arch. Mal. Coeur*, *61*, 1561-1594

Ministère de l'Agriculture (Ministry of Agriculture) (1980) *List of Oenological Practices* (Fr.) (*Circulaire No. DQ/SRF/C/80, No. 8043*), Paris, Service de la Répression des Fraudes et du Contrôle de la Qualité

Ministry of Agriculture, Fisheries and Food (1987) *Survey of Colour Usage in Food* (*Food Surveillance Paper No. 19*), London, Her Majesty's Stationery Office, p. 81

Misra, P.S., Lefèvre, A., Ishii, H., Rubin, E. & Lieber, C.S. (1971) Increase of ethanol, meprobamate and pentobarbital metabolism after chronic ethanol administration in man and in rats. *Am. J. Med.*, *51*, 346-351

Misselhorn, K. (1975) Formation of acetals in rum: a kinetic study. *Ann. Technol. agric.*, *24*, 371-381

Misslbeck, N.G., Campbell, T.C. & Roe, D.A. (1984) Effect of ethanol consumed in combination with high or low fat diets on the postinitiation phase of hepatocarcinogenesis in the rat. *J. Nutr.*, *114*, 2311-2323

Mistilis, S.P. & Garske, A. (1969) Induction of alcohol dehydrogenase in liver and gastro-intestinal tract. *Aust. Ann. Med.*, *18*, 227-231

Mitelman, F. & Wadstein, J. (1978) Chromosome aberrations in chronic alcoholics. *Lancet*, *i*, 216

Miyakawa, H., Iida, S., Leo, M.A., Greenstein, R.J., Zimmon, D.S. & Lieber, C.S. (1985) Pathogenesis of precirrhotic portal hypertension in alcohol-fed baboons. *Gastroenterology*, *88*, 143-150

Mizoi, Y., Ijiri, I., Tatsuno, Y., Kijima, T., Fujiwara, S., Adachi, J. & Hishida, S. (1979) Relationship between facial flushing and blood acetaldehyde levels after alcohol intake. *Pharmacol. Biochem. Behav.*, *10*, 303-311

Mohan, D., Sharma, H.K., Sundaram, K.R. & Neki, J.S. (1980) Pattern of alcohol consumption of rural Punjab males. *Indian J. med. Res.*, *72*, 702-711

Moldéus, P., Andersson, B. & Norling, A. (1978) Interaction of ethanol oxidation with glucuronidation in isolated hepatocytes. *Biochem. Pharmacol.*, *27*, 2583-2588

Møller, J., Brandt, N.J. & Tygstrup, I. (1979) Hepatic dysfunction in patient with fetal alcohol syndrome. *Lancet*, *i*, 605-606

Mommsen, S., Aagaard, J. & Sell, A. (1982) An epidemiological case-control study of bladder cancer in males from a predominantly rural district. *Eur. J. Cancer clin. Oncol.*, *18*, 1205-1210

Monson, R.R. & Lyon, J.L. (1975) Proportional mortality among alcoholics. *Cancer*, *36*, 1077-1079

Moore, M.H. & Gerstein, D.R., eds (1981) *Alcohol and Public Policy: Beyond the Shadow of Prohibition*, Washington DC, National Academy Press

Morgan, E.T., Devine, M. & Skett, P. (1981) Changes in the rat hepatic mixed function oxidase system associated with chronic ethanol vapor inhalation. *Biochem. Pharmacol.*, *30*, 595-600

Morgan, E.T., Koop, D.R. & Coon, M.J. (1982) Catalytic activity of cytochrome P-450 isozyme 3a isolated from liver microsomes of ethanol-treated rabbits. *J. biol. Chem.*, *257*, 13951-13957

Morgan, R.W. & Jain, M.G. (1974) Bladder cancer: smoking, beverages and artificial sweeteners. *Can. med. Assoc. J.*, *111*, 1067-1070

Morin, Y. & Daniel, P. (1967) Quebec beer-drinkers' cardiomyopathy: etiological considerations. *Can. med. Assoc. J.*, *97*, 926-928

Morpurgo, G., Bellincampi, D., Gualandi, G., Baldinelli, L. & Crescenzi, O.S. (1979) Analysis of mitotic nondisjunction with *Aspergillus nidulans*. *Environ. Health Perspect.*, *31*, 81-95

Mortelmans, K., Haworth, S., Lawlor, T., Speck, W., Tainer, B. & Zeiger, E. (1986) Salmonella mutagenicity tests: II. Results from the testing of 270 chemicals. *Environ. mol. Mutagenesis*, *8* (*Suppl. 7*), 1-119

Moser, J., ed. (1985) *Alcohol Policies in National Health and Development Planning* (*WHO Offset Publication No. 89*), Geneva, World Health Organization

Mukherjee, A.B. & Hodgen, G.D. (1982) Maternal ethanol exposure induces transient impairment of umbilical circulation and fetal hypoxia in monkeys. *Science*, *218*, 700-702

Müller, G., Spassowski, M. & Henschler, D. (1975) Metabolism of trichloroethylene in man. III. Interaction of trichloroethylene and ethanol. *Arch. Toxicol.*, *33*, 173-189

Murphy, S.E. & Hecht, S.S. (1986) Effects of chronic ethanol consumption on benzo(*a*)pyrene metabolism and glutathione S-transferase activities in Syrian golden hamster cheek pouch and liver. *Cancer Res.*, *46*, 141-146

Nagao, M., Takahashi, Y., Wakabayashi, K. & Sugimura, T. (1981) Mutagenicity of alcoholic beverages. *Mutat. Res.*, *88*, 147-154

Nakajima, T., Okuyama, S., Yonekura, I. & Sato, A. (1985) Effects of ethanol and phenobarbital administration on the metabolism and toxicity of benzene. *Chem.-biol. Interactions*, *55*, 23-38

Nakano, M. & Lieber, C.S. (1982) Ultrastructure of initial stages of perivenular fibrosis in alcohol-fed baboons. *Am. J. Pathol.*, *106*, 145-155

National Institute on Alcohol Abuse and Alcoholism (1987) *Sixth Special Report to the US Congress on Alcohol and Health from the Secretary of Health and Human Services* (*DHHS Publication No. (ADM) 87-1519*), Washington DC, US Government Printing Office, p. 2

Nayak, B.N. & Buttar, H.S. (1986) Induction of sister chromatid exchanges and chromosome damage by gossypol in bone marrow cells of mice. *Teratog. Carcinog. Mutagenesis*, *6*, 83-91

Nebert, D.W., Adesnik, M., Coon, M.J., Estabrook, R.W., Gonzalez, F.J., Guengerich, F.P., Gunsalus, I.C., Johnson, E.F., Kemper, B., Levin, W., Phillips, I.R., Sato, R. & Waterman, M.R. (1987) The P450 gene superfamily: recommended nomenclature. *DNA*, *6*, 1-11

Neis, J.M., te Brömmelstroet, B.W.J., van Gemert, P.J.L., Roelofs, H.M.J. & Henderson, P.T. (1985) Influence of ethanol induction on the metabolic activation of genetoxic agents by isolated rat hepatocytes. *Arch. Toxicol.*, *57*, 217-221

Nelson, B.K., Brightwell, W.S., MacKenzie, D.R., Khan, A., Burg, J.R., Weigel, W.W. & Goad, P.T. (1985a) Teratological assessment of methanol and ethanol at high inhalation levels in rats. *Fundam. appl. Toxicol.*, *5*, 727-736

Nelson, B.K., Brightwell, W.S. & Burg, J.R. (1985b) Comparison of behavioral teratogenic effects of ethanol and *n*-propanol administered by inhalation to rats. *Neurobehav. Toxicol. Teratol.*, *7*, 779-783

Nelson, R.L. & Samelson, S.L. (1985) Neither dietary ethanol nor beer augments experimental colon carcinogenesis in rats. *Dis. Colon Rectum*, *28*, 460-463

Nelson, R.R., Acree, T.E. & Butts, R.M. (1978) Isolation and identification of volatiles from Catawba wine. *J. agric. Food Chem.*, *26*, 1188-1190

Neugut, R.H. (1981) Epidemiological appraisal of the literature on the fetal alcohol syndrome in humans. *Early hum. Dev.*, *5*, 411-429

Newman, H.W. & Lehman, A.J. (1937) Rate of disappearance of alcohol from the blood stream in various species. *Arch. int. Pharmacodyn.*, *55*, 440-446

New York Heart Association Criteria Committee (1964) *Disease of the Heart and Blood Vessels*, Boston, Little, Brown & Co., p. 112

Nicholls, P., Edwards, G. & Kyle, E. (1974) Alcoholics admitted to four hospitals in England. II. General and cause-specific mortality. *Q. J. Stud. Alcohol*, *35*, 841-855

Nikkila, E.A. & Ojala, K. (1963) Role of hepatic L-a-glycerophosphate and triglyceride synthesis in production of fatty liver by ethanol. *Proc. Soc. exp. Biol. Med.*, *113*, 814-817

Nishimura, K. & Masuda, M. (1971) Minor constituents of whisky fusel oils. 1. Basic, phenolic and lactonic compounds. *J. Food Sci.*, *36*, 819-822

Nishimura, K. & Masuda, M. (1984) *Identification of some flavor characteristic compounds in alcoholic beverages.* In: Nykänen, L. & Lehtonen, P., eds, *Flavour Research of Alcoholic Beverages*, Vol. 3, *Instrumental and Sensory Analysis*, Helsinki, Foundation for Biotechnical and Industrial Fermentation Research, pp. 111-120

Nishimura, K., Ohnishi, M., Masuda, M., Koga, K. & Matsuyama, R. (1983) *Reactions of wood components during maturation.* In: Piggott, J.R., ed., *Flavour of Distilled Beverages: Origin and Development*, Chichester, Ellis Horweed, pp. 241-255

Noble, A.C., Orr, B.H., Cook, W.B. & Campbell, J.L. (1976) Trace element analysis of wine by proton-induced X-ray fluorescence spectrometry. *J. agric. Food Chem.*, *24*, 532-535

Nomura, F., Pikkarainen, P.H., Jauhonen, P., Arai, M., Gordon, E.R., Baraona, E. & Lieber, C.S. (1983) Effect of ethanol administration on the metabolism of ethanol in baboons. *J. Pharmacol. exp. Ther.*, *227*, 78-83

Norell, S.E., Ahlbom, A., Erwald, R., Jacobson, G., Lindberg-Navier, I., Olin, R., Törnberg, B. & Wiechel, K.-L. (1986) Diet and pancreatic cancer: a case-control study. *Am. J. Epidemiol.*, *124*, 894-902

Norton, R., Batey, R., Dwyer, T. & MacMahon, S. (1987) Alcohol consumption and the risk of alcohol related cirrhosis in women. *Br. med. J.*, *295*, 80-82

Nuutinen, H., Lindros, K.O. & Salaspuro, M. (1983) Determinants of blood acetaldehyde level during ethanol oxidation in chronic alcoholics. *Alcohol. clin. exp. Res.*, *7*, 163-168

Nuutinen, H.U., Salaspuro, M.P., Valle, M. & Lindros, K.O. (1984) Blood acetaldehyde concentration gradient between hepatic and antecubital venous blood in ethanol-intoxicated alcoholics and controls. *Eur. J. clin. Invest.*, *14*, 306-311

Nykänen, I. (1984) *The volatile compounds of* Hierochloe odorata. In: Nykänen, L. & Lehtonen, P., eds, *Flavour Research of Alcoholic Beverages*, Vol. 3, *Instrumental and Sensory Analysis*, Helsinki, Foundation for Biotechnical and Industrial Fermentation Research, pp. 131-139

Nykänen, L. (1984) *Aroma compounds liberated from oak chips and wooden casks by alcohol.* In: Nykänen, L. & Lehtonen, P., eds, *Flavour Research of Alcoholic Beverages*, Vol. 3, *Instrumental and Sensory Analysis*, Helsinki, Foundation for Biotechnical and Industrial Fermentation Research, pp. 141-148

Nykänen, L. (1986) Formation and occurrence of flavor compounds in wine and distilled alcoholic beverages. *Am. J. Enol. Viticult.*, *37*, 84-96

Nykänen, L. & Nykänen, I. (1977) Production of esters by different yeast strains in sugar fermentation. *J. Inst. Brew.*, *83*, 30-31

Nykänen, L. & Nykänen, I. (1983) *Rum flavour.* In: Piggott, J.R., ed., *Flavour of Distilled Beverages: Origin and Development*, Chichester, Ellis Horwood, pp. 49-63

Nykänen, L. & Suomalainen, H. (1983) *Aroma of Beer, Wine and Distilled Alcoholic Beverages*, Berlin, Akademie-Verlag

Nykänen, L., Puputti, E. & Suomalainen, H. (1968) Volatile fatty acids in some brands of whisky, cognac and rum. *J. Food Sci.*, *33*, 88-92

Nykänen, L., Nykänen, I. & Suomalainen, H. (1977) Distribution of esters produced during sugar fermentation between the yeast cell and the medium. *J. Inst. Brewing*, *83*, 32-34

Nykänen, L., Nykänen, I. & Moring, M. (1984) *Aroma compounds dissolved from oak chips by alcohol.* In: Adda, J., ed., *Progress in Flavour Research*, Amsterdam, Elsevier, pp. 339-346

Obe, G. (1986) *Epidemiological studies concerning chromosomal aberrations in alcoholics and smokers.* In: Ramel, C., Lambert, B. & Magnusson, J., eds, *Genetic Toxicology of Environmental Chemicals*, Part B, *Genetic Effects and Applied Mutagenesis*, New York, Alan R. Liss, pp. 315-326

Obe, G. & Anderson, D. (1987) Genetic effects of ethanol. *Mutat. Res.*, *186*, 177-200

Obe, G. & Beek, B. (1979) Mutagenic activity of aldehydes. *Drug Alcohol Depend.*, *4*, 91-94

Obe, G. & Ristow, H. (1977) Acetaldehyde, but not ethanol, induces sister chromatid exchanges in Chinese hamster cells *in vitro*. *Mutat. Res.*, *56*, 211-213

Obe, G. & Ristow, H. (1979) Mutagenic, cancerogenic and teratogenic effects of alcohol. *Mutat. Res.*, *65*, 229-259

Obe, G. & Salloch-Vogel, R.-R. (1985) Chromosomal mutations in alcoholics (Ger.). *Suchtgefahren*, *31*, 65-70

Obe, G., Ristow, H.J. & Herha, J. (1977) *Chromosomal damage by alcohol* in vitro *and* in vivo. In: Gross, M.M., ed., *Alcohol Intoxication and Withdrawal*, IIIa, *Biological Aspects of Ethanol*, New York, Plenum Press, pp. 47-70

Obe, G., Ristow, H. & Herha, J. (1978) *Mutagenic activity of alcohol in man.* In: *Mutations: Their Origin, Nature and Potential Relevance to Genetic Risk in Man*, Boppard, Harald Boldt, pp. 151-161

Obe, G., Natarajan, A.T., Meyers, M. & Den Hertog, A. (1979) Induction of chromosomal aberrations in peripheral lymphocytes of human blood *in vitro*, and of SCEs in bone-marrow cells of mice *in vivo* by ethanol and its metabolite acetaldehyde. *Mutat. Res.*, *68*, 291-294

Obe, G., Göbel, D., Engeln, H., Herha, J. & Natarajan, A.T. (1980) Chromosomal aberrations in peripheral lymphocytes of alcoholics. *Mutat. Res.*, *73*, 377-386

Obe, G., Brodmann, R., Fleischer, R., Engeln, H., Göbel, D. & Herha, J. (1985) Mutagenic and carcinogenic action of cultural materials (Ger.). In: Keup, W., ed., *Biology of Habits*, Berlin (West), Springer, pp. 31-43

Obe, G., Jonas, R. & Schmidt, S. (1986) Metabolism of ethanol *in vitro* produces a compound which induces sister-chromatid exchanges in human peripheral lymphocytes *in vitro*: acetaldehyde not ethanol is mutagenic. *Mutat. Res.*, *174*, 47-51

O'Connell, D.L., Hulka, B.S., Chambless, L.E., Wilkinson, W.E. & Deubner, D.C. (1987) Cigarette smoking, alcohol consumption, and breast cancer risk. *J. natl Cancer Inst.*, *78*, 229-234

Oisund, J.F., Fjorden, A.-E. & Mørland, J. (1978) Is moderate ethanol consumption teratogenic in the rat? *Acta pharmacol. toxicol.*, *43*, 145-155

Okanoue, T., Ou, O., Ohta, M., Yoshida, J., Horishi, M., Yuki, T., Okuno, T. & Takino, T. (1984) Effect of chronic ethanol administration on the cytoskeleton of rat hepatocytes — including morphometric analysis (Jpn.). *Acta hepatol. jpn.*, *25*, 210-213

Olegård, R., Sabel, K.-G., Aronsson, M., Sandin, B., Johansson, P.R., Carlsson, C., Kyllerman, M., Iversen, K. & Hrbek, A. (1979) Effects on the child of alcohol abuse during pregnancy. Retrospective and prospective studies. *Acta paediatr. scand.*, *Suppl. 275*, 112-121

Olsen, J., Sabroe, S. & Ipsen, J. (1985a) Effect of combined alcohol and tobacco exposure on risk of cancer of the hypopharynx. *J. Epidemiol. Commun. Health*, *39*, 304-307

Olsen, J., Sabroe, S. & Fasting, U. (1985b) Interaction of alcohol and tobacco as risk factors in cancer of the laryngeal region. *J. Epidemiol. Commun. Health*, *39*, 165-168

Olson, M.J., Pounds, J.G. & Casciano, D.A. (1984) Potentiation of dimethylnitrosamine genotoxicity in rat hepatocytes isolated following ethanol treatment *in vivo*. *Chem.-biol. Interactions*, *50*, 313-326

Ong, T.M., Whong, W.-Z., Stewart, J. & Brockman, H.E. (1986) Chlorophyllin: a potent antimutagen against environmental and dietary complex mixtures. *Mutat. Res.*, *173*, 111-115

Orme-Johnson, W.H. & Ziegler, D.M. (1965) Alcohol mixed function oxidase activity of mammalian liver microsomes. *Biochem. biophys. Res. Commun.*, *21*, 78-82

Oshima, A., Tsukuma, H., Hiyama, T., Fujimoto, I., Yamano, H. & Tanaka, M. (1984) Follow-up study of HBsAg-positive blood donors with special reference to effect of drinking and smoking on development of liver cancer. *Int. J. Cancer*, *34*, 775-779

Oshino, N., Oshino, R. & Chance, B. (1973) The characteristics of the 'peroxidatic' reaction of catalase in ethanol oxidation. *Biochem. J.*, *131*, 555-563

Ouellette, E.M., Rosett, H.L., Rosman, N.P. & Weiner, L. (1977) Adverse effects on offspring of maternal alcohol abuse during pregnancy. *New Engl. J. Med.*, *297*, 528-530

Ough, C.S. (1976a) Ethylcarbamate in fermented beverages and foods. I. Naturally occurring ethylcarbamate. *J. agric. Food Chem.*, *24*, 323-328

Ough, C.S. (1976b) Ethylcarbamate in fermented beverages and foods. II. Possible formation of ethylcarbamate from diethyl dicarbonate addition to wine. *J. agric. Food Chem.*, *24*, 328-331

Ough, C.S. (1984) *Volatile nitrogen compounds in fermented beverages*. In: Nykänen, L. & Lehtonen, P., eds, *Flavour Research of Alcoholic Beverages*, Vol. 3, *Instrumental and Sensory Analysis*, Helsinki, Foundation for Biotechnical and Industrial Fermentation Research, pp. 199-225

Ough, C.S. (1987) Chemicals used in making wine. *Chem. Eng. News*, 5 January, 19-28

Padmanabhan, R. & Muawad, W.M.R.A. (1985) Exencephaly and axial skeletal dysmorphogenesis induced by acute doses of ethanol in mouse fetuses. *Drug Alcohol Depend.*, *16*, 215-227

Padmanabhan, R., Hameed, M.S. & Sugathan, T.N. (1984) Effects of acute doses of ethanol on pre- and postnatal development in the mouse. *Drug Alcohol Depend.*, *14*, 197-208

Paganini-Hill, A. & Ross, R.K. (1983) Breast cancer and alcohol consumption. *Lancet*, *ii*, 626-627

Palamand, S.R., Hardwick, W.A. & Markl, K.S. (1969) Volatile amines in beer and their influence on beer flavor. *Am. Soc. Brew. Chem. Proc.*, 54-58

Palamand, S.R., Markl, K.S. & Hardwick, W.A. (1971) Trace flavor compounds of beer. *Am. Soc. Brew. Chem. Proc.*, 211-218

Palmer, K.R. & Jenkins, W.J. (1982) Impaired acetaldehyde oxidation in alcoholics. *Gut*, *23*, 729-733

Pantuck, E.J., Pantuck, C.B., Ryan, D.E. & Conney, A.H. (1985) Inhibition and stimulation of enflurane metabolism in the rat following a single dose or chronic administration of ethanol. *Anesthesiology*, *62*, 255-262

Parker, S., Udani, M., Gavaler, J.S. & Van Thiel, D.H. (1984) Adverse effects of ethanol upon the adult sexual behavior of male rats exposed *in utero*. *Neurobehav. Toxicol. Teratol.*, *6*, 289-293

Parl, F.F., Lev, R., Thomas, E. & Pitchumoni, C.S. (1979) Histologic and morphometric study of chronic gastritis in alcoholic patients. *Hum. Pathol.*, *10*, 45-56

Parrilla, R., Ohkawa, K., Lindros, K.O., Zimmerman, U.-J.P., Kobayashi, K. & Williamson, J.R. (1974) Functional compartmentation of acetaldehyde oxidation in rat liver. *J. biol. Chem.*, *249*, 4926-4933

Patschky, A. (1973) Chemical composition of imported Rumanian wines (Ger.). *Mitt. Rebe Wein Obstbau Früchteverwert. Klosterneuburg*, *23*, 101-116

Pauli, R.M. & Feldman, P.F. (1986) Major limb malformations following intrauterine exposure to ethanol: two additional cases and literature review. *Teratology*, *33*, 273-280

Peers, F.G. & Linsell, C.A. (1973) Dietary aflatoxins and liver cancer. A population-based study in Kenya. *Br. J. Cancer*, *27*, 473-484

Peiffer, J., Majewski, F., Fischbach, H., Bierich, J.R. & Volk, B. (1979) Alcohol embryo- and fetopathy. Neuropathology of 3 children and 3 fetuses. *J. neurol. Sci.*, *41*, 125-137

Pelkonen, O. & Sotaniemi, E. (1982) Drug metabolism in alcoholics. *Pharmacol. Ther.*, *16*, 261-268

Pell, S. & D'Alonzo, C.A. (1973) A five-year mortality study of alcoholics. *J. occup. Med.*, *15*, 120-125

Peng, R., Tu, Y.Y. & Yang, C.S. (1982) The induction and competitive inhibition of a high affinity microsomal nitrosodimethylamine demethylase by ethanol. *Carcinogenesis*, *3*, 1457-1461

Péquignot, G. & Cubeau, J. (1973) Methodological surveys comparing food consumption of individuals as estimated by questionnaire and by weighing food items (Fr.). *Rev. Epidémiol. Méd. soc. Santé publique*, *21*, 585-608

Péquignot, G., Tuyns, A.J. & Berta, J.L. (1978) Ascitic cirrhosis in relation to alcohol consumption. *Int. J. Epidemiol.*, *7*, 113-120

Péquignot, G., Crosignani, P., Terracini, B., Ascunce, N., Zubiri, A., Raymond, L., Estève, J. & Tuyns, A. (1988) A comparative study of smoking, drinking and dietary habits in population samples in France, Italy, Spain and Switzerland. III. Consumption of alcohol (Fr.). *Rev. Epidémiol. Méd. soc. Santé publique* (in press)

Perin, A., Scalabrino, G., Sessa, A. & Arnaboldi, A. (1974) In vitro inhibition of protein synthesis in rat liver as a consequence of ethanol metabolism. *Biochim. biophys. Acta*, *366*, 101-108

Perloff, J.K. (1971) The cardiomyopathies — current perspectives. *Circulation*, *44*, 942-949

Pernanen, K. (1974) *Validity of survey data on alcohol use*. In: Gibbins, R.J., Israel, Y., Kalant, H, Popham, R.E., Schmidt, W. & Smart, R.G., eds, *Research Advances in Alcohol and Drug Problems*, Vol. 1, New York, John Wiley & Sons, pp. 355-374

Phillips, M.J. (1982) Mallory bodies and the liver. *Lab. Invest.*, *47*, 311-313

Phillips, R.L., Garfinkel, L., Kuzma, J.W., Beeson, W.L., Lotz, T. & Brin, B. (1980) Mortality among California Seventh-day Adventists for selected cancer sites. *J. natl Cancer Inst.*, *65*, 1097-1107

Pieper, W.A. & Skeen, M.J. (1973) Changes in rate of ethanol elimination associated with chronic administration of ethanol to chimpanzees and rhesus monkeys. *Drug Metab. Disposition*, *1*, 634-641

Pierce, D.R. & West, J.R. (1986) Alcohol-induced microencephaly during the third trimester equivalent: relationship to dose and blood alcohol concentration. *Alcohol*, *3*, 185-191

Pikkarainen, P.H. & Lieber, C.S. (1980) Concentration dependency of ethanol elimination rates in baboons: effect of chronic alcohol consumption. *Alcohol. clin. exp. Res.*, *4*, 40-43

Pikkarainen, P.H., Gordon, E.R., Lebsack, M.E. & Lieber, C.S. (1981) Determinants of plasma free acetaldehyde levels during the oxidation of ethanol. Effects of chronic ethanol feeding. *Biochem. Pharmacol.*, *30*, 799-802

Pimstone, N.R. & French, S.W. (1984) Alcoholic liver disease. *Med. Clin. North Am.*, *68*, 39-56

Pollack, E.S., Nomura, A.M.Y., Heilbrun, L.K., Stemmermann, G.N. & Green, S.B. (1984) Prospective study of alcohol consumption and cancer. *New Engl. J. Med.*, *310*, 617-621

Popper, H. & Lieber, C.S. (1980) Histogenesis of alcoholic fibrosis and cirrhosis in the baboon. *Am. J. Pathol.*, *98*, 695-716

Porta, E.A., Markell, N. & Dorado, R.D. (1985) Chronic alcoholism enhances hepatocarcinogenicity of diethylnitrosamine in rats fed a marginally methyl-deficient diet. *Hepatology*, *5*, 1120-1125

Postel, W. & Adam, L. (1982) Gas chromatographic characterization and quantification of spirits. IV. Rum and arrak, and rum and arrak blends (Ger.). *Alkohol-Ind.*, *95*, 360, 362-363

Postel, W., Drawert, F. & Adam, L. (1972a) Gas chromatographic determination of volatile components of fermented beverages. II. The content of volatile components in beer (Ger). *Chem. mikrobiol. Technol. Lebensm.*, *1*, 169-182

Postel, W., Drawert, F. & Adam, L. (1972b) Gas chromatographic determination of volatile components of fermented beverages. III. Volatile components of wines (Ger.). *Chem. mikrobiol. Technol. Lebensm.*, *1*, 224-235

Postel, W., Drawert, F. & Adam, L. (1975) *Aroma compounds in spirits* (Ger.) In: Drawert, F., ed., *Odour and Taste Compounds*, Bad Pyrmont, Hans Nürnberg, pp. 99-111

Potter, J.D. & McMichael, A.J. (1986) Diet and cancer of the colon and rectum: a case-control study. *J. natl Cancer Inst.*, *76*, 557-569

Potter, J.D., McMichael, A.J. & Hartshorne, J.M. (1982) Alcohol and beer consumption in relation to cancers of bowel and lung: an extended correlation analysis. *J. chron. Dis.*, *35*, 833-842

Pottern, L.M., Morris, L.E., Blot, W.J., Ziegler, R.G. & Fraumeni, J.F., Jr (1981) Esophageal cancer among black men in Washington, DC. I. Alcohol, tobacco, and other risk factors. *J. natl Cancer Inst.*, *67*, 777-783

Pour, P.M., Reber, H.A. & Stepan, K. (1983) Modification of pancreatic carcinogenesis in the hamster model. XII. Dose-related effect of ethanol. *J. natl Cancer Inst.*, *71*, 1085-1087

Priscott, P.K. (1982) The effects of ethanol on rat embryos developing *in vitro*. *Biochem. Pharmacol.*, *31*, 3641-3643

Puech, J.-L. (1978) *Vieillissement des Eaux de Vie en Fûts de Chêne. Extraction et Evolution de la Lignine et de ses Produits de Dégradation* (Ageing of spirits in oak casks. Extraction and evolution of lignin and its degradation products), Thesis No. 2087, Toulouse, Université Paul Sabatier

Puputti, E. & Suomalainen, H. (1969) Biogenic amines in wine (Ger.). *Mitt. Rebe Wein Obstbau Früchteverwert. Klosterneuburg*, *19*, 184-192

Quazi, Q., Masakawa, A., Milman, D., McGann, B., Chua, A. & Haller, J. (1979) Renal anomalies in fetal alcohol syndrome. *Pediatrics*, *63*, 886-889

de Raat, W.K., Davis, P.B. & Bakker, G.L. (1983) Induction of sister-chromatid exchanges by alcohol and alcoholic beverages after metabolic activation by rat-liver homogenate. *Mutat. Res.*, *124*, 85-90

Rachamin, G., Macdonald, J.A., Wahid, S., Clapp, J.J., Khanna, J.M. & Israel, Y. (1980) Modulation of alcohol dehydrogenase and ethanol metabolism by sex hormones in the spontaneously hypertensive rat. Effect of chronic ethanol administration. *Biochem. J.*, *186*, 483-490

Racker, E. (1949) Aldehyde dehydrogenase, a diphosphopyridine nucleotide-linked enzyme. *J. biol. Chem.*, *177*, 883-892

Radike, M.J., Stemmer, K.L. & Bingham, E. (1981) Effect of ethanol on vinyl chloride carcinogenesis. *Environ. Health Perspect.*, *41*, 59-62

Räihä, N.C.R. & Oura, E. (1962) Effect of ethanol oxidation on levels of pyridine nucleotides in liver and yeast. *Proc. Soc. exp. Biol. Med.*, *109*, 908-910

Randall, C.L. & Taylor, W.J. (1979) Prenatal ethanol exposure in mice: teratogenic effects. *Teratology*, *19*, 305-312

Randall, C.L., Taylor, W.J. & Walker, D.W. (1977) Ethanol-induced malformations in mice. *Alcohol. clin. exp. Res.*, *1*, 219-224

Randall, C.L., Burling, T.A., Lochry, E.A. & Sutker, P.B. (1982) The effect of paternal alcohol consumption on fetal development in mice. *Drug Alcohol Depend.*, *9*, 89-95

Randall, C.L., Becker, H.C. & Middaugh, L.D. (1986) Effect of prenatal ethanol exposure on activity and shuttle avoidance behavior in adult C57 mice. *Alcohol Drug Res.*, *6*, 351-360

Rapp, A. & Mandery, H. (1986) Wine aroma. *Experientia*, *42*, 873-884

Rapp, A., Mandery, H. & Güntert, M. (1984) *Terpene compounds in wine*. In: Nykänen, L. & Lehtonen, P., eds, *Flavour Research of Alcoholic Beverages*, Vol. 3, *Instrumental and Sensory Analysis*, Helsinki, Foundation for Biotechnical and Industrial Fermentation Research, pp. 255-274

Rapp, A., Güntert, M. & Ullemeyer, H. (1985) Change in aroma substances during storage of white Riesling wines in bottles (Ger.). *Z. Lebensmitteluntersuch. Forsch.*, *180*, 109-116

Rasmussen, B.B. & Christensen, N. (1980) Teratogenic effect of maternal alcohol consumption in the mouse fetus: a histopathological study. *Acta pathol. microbiol. scand., Sect. A*, *88*, 285-289

Rasmussen, E.W. (1940) Effect of thirst on desorption of ethanol and ethanol content of blood after oral administration (Ger.). *Biochem. Z.*, *304*, 358-370

Raymond, L., Infante, F., Tuyns, A.J., Voirol, M. & Lowenfelds, A.B. (1987) Diet and pancreatic cancer (Fr.) *Gastroenterol. clin. biol.*, *11*, 488-492

Reazin, G.H. (1983) *Chemical analysis of whisky maturation*. In: Piggott, J.R., ed., *Flavour of Distilled Beverages: Origin and Development*, Chichester, Ellis Horwood, pp. 225-240

Reazin, G.H., Baldwin, S., Scales, H.S., Washington, H.W. & Andreasen, A.A. (1976) Determination of the congeners produced from ethanol during whisky maturation. *J. Assoc. off. anal. Chem.*, *59*, 770-776

Rebouças, G. & Isselbacher, K.J. (1961) Studies on the pathogenesis of the ethanol-induced fatty liver. I. Synthesis and oxidation of fatty acids by the liver. *J. clin. Invest.*, *40*, 1355-1362

Redmond, G. & Cohen, G. (1971) Induction of liver acetaldehyde dehydrogenase: possible role in ethanol tolerance after exposure to barbiturates. *Science*, *171*, 387-389

Regan, T.J., Wu, C.F., Weisse, A.B., Moschos, C.B., Ahmed, S.S. & Lyons, M.M. (1975) Acute myocardial infarction in toxic cardiomyopathy without coronary obstruction. *Circulation*, *51*, 453-461

Registrar General (1958) *Decennial Supplement for England and Wales, 1951. Occupational Mortality*, Part II, Vol. 2, Tables, London, Her Majesty's Stationery Office

Reinhard, C. (1977) Study of whisky (Ger.). *Dtsch. Lebensm.-Rundsch.*, *73*, 124-129

Reinke, L.A. & Moyer, M.J. (1985) *p*-Nitrophenol hydroxylation. A microsomal oxidation which is highly inducible by ethanol. *Drug Metab. Disposition*, *13*, 548-552

Reinke, L.A., Kauffman, F.C., Belinsky, S.A. & Thurman, R.G. (1980) Interactions between ethanol metabolism and mixed-function oxidation in perfused rat liver: inhibition of *p*-nitroanisole O-demethylation. *J. Pharmacol. exp. Ther.*, *213*, 70-78

Reinke, L.A., Moyer, M.J. & Notley, K.A. (1986) Diminished rates of glucuronidation and sulfation in perfused rat liver after chronic ethanol administration. *Biochem. Pharmacol.*, *35*, 439-447

Riboli, E., Caperle, M., Sabatino, C. & Crespi, M. (1986) Evaluation of dietary assessment methods. Pilot phase of a case-control study on colorectal polyps. *Ital. J. Gastroenterol.*, *18*, 245-248

Rieger, R. & Michaelis, A. (1960) *Radiomimetic effects of ethanol in Vicia faba* (Ger.). In: Stubbe, H., ed., *Chemical Mutagenesis. Erwin Baur Memorial Lectures*, I, July 1959, Berlin, Akademie-Verlag, pp. 54-65

Rieger, R. & Michaelis, A. (1961) Importance of ATP for the radiomimetic effect of ethanol in *Vicia faba* (Ger.). *Naturwissenschaften, 48*, 139

Rieger, R. & Michaelis, A. (1970) Intrachromosomal clustering of chromatid aberrations induced by maleic hydrazide and ethyl alcohol: studies with a new karyotype of *Vicia faba*. *Mutat. Res.*, *10*, 162-164

Rieger, R. & Michaelis, A. (1972) Effects of chromosome repatterning in *Vicia faba* L. I. Aberration distribution, aberration spectrum, and karyotype sensitivity after treatment with ethanol of differently reconstructed chromosome complements. *Biol. Zbl.*, *91*, 151-169

Rieger, R., Michaelis, A. & Nicoloff, H. (1982) Inducible repair processes in plant root tip meristems? 'Below-additivity effects' of unequally fractionated clastogen concentrations. *Biol. Zbl.*, *101*, 125-138

Rieger, R., Michaelis, A. & Schubert, I. (1985) Heat-shocks prior to treatment of *Vicia faba* root-tip meristems with maleic hydrazide or TEM reduce the yield of chromatid aberrations. *Mutat. Res.*, *143*, 79-82

Riihimäki, V., Savolainen, K., Pfäffli, P., Pekari, K., Sippel, H.W. & Laine, A. (1982) Metabolic interaction between m-xylene and ethanol. *Arch. Toxicol.*, *49*, 253-263

Ristow, H. & Obe, G. (1978) Acetaldehyde induces cross-links in DNA and causes sister-chromatid exchanges in human cells. *Mutat. Res.*, *58*, 115-119

Robinette, C.D., Hrubec, Z. & Fraumeni, J.F., Jr (1979) Chronic alcoholism and subsequent mortality in World War II veterans. *Am. J. Epidemiol.*, *109*, 687-700

Robles, E.A., Mezey, E., Halsted, C.H. & Schuster, M.M. (1974) Effect of ethanol on motility of the small intestine. *Johns Hopkins med. J.*, *135*, 17-24

Rockwood, G.A. & Riley, E.P. (1986) Suckling deficits in rat pups exposed to alcohol *in utero*. *Teratology*, *33*, 145-151

Rohan, T.E. & Potter, J.D. (1984) Retrospective assessment of dietary intake. *Am. J. Epidemiol.*, *120*, 876-887

Room, R. (1978) *Measurement and distribution of drinking patterns and problems in general population.* In: Edwards, G., Gross, M.M., Keller, M., Moser, J. & Room, R., eds, *Alcohol-related Disabilities* (*WHO Offset Publication No. 32*), Geneva, World Health Organization, pp. 61-87

Room, R. (1979) Measurements of drinking patterns in the general population and possible applications in studies of the role of alcohol in cancer. *Cancer Res.*, *39*, 2830-2833

Room, R. (1983) *Region and urbanization as factors in drinking practices and problems.* In: Kissin, B. & Begleiter, H., eds, *The Biology of Alcoholism*, Vol. 6, *The Pathogenesis of Alcoholism: Psychosocial Factors*, New York, Plenum Press, pp. 555-604

Room, R. (1984) Alcohol control and public health. *Ann. Rev. public Health*, *5*, 293-317

Root, A.W., Reiter, E.O., Andriola, M. & Duckett, G. (1975) Hypotholamic-pituitary function in the fetal alcohol syndrome. *J. Pediatr.*, *87*, 585-588

Rootman, I. & Moser, J. (1984) *Community Response to Alcohol-related Problems* (*DHHS Publication No. (ADM) 85-1371*), Washington DC, US Government Printing Office, pp. 79-81, 114-117

Rorabaugh, W.J. (1979) *The Alcoholic Republic: An American Tradition*, New York, Oxford University Press, pp. 61-92

Rosenberg, L., Slone, D., Shapiro, S., Kaufman, D.W., Helmrich, S.P., Miettinen, O.S., Stolley, P.D., Levy, M., Rosenshein, N.B., Schottenfeld, D. & Engle, R.L., Jr (1982) Breast cancer and alcoholic-beverage consumption. *Lancet*, *i*, 267-271

Rosenkranz, H.S. (1977) Mutagenicity of halogenated alkanes and their derivatives. *Environ. Health Perspect.*, *21*, 79-84

Rosovsky, H. (1986) Public health aspects of the production, marketing and control of alcoholic beverages in Mexico. *Contemp. Drug Probl.*, *12*, 659-678

Rothman, K.J. (1976) The estimation of synergy or antagonism. *Am. J. Epidemiol.*, *103*, 506-511

Rothman, K.J. (1978) The effect of alcohol consumption on risk of cancer of the head and neck. *Laryngoscope*, *88* (Suppl. 8), 125-129

Rothman, K.J. & Keller, A. (1972) The effect of joint exposure to alcohol and tobacco on risk of cancer of the mouth and pharynx. *J. chron. Dis.*, *25*, 711-716

Rubin, E. & Lieber, C.S. (1968) Hepatic microsomal enzymes in man and rat: induction and inhibition by ethanol. *Science*, *162*, 690-691

Rubin, E., Hutterer, F. & Lieber, C.S. (1968) Ethanol increases hepatic smooth endoplasmic reticulum and drug-metabolizing enzymes. *Science*, *159*, 1469-1470

Rubin, E., Gang, H., Misra, P.S. & Lieber, C.S. (1970) Inhibition of drug metabolism by acute ethanol intoxication. A hepatic microsomal mechanism. *Am. J. Med.*, *49*, 801-806

Rubin, E., Gang, H. & Lieber, C.S. (1971) Interaction of ethanol and pyrazole with hepatic microsomes. *Biochem. biophys. Res. Commun.*, *42*, 1-8

Rubin, E., Lieber, C.S., Altman, K., Gordon, G.G. & Southren, A.L. (1976) Prolonged ethanol consumption increases testosterone metabolism in the liver. *Science*, *191*, 563-564

Rudeen, P.K., Kappel, C.A. & Lear, K. (1986) Postnatal or in utero ethanol exposure reduction of the volume of the sexually dimorphic nucleus of the preoptic area in male rats. *Drug Alcohol Depend.*, *18*, 247-252

Rueff, J., Laires, A., Borba, H., Chaveca, T., Gomes, M.I. & Halpern, M. (1986) Genetic toxicology of flavonoids: the role of metabolic conditions in the induction of reverse mutation, SOS functions and sister-chromatid exchanges. *Mutagenesis*, *1*, 179-183

Rydberg, B. (1985) *Why do Swedish youth drink less alcohol?* In: Tongue, A. & Tongue, E., eds, *Proceedings of the 31st Meeting of the International Institute on the Prevention and Treatment of Alcoholism*, Lausanne, International Council on Alcohol and Addictions, Vol. 1, pp. 475-478

Saha, R.B., Middlekauff, J.E. & Hardwick, W.A. (1971) Quantitation of nucleic acid materials in beer and wort with particular reference to nucleosides and free bases. *Am. Soc. Brew. Chem. Proc.*, 206-210

Salaspuro, M.P. & Lieber, C.S. (1979) *Metabolic consequences of chronic alcohol consumption: attenuation of hepatic redox changes despite enhanced capacity to eliminate ethanol.* In: Galander, M., ed., *Currents in Alcoholism*, Vol. 5, New York, Grune & Stratton, pp. 109-118

Salaspuro, M.P. & Lieber, C.S. (1980) *Comparison of the detrimental effects of chronic alcohol intake in mammals and animals.* In: Eriksson, K., Sinclair, J.D. & Kiiaman, K., eds, *Animal Models in Alcohol Research*, London, Academic Press, pp. 359-376

Salaspuro, M.P. & Lindros, K. (1985) *Metabolism and toxicity of acetaldehyde.* In: Seitz, H.K. & Kommerell, B., eds, *Alcohol Related Diseases in Gastroenterology*, Berlin (West), Springer, pp. 106-123

Salaspuro, M.P. & Mäenpää, P.H. (1966) Influence of ethanol on the metabolism of perfused normal, fatty and cirrhotic rat livers. *Biochem. J.*, *100*, 768-774

Samson, H.H. (1981) Maternal ethanol consumption and fetal development in the rat: a comparison of ethanol exposure techniques. *Alcohol. clin. exp. Res.*, *5*, 67-74

Sanchis, R. & Guerri, C. (1986) Chronic ethanol intake in lactating rats: milk analysis. *Comp. Biochem. Physiol.*, *85C*, 107-110

Sandor, G.G.S., Smith, D.F. & MacLeod, P.M. (1981) Cardiac malformations in the fetal alcohol syndrome. *J. Pediatr.*, *98*, 771-773

Sandor, S., Fazakas-Todea, I. & Checiu, M. (1980) The effect of ethanol upon early development in mice and rats. II. In vitro effect upon early postimplantation rat embryos. *Morphol. Embryol.*, *26*, 315-320

Sarles, H. & Laugier, R. (1981) *Alcoholic pancreatitis.* In: Leevy, C.M., ed., *Clinics in Gastroenterology*, Vol. 10, *Alcohol and the GI Tract*, London, W.B. Saunders, pp. 401-415

Sato, A. & Nakajima, T. (1985) Enhanced metabolism of volatile hydrocarbons in rat liver following food deprivation, restricted carbohydrate intake, and administration of ethanol, phenobarbital, polychlorinated biphenyl and 3-methylcholanthrene: a comparative study. *Xenobiotica, 15*, 67-75

Sato, A., Nakajima, T. & Koyama, Y. (1981) Dose-related effects of a single dose of ethanol on the metabolism in rat liver of some aromatic and chlorinated hydrocarbons. *Toxicol. appl. Pharmacol., 60*, 8-15

Sato, A., Yonekura, I., Asakawa, M., Nakahara, H., Nakajima, T., Ohta, S., Shirai, T. & Ito, N. (1986) Augmentation of ethanol-induced enhancement of dimethylnitrosamine and diethylnitrosamine metabolism by lowered carbohydrate intake. *Jpn. J. Cancer Res. (Gann), 77*, 125-130

Sato, C., Matsuda, Y. & Lieber, C.S. (1981) Increased hepatotoxicity of acetaminophen after chronic ethanol consumption in the rat. *Gastroenterology, 80*, 140-148

Sato, C., Hasumura, Y. & Takeuchi, J. (1985) *Interaction of ethanol with drugs and xenobiotics*. In: Seitz, H.K. & Kommerell, B., eds, *Alcohol Related Diseases in Gastroenterology*, Berlin (West), Springer, pp. 172-184

Sato, M. & Lieber, C.S. (1981) Hepatic vitamin A depletion after chronic ethanol consumption in baboons and rats. *J. Nutr., 111*, 2015-2023

Schatzkin, A., Jones, D.Y., Hoover, R.N., Taylor, P.R., Brinton, L.A., Ziegler, R.G., Harvey, E.B., Carter, C.L., Licitra, L.M., Dufour, M.C. & Larson, D.B. (1987) Alcohol consumption and breast cancer in the epidemiologic follow-up study of the First National Health and Nutritional Examination Survey. *New Engl. J. Med., 316*, 1169-1173

Schmähl, D. (1976) Investigations on esophageal carcinogenicity by methylphenylnitrosamine and ethyl alcohol in rats. *Cancer Lett., 1*, 215-218

Schmähl, D., Thomas, C., Sattler, W. & Scheld, G.F. (1965) Experimental studies on syncarcinogenesis. III. Attempts to induce cancer in rats by administering diethylnitrosamine and CCl_4 (or ethyl alcohol) simultaneously. In addition, an experimental contribution regarding 'alcoholic cirrhosis' (Ger.). *Z. Krebsforsch., 66*, 526-532

Schmidt, W. & de Lint, J. (1972) Causes of death of alcoholics. *Q. J. Stud. Alcohol, 33*, 171-185

Schmidt, W. & Popham, R.E. (1981) The role of drinking and smoking in mortality from cancer and other causes in male alcoholics. *Cancer, 47*, 1031-1041

Schmidt, W., Popham, R.E. & Israel, Y. (1987) Dose-specific effects of alcohol on the lifespan of mice and the possible relevance to man. *Br. J. Addict., 82*, 775-788

Schmitt, A. (1972) Correlation between the content of compounds and sensorial properties of German wines in the province of Frankonia (Ger.). *Bayer. Landwirtsch. Jahrb., 49*, 259-330

Schnellmann, R.G., Wiersma, D.A., Randall, D.J., Smith, T.L. & Sipes, I.G. (1984) Hepatic mixed function oxygenase activity and glutathione *S*-transferase activity in mice following ethanol consumption and withdrawal. *Toxicology, 32*, 105-116

Schoeneman, R.L. & Dyer, R.H. (1973) Analytical profile of Scotch whiskies. *J. Assoc. off. anal. Chem., 56*, 1-10

Schoeneman, R.L., Dyer, R.H. & Earl, E.M. (1971) Analytical profile of straight bourbon whiskies. *J. Assoc. off. anal. Chem., 54*, 1247-1261

Scholz, R. & Nohl, H. (1976) Mechanism of the stimulatory effect of fructose on ethanol oxidation in perfused rat liver. *Eur. J. Biochem., 63*, 449-458

Schrauzer, G.N., McGinness, J.E., Ishmael, D. & Bell, L.J. (1979) Alcoholism and cancer. 1. Effects of long-term exposure to alcohol on spontaneous mammary adenocarcinoma and prolactin levels in C3H/St mice. *J. Stud. Alcohol*, *40*, 240-246

Schrauzer, G.N., Hamm, D., Kuehn, K. & Nakonecny, G. (1982) Effects of long term exposure to beer on the genesis and development of spontaneous mammary adenocarcinoma and prolactin levels in female virgin C_3H/St mice. *J. Am. Coll. Nutr.*, *1*, 285-291

Schreier, P. (1984) *Formation of wine aroma*. In: Nykänen, L. & Lehtonen, P., eds, *Flavour Research of Alcoholic Beverages*, Vol. 3, *Instrumental and Sensory Analysis*, Helsinki, Foundation for Biotechnical and Industrial Fermentation Research, pp. 9-37

Schreier, P. & Drawert, F. (1974) Gas chromatographic-mass spectrometric investigation of volatile constituents of wines. V. Alcohols, hydroxy-esters, lactones and other polar compounds of wine flavour (Ger.). *Chem. mikrobiol. Technol. Lebensm.*, *3*, 154-160

Schreier, P., Drawert, F. & Junker, A. (1975) Biosynthesis of aroma compounds by microorganisms. I. Formation of *N*-acetylamines by *Saccharomyces cerevisiae* (Ger.). *Z. Lebensmitteluntersuch. Forsch.*, *158*, 351-360

Schreier, P., Drawert, F. & Junker, A. (1976a) Gas chromatographic-mass spectrometric differentiation of the aroma compounds of different grape varieties of *Vitis vinefera* (Ger.). *Chem. mikrobiol. Technol. Lebensm.*, *4*, 154-157

Schreier, P., Drawert, F., Junker, A. & Reiner, L. (1976b) Application of the multiple discriminant analysis for the differentiation of grape varieties using the quantitative distribution of volatile wine constituents (Ger.). *Mitt. Rebe Wein Obstbau Früchteverwert. Klosterneuburg*, *26*, 225-234

Schreier, P., Drawert, F. & Schmid, M. (1978) Changes in the composition of neutral volatile components during the production of apple brandy. *J. Sci. Food Agric.*, *29*, 728-736

Schreier, P., Drawert, F. & Winkler, F. (1979) Composition of neutral volatile constituents in grape brandies. *J. agric. Food Chem.*, *27*, 365-372

Schubert, I., Sturelid, S., Döbel, P. & Rieger, R. (1979) Intra-chromosomal distribution patterns of mutagen-induced SCEs and chromatid aberrations in reconstructed karyotypes of *Vicia faba*. *Mutat. Res.*, *59*, 27-38

Schuller, P.L., Ockhuizen, T., Werringloer, J. & Marquardt, D. (1967) Aflatoxin B_1 and histamine in wine (Ger.). *Arzneimittelforschung*, *17*, 888-890

Schwartz, D., Denoix, P.F. & Anguera, G. (1957) Cancer sites associated with tobacco and alcohol in humans (Fr.). *Bull. Cancer*, *44*, 336-361

Schwartz, D., Lellouch, J., Flamant, R. & Denoix, P.F. (1962) Alcohol and cancer. Results of a retrospective study (Fr.). *Rev. fr. Etud. clin. biol.*, *7*, 590-604

Schwartz, J.L., Banda, M.J. & Wolff, S. (1982) 12-*O*-Tetradecanoylphorbol-13-acetate (TPA) induces sister-chromatid exchanges and delays in cell progression in Chinese hamster ovary and human cell lines. *Mutat. Res.*, *92*, 393-409

Schwarz, M., Buchmann, A., Wiesbeck, G. & Kunz, W. (1983) Effect of ethanol on early stages in nitrosamine carcinogenesis in rat liver. *Cancer Lett.*, *20*, 305-312

Schwarz, M., Buchmann, A., Moore, M. & Kunz, W. (1984) *The mechanism of cocarcinogenic action of ethanol in rat liver*. In: Börzsönyi, M., Lapis, K., Day, N.E. & Yamasaki, H., eds, *Models, Mechanisms and Etiology of Tumour Promotion* (*IARC Scientific Publications No. 56*), Lyon, International Agency for Research on Cancer, pp. 83-90

Schwetz, B.A., Smith, F.A. & Staples, R.E. (1978) Teratogenic potential of ethanol in mice, rats and rabbits. *Teratology, 18*, 385-392

Scott, W.J., Jr & Fradkin, R. (1984) The effects of prenatal ethanol in cynomolgus monkeys. *Teratology, 29*, 49-56

Seeff, L.B., Cuccherini, B.A., Zimmerman, H.J., Adler, E. & Benjamin, S.B. (1986) Acetaminophen hepatotoxicity in alcoholics. A therapeutic misadventure. *Ann. intern. Med., 104*, 399-404

Seitz, H.K. (1985) *Ethanol and carcinogenesis*. In: Seitz, H.K. & Kommerell, B., eds, *Alcohol Related Diseases in Gastroenterology*, Berlin (West), Springer, pp. 196-212

Seitz, H.K., Garro, A.J. & Lieber, C.S. (1978) Effect of chronic ethanol ingestion on intestinal metabolism and mutagenicity of benzo(*a*)pyrene. *Biochem. biophys. Res. Commun., 85*, 1061-1066

Seitz, H.K., Korsten, M.A. & Lieber, C.S. (1979) Ethanol oxidation by intestinal microsomes: increased activity after chronic ethanol administration. *Life Sci., 25*, 1443-1448

Seitz, H.K., Garro, A.J. & Lieber, C.S. (1981a) Sex dependent effect of chronic ethanol consumption in rats on hepatic microsome mediated mutagenicity of benzo[*a*]pyrene. *Cancer Lett., 13*, 97-102

Seitz, H.K., Garro, A.J. & Lieber, C.S. (1981b) Enhanced pulmonary and intestinal activation of procarcinogens and mutagens after chronic ethanol consumption in the rat. *Eur. J. clin. Invest., 11*, 33-38

Seitz, H.K., Bösche, J., Czygan, P., Veith, S. & Kommerell, B. (1982) Microsomal ethanol oxidation in the colonic mucosa of the rat. Effect of chronic ethanol ingestion. *Naunyn-Schmiedeberg's Arch. Pharmacol., 320*, 81-84

Seitz, H.K., Czygan, P., Waldherr, R., Veith, S., Raedsch, R., Kässmodel, H. & Kommerell, B. (1984) Enhancement of 1,2-dimethylhydrazine-induced rectal carcinogenesis following chronic ethanol consumption in the rat. *Gastroenterology, 86*, 886-891

Seitz, H.K., Czygan, P., Simanowski, U., Waldherr, R., Veith, S., Raedsch, R. & Kommerell, B. (1985) Stimulation of chemically induced rectal carcinogenesis by chronic ethanol ingestion. *Alcohol Alcohol., 20*, 427-433

Sen, N.P. (1969) Analysis and significance of tyramine in foods. *J. Food Sci., 34*, 22-26

Serbus, D.C., Stull, R.E. & Light, K.E. (1986) Neonatal ethanol exposure to rat pups: resultant alterations of cortical muscarinic and cerebellar H^1-histaminergic receptor binding dynamics. *Neuro Toxicol., 7*, 257-278

Seshadri, R., Baker, E. & Sutherland, G.R. (1982) Sister-chromatid exchange (SCE) analysis in mothers exposed to DNA-damaging agents and their newborn infants. *Mutat. Res., 97*, 139-146

Sharma, A. & Rawat, A.K. (1986) Teratogenic effects of lithium and ethanol in the developing fetus. *Alcohol, 3*, 101-106

Shaw, S., Jayatilleke, E., Ross, W.A., Gordon, E.R. & Lieber, C.S. (1981) Ethanol-induced lipid peroxidation: potentiation by long-term alcohol feeding and attenuation by methionine. *J. Lab. clin. Med., 98*, 417-424

Shibata, A., Hirohata, T., Toshima, H. & Tashiro, H. (1986) The role of drinking and cigarette smoking in the excess deaths from liver cancer. *Jpn. J. Cancer Res.* (*Gann*), *77*, 287-295

Shigeta, Y., Nomura, F., Iida, S., Leo, M.A., Felder, M.R. & Lieber, C.S. (1984) Ethanol metabolism *in vivo* by the microsomal ethanol-oxidizing system in deermice lacking alcohol dehydrogenase (ADH). *Biochem. Pharmacol., 33*, 807-814

Shimizu, J. & Watanabe, M. (1978) Gas chromatographic determination of diethyl esters of succinic, malic, and tartaric acid in wine (Jpn.). *Nippon Nogei Kagaku Kaishi*, *52*, 289-291 [*Chem. Abstr.*, *89*, 161476n]

Shinohara, T. & Watanabe, M. (1976) Gas chromatographic analysis of higher alcohols and ethyl acetate in table wines. *Agric. Biol. Chem. (Tokyo)*, *40*, 2475-2477

Sies, H. (1974) Biochemistry of the peroxisome of the liver cell. *Angew. Chem. int. Ed.*, *13*, 706-718

Simanowski, U.A., Seitz, H.K., Baier, B., Kommerell, B., Schmidt-Gayk, H. & Wright, N.A. (1986) Chronic ethanol consumption selectively stimulates rectal cell proliferation in the rat. *Gut*, *27*, 278-282

Simpson, R.F. & Miller, G.C. (1983) Aroma composition of aged Riesling wine. *Vitis*, *22*, 51-63

Simpson, R.F. & Miller, G.C. (1984) Aroma composition of Chardonnay wine. *Vitis*, *23*, 143-158

Sina, J.F., Bean, C.L., Dysart, G.R., Taylor, V.I. & Bradley, M.O. (1983) Evaluation of the alkaline elution/rat hepatocyte assay as a predictor of carcinogenic/mutagenic potential. *Mutat. Res.*, *113*, 357-391

Skog, O.-J. (1980) Is alcohol consumption lognormally distributed? *Br. J. Addict.*, *75*, 169-173

Skog, O.-J. (1985) The collectivity of drinking cultures: a theory of the distribution of alcohol consumption. *Br. J. Addict.*, *80*, 83-99

Slaughter, J.C. & Uvgard, A.R.A. (1971) Volatile amines of malt and beer. *J. Inst. Brew.*, *77*, 446-450

de Smedt, P., Liddle, P.A.P., Cresto, B. & Bossard, A. (1981) The analysis of non-volatile constituents of wine by glass capillary gas chromatography. *J. Inst. Brew.*, *87*, 349-351

Smith, B.A. & Gutmann, H.R. (1984) Differential effect of chronic ethanol consumption by the rat on microsomal oxidation of hepatocarcinogens and their activation to mutagens. *Biochem. Pharmacol.*, *33*, 2901-2910

Smith, D.I. (1987) Should the maximum alcohol content of beer sold in western Australia be restricted? *Aust. Drug Alcohol Rev.*, *6*, 93-104

Smith, D.M. & James, D.A. (1984) A comparison of alternative distributions of postimplantation death in the dominant lethal assay. *Mutat. Res.*, *128*, 195-206

Smith, I.E., Coles, C.D., Lancaster, J., Fernhoff, P.M. & Falek, A. (1986) The effect of volume and duration of prenatal ethanol exposure on neonatal physical and behavioral development. *Neurobehav. Toxicol. Teratol.*, *8*, 375-381

Smith, M.E. & Newman, H.W. (1959) The rate of ethanol metabolism in fed and fasting animals. *J. biol. Chem.*, *234*, 1544-1549

Smith, M., Hopkinson, D.A. & Harris, H. (1971) Developmental changes and polymorphism in human alcohol dehydrogenase. *Ann. hum. Genet.*, *34*, 251-271

Smith, M., Hopkinson, D.A. & Harris, H. (1973) Studies on the subunit structure and molecular size of the human alcohol dehydrogenase isozymes determined by the different loci, ADH_1, ADH_2 and ADH_3. *Ann. hum. Genet.*, *36*, 401-414

Smyth, H.F., Jr, Seaton, J. & Fischer, L. (1941) The single dose toxicity of some glycols and derivatives. *J. ind. Hyg. Toxicol.*, *23*, 259-268

Snyder, A.K., Singh, S.P. & Pullen, G.L. (1986) Ethanol-induced intrauterine growth retardation: correlation with placental glucose transfer. *Alcohol. clin. exp. Res.*, *10*, 167-170

Sobti, R.C., Krishan, A. & Pfaffenberger, C.D. (1982) Cytokinetic and cytogenetic effects of some agricultural chemicals on human lymphoid cells *in vitro*: organophosphates. *Mutat. Res.*, *102*, 89-102

Sobti, R.C., Krishan, A. & Davies, J. (1983) Cytokinetic and cytogenetic effect of agricultural chemicals on human lymphoid cells *in vitro*. II. Organochlorine pesticides. *Arch. Toxicol., 52*, 221-231

Sohn, O.S., Fiala, E.S., Puz, C., Hamilton, S.R. & Williams, G.M. (1987) Enhancement of rat liver microsomal metabolism of azoxymethane to methylazoxymethanol by chronic ethanol administration: similarity to the microsomal metabolism of *N*-nitrosodimethylamine. *Cancer Res., 47*, 3123-3129

Sokol, R.J., Miller, S.I. & Reed, G. (1980) Alcohol abuse during pregnancy: an epidemiologic study. *Alcohol. clin. exp. Res., 4*, 135-145

Song, B.-J., Gelboin, H.V., Park, S.-S., Yang, C.S. & Gonzalez, F.J. (1986) Complementary DNA and protein sequences of ethanol-inducible rat and human cytochrome P-450s. *J. biol. Chem., 261*, 16689-16697

Sorette, M.P., Maggio, C.A., Starpoli, A., Boissevain, A. & Greenwood, M.R.C. (1980) Maternal ethanol intake affects rat organ development despite adequate nutrition. *Neurobehav. Toxicol., 2*, 181-188

Sousa, J., Nath, J. & Ong, T.-M. (1985) Dietary factors affecting the urinary mutagenicity assay system. II. The absence of mutagenic activity in human urine following consumption of red wine or grape juice. *Mutat. Res., 156*, 171-176

Spalajkovic, M. (1976) Alcoholism and cancer of the larynx and hypopharynx (Fr.). *J. fr. Oto-rhino-laryngol., 25*, 49-50

Spector, W.S., ed. (1956) *Handbook of Toxicology*, Vol. 1, *Acute Toxicities of Solids, Liquids and Bases to Laboratory Animals*, Philadelphia, PA, W.B. Saunders, pp. 128-131

Spettoli, P. (1971) Histamine and other biogenic amines in some Italian wines (Ital.). *Ind. agrar., 9*, 1-5

Spiegel, P.G., Pekman, W.M., Rich, B.H., Versteeg, C.N., Nelson, V. & Dudnikov, M. (1979) The orthopedic aspects of the fetal alcohol syndrome. *Clin. Orthop., 139*, 58-63

Spiegelhalder, B. & Preussmann, R. (1985) In vivo nitrosation of amidopyrine in humans: use of 'ethanol effect' for biological monitoring of *N*-nitrosodimethylamine in urine. *Carcinogenesis, 6*, 545-548

Spiegelhalder, B., Eisenbrand, G. & Preussmann, R. (1979) Contamination of beer with trace quantities of *N*-nitrosodimethylamine. *Food Cosmet. Toxicol., 17*, 29-31

Spiegelhalder, B., Eisenbrand, G. & Preussmann, R. (1982) *Urinary excretion of N-nitrosamines in rats and humans*. In: Bartsch, H., O'Neill, I.K., Castegnaro, M. & Okada, M., eds, N-*Nitroso Compounds: Occurrence and Biological Effects* (*IARC Scientific Publications No. 41*), Lyon, International Agency for Research on Cancer, pp. 443-449

Sponholz, W.R. (1979) Monoethylester of tartaric and malic acid in wine (Ger.). *Dtsch. Lebensm.-Rundsch., 75*, 277-279

Stavric, B., Stoltz, D.R. & Klassen, R. (1983) Toxicants in foods with special emphasis on mutagens in beverages, fruits and vegetables. *Toxicon, Suppl. 3*, 409-412

Steele, C.M. & Ioannides, C. (1986) Different effects of chronic alcohol administration to rats on the activation of aromatic amines to mutagens in the Ames test. *Carcinogenesis, 7*, 825-829

Steiner, K., Schur, F. & Pfenninger, H. (1969) Determination of formaldehyde in beer (Ger.). *Brauwissenschaft, 22*, 87-90

Stemhagen, A., Slade, J., Altman, R. & Bill, J. (1983) Occupational risk factors and liver cancer. A retrospective case-control study of primary liver cancer in New Jersey. *Am. J. Epidemiol.*, *117*, 443-454

Stenbäck, F. (1969) The tumorigenic effect of ethanol. *Acta pathol. microbiol. scand.*, *77*, 325-326

Stocks, P. (1957) *Cancer incidence in North Wales and Liverpool region in relation to habits and environment.* In: *British Empire Cancer Campaign 35th Annual Report*, Part II (Suppl.), London

Stoltz, D.R., Stavric, B., Klassen, R. & Muise, T. (1982a) *The health significance of mutagens in foods.* In: Stich, H.F., ed., *Carcinogens and Mutagens in the Environment*, Vol. 1, *Food Products*, Boca Raton, FL, CRC Press, pp. 185-197

Stoltz, D.R., Stavric, B., Krewski, D., Klassen, R., Bendall, R. & Junkins, B. (1982b) Mutagenicity screening of foods. I. Results with beverages. *Environ. Mutagenesis*, *4*, 477-492

Stowell, A.R., Greenway, R.M. & Batt, R.D. (1977) Acetaldehyde formation during deproteinization of human blood samples containing ethanol. *Biochem. Med.*, *18*, 392-401

Strauss, C.R., Williams, P.J., Wilson, B. & Dimitriadis, E. (1984) *Formation and identification of aroma compounds from non-volatile precursors in grapes and wine.* In: Nykänen, L. & Lehtonen, P., eds, *Flavour Research of Alcoholic Beverages*, Vol. 3, *Instrumental and Sensory Analysis*, Helsinki, Foundation for Biotechnical and Industrial Fermentation Research, pp. 51-60

Streissguth, A.P. (1983) Alcohol and pregnancy: an overview and an update. *Subst. Alcohol Actions Misuse*, *4*, 149-173

Streissguth, A.P., Landesman-Dwyer, S., Martin, J.C. & Smith, D.W. (1980) Teratogenic effects of alcohol in humans and laboratory animals. *Science*, *209*, 353-361

Streissguth, A.P., Martin, D.C., Martin, J.C. & Barr, H.M. (1981) The Seattle longitudinal prospective study on alcohol and pregnancy. *Neurobehav. Toxicol. Teratol.*, *3*, 223-233

Streissguth, A.P., Clarren, S.K. & Jones, K.L. (1985) Natural history of the fetal alcohol syndrome: a 10-year follow-up of eleven patients. *Lancet*, *ii*, 85-91

Strömland, K. (1981) Eyeground malformations in the fetal alcohol syndrome. *Neuropediatrics*, *12*, 97-98

Strubelt, O., Obermeier, F. & Siegers, C.P. (1978) The influence of ethanol pretreatment on the effects of nine hepatotoxic agents. *Acta pharmacol. toxicol.*, *43*, 211-218

Strum, W.B. & Spiro, H.M. (1971) Chronic pancreatitis. *Ann. intern. Med.*, *74*, 264-277

Stuckey, E. & Berry, C.L. (1984) The effects of high dose sporadic (binge) alcohol intake in mice. *J. Pathol.*, *142*, 175-180

Subden, R.E., Krizus, A. & Rancourt, D. (1984) Mutagen content of table wines made from various grape species and hybrid cultivars. *Food chem. Toxicol.*, *22*, 309-313

Sulik, K.K. & Johnston, M.C. (1983) Sequence of developmental alterations following acute ethanol exposure in mice: craniofacial features of the fetal alcohol syndrome. *Am. J. Anat.*, *166*, 257-269

Sulik, K.K., Johnston, M.C. & Webb, M.A. (1981) Fetal alcohol syndrome: embryogenesis in a mouse model. *Science*, *214*, 936-938

Sundaram, K.R., Mohan, D., Advani, G.B., Sharma, H.K. & Bajaj, J.S. (1984) Alcohol abuse in a rural community in India. Part 1, epidemiological study. *Drug Alcohol Depend.*, *14*, 27-36

Sundby, P. (1967) *Alcoholism and Mortality*, Oslo, Universitetsforlaget

Sundheimer, D.W. & Brendel, K. (1984) Factors influencing sulfation in isolated rat hepatocytes. *Life Sci.*, *34*, 23-29

Suomalainen, H. & Nykänen, L. (1970) Investigations on the aroma of alcoholic beverages. *Noeringsmiddelindustrien*, *23*, 1-15

Swann, P.F. (1984) *Effect of ethanol on nitrosamine metabolism and distribution. Implications for the role of nitrosamines in human cancer and for the influence of alcohol consumption on cancer incidence.* In: O'Neill, I.K., von Borstel, R.C., Miller, C.T., Long, J. & Bartsch, H., eds, N-*Nitroso Compounds: Occurrence, Biological Effects and Relevance to Human Cancer* (*IARC Scientific Publications No. 57*), Lyon, International Agency for Research on Cancer, pp. 501-512

Swann, P.F., Coe, A.M. & Mace, R. (1984) Ethanol and dimethylnitrosamine and diethylnitrosamine metabolism and disposition in the rat. Possible relevance to the influence of ethanol on human cancer incidence. *Carcinogenesis*, *5*, 1337-1343

Sweeny, D.J. & Reinke, L.A. (1987) Effect of ethanol feeding on hepatic microsomal UDP-glucuronyltransferase activity. *Biochem. Pharmacol.*, *36*, 1381-1383

Swiatek, K.R., Dombrowski, G.J., Jr & Chao, K.-L. (1986) The inefficient transfer of maternally fed alcohol to nursing rats. *Alcohol*, *3*, 169-174

Switzer, B.R., Anderson, J.J.B. & Pick, J.R. (1986) Effects of dietary protein and ethanol intake on pregnant beagles fed purified diets. *J. Nutr.*, *116*, 689-697

Systembolaget (Swedish Alcoholic Retailing Monopoly) (1986) *Annual Report* (Swed.), Stockholm

Szilagyi, A. (1987) Thyroid hormones and alcoholic liver disease. *J. clin. Gastroenterol.*, *9*, 189-193

Takada, A., Nei, J., Takase, S. & Matsuda, Y. (1986) Effects of ethanol on experimental hepatocarcinogenesis. *Hepatology*, *6*, 65-72

Takahashi, D.M. (1974) Thin layer chromatographic determination of aflatoxins in wine. *J. Assoc. off. anal. Chem.*, *57*, 875-879

Takahashi, M., Hasegawa, R., Furukawa, F., Toyoda, K., Sato, H. & Hayashi, Y. (1986) Effects of ethanol, potassium metabisulfite, formaldehyde and hydrogen peroxide on gastric carcinogenesis in rats after initiation with *N*-methyl-*N'*-nitro-*N*-nitrosoguanidine. *Jpn. J. Cancer Res. (Gann)*, *77*, 118-124

Takehisa, S. & Kanaya, N. (1983) A comparison of *Vicia-faba*-root S10 and rat-liver S9 activation of ethanol, maleic hydrazide and cyclophosphamide as measured by sister-chromatid exchange induction in Chinese hamster ovary cells. *Mutat. Res.*, *124*, 145-151

Talamini, R., La Vecchia, C., Decarli, A., Franceschi, S., Grattoni, E., Grigoletto, E., Liberati, A. & Tognoni, G. (1984) Social factors, diet and breast cancer in a northern Italian population. *Br. J. Cancer*, *49*, 723-729

Tamura, G., Gold, C., Ferro-Luzzi, A. & Ames, B.N. (1980) Fecalase: a model for activation of dietary glycosides to mutagens by intestinal flora. *Proc. natl Acad. Sci. USA*, *77*, 4961-4965

Tates, A.D., de Vogel, N. & Neuteboom, I. (1980) Cytogenetic effects in hepatocytes, bone-marrow cells and blood lymphocytes of rats exposed to ethanol in the drinking water. *Mutat. Res.*, *79*, 285-288

Teschke, R., Minzlaff, M., Oldiges, H. & Frenzel, H. (1983) Effect of chronic alcohol consumption on tumor incidence due to dimethylnitrosamine administration. *J. Cancer Res. clin. Oncol.*, *106*, 58-64

Thieden, H.I.D. & Lundquist, F. (1967) The influence of fructose and its metabolites on ethanol metabolism *in vitro*. *Biochem. J.*, *102*, 177-180

Thieden, H.I.D., Grunnet, N., Damgaard, S.E. & Sestoft, L. (1972) Effect of fructose and glyceraldehyde on ethanol metabolism in human liver and rat liver. *Eur. J. Biochem.*, *30*, 250-261

Thiessen, D.D., Whitworth, N.S. & Rodgers, D.A. (1966) Reproductive variables and alcohol consumption of the C57BL/Crgl female mouse. *Q. J. Stud. Alcohol*, *27*, 591-595

Thomas, D.B., Uhl, C.N. & Hartge, P. (1983) Bladder cancer and alcoholic beverage consumption. *Am. J. Epidemiol.*, *118*, 720-727

Thomas, P.E., Bandiera, S., Maines, S.L., Ryan, D.E. & Levin, W. (1987) Regulation of cytochrome P-450j, a high-affinity *N*-nitrosodimethylamine demethylase, in rat hepatic microsomes. *Biochemistry*, *26*, 2280-2289

Thomson, A. & Majumdar, S.K. (1981) *The influence of ethanol on intestinal absorption and utilization of nutrients*. In: Leevy, C.M., ed., *Clinics in Gastroenterology*, Vol. 10, *Alcohol in the GI Tract*, London, W.B. Saunders, pp. 263-293

Thurman, R.G. (1977) Hepatic alcohol oxidation and its metabolic liability. *Fed. Proc.*, *36*, 1640-1646

Thurman, R.G., Glassman, E.B., Handler, J.A. & Forman, D. (1988) *The swift increase in alcohol metabolism (SIAM): a commentary on the regulation of alcohol metabolism in mammals*. In: Crow, C. & Batt, B., eds, *Human Alcohol Metabolism*, Boca Raton, FL, CRC Press (in press)

Tillner, I. & Majewski, F. (1978) Furrows and dermal ridges of the hand in patients with alcohol embryopathy. *Hum. Genet.*, *42*, 307-314

Tobon, F. & Mezey, E. (1971) Effect of ethanol administration on hepatic ethanol and drug-metabolizing enzymes and on rates of ethanol degradation. *J. Lab. clin. Med.*, *77*, 110-121

Tomera, J.F., Skipper, P.L., Wishnok, J.S., Tannenbaum, S.R. & Brunengraber, H. (1984) Inhibition of *N*-nitrosodimethylamine metabolism by ethanol and other inhibitors in the isolated perfused rat liver. *Carcinogenesis*, *5*, 113-116

Topham, J.C. (1980) The detection of carcinogen-induced sperm head abnormalities in mice. *Mutat. Res.*, *69*, 149-155

Topham, J.C. (1983) *Chemically induced changes in sperm in animals and humans*. In: de Serres, F.J., ed., *Chemical Mutagens. Principles and Methods for Their Detection*, Vol. 8, New York, Plenum Press, pp. 201-234

de Torok, D. (1972) Chromosomal irregularities in alcoholics. *Ann. N.Y. Acad. Sci.*, *197*, 90-100

Toskulkao, C. & Glinsukon, T. (1986) Effect of ethanol on the in vivo covalent binding and in vitro metabolism of aflatoxin B_1 in rats. *Toxicol. Lett.*, *30*, 151-157

Tottmar, S.O.C., Kiessling, K.-H. & Forsling, M. (1974) Effects of phenobarbital and ethanol on rat liver aldehyde dehydrogenases. *Acta pharmacol. toxicol.*, *35*, 270-276

Traiger, G.J. & Plaa, G.L. (1971) Differences in the potentiation of carbon tetrachloride in rats by ethanol and isopropanol pretreatment. *Toxicol. appl. Pharmacol.*, *20*, 105-112

Treml, V.G. (1982) *Alcohol in the USSR: A Statistical Study*, Durham, NC, Duke Press Policy Studies

Tressl, R., Kossa, T. & Renner, R. H. (1975a) *Gas chromatographic-mass spectrometric analysis of volatile compounds of hops, wort and beer and their genesis. II. Phenols and oxygen-containing heterocyclic components in wort and beer* (Ger.). In: *Proceedings of the European Brewery Convention, Nice*, pp. 737-756

Tressl, R., Kossa, T., Renner, R. & Köppler, H. (1975b) Gas chromatographic-mass spectrometric analysis of volatile compounds of hops, wort and beer and their genesis. I. Organic acids in wort and beer (Ger.). *Montasschr. Brau.*, *28*, 109-118

Tressl, R., Renner, R. & Apetz, M. (1976) Volatile phenolic compounds in beer, smoked beer and sherry (Ger.). *Z. Lebensmitteluntersuch. Forsch.*, *162*, 115-122

Tressl, R., Renner, R., Kossa, T. & K 2vppler, H. (1977) *Gas chromatographic-mass spectrometric analysis of volatile compounds in hops, wort and beer and their genesis. III. Nitrogen-containing aroma components in malt and beer (Ger.).* In: *Proceedings in the 16th European Brewery Convention Congress, Amsterdam*, pp. 639-707

Tressl, R., Friese, L., Fendesack, F. & Köppler, H. (1978) Gas chromatographic-mass spectrometric investigation of hop aroma constituents in beer. *J. agric. Food Chem.*, *26*, 1422-1426

Trichopoulos, D., Ouranos, G., Day, N.E., Tzonou, A., Manousos, O., Papadimitriou, C. & Trichopoulos, A. (1985) Diet and cancer of the stomach: a case-control study in Greece. *Int. J. Cancer*, *36*, 291-297

Trichopoulos, D., Day, N.E., Kaklamani, E., Tzonou, A., Muñoz, N., Zavitsanos, X., Koumantaki, Y. & Trichopoulos, A. (1987) Hepatitis B virus, tobacco smoking and ethanol consumption in the etiology of hepatocellular carcinomas. *Int. J. Cancer*, *39*, 45-49

Truitt, E.B., Jr (1971) *Blood acetaldehyde levels after alcohol consumption by alcoholic and nonalcoholic subjects.* In: Roach, M.K., McIsaac, W.M. & Creaven, P.J., eds, *Biological Aspects of Alcohol*, Austin, TX, University of Texas, pp. 212-232

Tsukamoto, H., French, S.W., Benson, N., Delgado, G., Rao, G.A., Larkin, E.C. & Largman, C. (1985) Severe and progressive steatosis and focal necrosis in rat liver induced by continuous intragastric infusion of ethanol and low fat diet. *Hepatology*, *5*, 224-232

Tsukamoto, H., Towner, S.J., Ciofalo, L.M. & French, S.W. (1986) Ethanol-induced liver fibrosis in rats fed high fat diet. *Hepatology*, *6*, 814-822

Tuma, D.J., Zetterman, R.K. & Sorrell, M.F. (1980) Inhibition of glycoprotein secretion by ethanol and acetaldehyde in rat liver slices. *Biochem. Pharmacol.*, *29*, 35-38

Tuttas, R. & Beye, F. (1977) The genuine compounds of *Cerasus avium* and their taste from the fruit to the distillate (Ger.). *Branntweinwirtschaft*, *117*, 349-355

Tuyns, A.J. (1970) Cancer of the esophagus: further evidence of the relation to drinking habits in France. *Int. J. Cancer*, *5*, 152-156

Tuyns, A.J. (1983) Oesophageal cancer in non-smoking drinkers and in non-drinking smokers. *Int. J. Cancer*, *32*, 443-444

Tuyns, A.J. & Massé, G. (1975) Cancer of the oesophagus in Brittany: an incidence study in Ille-et-Vilaine. *Int. J. Epidemiol.*, *4*, 55-59

Tuyns, A.J. & Péquignot, G. (1984) Greater risk of ascitic cirrhosis in females in relation to alcohol consumption. *Int. J. Epidemiol.*, *13*, 53-57

Tuyns, A.J., Péquignot, G. & Jensen, O.M. (1977) Oesophageal cancer in Ille-et-Vilaine in relation to alcohol and tobacco consumption: multiplicative risks (Fr.). *Bull. Cancer*, *64*, 45-60

Tuyns, A.J., Péquignot, G. & Abbatucci, J.S. (1979) Oesophageal cancer and alcohol consumption: importance of type of beverage. *Int. J. Cancer*, *23*, 443-447

Tuyns, A.J., Castegnaro, M., Toussaint, G., Walker, E.A., Griciute, L., Le Talaer, L.Y., Loquet, C., Guérain, J. & Drilleau, J.F. (1980) Research on etiological factors for oesophageal cancer in the west of France (Fr.). *Bull. Cancer*, *67*, 15-28

Tuyns, A.J., Péquignot, G., Gignoux, M. & Valla, A. (1982) Cancers of the digestive tract, alcohol and tobacco. *Int. J. Cancer*, *30*, 9-11

Tuyns, A.J., Hu, M.X. & Péquignot, G. (1983) Alcohol consumption patterns in the department of Calvados (France). *Rev. Epidémiol. Santé publique*, *31*, 179-197

Tuyns, A.J., Riboli, E., Doornbos, G. & Péquignot, G. (1987) Diet and esophageal cancer in Calvados (France). *Nutr. Cancer*, *9*, 81-92

Tuyns, A.J., Estève, J., Raymond, L., Berrino, F., Benhamou, E., Blanchet, F., Boffetta, P., Crosignani, P., del Moral, A., Lehmann, W., Merletti, F., Péquignot, G., Riboli, E., Sancho-Garnier, H., Terracini, B., Zubiri, A. & Zubiri, Z. (1988) Cancer of the larynx/hypopharynx, tobacco and alcohol. *Int. J. Cancer*, *41*, 483-491

Tweedie, J.H., Reber, H.A., Pour P. & Ponder, D.M. (1981) Protective effect of ethanol on the development of pancreatic cancer. *Surg. Forum*, *32*, 222-224

Tze, W.J., Friesen, H.G. & MacLeod, P.M. (1976) Growth hormone response in fetal alcohol syndrome. *Arch. Dis. Child.*, *51*, 703-706

Udani, M., Parker, S., Gavaler, J. & Van Thiel, D.H. (1985) Effects of in utero exposure to alcohol upon male rats. *Alcohol. clin. exp. Res.*, *9*, 355-359

Ueng, T.-H., Friedman, F.K., Miller, H., Park, S.S., Gelboin, H.V. & Alvares, A.P. (1987) Studies on ethanol-inducible cytochrome P-450 in rabbit liver, lungs and kidneys. *Biochem. Pharmacol.*, *36*, 2689-2691

Ugarte, G., Pereda, T., Pino, M.E. & Iturriaga, H. (1972) Influence of alcohol intake, length of abstinence and meprobamate on the rate of ethanol metabolism in man. *Q. J. Stud. Alcohol*, *33*, 698-705

Ugarte, G., Iturriaga, H. & Pereda, T. (1977) Possible relationship between the rate of ethanol metabolism and the severity of hepatic damage in chronic alcoholics. *Dig. Dis.*, *22*, 406-410

United Nations (1961) *Standard International Trade Classification*, rev., New York

Väänänen, H., Salaspuro, M. & Lindros, K. (1984) The effect of chronic ethanol ingestion on ethanol metabolizing enzymes in isolated periportal and perivenous rat hepatocytes. *Hepatology*, *4*, 862-866

Valenzuela, A., Fernandez, N., Fernandez, V., Ugarte, G. & Videla, L.A. (1980) Effect of acute ethanol ingestion on lipoperoxidation and on the activity of the enzymes related to peroxide metabolism in rat liver. *FEBS Lett.*, *111*, 11-13

Välimäki, M., Salaspuro, M., Härkönen, M. & Ylikahri, R. (1982) Liver damage and sex hormones in chronic male alcoholics. *Clin. Endocrinol.*, *17*, 469-477

Van Buren, J.P., Bertino, J.J., Einset, J., Remaily, G.W. & Robinson, W.B. (1970) A comparative study of the antocyanin pigment composition in wines derived from hybrid grapes. *Am. J. Enol. Vitic.*, *21*, 117-130

Van Thiel, D.H. & Gavaler, J.S. (1985) *Ethanol and the endocrine system.* In: Seitz, H.K. & Kommerell, B., eds, *Alcohol Related Diseases in Gastroenterology*, Berlin (West), Springer, pp. 324-341

Van Thiel, D.H. & Lester, R. (1977) Therapy of sexual dysfunction in alcohol abusers: a Pandora's box. *Gastroenterology*, *72*, 1354-1356

Van Thiel, D.H., Gavaler, J.S. & Lester, R. (1978) Alcohol-induced ovarian failure in the rat. *J. clin. Invest.*, *61*, 624-632

Van Thiel, D.H., Gavaler, J.S., Cobb, C.F., Santucci, L. & Graham, T.O. (1983) Ethanol, a Leydig cell toxin: evidence obtained *in vivo* and *in vitro*. *Pharmacol. Biochem. Behav.*, *18*, 317-323

Varma, P.K. & Persaud, T.V.N. (1979) Influence of pyrazole, an inhibitor of alcohol dehydrogenase on the prenatal toxicity of ethanol in the rat. *Res. Commun. chem. Pathol. Pharmacol.*, *26*, 65-73

Vassallo, A., Correa, P., De Stéfani, E., Cendán, M., Zavala, D., Chen, V., Carzoglio, J. & Deneo-Pellegrini, H. (1985) Oesophageal cancer in Uruguay: a case-control study. *J. natl Cancer Inst.*, *75*, 1005-1009

Véghelyi, P.V. & Osztovics, M. (1978) The alcohol syndromes: the intrarecombinogenic effect of acetaldehyde. *Experientia*, *34*, 195-196

Véghelyi, P.V., Osztovics. M., Kardos, G., Leisztner, L., Szaszovsky, E., Igali, S. & Imrei, J. (1978) The fetal alcohol syndrome: symptoms and pathogenesis. *Acta pediat. acad. sci. hung.*, *19*, 171-189

Velema, J.P., Walker, A.M. & Gold, E.B. (1986) Alcohol and pancreatic cancer. Insufficient epidemiologic evidence for a causal relationship. *Epidemiol. Rev.*, *8*, 28-41

Versluys, J.J. (1949) Cancer and occupation in the Netherlands. *Br. J. Cancer*, *3*, 161-185

Verzele, M. (1986) Centenary review, 100 years of hop chemistry and its relevance to brewing. *J. Inst. Brew.*, *92*, 32-48

Vesell, E.S., Page, J.G. & Passananti, G.T. (1971) Genetic and environmental factors affecting ethanol metabolism in man. *Clin. Pharmacol. Ther.*, *12*, 192-201

Victoria, C.G., Muñoz, N., Day, N.E., Barcelos, L.B., Peccin, D.A. & Braga, N.M. (1987) Hot beverages and oesophageal cancer in southern Brazil: a case-control study. *Int. J. Cancer*, *39*, 710-716

Videla, L.A., Fernandez, V., Ugarte, G. & Valenzuela, A. (1980) Effect of acute ethanol intoxication on the content of reduced glutathione of the liver in relation to its lipoperoxidative capacity in the rat. *FEBS Lett.*, *111*, 6-10

Viirre, E., Cain, D.P. & Ossenkopp, K.-P. (1986) Prenatal ethanol exposure alters rat brain morphology but does not affect amygdaloid kindling. *Neurobehav. Toxicol. Teratol.*, *8*, 615-620

Villeneuve, J.-P., Mavier, P. & Joly, J.-G. (1976) Ethanol-induced cytochrome P-450: catalytic activity after partial purification. *Biochem. biophys. Res. Commun.*, *70*, 723-728

Vincent, R.G. & Marchetta, F. (1963) The relationship of the use of tobacco and alcohol to cancer of the oral cavity, pharynx or larynx. *Am. J. Surg.*, *106*, 501-505

Visser, M.K. & Lindsay, R.C. (1971) Ester precursors of aldehydes associated with staling of beer. *Tech. Q. Master Brew. Assoc. Am.*, *8*, 123-128

Vogel, E. (1972) Investigations on the mutagenicity of DDT and the DDT-metabolites DDE, DDD, DDOM and DDA in *Drosophila melanogaster* (Ger.). *Mutat. Res.*, *16*, 157-164

Vogel, E. & Chandler, J.L.R. (1974) Mutagenicity testing of cyclamate and some pesticides in *Drosophila melanogaster*. *Experientia*, *30*, 621-623

Vogel, E.W., Zijlstra, J.A. & Blijleven, W.G.H. (1983) Mutagenic activity of selected aromatic amines and polycyclic hydrocarbons in *Drosophila melanogaster*. *Mutat. Res.*, *107*, 53-77

Voirol, M., Infante, F., Raymond, L., Hollenweger, V., Conti, M.C. & Loizeau, E. (1980) *Alcohol, food and tobacco consumption in pancreatic diseases*. In: *Alcohol and the Gastrointestinal Tract* (*Les Colloques de l'INSERM 95*), Paris, Institut National de Science et de la Recherche Médicale, pp. 59-62

Vorhees, C.V. & Fernandez, K. (1986) Effects of short-term prenatal alcohol exposure on maze, activity, and olfactory orientation performance in rats. *Neurobehav. Toxicol. Teratol.*, *8*, 23-28

Wackerbauer, K., Kossa, T. & Tressl, R. (1977) *Formation of phenols by yeasts* (Ger.). In: *Proceedings of the European Brewery Convention, Amsterdam*, pp. 495-505

Wahi, P.N. (1968) The epidemiology of oral and oropharyngeal cancer. A report of the study in Mainpuri district, Uttar Pradesh, India. *Bull. World Health Org.*, *38*, 495-521

Wainright, T. (1986a) The chemistry of nitrosamine formation: relevance to malting and brewing. *J. Inst. Brew.*, *92*, 49-64

Wainright, T. (1986b) Nitrosamines in malt and beer. *J. Inst. Brew.*, *92*, 73-80

Walker, R.M., McElligott, T.F., Power, E.M., Massey, T.E. & Racz, W.J. (1983) Increased acetaminophen-induced hepatotoxicity after chronic ethanol consumption in mice. *Toxicology*, *28*, 193-206

Wallén, M., Näslund, P.H. & Nordqvist, M.B. (1984) The effects of ethanol on the kinetics of toluene in man. *Toxicol. appl. Pharmacol.*, *76*, 414-419

Wallgren, H. & Barry, H., III (1970) *Actions of Alcohol*, Vol. 1, *Biochemical, Physiological and Psychological Aspects*, Amsterdam, Elsevier

Wallgren, H. & Hillbom, M.E. (1969) Depressed lung evaporation and gastric evacuation of ethanol after intraperitoneal injection of glucose to rats (Abstract). *Scand. J. clin. Lab. Invest.*, *23* (Suppl. 108), 58

Walsh, B. & Grant, M. (1985) *Public Health Implications of Alcohol Production and Trade* (*WHO Offset Publication No. 88*), Geneva, World Health Organization

Walter, S.D. & Iwane, M. (1983) Interaction of alcohol and tobacco in laryngeal cancer. *Am. J. Epidemiol.*, *117*, 639-641

Warner, R.H. & Rosett, H.L. (1975) The effects of drinking on offspring. An historical survey of the American and British literature. *Q. J. Stud. Alcohol*, *36*, 1395-1420

von Wartburg, J.P. & Schürch, P.M. (1968) Atypical human liver alcohol dehydrogenase. *Ann. N.Y. Acad. Sci.*, *151*, 936-946

von Wartburg, J.-P., Papenberg, J. & Aebi, H. (1965) An atypical human alcohol dehydrogenase. *Can. J. Biochem.*, *43*, 889-898

Washington, W.J., Cain, K.T., Cacheiro, N.L.A. & Generoso, W.M. (1985) Ethanol-induced late fetal death in mice exposed around the time of fertilization. *Mutat. Res.*, *147*, 205-210

Watanabe, M., Honda, S., Hayashi, M. & Matsuda, T. (1982) Mutagenic effects of combinations of chemical carcinogens and environmental pollutants in mice as shown by the micronucleus test. *Mutat. Res.*, *97*, 43-48

Weatherall, D.J., Ladingham, J.G.G. & Warrell, D.A. (1983) *Oxford Textbook of Medicine*, Vol. 1, Oxford, Oxford University Press

Webster, L.A., Layde, P.M., Wingo, P.A. & Dry, H.W. (1983) Alcohol consumption and risk of breast cancer. *Lancet*, *ii*, 724-726

Webster, W.S., Walsh, D.A., Lipson, A.H. & McEwen, S.E. (1980) Teratogenesis after acute alcohol exposure in inbred and outbred mice. *Neurobehav. Toxicol.*, *2*, 227-234

Webster, W.S., Walsh, D.A., McEwen, S.E. & Lipson, A.H. (1983) Some teratogenic properties of ethanol and acetaldehyde in C57BL/6J mice: implications for the study of the fetal alcohol syndrome. *Teratology*, *27*, 231-243

Webster, W.S., Germain, M.-A., Lipson, A. & Walsh, D.A. (1984) Alcohol and congenital heart defects: an experimental study in mice. *Cardiovasc. Res.*, *18*, 335-338

Wehman, H.J. & Plantholt, B.A. (1974) Asbestos fibrils in beverages. I. Gin. *Bull environ. Contam. Toxicol.*, *4*, 267-272

Weinberg, J. (1985) Effects of ethanol and maternal nutritional status on fetal development. *Alcohol. clin. exp. Res.*, *9*, 49-55

Wendell, G.D. & Thurman, R.G. (1979) Effect of ethanol concentration on rates of ethanol elimination in normal and alcohol-treated rats *in vivo*. *Biochem. Pharmacol.*, *28*, 273-279

Wendt, V.E., Ajluni, R., Bruce, T.A., Prasad, A.S. & Bing, R.J. (1966) Acute effects of alcohol on human myocardium. *Am. J. Cardiol.*, *17*, 804-812

West, J.R., Black, A.C., Jr, Reimann, P.C. & Alkana, R.L. (1981a) Polydactyly and polysyndactyly induced by prenatal exposure to ethanol. *Teratology*, *24*, 13-18

West, J.R., Hodges, C.A. & Black, A.C., Jr (1981b) Prenatal exposure to ethanol alters the organization of hippocampal mossy fibers in rats. *Science*, *211*, 957-959

West, R.O. (1966) Epidemiologic study of malignancies of the ovaries. *Cancer*, *19*, 1001-1007

White, F.H. & Wainwright, T. (1975) Analysis of diacetyl and related compounds in fermentations. *J. Inst. Brew.*, *81*, 37-45

Wiberg, G.S., Trenholm, H.L. & Coldwell, B.B. (1970) Increased ethanol toxicity in old rats: changes in LD50, in vivo and in vitro metabolism, and liver alcohol dehydrogenase activity. *Toxicol. appl. Pharmacol.*, *16*, 718-727

Wickramasinghe, S.N., Barden, G. & Levy, L. (1987) The capacity of macrophages from different murine tissues to metabolise ethanol and generate an ethanol-dependent non-dialysable cytotoxic activity *in vitro*. *Alcohol Alcohol.*, *22*, 31-39

Wienbeck, M. & Berges, W. (1985) *Esophageal and gastric lesions in the alcoholic*. In: Seitz, A.K. & Kommerell, B., eds, *Alcohol Related Diseases in Gastroenterology*, Berlin (West), Springer, pp. 361-375

Willems, G., Vansteekiste, Y. & Smets, P.H. (1971) Effects of ethanol on the cell proliferation kinetics in the fundic mucosa of dogs. *Am. J. dig. Dis.*, *16*, 1057-1063

Willett, W.C., Stampfer, M.J., Colditz, G.A., Rosner, B.A., Hennekens, C.H. & Speizer, F.E. (1987) Moderate alcohol consumption and the risk of breast cancer. *New Engl. J. Med.*, *316*, 1174-1180

Williams, A.A. (1982) Recent developments in the field of wine flavour research. *J. Inst. Brew.*, *88*, 43-53

Williams, P.J., Strauss, C.R., Wilson, B. & Dimitriadis, E. (1985) *Recent studies into grape terpene glycosides*. In: Adda, J., ed., *Progress in Flavour Research 1984*, Amsterdam, Elsevier, pp. 349-357

Williams, R.R. & Horm, J.W. (1977) Association of cancer sites with tobacco and alcohol consumption and socioeconomic status of patients: interview study from the Third National Cancer Survey. *J. natl Cancer Inst.*, *58*, 525-547

Wilson, B., Strauss, C.R. & Williams, P.J. (1984) Changes in free and glycosidically bound monoterpenes in developing muscat grapes. *J. agric. Food Chem.*, *32*, 919-924

Wilson, B., Strauss, C.R. & Williams, P.J. (1986) The distribution of free and glycosidically-bound monoterpenes among skin, juice, and pulp fractions of some white grape varieties. *Am. J. Enol. Vitic.*, *37*, 107-111

Wilson, F.A. & Hoyumpa, A.M., Jr (1979) Ethanol and small intestinal transport. *Prog. Gastroenterol.*, *76*, 388-403

Wilson, J.S., Korsten, M.A. & Lieber, C.S. (1986) The combined effects of protein deficiency and chronic ethanol administration on rat ethanol metabolism. *Hepatology*, *6*, 823-829

Windholz, M. (1983) *The Merck Index*, 10th ed., Rahway, NJ, Merck & Co., pp. 34-35

Winship, D.H., Caflish, C.R., Zboralske, F.F. & Hogan, W.J. (1968) Deterioration of esophageal peristalsis in patients with alcoholic neuropathy. *Gastroenterology*, *55*, 173-178

Wisniewski, K., Dambska, M., Sher, J.H. & Quazi, Q. (1983) A clinical neuropathological study of the fetal alcohol syndrome. *Neuropediatrics*, *14*, 197-201

Withycombe, D.A. & Lindsay, R.C. (1973) Determination of trans-2-nonenal in stale beer. *Tech. Q. Master Brew. Assoc. Am.*, *10*, XIX-XX

Wohleb, R., Jennings, W.G. & Lewis, M.J. (1972) Some observations on *trans*-2-nonenal in beer as determined by a headspace sampling technique for gas-liquid chromatography. *Am. Soc. Brew. Chem. Proc.*, 1-3

Woidich, H., Pfannhauser, W., Blaicher, G. & Pechaner, U. (1980) Investigations concerning biogenic amines in red and white wines (Ger.) *Mitt. Rebe Wein Obstbau Früchteverwert. Klosterneuburg*, *30*, 27-31

Wolf, E. (1982) *Europe and the People Without History*, Berkeley-Los Angeles, CA, University of California Press

Woodhouse, K.W., Williams, F.M., Mutch, E., Wright, P., James, O.F.W. & Rawlins, M.D. (1983) The effect of alcoholic cirrhosis on the activities of microsomal aldrin epoxidase, 7-ethoxycoumarin *O*-de-ethylase and epoxide hydrolase, and on the concentrations of reduced glutathione in human liver. *Br. J. clin. Pharmacol.*, *15*, 667-672

Woodruff, R.C., Mason, J.M., Valencia, R. & Zimmering, S. (1984) Chemical mutagenesis testing in *Drosophila*: I. Comparison of positive and negative control data for sex-linked recessive lethal mutations and reciprocal translocations in three laboratories. *Environ. Mutagenesis*, *6*, 189-202

World Health Organization (1980) *Problems Related to Alcohol Consumption: Report of a WHO Expert Committee* (*WHO Technical Report Series No. 650*), Geneva

Woutersen, R.A., van Garderen-Hoetmer, A., Bax, J., Feringa, A.W. & Scherer, E. (1986) Modulation of putative preneoplastic foci in exocrine pancreas of rats and hamsters. I. Interaction of dietary fat and ethanol. *Carcinogenesis*, *7*, 1587-1593

Wright, J.T., Macrae, K.D., Barrison, I.G. & Waterson, E.J. (1984) *Effects of moderate alcohol consumption and smoking on fetal outcome*. In: *Mechanisms of Alcohol Damage In Utero* (*Ciba Foundation Symposium 105)*, London, Pitman, pp. 240-253

Wu, A.H., Paganini-Hill, A., Ross, R.K. & Henderson, B.E. (1987) Alcohol, physical activity and other risk factors for colorectal cancer: a prospective study. *Br. J. Cancer*, *55*, 687-694

Wucherpfennig, K. & Semmler, G. (1972) On the SO_2 needs of wine from various wine growing areas in the world and its dependence on the treatment of grapes (Ger.). *Alimenta*, *11*, 31-42

Wucherpfennig, K. & Semmler, G. (1973) On the SO_2 needs of wine from various wine growing areas in the world and its dependence on formation of acetaldehyde in the process of fermentation (Ger.). *Dtsch. Weinbau*, *24*, 846, 851-855

Wynder, E.L. & Bross, I.J. (1957) Etiological factors in mouth cancer. An approach to its prevention. *Br. med. J.*, *i*, 1137-1143

Wynder, E.L. & Bross, I.J. (1961) A study of etiological factors in cancer of the esophagus. *Cancer*, *14*, 389-413

Wynder, E.L. & Shigematsu, T. (1967) Environmental factors of cancer of the colon and rectum. *Cancer*, *20*, 1520-1561

Wynder, E.L., Bross, I.J. & Day, E. (1956) A study of environmental factors in cancer of the larynx. *Cancer*, *9*, 86-110

Wynder, E.L., Bross, I.J. & Feldman, R.M. (1957a) A study of etiological factors in cancer of the mouth. *Cancer*, *10*, 1300-1323

Wynder, E.L., Hultberg, S., Jacobsson, F. & Bross, I.J. (1957b) Environmental factors in cancer of the upper alimentary tract. A Swedish study with special reference to Plummer-Vinson (Paterson-Kelly) syndrome. *Cancer*, *10*, 470-487

Wynder, E.L., Lemon, F.R. & Bross, I.J. (1959) Cancer and coronary artery disease among Seventh-day Adventists. *Cancer*, *12*, 1016-1028

Wynder, E.L., Kmet, J., Dungal, N. & Segi, M. (1963a) An epidemiological investigation of gastric cancer. *Cancer*, *16*, 1461-1497

Wynder, E.L., Onderdonk, J. & Mantel, N. (1963b) An epidemiological investigation of cancer of the bladder. *Cancer*, *16*, 1388-1407

Wynder, E.L., Mabuchi, K. & Whitmore, W.F., Jr (1971) Epidemiology of cancer of the prostate. *Cancer*, *28*, 344-360

Wynder, E.L., Mabuchi, K., Maruchi, N. & Fortner, J.G. (1973a) A case-control study of cancer of the pancreas. *Cancer*, *31*, 641-648

Wynder, E.L., Mabuchi, K., Maruchi, N. & Fortner, J.G. (1973b) Epidemiology of cancer of the pancreas. *J. natl Cancer Inst.*, *50*, 645-667

Wynder, E.L., Covey, L.S., Mabuchi, K. & Mushinski, M. (1976) Environmental factors in cancer of the larynx. A second look. *Cancer*, *38*, 1591-1601

Wynder, E.L., Hall, N.E.L. & Polansky, M. (1983) Epidemiology of coffee and pancreatic cancer. *Cancer Res.*, *43*, 3900-3906

Wynter, J.M., Walsh, D.A., Webster, W.S., McEwen, S.E. & Lipson, A.H. (1983) Teratogenesis after acute alcohol exposure in cultured rat embryos. *Teratog. Carcinog. Mutagenesis*, *3*, 421-428

Yamamoto, R.S., Korzis, J. & Weisburger, J.H. (1967) Chronic ethanol ingestion and the hepatocarcinogenicity of *N*-hydroxy-*N*-2-fluorenylacetamide. *Int. J. Cancer*, *2*, 337-343

Yanai, J. & Ginsburg, B.E. (1976) Audiogenic seizures in mice whose parents drank alcohol. *Q. J. Stud. Alcohol*, *37*, 1564-1571

Yang, C.S., Koop, D.R., Wang, T. & Coon, M.J. (1985a) Immunochemical studies on the metabolism of nitrosamines by ethanol-inducible cytochrome P-450. *Biochem. biophys. Res. Commun.*, *128*, 1007-1013

Yang, C.S., Tu, Y.Y., Koop, D.R. & Coon, M.J. (1985b) Metabolism of nitrosamines by purified rabbit liver cytochrome P-450 isozymes. *Cancer Res.*, *45*, 1140-1145

Ylikahri, R.H., Huttunen, M.O. & Härkönen, M. (1980) Hormonal changes during alcohol intoxication and withdrawal. *Pharmacol. Biochem. Behav.*, *13* Suppl. 1, 131-137

Yoshida, A., Impraim, C.C. & Huang, I.-Y. (1981) Enzymatic and structural differences between usual and atypical human liver alcohol dehydrogenases. *J. biol. Chem.*, *256*, 12430-12436

Yost, G.S. & Finley, B.L. (1983) Ethanol as an inducer of UDP-glucuronyltransferase: a comparison with phenobarbital and 3-methylcholanthrene induction in rabbit hepatic microsomes. *Biochem. biophys. Res. Commun.*, *111*, 219-223

Younes, M., Schlichting, R. & Siegers, C.-P. (1980) Glutathione S-transferase activities in rat liver: effect of some factors influencing the metabolism of xenobiotics. *Pharmacol. Res. Commun.*, *12*, 115-129

Young, M. & Russell, W.T. (1926) *An Investigation into the Statistics of Cancer in Different Trades and Professions*, London, Her Majesty's Stationery Office

Yu, C.-L., Swaminathan, B., Butler, L.G. & Pratt, D.E. (1986) Isolation and identification of rutin as the major mutagen of red wine. *Mutat. Res.*, *170*, 103-113

Yu, M.C., Mack, T., Hanisch, R., Peters, R.L., Henderson, B.E. & Pike, M.C. (1983) Hepatitis, alcohol consumption, cigarette smoking, and hepatocellular carcinoma in Los Angeles. *Cancer Res.*, *43*, 6077-6079

Yuki, T. & Thurman, R.G. (1980) The swift increase in alcohol metabolism. Time course for the increase in hepatic oxygen uptake and the involvement of glycolysis. *Biochem. J.*, *186*, 119-126

Zagraniski, R.T., Kelsey, J.L. & Walter, S.D. (1986) Occupational risk factors for laryngeal carcinoma, Connecticut, 1975-1980. *Am. J. Epidemiol.*, *124*, 67-76

Ziegler, L. & Piendl, A. (1976) Nucleobases and nucleosides in beer. *Tech. Q. Master Brew. Assoc. Am.*, *13*, 177-181

Ziegler, R.G. (1986) Alcohol-nutrient interactions in cancer etiology. *Cancer*, *58*, 1942-1948

Zimmerberg, B., Riley, E.P. & Glick, S.D. (1986) Differential effects of prenatal exposure to alcohol on activity and circling behavior in rats. *Pharmacol. Biochem. Behav.*, *25*, 1021-1025

Zimmerman, H.J. (1986) Effects of alcohol on other hepatotoxins. *Alcohol. clin. exp. Res.*, *10*, 3-15

APPENDICES

Appendix 1
Occurrence of flavour compounds and some other compounds in alcoholic beverages

Appendix 1. Occurrence of flavour compounds and some other compounds in alcoholic beverages[a]

Compound	Molecular formula	Identified in		
		Beer	Wine	Spirits
FLAVOUR COMPOUNDS				
Aliphatic monohydric alcohols				
Methanol	CH_4O			+
Allyl alcohol (2-Propen-1-ol)	C_3H_6O			+
1-Propanol	C_3H_8O	+	+	+
Isopropyl alcohol (IARC, 1977b, 1987a)	C_3H_8O	+	+	+
2-Methyl-1-propanol	$C_4H_{10}O$	+	+	+
n-Butyl alcohol (1-Butanol)	$C_4H_{10}O$	+	+	+
sec-Butyl alcohol (2-Butanol)	$C_4H_{10}O$	+	+	+
tert-Butyl alcohol (2-Methyl-2-propanol)	$C_4H_{10}O$		+	
Methylbutenol	$C_5H_{10}O$			+
2-Methyl-3-buten-2-ol	$C_5H_{10}O$	+		
2-Methyl-1-butanol	$C_5H_{12}O$	+	+	+
Pentyl alcohol (1-Pentanol)	$C_5H_{12}O$	+	+	+
3-Methyl-1-butanol	$C_5H_{12}O$	+	+	+
tert-Pentyl alcohol (2-Methyl-2-butanol)	$C_5H_{12}O$	+	+	+
2-Pentanol	$C_5H_{12}O$	+	+	+
3-Pentanol	$C_5H_{12}O$		+	+
2,4-Hexadien-1-ol, *trans,trans-*	$C_6H_{10}O$		+	
2-Hexen-1-ol	$C_6H_{12}O$	+		
2-Hexen-1-ol, *cis-*				+
2-Hexen-1-ol, *trans-*		+	+	+
3-Hexenol	$C_6H_{12}O$	+		
3-Hexenol, *cis-*		+	+	+
3-Hexenol, *trans-*			+	+
3-Methyl-1-pentanol	$C_6H_{14}O$		+	+
4-Methyl-1-pentanol	$C_6H_{14}O$		+	+
N-Hexyl alcohol (1-Hexanol)	$C_6H_{14}O$	+	+	+
4-Methyl-2-pentanol	$C_6H_{14}O$			+
2-Hexanol	$C_6H_{14}O$	+	+	+
3-Hexanol	$C_6H_{14}O$			+
2-Hepten-1-ol, *trans-*	$C_7H_{14}O$			+
1-Hepten-3-ol	$C_7H_{14}O$	+		+
5-Methyl-1-hexanol	$C_7H_{16}O$			+
n-Heptyl alcohol (1-Heptanol)	$C_7H_{16}O$	+	+	+
2-Heptanol	$C_7H_{16}O$	+	+	+
3-Heptanol	$C_7H_{16}O$			+

Appendix 1 (contd)

Compound	Molecular formula	Identified in		
		Beer	Wine	Spirits
4-Heptanol	$C_7H_{16}O$			+
2-Octen-1-ol, *trans-*	$C_8H_{16}O$			+
1-Octen-3-ol	$C_8H_{16}O$	+	+	+
6-Methyl-1-heptanol	$C_8H_{18}O$		+	
2-Ethyl-1-hexanol	$C_8H_{18}O$	+	+	+
n-Octyl alcohol (1-Octanol)	$C_8H_{18}O$	+	+	+
2-Octanol	$C_8H_{18}O$	+	+	+
3-Octanol	$C_8H_{18}O$		+	+
2-Nonen-1-ol,*trans-*	$C_9H_{18}O$			+
2,6-Dimethyl-4-heptanol	$C_9H_{20}O$			+
n-Nonyl alcohol (1-Nonanol)	$C_9H_{20}O$	+	+	+
2-Nonanol	$C_9H_{20}O$	+	+	+
9-Decen-1-ol	$C_{10}H_{20}O$			+
n-Decyl alcohol (1-Decanol)	$C_{10}H_{22}O$	+	+	+
2-Decanol	$C_{10}H_{22}O$	+	+	+
3-Decanol	$C_{10}H_{22}O$			+
6-Undecen-2-ol	$C_{11}H_{22}O$			
6-Undecen-2-ol, *cis-*				+
6-Undecen-2-ol, *trans-*				+
n-Undecyl alcohol (1-Undecanol)	$C_{11}H_{24}O$		+	+
2-Undecanol	$C_{11}H_{24}O$		+	+
n-Dodecyl alcohol (1-Dodecanol)	$C_{12}H_{26}O$	+	+	+
2-Dodecanol	$C_{12}H_{26}O$	+	+	
1-Tetradecanol	$C_{14}H_{30}O$		+	+
1-Pentadecanol	$C_{15}H_{32}O$		+	
1-Hexadecanol	$C_{16}H_{34}O$			+
Octadecanol	$C_{18}H_{38}O$			+
Aliphatic aldehydes				
Formaldehyde (IARC, 1982a, 1987a)	CH_2O	+	+	+
Glyoxal	$C_2H_2O_2$	+		+
Acetaldehyde (IARC, 1985, 1987a)	C_2H_4O	+	+	+
Glycolic aldehyde	$C_2H_4O_2$		+	
Acrolein (IARC, 1985, 1987a)	C_3H_4O	+		+
Pyruvaldehyde	$C_3H_4O_2$	+		+
Malonaldehyde (IARC, 1985, 1987a)	$C_3H_4O_2$	+		
Propionaldehyde	C_3H_6O	+	+	+
Glyceraldehyde	$C_3H_6O_3$	+		
2-Methyl-2-propenal	C_4H_6O			+
Crotonaldehyde	C_4H_6O	+		+
Isobutyraldehyde	C_4H_8O	+	+	+
Butyraldehyde	C_4H_8O	+	+	+
3-Hydroxybutyraldehyde	$C_4H_8O_2$	+		
Pentadienal	C_5H_6O	+		
2-Methyl-2-butenal, *cis-*	C_5H_8O			+

Appendix 1 (contd)

Compound	Molecular formula	Identified in		
		Beer	Wine	Spirits
3-Methyl-2-butenal	C_5H_8O			+
2-Pentenal	C_5H_8O			+
2-Pentenal, *trans-*				+
Glutaraldehyde	$C_5H_8O_2$	+		
2-Methylbutyraldehyde	$C_5H_{10}O$	+	+	+
Isovaleraldehyde	$C_5H_{10}O$	+	+	+
Valeraldehyde	$C_5H_{10}O$	+	+	+
2-Ethoxypropionaldehyde	$C_5H_{10}O_2$			+
3-Ethoxypropionaldehyde	$C_5H_{10}O_2$			+
5-Hydroxyvaleraldehyde	$C_5H_{10}O_2$	+		
Hexadienal	C_6H_8O	+		
2,4-Hexadienal	C_6H_8O	+		
2,4-Hexadienal, *trans,trans-*		+		
2-Methyl-2-pentenal, *trans-*	$C_6H_{10}O$			+
2-Hexenal	$C_6H_{10}O$	+	+	
2-Hexenal, *trans-*		+		+
3-Methylvaleraldehyde	$C_6H_{12}O$	+		
Hexanal	$C_6H_{12}O$	+	+	+
1-Cyclohexene-1-carboxaldehyde	$C_7H_{10}O$			+
2-Heptenal, *trans-*	$C_7H_{12}O$	+		+
4-Heptenal	$C_7H_{12}O$	+		
Octadienal	$C_8H_{12}O$	+		
Octadienal, *trans,trans-*		+		
2-Octenal, *trans-*	$C_8H_{14}O$			+
Octanal	$C_8H_{16}O$	+	+	+
2,4-Nonadienal, *trans,trans-*	$C_9H_{14}O$	+		+
2,6-Nonadienal, *trans,cis-*	$C_9H_{14}O$	+		
2-Nonenal	$C_9H_{16}O$	+		
2-Nonenal, *trans-*		+		+
Nonanal	$C_9H_{18}O$	+	+	+
2,2,3-Trimethyl-3-cyclopentenyl-1-acetaldehyde	$C_{10}H_{16}O$			+
Decadienal	$C_{10}H_{16}O$	+		
2,4-Decadienal, *trans,trans-*	$C_{10}H_{16}O$			+
2-Decenal, *trans-*	$C_{10}H_{18}O$			+
Decanal	$C_{10}H_{20}O$	+	+	+
Undecanal	$C_{11}H_{22}O$		+	+
Lauraldehyde	$C_{12}H_{24}O$	+	+	+
Myristaldehyde	$C_{14}H_{28}O$		+	
Aliphatic ketones				
Acetone	C_3H_6O	+	+	+
1-Hydroxy-2-propanone	$C_3H_6O_2$	+	+	+
Dihydroxyacetone	$C_3H_6O_3$		+	
2,3-Butanedione (Diacetyl)	$C_4H_6O_2$	+	+	+
2-Butanone	C_4H_8O	+	+	+

Appendix 1 (contd)

Compound	Molecular formula	Identified in		
		Beer	Wine	Spirits
3-Hydroxy-2-butanone	$C_4H_8O_2$	+	+	+
1,2-Cyclopentanedione	$C_5H_6O_2$			+
Cyclopentanone	C_5H_8O			+
3-Penten-2-one	C_5H_8O			+
3-Penten-2-one, *trans-*				+
2,3-Pentanedione	$C_5H_8O_2$	+	+	+
3-Methyl-2-butanone	$C_5H_{10}O$	+		+
2-Pentanone	$C_5H_{10}O$	+	+	+
3-Pentanone	$C_5H_{10}O$	+	+	
3-Hydroxy-2-pentanone	$C_5H_{10}O_2$	+		
2-Hydroxy-3-methyl-2-cyclopenten-1-one	$C_6H_8O_2$	+		
5-Methyl-1,2-cyclopentanedione	$C_6H_8O_2$			+
2-Methyl-1,3-cyclopentanedione	$C_6H_8O_2$	+		
4-Methyl-3-penten-2-one	$C_6H_{10}O$		+	+
5-Hexen-2-one	$C_6H_{10}O$	+		
2-Methylcyclopentanone	$C_6H_{10}O$			+
2,3-Hexanedione	$C_6H_{10}O_2$	+		
2,5-Hexanedione	$C_6H_{10}O_2$	+		
3-Methyl-2-pentanone	$C_6H_{12}O$	+		
4-Methyl-2-pentanone	$C_6H_{12}O$	+		+
2-Hexanone	$C_6H_{12}O$	+	+	+
3-Hexanone	$C_6H_{12}O$	+	+	+
4-Ethoxy-2-butanone	$C_6H_{12}O_2$			+
4-Hydroxy-4-methyl-2-pentanone	$C_6H_{12}O_2$			+
2-Methyl-1,3-cyclohexanedione	$C_7H_{10}O_2$	+		
2-Hepten-4-one	$C_7H_{12}O$	+		
2,3-Heptanedione	$C_7H_{12}O_2$	+		
2,4-Dimethyl-3-pentanone	$C_7H_{14}O$			+
2-Heptanone	$C_7H_{14}O$	+	+	+
3-Heptanone	$C_7H_{14}O$			+
4-Ethoxy-2-pentanone	$C_7H_{14}O_2$			+
6-Methyl-3,4-heptadien-2-one	$C_8H_{12}O$			
6-Methyl-3,4-heptadien-2-one, *cis-*				+
6-Methyl-3,4-heptadien-2-one, *trans-*				+
6-Methyl-5-hepten-2-one	$C_8H_{14}O$	+	+	+
1-Octen-3-one	$C_8H_{14}O$		+	
2-Octanone	$C_8H_{16}O$	+	+	+
3-Octanone	$C_8H_{16}O$		+	+
3,5,5-Trimethyl-2-cyclohexene-1,4-dione	$C_9H_{12}O_2$			+
3-Nonen-2-one, *trans-*	$C_9H_{16}O$			+
2-Nonen-4-one, *trans-*	$C_9H_{16}O$			+
2-Nonanone	$C_9H_{18}O$	+	+	+
2-Decanone	$C_{10}H_{20}O$	+	+	+
2-Undecen-4-one, *trans-*	$C_{11}H_{20}O$			+
2-Undecanone	$C_{11}H_{22}O$	+	+	+

Appendix 1 (contd)

Compound	Molecular formula	Identified in		
		Beer	Wine	Spirits
2-Dodecanone	$C_{12}H_{24}O$			+
2-Tridecanone	$C_{13}H_{26}O$			+
2-Tetradecanone	$C_{14}H_{28}O$			+
Acetals				
Formaldehyde dimethyl acetal	$C_3H_8O_2$	+		
2,4-Dimethyl-1,3-dioxolane	$C_5H_{10}O_2$		+	
5-Hydroxy-2-methyl-1,3-dioxane	$C_5H_{10}O_3$			
5-Hydroxy-2-methyl-1,3-dioxane, *cis-*			+	
5-Hydroxy-2-methyl-1,3-dioxane, *trans-*			+	
4-Hydroxymethyl-2-methyl-1,3-dioxolane	$C_5H_{10}O_3$			
4-Hydroxymethyl-2-methyl-1,3-dioxolane, *cis-*			+	
4-Hydroxymethyl-2-methyl-1,3-dioxolane, *trans-*			+	
Formaldehyde diethyl acetal	$C_5H_{12}O_2$			+
Acetaldehyde methyl ethyl acetal	$C_5H_{12}O_2$		+	+
2,4,5-Trimethyl-1,3-dioxolane	$C_6H_{12}O_2$		+	+
Acetaldehyde acetyl ethyl acetal	$C_6H_{12}O_3$			+
Acetaldehyde diethyl acetal (Acetal)	$C_6H_{14}O_2$	+	+	+
Acetaldehyde methyl propyl acetal	$C_6H_{14}O_2$		+	
2,4-Dimethyl-5-ethyl-1,3-dioxolane	$C_7H_{14}O_2$		+	
2-Isopropyl-4-methyl-1,3-dioxolane	$C_7H_{14}O_2$		+	
Acrolein diethyl acetal	$C_7H_{14}O_2$			+
Pyruvaldehyde diethyl acetal	$C_7H_{14}O_3$		+	+
Acetaldehyde ethyl propyl acetal	$C_7H_{16}O_2$		+	+
Propionaldehyde diethyl acetal	$C_7H_{16}O_2$			+
Acetaldehyde diallyl acetal	$C_8H_{14}O_2$			+
2-Isobutyl-4-methyl-1,3-dioxolane	$C_8H_{16}O_2$			
2-Isobutyl-4-methyl-1,3-dioxolane, *cis-*			+	
2-Isobutyl-4-methyl-1,3-dioxolane, *trans-*			+	
2,3-Butanedione diethyl acetal	$C_8H_{16}O_3$			+
Acetaldehyde ethyl isobutyl acetal	$C_8H_{18}O_2$			+
Acetaldehyde ethyl butyl acetal	$C_8H_{18}O_2$			+
Acetaldehyde dipropyl acetal	$C_8H_{18}O_2$		+	+
Isobutyraldehyde diethyl acetal	$C_8H_{18}O_2$			+
Butyraldehyde diethyl acetal	$C_8H_{18}O_2$			+
Hexanaldehyde dimethyl acetal	$C_8H_{18}O_2$			+
Ethoxyacetaldehyde diethyl acetal	$C_8H_{18}O_3$		+	
2-Ethoxyacetaldehyde diethyl acetal	$C_8H_{18}O_3$			+
2-Pentyl-4-methyl-1,3-dioxolane, *trans-*	$C_9H_{18}O_2$		+	
Acetaldehyde ethyl 2-methylbutyl acetal	$C_9H_{20}O_2$		+	+
Acetaldehyde ethyl isopentyl acetal	$C_9H_{20}O_2$		+	+
Acetaldehyde ethyl pentyl acetal	$C_9H_{20}O_2$			+
Priopionaldehyde ethyl isobutyl acetal	$C_9H_{20}O_2$			+
Isobutyraldehyde ethyl propyl acetal	$C_9H_{20}O_2$			+
2-Methylbutyraldehyde diethyl acetal	$C_9H_{20}O_2$			+

Appendix 1 (contd)

Compound	Molecular formula	Identified in		
		Beer	Wine	Spirits
Isovaleraldehyde diethyl acetal	$C_9H_{20}O_2$			+
Valeraldehyde diethyl acetal	$C_9H_{20}O_2$		+	+
3-Ethoxypropionaldehyde diethyl acetal	$C_9H_{20}O_3$			+
Acetaldehyde ethyl 3-hexenyl acetal	$C_{10}H_{20}O_2$			+
Acetaldehyde ethyl hexyl acetal	$C_{10}H_{20}O_2$			+
Acetaldehyde isopentyl propyl acetal	$C_{10}H_{20}O_2$			+
Acetaldehyde diisobutyl acetal	$C_{10}H_{20}O_2$		+	+
Acetaldehyde dibutyl acetal	$C_{10}H_{20}O_2$		+	
Propionaldehyde ethyl isopentyl acetal	$C_{10}H_{20}O_2$			+
Isobutyraldehyde ethyl isobutyl acetal	$C_{10}H_{22}O_2$			+
Hexanaldehyde diethyl acetal	$C_{10}H_{22}O_2$			+
3-Hydroxypropionaldehyde ethyl isopentyl acetal	$C_{10}H_{22}O_3$			+
3-Ethoxy-2-methylpropionaldehyde diethyl acetal	$C_{10}H_{22}O_3$			+
3-Ethoxybutyraldehyde diethyl acetal	$C_{10}H_{22}O_3$			+
Acetaldehyde ethyl benzyl acetal	$C_{11}H_{16}O_2$			+
Acetaldehyde isobutyl isopentyl acetal	$C_{11}H_{24}O_2$		+	+
Acetaldehyde butyl isopentyl acetal	$C_{11}H_{24}O_2$			+
Acetaldehyde butyl pentyl acetal	$C_{11}H_{24}O_2$			+
Propionaldehyde propyl isopentyl acetal	$C_{11}H_{24}O_2$			+
Propionaldehyde diisobutyl acetal	$C_{11}H_{24}O_2$			+
Isobutyraldehyde ethyl isopentyl acetal	$C_{11}H_{24}O_2$			+
Isobutyraldehyde propyl isobutyl acetal	$C_{11}H_{24}O_2$			+
Butyraldehyde ethyl isopentyl acetal	$C_{11}H_{24}O_2$			+
Butyraldehyde ethyl pentyl acetal	$C_{11}H_{24}O_2$			+
Isovaleraldehyde ethyl isobutyl acetal	$C_{11}H_{24}O_2$			+
Isovaleraldehyde dipropyl acetal	$C_{11}H_{24}O_2$			+
Valeraldehyde ethyl isobutyl acetal	$C_{11}H_{24}O_2$			+
Acetaldehyde ethyl phenethyl acetal	$C_{12}H_{18}O_2$		+	+
2-Phenylacetaldehyde diethyl acetal	$C_{12}H_{18}O_2$		+	+
Acetaldehyde di(2-methylbutyl) acetal	$C_{12}H_{26}O_2$		+	+
Acetaldehyde isopentyl 2-methylbutyl acetal	$C_{12}H_{26}O_2$		+	+
Acetaldehyde diisopentyl acetal	$C_{12}H_{26}O_2$		+	+
Acetaldehyde isopentyl pentyl acetal	$C_{12}H_{26}O_2$			+
Isobutyraldehyde propyl isopentyl acetal	$C_{12}H_{26}O_2$			+
Isobutyraldehyde diisobutyl acetal	$C_{12}H_{26}O_2$			+
Isovaleraldehyde ethyl isopentyl acetal	$C_{12}H_{26}O_2$			+
Isovaleraldehyde propyl isobutyl acetal	$C_{12}H_{26}O_2$			+
Valeraldehyde ethyl pentyl acetal	$C_{12}H_{26}O_2$			+
3-Ethoxypropionaldehyde ethyl isopentyl acetal	$C_{12}H_{26}O_3$			+
Acetaldehyde isopentyl hexyl acetal	$C_{13}H_{28}O_2$		+	
Isobutyraldehyde isobutyl isopentyl acetal	$C_{13}H_{28}O_2$			+
Isovaleraldehyde isopentyl propyl acetal	$C_{13}H_{28}O_2$			+
Isovaleraldehyde diisobutyl acetal	$C_{13}H_{28}O_2$			+
Valeraldehyde diisobutyl acetal	$C_{13}H_{28}O_2$			+
Acetaldehyde dihexyl acetal	$C_{14}H_{30}O_2$		+	

Appendix 1 (contd)

Compound	Molecular formula	Identified in		
		Beer	Wine	Spirits
Isobutyraldehyde diisopentyl acetal	$C_{14}H_{30}O_2$			+
Isovaleraldehyde isobutyl isopentyl acetal	$C_{14}H_{30}O_2$			+
Ethoxyacetaldehyde dipentyl acetal	$C_{14}H_{30}O_3$		+	
Acetaldehyde 2-methylbutyl phenethyl acetal	$C_{15}H_{24}O_2$		+	
Acetaldehyde isopentyl phenethyl acetal	$C_{15}H_{24}O_2$		+	
Isovaleraldehyde diisopentyl acetal	$C_{15}H_{32}O_2$			+
Hexoxyacetaldehyde dipentyl acetal	$C_{18}H_{38}O_3$		+	
Aliphatic monocarboxylic acids				
Formic acid	CH_2O_2	+	+	
Acetic acid	$C_2H_4O_2$	+	+	+
Propionic acid	$C_3H_6O_2$	+	+	+
Crotonic acid	$C_4H_6O_2$	+		
Isobutyric acid	$C_4H_8O_2$	+	+	+
Butyric acid	$C_4H_8O_2$	+	+	+
Pentenoic acid	$C_5H_8O_2$	+		
2-Methylbutyric acid	$C_5H_{10}O_2$	+	+	+
Isovaleric acid	$C_5H_{10}O_2$	+	+	+
Valeric acid	$C_5H_{10}O_2$	+	+	+
3-Ethoxypropionic acid	$C_5H_{10}O_3$			+
Sorbic acid	$C_6H_8O_2$		+	
4-Methyl-3-pentenoic acid	$C_6H_{10}O_2$	+	+	
Hexenoic acid	$C_6H_{10}O_2$	+	+	
2-Hexenoic acid	$C_6H_{10}O_2$	+		
3-Hexenoic acid	$C_6H_{10}O_2$	+	+	
3-Hexenoic acid, *cis*-			+	
4-Methylvaleric acid	$C_6H_{12}O_2$	+		+
Hexanoic acid	$C_6H_{12}O_2$	+	+	+
Heptenoic acid	$C_7H_{12}O_2$	+		+
2-Heptenoic acid	$C_7H_{12}O_2$	+		
2-Ethyl-3-methylbutanoic acid	$C_7H_{14}O_2$			+
2-Methylhexanoic acid	$C_7H_{14}O_2$			+
Heptanoic acid	$C_7H_{14}O_2$	+	+	+
2-Octenoic acid	$C_8H_{14}O_2$	+		
2-Ethylhexanoic acid	$C_8H_{16}O_2$		+	
6-Methylheptanoic acid	$C_8H_{16}O_2$			+
Octanoic acid	$C_8H_{16}O_2$	+	+	+
2-Nonenoic acid	$C_9H_{16}O_2$	+		
Nonanoic acid	$C_9H_{18}O_2$	+	+	+
3,7-Dimethyl-2,6-octadienoic acid	$C_{10}H_{16}O_2$		+	
Decadienoic acid	$C_{10}H_{16}O_2$	+		
4,8-Decadienoic acid	$C_{10}H_{16}O_2$	+		
Decenoic acid	$C_{10}H_{18}O_2$	+		
4-Decenoic acid	$C_{10}H_{18}O_2$	+		
9-Decenoic acid	$C_{10}H_{18}O_2$		+	

Appendix 1 (contd)

Compound	Molecular formula	Identified in		
		Beer	Wine	Spirits
Decanoic acid	$C_{10}H_{20}O_2$	+	+	+
10-Undecenoic acid	$C_{11}H_{20}O_2$		+	+
9-Methyldecanoic acid	$C_{11}H_{22}O_2$	+		
Undecanoic acid	$C_{11}H_{22}O_2$	+	+	+
Dodecenoic acid	$C_{12}H_{22}O_2$	+		
Lauric acid	$C_{12}H_{24}O_2$	+	+	+
Methyllauric acid	$C_{13}H_{26}O_2$	+		
Tridecanoic acid	$C_{13}H_{26}O_2$	+	+	+
Tetradecenoic acid	$C_{14}H_{26}O_2$	+		
Myristic acid	$C_{14}H_{28}O_2$	+	+	+
Pentadecanoic acid	$C_{15}H_{30}O_2$	+	+	+
9-Hexadecenoic acid	$C_{16}H_{30}O_2$	+	+	+
Palmitic acid	$C_{16}H_{32}O_3$	+	+	+
Heptadecanoic acid	$C_{17}H_{34}O_2$	+	+	+
Linolenic acid	$C_{18}H_{30}O_2$	+		+
Linoleic acid	$C_{18}H_{32}O_2$	+		+
Oleic acid	$C_{18}H_{34}O_2$	+	+	+
Stearic acid	$C_{18}H_{36}O_2$	+	+	+
Docosanoic acid	$C_{22}H_{44}O_2$	+		
Hexacosanoic acid	$C_{26}H_{52}O_2$	+		
Aliphatic monobasic hydroxy acids				
Glycolic acid	$C_2H_4O_3$	+	+	
Lactic acid	$C_3H_6O_3$	+	+	+
D-Lactic acid		+	+	
L-Lactic acid		+	+	
2-Methyllactic acid	$C_4H_8O_3$		+	
2-Hydroxybutyric acid	$C_4H_8O_3$		+	
2-Hydroxy-2-methylbutyric acid	$C_5H_{10}O_3$		+	
2-Hydroxy-3-methylbutyric acid	$C_5H_{10}O_3$	+	+	
2,3-Dihydroxy-2-methylbutyric acid	$C_5H_{10}O_4$		+	
2,3-Dihydroxy-3-methylbutyric acid	$C_5H_{10}O_4$		+	
2-Hydroxy-3-methylvaleric acid	$C_6H_{12}O_3$	+	+	
D-2-Hydroxy-3-methylvaleric acid			+	
L-2-Hydroxy-3-methylvaleric acid			+	
Hydroxy-4-methylvaleric acid	$C_6H_{12}O_3$	+	+	
2-Hydroxyhexanoic acid	$C_6H_{12}O_3$		+	
2-Hydroxyheptanoic acid	$C_7H_{14}O_3$	+		
2-Hydroxyoctanoic acid	$C_8H_{16}O_3$	+		
3-Hydroxyoctanoic acid	$C_8H_{16}O_3$	+	+	
3-Hydroxydecanoic acid	$C_{10}H_{20}O_3$	+		
2-Hydroxylauric acid	$C_{12}H_{24}O_3$		+	
9,10,11-Trihydroxy-12-octadecenoic acid, *trans-*	$C_{18}H_{34}O_5$	+		
9,10,13-Trihydroxy-11-octadecenoic acid, *trans-*	$C_{18}H_{34}O_5$	+		
9,12,13-Trihydroxy-11-octadecenoic acid, *trans-*	$C_{18}H_{34}O_5$	+		

Appendix 1 (contd)

Compound	Molecular formula	Identified in		
		Beer	Wine	Spirits
Aldonic and uronic acids				
Ascorbic acid	$C_6H_8O_6$		+	
arabino-Hexulosonic acid (2-Ketogluconic acid)	$C_6H_{10}O_7$	+		
Glucuronic acid	$C_6H_{10}O_7$	+	+	
Galacturonic acid	$C_6H_{10}O_7$	+	+	
Galactaric acid	$C_6H_{10}O_8$		+	
Gluconic acid	$C_6H_{12}O_7$	+	+	
Aliphatic monobasic oxo acids				
Glyoxylic acid	$C_2H_2O_3$	+	+	
Glyoxylic acid, *syn-*		+		
Glyoxylic acid, *anti-*		+		
Pyruvic acid	$C_3H_4O_3$	+	+	
Pyruvic acid, *syn-*		+		
Pyruvic acid, *anti-*		+		
2-Oxobutyric acid	$C_4H_6O_3$	+		
Acetoacetic acid	$C_4H_6O_3$		+	
3-Methyl-2-oxobutyric acid	$C_5H_8O_3$	+		
Levulinic acid	$C_5H_8O_3$	+	+	
2-Hydroxy-2-methylacetoacetic acid	$C_5H_8O_4$	+		
3-Methyl-2-oxovaleric acid	$C_6H_{10}O_3$	+		
4-Methyl-2-oxovaleric acid	$C_6H_{10}O_3$	+	+	
2-Oxohexanoic acid	$C_6H_{10}O_3$	+	+	
5-Oxohexanoic acid	$C_6H_{10}O_3$	+		
2-Ethyl-2-hydroxyacetoacetic acid	$C_6H_{10}O_4$	+		
7-Oxoheptanoic acid	$C_7H_{12}O_3$	+		
Aliphatic di- and tricarboxylic acids				
Oxalic acid	$C_2H_2O_4$	+	+	
Mesoxalic acid	$C_2H_2O_5$		+	
Malonic acid	$C_3H_4O_4$	+	+	
Fumaric acid	$C_4H_4O_4$	+	+	
Oxalacetic acid	$C_4H_4O_5$	+	+	
Succinic acid	$C_4H_6O_4$	+	+	
Malic acid	$C_4H_6O_5$	+	+	
Tartaric acid	$C_4H_6O_6$	+	+	
Mesaconic acid	$C_5H_6O_4$	+	+	
Citraconic acid	$C_5H_6O_4$	+	+	
Methylenesuccinic acid	$C_5H_6O_4$		+	
Glutaconic acid	$C_5H_6O_4$		+	
2-Oxoglutaric acid	$C_5H_6O_5$	+	+	
Methylsuccinic acid	$C_5H_8O_4$		+	
Glutaric acid	$C_5H_8O_4$	+	+	
2-Methylmalic acid	$C_5H_8O_5$	+	+	
2-Hydroxyglutaric acid	$C_5H_8O_5$	+	+	

Appendix 1 (contd)

Compound	Molecular formula	Identified in		
		Beer	Wine	Spirits
1-Propene-1,2,3-tricarboxylic acid	$C_6H_6O_6$	+	+	
1-Propene-1,2,3-tricarboxylic acid, *cis-*			+	
1-Oxo-1,2,3-propanetricarboxylic acid	$C_6H_6O_7$	+		
1,2,3-Propanetricarboxylic acid	$C_6H_8O_6$		+	
Isocitric acid	$C_6H_8O_7$	+	+	
Citric acid	$C_6H_8O_7$	+	+	
3-Methylglutaric acid	$C_6H_{10}O_4$		+	
Adipic acid	$C_6H_{10}O_4$		+	
Galactaric acid	$C_6H_{10}O_8$		+	
Pimelic acid	$C_7H_{12}O_4$	+	+	
2-Isopropylmalic acid	$C_7H_{12}O_5$	+	+	
Suberic acid	$C_8H_{14}O_4$	+	+	
3-Ethylheptanedioic acid	$C_9H_{16}O_4$			+
Azelaic acid	$C_9H_{16}O_4$	+	+	
Sebacic acid	$C_{10}H_{18}O_4$	+	+	
Undecanedioic acid	$C_{11}H_{20}O_4$	+		
Dodecanedioic acid	$C_{12}H_{22}O_4$	+		
Esters of aliphatic monocarboxylic acids				
Methyl formate	$C_2H_4O_2$	+	+	+
Ethyl formate	$C_3H_6O_2$	+	+	+
Methyl acetate	$C_3H_6O_2$	+	+	+
Vinyl acetate (IARC, 1986b, 1987a)	$C_4H_6O_2$			+
Isopropyl formate	$C_4H_8O_2$		+	
Propyl formate	$C_4H_8O_2$		+	
Ethyl acetate	$C_4H_8O_2$	+	+	+
Methyl propionate	$C_4H_8O_2$		+	+
Acetonyl acetate	$C_5H_8O_3$	+		
Isobutyl formate	$C_5H_{10}O_2$	+		+
Butyl formate	$C_5H_{10}O_2$		+	
Isopropyl acetate	$C_5H_{10}O_2$	+	+	+
Propyl acetate	$C_5H_{10}O_2$	+	+	+
Ethyl propionate	$C_5H_{10}O_2$	+	+	+
Methyl isobutyrate	$C_5H_{10}O_2$		+	+
Methyl butyrate	$C_5H_{10}O_2$		+	+
1,3-Propanediol monoacetate	$C_5H_{10}O_3$		+	
Furfuryl formate	$C_6H_6O_3$	+		
Ethyl methacrylate	$C_6H_{10}O_2$		+	
Ethyl 2-butenoate	$C_6H_{10}O_2$		+	
Ethyl 2-butenoate, *trans-*			+	
2-Methylbutyl formate	$C_6H_{12}O_2$		+	
Isopentyl formate	$C_6H_{12}O_2$	+	+	+
Pentyl formate	$C_6H_{12}O_2$			+
tert-Butyl acetate	$C_6H_{12}O_2$			+
Isobutyl acetate	$C_6H_{12}O_2$	+	+	+

Appendix 1 (contd)

Compound	Molecular formula	Identified in		
		Beer	Wine	Spirits
Butyl acetate	$C_6H_{12}O_2$	+	+	+
sec-Butyl acetate	$C_6H_{12}O_2$	+		+
Isopropyl propionate	$C_6H_{12}O_2$		+	
Propyl propionate	$C_6H_{12}O_2$		+	+
Ethyl isobutyrate	$C_6H_{12}O_2$	+	+	+
Ethyl butyrate	$C_6H_{12}O_2$	+	+	+
Methyl valerate	$C_6H_{12}O_2$		+	
Ethoxyethyl acetate	$C_6H_{12}O_3$			+
2-Butanediol monoacetate	$C_6H_{12}O_3$		+	
2-Butanediol monoacetate, *threo-*			+	
2-Butanediol monoacetate, *erythro-*			+	
Furfuryl acetate	$C_7H_8O_3$	+		+
Methyl 2,4-hexadienoate	$C_7H_{10}O_2$		+	
Hexenyl formate	$C_7H_{12}O_2$			+
Methyl hexenoate	$C_7H_{12}O_2$	+		
Isopentyl acetate	$C_7H_{14}O_2$	+	+	+
2-Methylbutyl acetate	$C_7H_{14}O_2$		+	
Pentyl acetate	$C_7H_{14}O_2$	+	+	+
1-Methylbutyl acetate	$C_7H_{14}O_2$		+	
Isobutyl propionate	$C_7H_{14}O_2$		+	+
sec-Butyl propionate	$C_7H_{14}O_2$		+	
tert-Butyl propionate	$C_7H_{14}O_2$			+
Butyl propionate	$C_7H_{14}O_2$			+
Isopropyl isobutyrate	$C_7H_{14}O_2$		+	
Isopropyl butyrate	$C_7H_{14}O_2$		+	
Propyl butyrate	$C_7H_{14}O_2$		+	+
Ethyl 2-methylbutyrate	$C_7H_{14}O_2$	+	+	+
Ethyl isovalerate	$C_7H_{14}O_2$	+	+	+
Ethyl valerate	$C_7H_{14}O_2$		+	+
Methyl 3-methylvalerate	$C_7H_{14}O_2$		+	
Methyl hexanoate	$C_7H_{14}O_2$	+	+	+
Ethyl 3-ethoxypropionate	$C_7H_{14}O_3$			+
Triethyl *ortho*-formate	$C_7H_{16}O_3$		+	+
Benzyl formate	$C_8H_8O_2$			+
Ethyl sorbate	$C_8H_{12}O_2$		+	+
Cyclohexyl acetate	$C_8H_{14}O_2$		+	
2-Hexenyl acetate, *trans-*	$C_8H_{14}O_2$			+
3-Hexenyl acetate	$C_8H_{14}O_2$		+	
3-Hexenyl acetate, *cis-*			+	+
3-Hexenyl acetate, *trans-*			+	+
Ethyl 4-methyl-3-pentenoate	$C_8H_{14}O_2$		+	
Ethyl hexenoate	$C_8H_{14}O_2$	+		
Ethyl 2-hexenoate	$C_8H_{14}O_2$		+	
Ethyl 2-hexenoate, *trans-*				+
Ethyl 3-hexenoate, *cis-*	$C_8H_{14}O_2$	+	+	

Appendix 1 (contd)

Compound	Molecular formula	Identified in		
		Beer	Wine	Spirits
Methyl 4-methyl-2-hexenoate	$C_8H_{14}O_2$	+		
Methyl heptenoate	$C_8H_{14}O_2$	+		
Heptyl formate	$C_8H_{16}O_2$		+	
Hexyl acetate	$C_8H_{16}O_2$	+	+	+
2-Methylbutyl propionate	$C_8H_{16}O_2$		+	
Isopentyl propionate	$C_8H_{16}O_2$	+	+	+
Pentyl propionate	$C_8H_{16}O_2$		+	
Isobutyl isobutyrate	$C_8H_{16}O_2$		+	+
Butyl isobutyrate	$C_8H_{16}O_2$			+
Isobutyl butyrate	$C_8H_{16}O_2$			+
Butyl butyrate	$C_8H_{16}O_2$		+	+
Ethyl hexanoate	$C_8H_{16}O_2$	+	+	+
Methyl heptanoate	$C_8H_{16}O_2$		+	
Diethoxyethyl acetate	$C_8H_{16}O_4$			+
Phenethyl formate	$C_9H_{10}O_2$	+	+	+
Benzyl acetate (IARC, 1986c, 1987a)	$C_9H_{10}O_2$		+	+
Ethyl heptenoate	$C_9H_{16}O_2$	+		+
Heptyl acetate	$C_9H_{18}O_2$	+	+	+
2-Methylbutyl isobutyrate	$C_9H_{18}O_2$	+	+	
Isopentyl isobutyrate	$C_9H_{18}O_2$	+	+	+
2-Methylbutyl butyrate	$C_9H_{18}O_2$		+	+
Isopentyl butyrate	$C_9H_{18}O_2$	+	+	+
Pentyl butyrate	$C_9H_{18}O_2$	+		
Isobutyl 2-methylbutyrate	$C_9H_{18}O_2$		+	+
Isobutyl isovalerate	$C_9H_{18}O_2$		+	
Isobutyl valerate	$C_9H_{18}O_2$		+	+
Butyl valerate	$C_9H_{18}O_2$		+	
Propyl hexanoate	$C_9H_{18}O_2$		+	+
Ethyl 5-methylhexanoate	$C_9H_{18}O_2$	+		
Ethyl heptanoate	$C_9H_{18}O_2$	+	+	+
Methyl octanoate	$C_9H_{18}O_2$	+	+	+
Phenethyl acetate	$C_{10}H_{12}O_2$	+	+	+
Ethyl phenyl acetate	$C_{10}H_{12}O_2$		+	
Benzyl propionate	$C_{10}H_{12}O_2$			+
4-Hydroxyphenethyl acetate	$C_{10}H_{12}O_3$	+	+	
Octyl acetate	$C_{10}H_{20}O_2$	+	+	+
Hexyl isobutyrate	$C_{10}H_{12}O_2$	+	+	+
Hexyl butyrate	$C_{10}H_{12}O_2$	+	+	+
Isopentyl 2-methylbutyrate	$C_{10}H_{12}O_2$		+	+
Isopentyl isovalerate	$C_{10}H_{12}O_2$	+	+	+
Pentyl isovalerate	$C_{10}H_{12}O_2$	+		
2-Methylbutyl valerate	$C_{10}H_{12}O_2$		+	
Isopentyl valerate	$C_{10}H_{12}O_2$		+	+
Pentyl valerate	$C_{10}H_{12}O_2$		+	
Isobutyl hexanoate	$C_{10}H_{12}O_2$	+	+	+

Appendix 1 (contd)

Compound	Molecular formula	Identified in		
		Beer	Wine	Spirits
Butyl hexanoate	$C_{10}H_{12}O_2$	+	+	+
Ethyl octanoate	$C_{10}H_{12}O_2$	+	+	+
Methyl nonanoate	$C_{10}H_{12}O_2$		+	
Phenethyl propionate	$C_{11}H_{14}O_2$	+	+	
Methyl 2,4,7-decatrienoate,	$C_{11}H_{16}O_2$			
trans,cis,cis-				+
trans,trans,cis-				+
Methyl 2,4-decadienoate,	$C_{11}H_{18}O_2$			
trans,cis-				+
trans,trans-				+
Methyl 4,8-decadienoate	$C_{11}H_{18}O_2$	+		
Ethyl nonenoate	$C_{11}H_{20}O_2$	+		
Methyl 4-decenoate	$C_{11}H_{20}O_2$	+		
Methyl 4-decenoate, *cis-*	$C_{11}H_{20}O_2$		+	
Nonyl acetate	$C_{11}H_{22}O_2$	+	+	
1-Methylhexyl butyrate	$C_{11}H_{22}O_2$	+		
Hexyl 2-methylbutyrate	$C_{11}H_{22}O_2$			+
Hexyl isovalerate	$C_{11}H_{22}O_2$		+	
Hexyl valerate	$C_{11}H_{22}O_2$		+	+
2-Methylbutyl hexanoate	$C_{11}H_{22}O_2$		+	+
Isopentyl hexanoate	$C_{11}H_{22}O_2$	+	+	+
Pentyl hexanoate	$C_{11}H_{22}O_2$	+	+	+
1-Methylbutyl hexanoate	$C_{11}H_{22}O_2$	+		
Isobutyl heptanoate	$C_{11}H_{22}O_2$			+
Butyl heptanoate	$C_{11}H_{22}O_2$			+
Propyl octanoate	$C_{11}H_{22}O_2$		+	+
Ethyl nonanoate	$C_{11}H_{22}O_2$	+	+	+
Methyl decanoate	$C_{11}H_{22}O_2$	+	+	+
Phenethyl isobutyrate	$C_{12}H_{16}O_2$	+	+	+
Phenethyl butyrate	$C_{12}H_{16}O_2$	+	+	+
Ethyl 2,4,7-decatrienoate,	$C_{12}H_{18}O_2$			
trans,cis,cis-				+
trans,trans,cis-				+
Ethyl decadienoate	$C_{12}H_{20}O_2$	+	+	
Ethyl 2,4-decadienoate,	$C_{12}H_{20}O_2$			
trans,cis-				+
trans,trans-				+
Ethyl 4,8-decadienoate	$C_{12}H_{20}O_2$	+		
Ethyl decenoate	$C_{12}H_{22}O_2$	+	+	
Ethyl 2-decenoate, *trans-*	$C_{12}H_{22}O_2$			+
Ethyl 4-decenoate	$C_{12}H_{22}O_2$	+		
Ethyl 4-decenoate, *cis-*				+
Ethyl 9-decenoate	$C_{12}H_{22}O_2$	+	+	+
Decyl acetate	$C_{12}H_{24}O_2$		+	+
Octyl butyrate	$C_{12}H_{24}O_2$	+		

Appendix 1 (contd)

Compound	Molecular formula	Identified in		
		Beer	Wine	Spirits
Hexyl hexanoate	$C_{12}H_{24}O_2$	+	+	+
Isopentyl heptanoate	$C_{12}H_{24}O_2$	+		
Isobutyl octanoate	$C_{12}H_{24}O_2$		+	+
Butyl octanoate	$C_{12}H_{24}O_2$	+	+	+
Ethyl decanoate	$C_{12}H_{24}O_2$	+	+	+
Phenethyl isovalerate	$C_{13}H_{18}O_2$	+		
Phenethyl valerate	$C_{13}H_{18}O_2$		+	
Propyl 2,4-decadienoate, *trans,cis-*	$C_{13}H_{22}O_2$			+
Methyl 2,6-dodecadienoate, *trans,cis-*	$C_{13}H_{22}O_2$			+
Heptyl hexanoate	$C_{13}H_{26}O_2$		+	
Hexyl heptanoate	$C_{13}H_{26}O_2$		+	+
2-Methylbutyl octanoate	$C_{13}H_{26}O_2$	+	+	+
Isopentyl octanoate	$C_{13}H_{26}O_2$	+	+	+
Pentyl octanoate	$C_{13}H_{26}O_2$		+	
Isobutyl nonanoate	$C_{13}H_{26}O_2$			+
Propyl decanoate	$C_{13}H_{26}O_2$		+	+
Ethyl undecanoate	$C_{13}H_{26}O_2$		+	+
Methyl laurate	$C_{13}H_{26}O_2$		+	+
Phenethyl hexenoate	$C_{14}H_{18}O_2$	+		
Phenethyl hexanoate	$C_{14}H_{20}O_2$	+	+	+
Butyl 2,4-decadienoate, *trans,cis-*	$C_{14}H_{24}O_2$			+
Ethyl dodecadienoate	$C_{14}H_{24}O_2$			+
Ethyl 2,6-dodecadienoate, *trans,cis-*	$C_{14}H_{24}O_2$			+
Isobutyl decenoate	$C_{14}H_{26}O_2$		+	
Ethyl dodecenoate	$C_{14}H_{26}O_2$			+
Ethyl 2-dodecenoate, *trans-*	$C_{14}H_{26}O_2$			+
Ethyl 6-dodecenoate, *cis-*	$C_{14}H_{26}O_2$			+
Dodecyl acetate	$C_{14}H_{28}O_2$			+
Octyl hexanoate	$C_{14}H_{28}O_2$	+		
1-Methylheptyl hexanoate	$C_{14}H_{28}O_2$	+		
Hexyl octanoate	$C_{14}H_{28}O_2$	+	+	+
Isopentyl nonanoate	$C_{14}H_{28}O_2$	+		+
Isobutyl decanoate	$C_{14}H_{28}O_2$		+	+
Butyl decanoate	$C_{14}H_{28}O_2$		+	
Ethyl laurate	$C_{14}H_{28}O_2$	+	+	+
Methyl 5,8-tetradecadienoate, *cis,cis-*	$C_{15}H_{26}O_2$			+
2-Methylbutyl 9-decenoate	$C_{15}H_{28}O_2$		+	
Isopentyl decenoate	$C_{15}H_{28}O_2$		+	
Isopentyl 4-decenoate	$C_{15}H_{28}O_2$	+		
Isopentyl 9-decenoate	$C_{15}H_{28}O_2$		+	
2-Methylbutyl decanoate	$C_{15}H_{30}O_2$	+	+	+
Isopentyl decanoate	$C_{15}H_{30}O_2$	+	+	+
Pentyl decanoate	$C_{15}H_{30}O_2$			+
Propyl laurate	$C_{15}H_{30}O_2$		+	+
Methyl myristate	$C_{15}H_{30}O_2$			+

Appendix 1 (contd)

Compound	Molecular formula	Identified in		
		Beer	Wine	Spirits
Phenethyl octanoate	$C_{16}H_{24}O_2$	+	+	+
Ethyl 5,8-tetradecadienoate, *cis,cis-*	$C_{16}H_{28}O_2$			+
Hexyl decenoate	$C_{16}H_{30}O_2$		+	
Ethyl 5-tetradecenoate, *cis-*	$C_{16}H_{30}O_2$			+
Hexyl decanoate	$C_{16}H_{32}O_2$	+	+	
Isopentyl undecanoate	$C_{16}H_{32}O_2$			+
Isobutyl laurate	$C_{16}H_{32}O_2$	+	+	+
Ethyl myristate	$C_{16}H_{32}O_2$	+	+	+
2-Methylbutyl laurate	$C_{17}H_{34}O_2$		+	+
Isopentyl laurate	$C_{17}H_{34}O_2$	+	+	+
Isobutyl tridecanoate	$C_{17}H_{34}O_2$			+
Isopropyl myristate	$C_{17}H_{34}O_2$			+
Ethyl pentadecanoate	$C_{17}H_{34}O_2$		+	+
Methyl palmitate	$C_{17}H_{34}O_2$			+
Phenethyl decanoate	$C_{18}H_{28}O_2$			+
Ethyl 9-hexadecenoate	$C_{18}H_{34}O_2$			+
Isopentyl tridecanoate	$C_{18}H_{36}O_2$			+
Isobutyl myristate	$C_{18}H_{36}O_2$			+
Ethyl palmitate	$C_{18}H_{36}O_2$		+	+
Methyl linoleate	$C_{19}H_{34}O_2$			+
Methyl oleate	$C_{19}H_{36}O_2$			+
2-Methylbutyl myristate	$C_{19}H_{38}O_2$		+	+
Isopentyl myristate	$C_{19}H_{38}O_2$		+	+
Propyl palmitate	$C_{19}H_{38}O_2$			+
Ethyl heptadecanoate	$C_{19}H_{38}O_2$			+
Ethyl linolenate	$C_{20}H_{34}O_2$	+		+
Ethyl linoleate	$C_{20}H_{36}O_2$	+		+
Ethyl oleate	$C_{20}H_{38}O_2$	+		+
Hexyl myristate	$C_{20}H_{40}O_2$			+
Isopentyl pentadecanoate	$C_{20}H_{40}O_2$			+
Isobutyl palmitate	$C_{20}H_{40}O_2$			+
Ethyl stearate	$C_{20}H_{40}O_2$		+	+
2-Methylbutyl palmitate	$C_{21}H_{42}O_2$		+	+
Isopentyl palmitate	$C_{21}H_{42}O_2$		+	+
Ethyl nonadecanoate	$C_{21}H_{42}O_2$			+
Isobutyl stearate	$C_{22}H_{44}O_2$			+
Ethyl eicosanoate	$C_{22}H_{44}O_2$			+
Ethyl heneicosanoate	$C_{23}H_{46}O_2$			+
Isobutyl eicosanoate	$C_{24}H_{48}O_2$			+
Ethyl docosanoate	$C_{24}H_{48}O_2$			+
Ethyl tricosanoate	$C_{25}H_{50}O_2$			+
Ethyl tetracosanoate	$C_{26}H_{52}O_2$			+
Esters of aliphatic monobasic hydroxy and oxo acids				
Methyl lactate	$C_4H_8O_3$		+	

Appendix 1 (contd)

Compound	Molecular formula	Identified in		
		Beer	Wine	Spirits
Ethyl pyruvate	$C_5H_8O_3$		+	+
Ethyl lactate	$C_5H_{10}O_3$	+	+	+
Ethyl hydracrylate	$C_5H_{10}O_3$		+	
Ethyl acetoacetate	$C_6H_{10}O_3$		+	
Propyl lactate	$C_6H_{12}O_3$		+	
Ethyl 2-hydroxybutyrate	$C_6H_{12}O_3$		+	+
Ethyl 3-hydroxybutyrate	$C_6H_{12}O_3$		+	+
Ethyl 4-hydroxybutyrate	$C_6H_{12}O_3$		+	
Ethyl levulinate	$C_7H_{12}O_3$	+	+	+
Isobutyl lactate	$C_7H_{14}O_3$		+	+
Butyl lactate	$C_7H_{14}O_3$			+
Ethyl 2-hydroxy-2-methylbutyrate	$C_7H_{14}O_3$		+	
Ethyl 2-hydroxy-3-methylbutyrate	$C_7H_{14}O_3$		+	+
Ethyl 4-hydroxyvalerate	$C_7H_{14}O_3$		+	
Isopentyl lactate	$C_8H_{16}O_3$	+	+	+
Ethyl 2-hydroxy-3-methylvalerate	$C_8H_{16}O_3$		+	+
Ethyl 2-hydroxy-4-methylvalerate	$C_8H_{16}O_3$		+	+
2,4-Hexadienyl lactate, *trans,trans-*	$C_9H_{14}O_3$		+	
3-Hexenyl lactate, *cis-*	$C_9H_{16}O_3$			+
Hexyl lactate	$C_9H_{18}O_3$		+	+
Methyl 3-hydroxyoctanoate	$C_9H_{18}O_3$			+
Ethyl 2,2-diethoxypropionate	$C_9H_{18}O_4$		+	+
Ethyl 3-hydroxyoctanoate	$C_{10}H_{20}O_3$			+
Esters of aliphatic di- and tricarboxylic acids				
Diethyl oxalate	$C_6H_{10}O_4$		+	+
Ethyl hydrogen succinate	$C_6H_{10}O_4$	+	+	+
Dimethyl malate	$C_6H_{10}O_5$		+	
Ethyl hydrogen malate	$C_6H_{10}O_5$		+	
Ethyl hydrogen tartrate	$C_6H_{10}O_6$		+	
Diethyl malonate	$C_7H_{12}O_4$		+	+
Ethyl methyl succinate	$C_7H_{12}O_4$		+	+
Propyl hydrogen succinate	$C_7H_{12}O_4$		+	
Ethyl hydrogen glutarate	$C_7H_{12}O_4$		+	
Ethyl methyl malate	$C_7H_{12}O_5$		+	
Ethyl hydrogen 2-methylmalate	$C_7H_{12}O_5$		+	
Diethyl fumarate	$C_8H_{12}O_4$		+	+
Diethyl maleate	$C_8H_{12}O_4$		+	
Ethyl dihydrogen citrate	$C_8H_{12}O_7$			+
Diethyl succinate	$C_8H_{14}O_4$	+	+	+
Isobutyl hydrogen succinate	$C_8H_{14}O_4$		+	
Butyl hydrogen succinate	$C_8H_{14}O_4$		+	
Ethyl methyl glutarate	$C_8H_{14}O_4$			+
Diethyl malate	$C_8H_{14}O_5$		+	+
Diethyl tartrate	$C_8H_{14}O_6$		+	+

Appendix 1 (contd)

Compound	Molecular formula	Identified in		
		Beer	Wine	Spirits
Ethyl propyl succinate	$C_9H_{16}O_4$		+	+
Isopentyl hydrogen succinate	$C_9H_{16}O_4$		+	
Diethyl methylsuccinate	$C_9H_{16}O_4$		+	+
Diethyl glutarate	$C_9H_{16}O_4$		+	+
Diethyl 2-methylmalate	$C_9H_{16}O_5$		+	
Ethyl hydrogen 2-isopropylmalate	$C_9H_{16}O_5$		+	
Diethyl 2-hydroxyglutarate	$C_9H_{16}O_5$		+	
Ethyl isobutyl succinate	$C_{10}H_{18}O_4$		+	+
Butyl ethyl succinate	$C_{10}H_{18}O_4$			+
Dipropyl succinate	$C_{10}H_{18}O_4$		+	
Diethyl adipate	$C_{10}H_{18}O_4$			+
Ethyl 2-methylbutyl succinate	$C_{11}H_{20}O_4$		+	
Ethyl isopentyl succinate	$C_{11}H_{20}O_4$		+	+
Ethyl pentyl succinate	$C_{11}H_{20}O_4$			+
Ethyl hydrogen azelate	$C_{11}H_{20}O_4$		+	
Ethyl hexyl succinate	$C_{12}H_{22}O_4$			+
Diethyl suberate	$C_{12}H_{22}O_4$			+
Diethyl azelate	$C_{13}H_{24}O_4$			+
Diisopentyl succinate	$C_{14}H_{26}O_4$		+	+
Tributyl 1-propene-1,2,3-tricarboxylate	$C_{18}H_{30}O_6$		+	
Amines and amides				
Ammonia	H_3N	+		
Methylamine	CH_5N	+	+	
N-Nitrosodimethylamine (IARC, 1978, 1987a)	$C_2H_6N_2O$	+	+	+
Ethylamine	C_2H_7N	+	+	
Dimethylamine	C_2H_7N	+	+	
2-Aminoethanol	C_2H_7NO	+	+	
Ethylenediamine	$C_2H_8N_2$		+	
N,N-Dimethylformamide	C_3H_7NO	+		
N-Methylacetamide	C_3H_7NO	+		
Ethyl carbamate (Urethane) (IARC, 1974, 1987a)	$C_3H_7NO_2$		+	+
Trimethylamine	C_3H_9N	+		
Isopropylamine	C_3H_9N	+	+	
Propylamine	C_3H_9N	+	+	
3-Amino-1-propanol	C_3H_9NO	+	+	
1,3-Propanediamine	$C_3H_{10}N_2$	+	+	
N-Nitrosopyrrolidine (IARC, 1978, 1987a)	$C_4H_8N_2O$	+		
N,N-Dimethylacetamide	C_4H_9NO	+		
N-Ethylacetamide	C_4H_9NO	+	+	
N-Nitrosodiethylamine (IARC, 1978, 1987a)	$C_4H_{10}N_2O$	+	+	+
Isobutylamine	$C_4H_{11}N$	+	+	
Butylamine	$C_4H_{11}N$	+	+	
sec-Butylamine	$C_4H_{11}N$	+		
1,4-Butanediamine	$C_4H_{12}N_2$	+	+	

Appendix 1 (contd)

Compound	Molecular formula	Identified in		
		Beer	Wine	Spirits
N-Nitrosoproline (IARC, 1978, 1987a)	$C_5H_8N_2O_3$	+		
Betaine	$C_5H_{11}NO_2$		+	
Isopentylamine	$C_5H_{13}N$	+	+	
Pentylamine	$C_5H_{13}N$	+	+	
1,5-Pentanediamine	$C_5H_{14}N_2$	+	+	
Choline	$C_5H_{15}NO_2$	+		
2-(Diacetylamino)ethanol	$C_6H_{11}NO_3$		+	
N-Isobutylacetamide	$C_6H_{13}NO$		+	
N-[3-(Methylthio)propyl]acetamide	$C_6H_{13}NOS$		+	
N-Nitrosodi-*n*-propylamine (IARC, 1978, 1987a)	$C_6H_{14}N_2O$		+	+
N,*N*-Dimethylbutylamine	$C_6H_{15}N$	+		
Hexylamine	$C_6H_{15}N$	+	+	
para-(Aminomethyl)phenol	C_7H_9NO	+		
N-Furfurylacetamide	$C_7H_9NO_2$	+		
N-Methyl-*N*-butylacetamide	$C_7H_{15}NO$		+	
N-(2-Methylbutyl)acetamide	$C_7H_{15}NO$	+	+	
N-Isopentylacetamide	$C_7H_{15}NO$	+	+	
Choline acetate	$C_7H_{17}NO_3$		+	
N-(3-Aminopropyl)-1,4-butanediamine	$C_7H_{19}N_3$	+	+	
Phenylacetonitrile	C_8H_7N			+
2′-Aminoacetophenone	C_8H_9NO	+		
Methyl anthranilate	$C_8H_9NO_2$		+	
Phenethylamine	$C_8H_{11}N$	+	+	
para-(2-Aminoethyl)phenol	$C_8H_{11}NO$	+	+	
Diisobutylamine	$C_8H_{19}N$	+		
N-Methylphenylethylamine	$C_9H_{13}N$	+	+	
para-[2-(Methylamino)]phenol	$C_9H_{13}NO$	+		
Tripropylamine	$C_9H_{21}N$	+		
N-Phenethylacetamide	$C_{10}H_{13}NO$	+	+	
para-[2-(Dimethylamino)ethyl]phenol	$C_{10}H_{15}NO$	+		
N,*N*′-Bis(3-aminopropyl)-1,4-butanediamine	$C_{10}H_{26}N_4$	+		
2-Amino-4-octadecene-1,3-diol	$C_{18}H_{37}NO_2$		+	
N-*Heterocyclics*				
Thiazole	C_3H_3NS	+		+
Pyrazine	$C_4H_4N_2$	+		
Uracil	$C_4H_4N_2O_2$	+	+	
Pyrrole	C_4H_5N	+		
Cytosine	$C_4H_5N_3O$	+	+	
2-Pyrrolidone	C_4H_7NO	+		
Pyrrolidine	C_4H_9N	+	+	
Hypoxanthine	$C_5H_4N_4O$	+	+	
Xanthine	$C_5H_4N_4O_2$	+	+	
Pyridine	C_5H_5N	+		+
Pyrrole-2-carboxaldehyde	C_5H_5NO	+		

Appendix 1 (contd)

Compound	Molecular formula	Identified in		
		Beer	Wine	Spirits
2-Acetylthiazole	C_5H_5NOS	+		
Adenine	$C_5H_5N_5$	+	+	
Guanine	$C_5H_5N_5O$	+		
Methylpyrazine	$C_5H_6N_2$	+		+
Thymine	$C_5H_6N_2O_2$	+	+	
1-Methylpyrrole	C_5H_7N	+		
2-Methylpyrrole	C_5H_7N	+		
5-Oxoproline	$C_5H_7NO_3$	+		
1-Methyl-2-pyrrolidone	C_5H_9NO	+		
Histamine	$C_5H_9N_3$	+	+	
Piperidine	$C_5H_{11}N$		+	
Nicotinic acid	$C_6H_5NO_2$		+	
Picoline	C_6H_7N		+	
α-Picoline	C_6H_7N			+
β-Picoline	C_6H_7N			+
γ-Picoline	C_6H_7N			+
1-Methylpyrrole-2-carboxaldehyde	C_6H_7NO			+
5-Methylpyrrole-2-carboxaldehyde	C_6H_7NO	+		
Methyl 1-pyrrolyl ketone	C_6H_7NO	+		
Methyl 2-pyrrolyl ketone	C_6H_7NO	+		
4-Methyl-4-vinylthiazole	C_6H_7NS			+
2,3-Dimethylpyrazine	$C_6H_8N_2$	+		+
2,5-Dimethylpyrazine	$C_6H_8N_2$	+		+
2,6-Dimethylpyrazine	$C_6H_8N_2$	+		+
Ethylpyrazine	$C_6H_8N_2$	+		+
5-Hydroxyethyl-4-methylthiazole	C_6H_9NOS	+		
4-Methyl-5-(β-hydroxyethyl)thiazole	C_6H_9NOS			+
Histidine	$C_6H_9N_3O_2$		+	
2-Benzothiazolol	C_7H_5NOS		+	
Benzothiazole	C_7H_5NS	+		
Methyl 2-pyridyl ketone	C_7H_7NO	+		
Methyl 3-pyridyl ketone	C_7H_7NO	+		
Methyl nicotinate	$C_7H_7NO_2$	+		
2-Methyl-6-vinylpyrazine	$C_7H_8N_2$			+
6,7-Dihydro-5*H*-cyclopentapyrazine	$C_7H_8N_2$	+		
2,5-Lutidine	C_7H_9N			+
2,6-Lutidine	C_7H_9N		+	+
3,5-Lutidine	C_7H_9N			+
2-Ethylpyridine	C_7H_9N			+
4-Ethylpyridine	C_7H_9N			+
1-Ethylpyrrole-2-carboxaldehyde	C_7H_9NO			+
Methyl 5-methyl-2-pyrrolyl ketone	C_7H_9NO	+		
Trimethylpyrazine	$C_7H_{10}N_2$	+		+
3-Ethyl-2-methylpyrazine	$C_7H_{10}N_2$	+		+
5-Ethyl-2-methylpyrazine	$C_7H_{10}N_2$	+		+

Appendix 1 (contd)

Compound	Molecular formula	Identified in		
		Beer	Wine	Spirits
6-Ethyl-2-methylpyrazine	$C_7H_{10}N_2$	+		+
5-Oxoproline ethyl ester	$C_7H_{11}NO_3$		+	
2-Furylpyrazine	$C_8H_6N_2O$	+		
Indone	C_8H_7N	+	+	
5-Methylcyclopentapyrazine	$C_8H_8N_2$	+		
Ethyl nicotinate	$C_8H_9NO_2$	+		
6,7-Dihydro-2-methyl-5*H*-cyclopentapyrazine	$C_8H_{10}N_2$	+		
6,7-Dihydro-5-methyl-5*H*-cyclopentapyrazine	$C_8H_{10}N_2$	+		
5-Ethyl-2-methylpyridine	$C_8H_{11}N$			+
2-Isopropylpyridine	$C_8H_{11}N$			+
Tetramethylpyrazine	$C_8H_{12}N_2$	+		+
3,5-Dimethyl-2-ethylpyrazine	$C_8H_{12}N_2$	+		+
2,5-Dimethyl-3-ethylpyrazine	$C_8H_{12}N_2$	+		+
5,6-Dimethyl-2-ethylpyrazine	$C_8H_{12}N_2$	+		
2,5-Diethylpyrazine	$C_8H_{12}N_2$			+
Quinoline	C_9H_7N			+
2-(2′-Furyl)methylpyrazine	$C_9H_8N_2O$	+		
1-Furfurylpyrrole	C_9H_9NO	+		
2,4-Dimethyl-3-propylpyrazine	$C_9H_{14}N_2$			+
Quinaldine	$C_{10}H_9N$			+
6-Methylquinoline	$C_{10}H_9N$			+
N-Furfurylpyrrol-2-aldehyde	$C_{10}H_9NO_2$	+		
3-Indolylacetic acid	$C_{10}H_9NO_2$		+	
5-Methoxy-2-indolylcarboxylic acid	$C_{10}H_9NO_3$		+	
2-(2′-Furyl)dimethylpyrazine	$C_{10}H_{10}N_2O$	+		
Ethylindole	$C_{10}H_{11}N$		+	
Indole-3-ethanol	$C_{10}H_{11}NO$	+	+	
3-(2-Aminoethyl)indole	$C_{10}H_{12}N_2$	+		
3-(2-Aminoethyl)indol-5-ol	$C_{10}H_{12}N_2O$	+		
1-Isopentylpyrrole-2-carboxaldehyde	$C_{10}H_{15}NO$			+
3-(3-Indolyl)propenoic acid	$C_{11}H_9NO_2$		+	
Isopentyl nicotinate	$C_{11}H_{15}NO_2$	+		
Phenethyl nicotinate	$C_{14}H_{13}NO_2$	+		
Sulphur compounds				
Thioformaldehyde	CH_2S	+		
Methanethiol	CH_4S	+		+
Carbon disulphide	CS_2		+	+
Dithioformaldehyde	$C_2H_4S_2$	+		
Ethanethiol	C_2H_6S	+	+	+
Methyl sulphide	C_2H_6S	+	+	+
Methyl disulphide	$C_2H_6S_2$	+	+	+
Dimethyl trisulphide	$C_2H_6S_3$	+	+	+
Thiazole	C_3H_3NS	+		+
S-Methyl thioacetate	C_3H_6OS	+	+	

Appendix 1 (contd)

Compound	Molecular formula	Identified in		
		Beer	Wine	Spirits
(Methylthio)acetic acid	$C_3H_6O_2S$	+		
2-Propanethione	C_3H_6S	+		
2-Propene-1-thiol	C_3H_6S	+		
Ethyl methyl sulphide	C_3H_8S	+		
Ethyl methyl disulphide	$C_3H_8S_2$	+		
3-(Methylthio)propionaldehyde	C_3H_8OS	+		
S-Ethyl thioacetate	C_4H_8OS	+	+	
3-(Methylthio)propionic acid	$C_4H_8O_2S$	+	+	
Tetrahydrothiophene	C_4H_8S		+	
3-(Methylthio)-1-propanol	$C_4H_{10}OS$	+	+	+
Diethyl sulphite	$C_4H_{10}O_3S$			+
2-Methyl-2-propanethiol	$C_4H_{10}S$	+		
2-Methyl-2-propanethiol	$C_4H_{10}S$	+		
Ethyl sulphide	$C_4H_{10}S$	+		+
Ethyl disulphide	$C_4H_{10}S_2$	+		+
2-Thiophenecarboxaldehyde	C_5H_4OS	+		+
2-Thiophenecarboxylic acid	$C_5H_4O_2S$	+		
Dihydro-2-methyl-3(2*H*)-thiophenone	C_5H_8OS	+	+	
Methyl 3-(methylthio)propionate	$C_5H_{10}O_2S$		+	
3-Methyl-2-butene-1-thiol	$C_5H_{10}S$	+		
3-(Ethylthio)-1-propanol	$C_5H_{12}OS$		+	
1-Pentanethiol	$C_5H_{12}S$	+		
Butyl methyl sulphide	$C_5H_{12}S$	+		
Ethyl propyl sulphide	$C_5H_{12}S$	+		
1-(2-Thienyl)ethanone	C_6H_6OS	+		
2-Methyl-2-thiophenecarboxaldehyde	C_6H_6OS	+		+
Allyl sulphide	$C_6H_{10}S$			+
N,*S*-Diacetyl-2-aminoethanethiol	$C_6H_{11}NO_2S$		+	
3-(Methylthio)propyl acetate	$C_6H_{12}O_2S$	+	+	+
Ethyl 3-(methylthio)propionate	$C_6H_{12}O_2S$	+	+	+
N-[3-(Methylthio)propyl]acetamide	$C_6H_{13}NOS$		+	
Butyl ethyl sulphide	$C_6H_{14}S$	+		+
Isopropyl sulphide	$C_6H_{14}S$	+		+
Isopropyl disulphide	$C_6H_{14}S_2$			+
2-Benzothiazolol	C_7H_5NOS		+	
Benzothiazole	C_7H_5NS	+		
Ethyl 2-thiophenecarboxylate	$C_7H_8O_2S$			+
S-Methyl 4-methylpentanethioate	$C_7H_{14}OS$	+		
5-Methyl hexanethioate	$C_7H_{14}OS$	+		
2-(Methylthio)benzothiazole	$C_8H_7NS_2$			+
tert-Butyl sulphide	$C_8H_{18}S$	+		
Isobutyl sulphide	$C_8H_{18}S$	+		
4-(4-Methyl-3-pentenyl)-3,6-dihydro-1,2-dithiin	$C_{10}H_{16}S_2$	+		
Isopentyl sulphide	$C_{10}H_{22}S$			+
Hydrogen sulphide	H_2S	+	+	+

Appendix 1 (contd)

Compound	Molecular formula	Identified in		
		Beer	Wine	Spirits
Terpenoids				
7,7-Dimethyl-6,8-dioxabicyclo[3.2.1]octane	$C_8H_{14}O_2$	+		
para-Cymene	$C_{10}H_{14}$		+	+
para-Isopropylbenzyl alcohol (Cuminyl alcohol)	$C_{10}H_{14}O$			+
meta-Cymenol	$C_{10}H_{14}O$			+
para-Cymenol	$C_{10}H_{14}O$			+
para-Mentha-6,8-dien-2-one (*d*-Carvone)	$C_{10}H_{14}O$	+		+
2(10)-Pinen-3-one (Pinocarvone)	$C_{10}H_{14}O$			+
1,7,7-Trimethyltricyclo[2.2.1.0^{26}]heptane (Tricyclene)	$C_{10}H_{16}$			+
7-Methyl-3-methylene-1,6-octadiene (Myrcene)	$C_{10}H_{16}$	+	+	+
para-Mentha-1(7),2-diene (β-Phellandrene)	$C_{10}H_{16}$			+
para-Mentha-1,3-diene (α-Terpinene)	$C_{10}H_{16}$			+
para-Mentha-1,4-diene (γ-Terpinene)	$C_{10}H_{16}$			+
para-Mentha-1,4(8)-diene (Terpinolene)	$C_{10}H_{16}$			+
para-Mentha-1,5-diene (α-Phellandrene)	$C_{10}H_{16}$			+
para-Mentha-1,8-diene (Limonene)	$C_{10}H_{16}$	+	+	+
3-Thujene (α-Thujene)	$C_{10}H_{16}$			+
4(10)-Thujene (Sabinene)	$C_{10}H_{16}$			+
2-Pinene (α-Pinene)	$C_{10}H_{16}$	+		+
2(10)-Pinene (β-Pinene)	$C_{10}H_{16}$			+
Camphene	$C_{10}H_{16}$			+
3-Carene	$C_{10}H_{16}$			+
3,7-Dimethyl-1,5,7-octatrien-3-ol (Ho-trienol)	$C_{10}H_{16}O$		+	+
3,7-Dimethyl-2,6-octadienal (Citral)	$C_{10}H_{16}O$	+	+	
2-Methyl-6-methylene-7-octen-2-ol (Myrcenol)	$C_{10}H_{16}O$			+
2,6,6-Trimethyl-1-cyclohexene-1-carboxaldehyde (β-Cyclocitral)	$C_{10}H_{16}O$			+
4-Isopropyl-1-cyclohexene-1-carboxaldehyde (Phellandral)	$C_{10}H_{16}O$			+
8,8-Dimethyl-2-methylene-6-oxabicyclo-[3.2.1]octane (Karahana ether)	$C_{10}H_{16}O$	+		
Hexahydro-1,1-dimethyl-4-methylene-1*H*-cyclopenta[*c*]furan (Hop ether)	$C_{10}H_{16}O$	+		
Tetrahydro-5-isopropenyl-2-methyl-2-vinylfuran	$C_{10}H_{16}O$			+
3,6-Dihydro-4-methyl-2-(2-methyl-1-propenyl)-2*H*-pyran (Nerol oxide)	$C_{10}H_{16}O$		+	+
para-Mentha-1(7),8-dien-2-ol, *trans*-	$C_{10}H_{16}O$			+
para-Menth-3-en-2-one (Carvenone)	$C_{10}H_{16}O$			+
6,8-Epoxy-*para*-menth-1-ene (Pinol)	$C_{10}H_{16}O$			+
2(10)-Pinen-3-ol, *trans*- (*trans*-Pinocarveol)	$C_{10}H_{16}O$			+
2-Pinen-10-ol (Myrtenol)	$C_{10}H_{16}O$			+
1,3,3-Trimethyl-2-norbornanone (Fenchone)	$C_{10}H_{16}O$			+
2-Bornanone (Camphor)	$C_{10}H_{16}O$			+
3,7-Dimethyl-1,6-octadien-3-ol (Linalool)	$C_{10}H_{18}O$	+	+	+

Appendix 1 (contd)

Compound	Molecular formula	Identified in		
		Beer	Wine	Spirits
Geraniol	$C_{10}H_{18}O$			
Geraniol, *cis-* (Nerol)		+	+	+
Geraniol, *trans-* (Geraniol)		+	+	+
Tetrahydro-4-methyl-2-(2-methyl-1-propenyl)-2*H*-pyran (Rose oxide)	$C_{10}H_{18}O$			
Rose oxide, *cis-*			+	+
Rose oxide, *trans-*			+	+
Terpineol	$C_{10}H_{18}O$	+		+
para-Menth-3-en-1-ol (3-Terpinen-1-ol)	$C_{10}H_{18}O$			+
para-Menth-4(8)-en-1-ol (γ-Terpineol)	$C_{10}H_{18}O$			+
para-Menth-8-en-1-ol, *trans-* (β-Terpineol)	$C_{10}H_{18}O$			+
para-Menth-6-en-2-ol, (2*S*,4*S*)-(*P*)-(*cis*-Carvotanacetol)	$C_{10}H_{18}O$			+
para-Menth-8-en-3-ol, (1*R*,3*R*,4*S*)-(*M*)-(Isopulegol)	$C_{10}H_{18}O$			+
para-Menth-1-en-4-ol (4-Terpineol)	$C_{10}H_{18}O$	+	+	+
para-Menth-1-en-8-ol (α-Terpineol)	$C_{10}H_{18}O$	+	+	+
para-Menth-1-en-9-ol	$C_{10}H_{18}O$			+
para-Menthan-2-one, *trans-* (Carvomenthone)	$C_{10}H_{18}O$			+
1,4-Epoxy-*para*-menthane (1,4-Cineole)	$C_{10}H_{18}O$			+
1,8-Epoxy-*para*-menthane (1,8-Cineole)	$C_{10}H_{18}O$	+		+
Isoborneol (*exo*-2-Bornanol)	$C_{10}H_{18}O$			+
Borneol (*endo*-2-Bornanol)	$C_{10}H_{18}O$			+
1,3,3-Trimethyl-2-norbornanol (Fenchol)	$C_{10}H_{18}O$	+		
1,3,3-Trimethyl-2-norbornanol, *endo-* (α-Fenchol)	$C_{10}H_{18}O$			+
3,7-Dimethylocta-1,5-dien-3,7-diol	$C_{10}H_{18}O_2$		+	
Tetrahydro-α,α,5-trimethyl-5-vinyl-furfuryl alcohol (Linalool oxide)	$C_{10}H_{18}O_2$			
Linalool oxide, *cis-*			+	+
Linalool oxide, *trans-*		+	+	+
Linalool oxide, crystalline			+	
3,7-Dimethyl-6-octen-1-ol (Citronellol)	$C_{10}H_{20}O$	+		+
Menthol	$C_{10}H_{20}O$			+
3-Methyl-2-(2-pentenyl)-2-cyclopenten-1-one, *cis-* (Jasmone)	$C_{11}H_{16}O$	+		
2,2,7,7-Tetramethyl-1,6-dioxaspiro[4,4]-nona-3,8-diene	$C_{11}H_{16}O_2$	+		
2,2,7,7-Tetramethyl-1,6-dioxaspiro[4,4]-non-3-ene	$C_{11}H_{18}O_2$	+		
Linalyl acetate	$C_{12}H_{20}O_2$			+
Geranyl acetate	$C_{12}H_{20}O_2$			+
Bornyl acetate	$C_{12}H_{20}O_2$			+
Ethyl geranyl ether	$C_{12}H_{22}O$			+

Appendix 1 (contd)

Compound	Molecular formula	Identified in		
		Beer	Wine	Spirits
1-(6,6-Dimethyl-2-methylene-3-cyclohexen-yl)-1-buten-3-one, *trans-*	$C_{13}H_{18}O$			+
1-(2,6,6-Trimethyl-1,3-cyclohexadien-1-yl)-2-buten-1-one (Damascenone)	$C_{13}H_{18}O$	+	+	+
Damascenone, *cis-*				+
Damascenone, *trans-*				+
Ionone	$C_{13}H_{20}O$			+
4-(2,6,6-Trimethyl-2-cyclohexen-1-yl)-3-buten-2-one, *trans-* (α-Ionone)	$C_{13}H_{20}O$	+	+	+
4-(2,6,6-Trimethyl-1-cyclohexen-1-yl)-3-buten-2-one (β-Ionone)	$C_{13}H_{20}O$	+	+	+
3,5,6,8a-Tetrahydro-2,5,5,8a-tetramethyl-2*H*-1-benzopyran, *trans-* (*trans*-Edulan; Edulan I)	$C_{13}H_{20}O$			+
3,4,4a,5,6,8a-Hexahydro-2,5,5,8-tetramethyl-4,4a-epoxy-2*H*-1-benzopyran (4,4a-Epoxyedulan)	$C_{13}H_{20}O$			+
Geranylacetone	$C_{13}H_{22}O$			+
5-(1-Hydroxy-2,6,6-trimethyl-4-oxo-2-cyclohexen-1-yl)-3-methyl-2,4-pentadienoic acid (Abscisic acid)	$C_{15}H_{20}O_4$		+	
3,7,11-Trimethyl-1,3,6,10-dodecatetraene (Farnesene; α-Farnesene)	$C_{15}H_{24}$	+		+
7,11-Dimethyl-3-methylene-1,8,10-dodecatriene (β-Farnesene)	$C_{15}H_{24}$			+
2,6,6,9-Tetramethyl-1,4,8-cycloundecatriene *trans,trans,trans-* (Humulene; α-Caryophyllene)	$C_{15}H_{24}$	+		+
4,11,11-Trimethyl-8-methylenebicyclo[7.2.0]-undec-4-ene,	$C_{15}H_{24}$			
,*cis*-(1*R*,9*S*)-(*M*)- (Isocaryophyllene)		+		
,*trans*-(1*R*,9*S*)-(*M*)- (Caryophyllene; β-Caryophyllene)		+		+
1,3-Dimethyl-8-isopropyltricyclo-[4.4.0.0^{2,7}]dec-3-ene (α-Copaene)	$C_{15}H_{24}$			+
1,2,3,5,6,8a-Hexahydro-4,7-dimethyl-1-iso-propylnaphthalene (δ-Cadinene)	$C_{15}H_{24}$			+
1,2,4a,5,6,8a-Hexahydro-4,7-dimethyl-1-isopropyl-naphthalene, (1*S*)-(1,4aα,8aα)-(α-Muurolene)	$C_{15}H_{24}$			+
1,2,3,4,4a,5,6,8a-Octahydro-7-methyl-4-methylene-1-isopropylnaphthalene,	$C_{15}H_{24}$			
,(1α,4aα,8aα)- (γ-Muurolene),				+
,(1α,4aα,8aα)- (γ-Cadinene)				+
3a,3b,4,5,6,7-Hexahydro-4-isopropyl-3,7-dimethyl-1*H*-cyclopenta(1,3)cyclopropa(1,2)benzene, (3α,3bα,4α,7β)-(*M*)- (α-Cubebene)	$C_{15}H_{24}$			+
3,3,7-Trimethyl-11-methylene-4,7-cycloundecadien-1-ol, *trans,trans*-(*R*)-(*P*)- (Humulenol I)	$C_{15}H_{24}O$	+		

Appendix 1 (contd)

Compound	Molecular formula	Identified in		
		Beer	Wine	Spirits
6,6,9-Trimethyl-2-methylene-4,8-cycloundecadien-1-ol, *trans,trans*-(*R*)-(*P*)- (Humulenol; Humulenol II)	$C_{15}H_{24}O$	+		
2,6,6,9-Tetramethyl-4,8-cycloundecadien-1-one, *trans,trans*-(*P*)- (Humuladienone)	$C_{15}H_{24}O$	+		
4,11,11-Trimethyl-8-methylenebicyclo-[7.2.0]undec-3-en-5-ol (Caryophyllenol)	$C_{15}H_{24}O$	+		
1,5,5,8-Tetramethyl-12-oxabicyclo[9.1.0]-dodeca-3,7-diene, *trans,trans*-(1*R*,11*R*)-(*M*)- (Humulene epoxide II)	$C_{15}H_{24}O$	+		
1,5,9,9-Tetramethyl-12-oxabicyclo[9.1.0]-dodeca-4,7-diene, *trans,trans*-(1*R*,11*R*)-(*M*)- (Humulene epoxide; Humulene epoxide I)	$C_{15}H_{24}O$	+		
1,3-Dimethyl-3,4-epoxy-8-isopropyltricyclo-[4.4.0.0^{2,7}]decane (α-Copaene epoxide)	$C_{15}H_{24}O$			+
4,12,12-Trimethyl-9-methylene-5-oxatricy-clo[8.2.0.0^{4,6}]dodecane, (1*R*,4*R*,6*R*,10*S*)- (Caryophyllene epoxide)	$C_{15}H_{24}O$	+		
1-(2,6,6-Trimethyl-1,3-cyclohexadien-1-yl)-3-ethoxybutan-1-one	$C_{15}H_{24}O_2$			+
3,7,11-Trimethyl-1,6,10-dodecatrien-3-ol (Nerolidol)	$C_{15}H_{26}O$	+		+
3,7,11-Trimethyl-2,6,10-dodecatrien-1-ol (Farnesol)	$C_{15}H_{26}O$		+	
Farnesol, *cis-*			+	
Farnesol, *trans-*			+	
1,5,5,8-Tetramethyl-3,7-cycloundecadien-1-ol, *trans,trans*-(*M*)- (Humulol)	$C_{15}H_{26}O$	+		
4,4,8-Trimethyltricyclo[6.3.1.0^{2,5}]dodecan-1-ol- (Caryolan-1-ol)	$C_{15}H_{26}O$	+		
1,3,4,5,6,8a-Hexahydro-4,7-dimethyl-1-iso-propyl-4a(2*H*)-naphthalenol, (1*S*)-(1α,4β,4aα,8aα)- (Epicubenol)	$C_{15}H_{26}O$	+		
Cadinol	$C_{15}H_{26}O$	+		
1,2,3,4,4a,7,8,8a-Octahydro-1,6-dimethyl-4-isopropyl-1-naphthalenol	$C_{15}H_{26}O$			
, (1*R*)-(1α,4β,4aα,8aα)- (α-Cadinol)				+
, (1*S*)-(1α,4α,4aα,8aβ)- (δ-Cadinol)		+		+
, (1*S*)-(1α,4α,4aα,8aβ)- (τ-Cadinol)		+		
Decahydro-4a-methyl-8-methylene-2-isopro-pyl-1-naphthalenol, (1*S*)-(1α,2β,4aβ,8aα)- (Junenol)	$C_{15}H_{26}O$	+		
Phenols and phenyl ethers				
Phenol	C_6H_6O	+	+	+

Appendix 1 (contd)

Compound	Molecular formula	Identified in		
		Beer	Wine	Spirits
Pyrocatechol	$C_6H_6O_2$	+	+	
Resorcinol (IARC, 1977b, 1987a)	$C_6H_6O_2$	+	+	
Pyrogallol	$C_6H_6O_3$	+	+	
Phloroglucinol	$C_6H_6O_3$	+	+	
Cresol	C_7H_8O	+		
ortho-Cresol	C_7H_8O	+	+	+
meta-Cresol	C_7H_8O	+	+	+
para-Cresol	C_7H_8O	+	+	+
5-Methylresorcinol	$C_7H_8O_2$	+	+	
ortho-Methoxyphenol	$C_7H_8O_2$	+	+	+
para-Vinylphenol	C_8H_8O	+	+	+
2,5-Xylenol	$C_8H_{10}O$			+
2,6-Xylenol	$C_8H_{10}O$			+
3,5-Xylenol	$C_8H_{10}O$			+
Ethylphenol	$C_8H_{10}O$			+
ortho-Ethylphenol	$C_8H_{10}O$		+	+
meta-Ethylphenol	$C_8H_{10}O$			+
para-Ethylphenol	$C_8H_{10}O$	+	+	+
ortho-Dimethoxybenzene	$C_8H_{10}O_2$	+		+
meta-Dimethoxybenzene	$C_8H_{10}O_2$			+
2-Methoxy-4-methylphenol	$C_8H_{10}O_2$	+	+	+
2-Methoxy-6-methylphenol	$C_8H_{10}O_2$			+
4-Ethylpyrocatechol	$C_8H_{10}O_2$		+	
2,6-Dimethoxyphenol	$C_8H_{10}O_3$	+	+	+
Vanillyl alcohol	$C_8H_{10}O_3$	+		
para-Allylphenol	$C_9H_{10}O$		+	
para-Propenylphenol	$C_9H_{10}O$		+	
Vinyl-2-methoxyphenol	$C_9H_{10}O_2$	+		
4-Vinyl-2-methoxyphenol	$C_9H_{10}O_2$	+	+	+
2,3,5-Trimethylphenol	$C_9H_{12}O$			+
2,4,5-Trimethylphenol	$C_9H_{12}O$			+
Mesitol	$C_9H_{12}O$			+
ortho-Isopropylphenol	$C_9H_{12}O$			+
para-Propylphenol	$C_9H_{12}O$	+		
Ethyl-2-methoxyphenol	$C_9H_{12}O_2$			+
4-Ethyl-2-methoxyphenol	$C_9H_{12}O_2$	+	+	+
2,6-Dimethoxy-4-methylphenol	$C_9H_{12}O_3$	+		
Trimethoxyphenol	$C_9H_{12}O_4$		+	
1-Naphthol	$C_{10}H_8O$		+	
1-Allyl-methoxybenzene	$C_{10}H_{12}O$		+	
2-Methoxy-4-propenylphenol	$C_{10}H_{12}O_2$	+	+	+
4-Allyl-2-methoxyphenol (Eugenol) (IARC, 1985, 1987a)	$C_{10}H_{12}O_2$	+	+	+

Appendix 1 (contd)

Compound	Molecular formula	Identified in		
		Beer	Wine	Spirits
3-(4-Hydroxy-3-methoxyphenyl)-2-propen-1-ol	$C_{10}H_{12}O_3$			+
4-Vinyl-2,6-dimethoxyphenol	$C_{10}H_{12}O_3$	+		+
Tetramethylphenol	$C_{10}H_{14}O$			+
Carvacrol	$C_{10}H_{14}O$	+		+
Thymol	$C_{10}H_{14}O$			+
Propyl-2-methoxyphenol	$C_{10}H_{14}O_2$			+
2-Methoxy-4-propylphenol	$C_{10}H_{14}O_2$			+
1-Ethoxy-1-(4-methoxyphenyl)ethane	$C_{10}H_{14}O_2$			+
Ethyl 4-methoxybenzyl ether	$C_{10}H_{14}O_2$			+
4-Ethyl-2,6-dimethoxyphenol	$C_{10}H_{14}O_3$	+	+	+
Ethyl vanillyl ether	$C_{10}H_{14}O_3$			+
4-Allyl-1,2-dimethoxybenzene	$C_{11}H_{14}O_2$		+	
Methyl-4-allyl-2-methoxyphenol	$C_{11}H_{14}O_2$			+
4-Propenyl-2,6-dimethoxyphenol	$C_{11}H_{14}O_3$	+		
4-Allyl-2,6-dimethoxyphenol	$C_{11}H_{14}O_3$	+		
Isopropyl-2,6-dimethoxyphenol	$C_{11}H_{16}O_3$		+	
2,6-Di-*tert*-butyl-4-methylphenol	$C_{15}H_{24}O$		+	
Aromatic alcohols				
Benzyl alcohol	C_7H_8O	+	+	+
1-Phenylethyl alcohol	$C_8H_{10}O$		+	+
Phenethyl alcohol	$C_8H_{10}O$	+	+	+
Tyrosol	$C_8H_{10}O_2$	+	+	
Cinnamyl alcohol	$C_9H_{10}O$			+
3-Phenylpropanol	$C_9H_{12}O$		+	
Methoxytyrosol	$C_9H_{12}O_3$		+	
Aromatic aldehydes and ketones				
Benzaldehyde	C_7H_6O	+	+	+
Salicylaldehyde	$C_7H_6O_2$	+	+	+
para-Hydroxybenzaldehyde	$C_7H_6O_2$	+	+	+
Protocatechualdehyde	$C_7H_6O_3$	+	+	+
Piperonal	$C_8H_6O_3$	+	+	
ortho-Tolualdehyde	C_8H_8O			+
meta-Tolualdehyde	C_8H_8O			+
para-Tolualdehyde	C_8H_8O	+		
Phenylacetaldehyde	C_8H_8O	+	+	+
Acetophenone	C_8H_8O		+	+
Hydroxymethylbenzaldehyde	$C_8H_8O_2$			+
para-Anisaldehyde	$C_8H_8O_2$	+		+
2′-Hydroxyacetophenone	$C_8H_8O_2$		+	
4′-Hydroxyacetophenone	$C_8H_8O_2$	+	+	
Vanillin	$C_8H_8O_3$	+	+	+
Cinnamaldehyde	C_9H_8O	+	+	+
1-Indanone	C_9H_8O	+		+
2,4-Dimethylbenzaldehyde	$C_9H_{10}O$			+

Appendix 1 (contd)

Compound	Molecular formula	Identified in		
		Beer	Wine	Spirits
Ethylbenzaldehyde	$C_9H_{10}O$		+	
4-Ethylbenzaldehyde	$C_9H_{10}O$		+	
Hydrocinnamaldehyde	$C_9H_{10}O$	+		
3-Phenyl-2-propanone	$C_9H_{10}O$			+
4′-Methylacetophenone	$C_9H_{10}O$			+
2′-Hydroxy-5′-methylacetophenone	$C_9H_{10}O_2$			+
2-Ethoxybenzaldehyde	$C_9H_{10}O_2$			+
4′-Hydroxy-3′-methoxyacetophenone	$C_9H_{10}O_3$	+	+	+
4-Hydroxy-3,5-dimethoxybenzaldehyde	$C_9H_{10}O_4$	+	+	+
4-Hydroxy-3-methoxycinnamaldehyde	$C_{10}H_{10}O_3$			+
Ethylacetophenone	$C_{10}H_{12}O$		+	
4′-Ethylacetophenone	$C_{10}H_{12}O$		+	
para-Isopropylbenzaldehyde	$C_{10}H_{12}O$			+
3-Hydroxy-4-phenyl-2-butanone	$C_{10}H_{12}O_2$		+	
4-Acetonyl-2-methoxyphenol	$C_{10}H_{12}O_3$	+		
4′-Hydroxy-3′-methoxypropiophenone	$C_{10}H_{12}O_3$			+
4′-Hydroxy-3′,5′-dimethoxyacetophenone	$C_{10}H_{12}O_4$	+	+	+
4-Hydroxy-3,5-dimethoxycinnamaldehyde	$C_{11}H_{12}O_4$			+
4-Acetonyl-2,6-dimethoxyphenol	$C_{11}H_{14}O_4$	+		
4′-Hydroxy-3′,5′-dimethoxypropiophenone	$C_{11}H_{14}O_4$			+
2′-Methyl-5′-isopropylacetophenone	$C_{12}H_{16}O$			+
1-(2,3,6-Trimethylphenyl)-2-buten-1-one	$C_{13}H_{16}O$			
, *cis-*				+
, *trans-*				+
4-(2,3,6-Trimethylphenyl)-3-buten-2-one	$C_{13}H_{16}O$			+
Aromatic and other carboxylic acids				
Benzoic acid	$C_7H_6O_2$	+	+	+
Salicylic acid	$C_7H_6O_2$	+	+	+
para-Hydroxybenzoic acid	$C_7H_6O_3$	+	+	+
ortho-Pyrocatechuic acid	$C_7H_6O_4$	+	+	
α-Resorcylic acid	$C_7H_6O_4$	+	+	
β-Resorcylic acid	$C_7H_6O_4$	+	+	
γ-Resorcylic acid	$C_7H_6O_4$	+	+	
Gentisic acid	$C_7H_6O_4$	+	+	+
Protocatechuic acid	$C_7H_6O_4$	+	+	+
Gallic acid	$C_7H_6O_5$	+	+	+
2,4,6-Trihydroxybenzoic acid	$C_7H_6O_5$		+	
3,4,5-Trihydroxy-1-cyclohexene-1-carboxylic acid	$C_7H_{10}O_5$	+	+	
1,3,4,5-Tetrahydroxycyclohexanecarboxylic acid	$C_7H_{12}O_6$	+	+	+
Phenylglyoxylic acid	$C_8H_6O_3$	+		
Phthalic acid	$C_8H_6O_4$	+	+	+
para-Toluic acid	$C_8H_8O_2$		+	
Phenylacetic acid	$C_8H_8O_2$	+	+	+
para-Hydroxyphenylacetic acid	$C_8H_8O_3$	+	+	

Appendix 1 (contd)

Compound	Molecular formula	Identified in		
		Beer	Wine	Spirits
Vanillic acid	$C_8H_8O_4$	+	+	+
Cinnamic acid	$C_9H_8O_3$	+	+	+
Cinnamic acid, *cis-*		+		
Cinnamic acid, *trans-*		+		
ortho-Hydroxycinnamic acid	$C_9H_8O_3$	+	+	
meta-Hydroxycinnamic acid	$C_9H_8O_3$	+	+	
para-Hydroxycinnamic acid	$C_9H_8O_3$	+	+	+
para-Hydroxycinnamic acid, *cis-*		+	+	
para-Hydroxycinnamic acid, *trans-*		+	+	
Phenylpyruvic acid	$C_9H_8O_3$	+	+	
3,4-Dihydroxycinnamic acid	$C_9H_8O_4$	+	+	+
3,4-Dihydroxycinnamic acid, *cis-*			+	
3,4-Dihydroxycinnamic acid, *trans-*			+	
para-Hydroxyphenylpyruvic acid	$C_9H_8O_4$		+	
Phenylpropionic acid	$C_9H_{10}O_2$	+	+	+
Hydratropic acid	$C_9H_{10}O_2$		+	
Hydrocinnamic acid	$C_9H_{10}O_2$	+	+	+
para-Hydroxyphenylpropionic acid	$C_9H_{10}O_3$	+	+	
Phenyllactic acid	$C_9H_{10}O_3$	+		
3-Phenyllactic acid	$C_9H_{10}O_3$		+	
Veratric acid	$C_9H_{10}O_4$	+	+	
4-Hydroxy-3-methoxyphenylacetic acid	$C_9H_{10}O_4$		+	
3,4-Dihydroxyhydrocinnamic acid	$C_9H_{10}O_4$		+	
4-Hydroxy-3,5-dimethoxybenzoic acid	$C_9H_{10}O_5$	+	+	+
4-Hydroxy-3-methoxycinnamic acid	$C_{10}H_{10}O_4$	+	+	+
4-Hydroxy-3-methoxycinnamic acid, *cis-*		+		
4-Hydroxy-3-methoxycinnamic acid, *trans*		+		
para-Hydroxyphenylbutyric acid	$C_{10}H_{12}O_3$		+	
4-Hydroxy-3,5-dimethoxycinnamic acid	$C_{10}H_{12}O_5$	+	+	
Tartaric acid mono(4-hydroxycinnamate)	$C_{13}H_{12}O_8$		+	
, *cis-*			+	
, *trans-*			+	
Tartaric acid mono(3,4-dihydroxycinnamate)	$C_{13}H_{12}O_9$		+	
, *trans-*			+	
Tartaric acid mono(4-hydroxy-3-methoxy-cinnamate)	$C_{14}H_{14}O_9$		+	
1,3,4,5-Tetrahydroxycyclohexanecarboxylic acid mono[3-(*para*-hydroxycinnamate)]	$C_{16}H_{18}O_8$		+	
Chlorogenic acid	$C_{16}H_{18}O_9$	+	+	+
Isochlorogenic acid	$C_{16}H_{18}O_9$	+	+	
Neochlorogenic acid	$C_{16}H_{18}O_9$	+	+	
Esters of aromatic acids				
Methyl benzoate	$C_8H_8O_2$			+
Methyl salicylate	$C_8H_8O_3$			+

Appendix 1 (contd)

Compound	Molecular formula	Identified in		
		Beer	Wine	Spirits
Methyl anthranilate	$C_8H_9NO_2$		+	
Ethyl benzoate	$C_9H_{10}O_2$	+	+	+
Methyl phenylacetate	$C_9H_{10}O_2$			+
Ethyl salicylate	$C_9H_{10}O_3$		+	+
Ethyl *para*-hydroxybenzoate	$C_9H_{10}O_3$		+	
Dimethyl phthalate	$C_{10}H_{10}O_4$		+	+
Ethyl hydrogen phthalate	$C_{10}H_{10}O_4$		+	
Ethyl phenylacetate	$C_{10}H_{12}O_2$	+	+	+
Ethyl vanillate	$C_{10}H_{12}O_4$		+	+
Ethyl cinnamate	$C_{11}H_{12}O_2$	+	+	+
Isobutyl benzoate	$C_{11}H_{14}O_2$	+	+	
Ethyl 2-phenylpropionate	$C_{11}H_{14}O_2$			+
Ethyl hydrocinnamate	$C_{11}H_{14}O_2$			+
Ethyl 3-phenyllactate	$C_{11}H_{14}O_3$		+	
Ethyl 4-hydroxy-3,5-dimethoxybenzoate	$C_{11}H_{14}O_5$		+	+
Ethyl 4-phenyl-3-butenoate	$C_{12}H_{14}O_2$		+	
Diethyl phthalate	$C_{12}H_{14}O_2$		+	+
Isopentyl benzoate	$C_{12}H_{16}O_2$	+		
Pentyl benzoate	$C_{12}H_{16}O_2$	+		
Isopentyl salicylate	$C_{12}H_{16}O_3$			+
Diisobutyl phthalate	$C_{16}H_{22}O_4$		+	
Dibutyl phthalate	$C_{16}H_{22}O_4$		+	+
Lactones				
Dihydro-2(3*H*)-furanone (γ-Butyrolactone) (IARC, 1976b, 1987a)	$C_4H_6O_2$	+	+	+
Tetrahydro-5-oxo-2-furoic acid	$C_5H_6O_4$		+	
Dihydro-3-methyl-2(3*H*)-furanone	$C_5H_8O_2$		+	
Dihydro-5-methyl-2(3*H*)-furanone	$C_5H_8O_2$	+	+	
Tetrahydro-2*H*-pyran-2-one	$C_5H_8O_2$	+		
5,5-Dimethyl-2(5*H*)-furanone	$C_6H_8O_2$	+		
4-Acetyldihydro-2(3*H*)-furanone	$C_6H_8O_3$		+	
4,5-Dimethyl-2,3-tetrahydrofurandione	$C_6H_8O_3$		+	+
6-Methyldihydro-2,5(3*H*)-pyrandione	$C_6H_8O_3$		+	
Dihydro-5,5-dimethyl-2(3*H*)-furanone	$C_6H_{10}O_2$	+		
Tetrahydro-5-methyl-2*H*-pyran-2-one	$C_6H_{10}O_2$	+		
5-Ethyldihydro-2(3*H*)-furanone	$C_6H_{10}O_2$	+	+	+
Dihydro-3-hydroxy-4,4-dimethyl-2(3*H*)-furanone	$C_6H_{10}O_3$		+	
Dihydro-5-ethoxy-2(3*H*)-furanone	$C_6H_{10}O_3$		+	
Dihydro-5-(1-hydroxyethyl)-2(3*H*)-furanone	$C_6H_{10}O_3$		+	
Dihydro-5-methyl-5-vinyl-2(3*H*)-furanone	$C_7H_{10}O_2$		+	
5-Carbethoxydihydro-2(3*H*)-furanone	$C_7H_{10}O_4$		+	
Dihydro-5-propyl-2(3*H*)-furanone	$C_7H_{12}O_2$	+		
Phthalide	$C_8H_6O_2$		+	
5-Butyldihydro-2(3*H*)-furanone	$C_8H_{14}O_2$	+		+

Appendix 1 (contd)

Compound	Molecular formula	Identified in		
		Beer	Wine	Spirits
Tetrahydro-6-propyl-2*H*-pyran-2-one	$C_8H_{14}O_2$			+
Coumarin (IARC, 1976b, 1987a)	$C_9H_6O_2$		+	+
7-Hydroxycoumarin	$C_9H_6O_3$	+	+	
7,8-Dihydroxycoumarin	$C_9H_6O_4$	+	+	
5-Butyl-4-methyldihydro-2(3*H*)-furanone	$C_9H_{16}O_2$		+	+
, *cis*-			+	+
, *trans*-			+	+
Hydroxynonanoic acid lactone	$C_9H_{16}O_2$	+		
Dihydro-5-pentyl-2(3*H*)-furanone	$C_9H_{16}O_2$	+	+	+
6-Butyltetrahydro-2*H*-pyran-2-one	$C_9H_{16}O_2$			+
6-Methylcoumarin	$C_{10}H_8O_2$			+
7-Hydroxy-6-methoxycoumarin	$C_{10}H_8O_4$	+	+	+
Dihydro-4-methyl-5-pentyl-2(3*H*)-furanone	$C_{10}H_{18}O_2$			+
5-Hexyldihydro-2(3*H*)-furanone	$C_{10}H_{18}O_2$	+	+	+
Tetrahydro-6-pentyl-2*H*-pyran-2-one	$C_{10}H_{18}O_2$		+	+
Tetrahydro-4,4,7a-trimethyl-2(4*H*)-benzofuranone	$C_{11}H_{16}O_2$	+		
5-Heptyldihydro-2(3*H*)-furanone	$C_{11}H_{20}O_2$			+
Dihydro-5-octyl-2(3*H*)-furanone	$C_{12}H_{22}O_2$	+		+
6-Heptyltetrahydro-2*H*-pyran-2-one	$C_{12}H_{22}O_2$			+
2,3,7,8-Tetrahydroxy[1]benzopyrano[5,4,3-*cde*]-[1]-benzopyran-5,10-dione (Ellagic acid)	$C_{14}H_6O_8$	+	+	+
O-*Heterocyclics* (see also lactones and terpenoids)				
Dihydrofuran	C_4H_6O			+
2-Furaldehyde	$C_5H_4O_2$	+	+	+
2-Furoic acid	$C_5H_4O_3$	+	+	+
3-Furoic acid	$C_5H_4O_3$			+
2-Methylfuran	C_5H_6O			+
Furfuryl alcohol	$C_5H_6O_2$	+	+	+
Dihydro-2-methyl-3(2*H*)-furanone	$C_5H_8O_2$	+		+
2-Methyltetrahydrofuran	$C_5H_{10}O$			+
Furan-3,4-dicarboxylic acid	$C_6H_4O_5$		+	
3-Methyl-2-furaldehyde	$C_6H_6O_2$			+
5-Methyl-2-furaldehyde	$C_6H_6O_2$	+	+	+
Furyl methyl ketone	$C_6H_6O_2$	+		+
2-Furyl methyl ketone	$C_6H_6O_2$	+		+
3-Furyl methyl ketone	$C_6H_6O_2$			+
Methyl 2-furoate	$C_6H_6O_3$			+
Hydroxymethyl-2-furaldehyde	$C_6H_6O_3$	+	+	+
5-Hydroxymethyl-2-furaldehyde	$C_6H_6O_3$	+		
2-Acetyl-3-hydroxyfuran	$C_6H_6O_3$	+		
3-Hydroxy-2-methyl-4*H*-pyran-4-one	$C_6H_6O_3$	+		
5-Hydroxy-2-(hydroxymethyl)-4*H*-pyran-4-one	$C_6H_6O_4$	+		
3,5-Dihydroxy-2-methyl-4*H*-pyran-4-one	$C_6H_6O_4$	+		
5-Methylfurfuryl alcohol	$C_6H_8O_2$	+		

Appendix 1 (contd)

Compound	Molecular formula	Identified in		
		Beer	Wine	Spirits
5-Hydroxymethylfurfuryl alcohol	$C_6H_8O_3$	+		
4-Hydroxy-2,5-dimethyl-3(2*H*)-furanone	$C_6H_8O_3$	+		
2,5-Di(hydroxymethyl)furan	$C_6H_8O_3$	+		
3,5-Dihydroxy-2-methyl-5,6-dihydro-4*H*-pyran-4-one	$C_6H_8O_4$	+		
2,5-Dimethoxytetrahydrofuran	$C_6H_{12}O_3$			+
5-Methyl-2-acetylfuran	$C_7H_8O_2$	+		+
1-(2-Furyl)-1-propanone	$C_7H_8O_2$	+		+
Ethyl furoate	$C_7H_8O_3$		+	
Ethyl 2-furoate	$C_7H_8O_3$	+	+	+
Ethyl furfuryl ether	$C_7H_{10}O_2$		+	+
Propyl tetrahydrofuryl ether	$C_7H_{14}O_2$		+	
1-(2-Furyl)-2-buten-1-one	$C_8H_8O_2$			+
3-Acetyl-4-hydroxy-6-methyl-2*H*-pyran-2-one	$C_8H_8O_4$			+
Propyl furoate	$C_8H_{10}O_3$		+	
2-Acetyl-4,5-dimethylfuran	$C_8H_{10}O_2$			+
2-Acetyl-5-ethylfuran	$C_8H_{10}O_2$			+
1-(2-Furyl)-1-penten-3-one	$C_9H_{10}O_2$			+
Ethyl 3-(2-furyl)acrylate	$C_9H_{10}O_3$			+
Isobutyl 2-furoate	$C_9H_{12}O_3$			+
Butylfuryl alcohol	$C_9H_{14}O_2$		+	
Isopentyl 2-furoate	$C_{10}H_{14}O_3$			+
Tetrahydro-2,6,6-trimethyl-2-vinyl-4-hydroxypyran	$C_{10}H_{18}O_2$		+	
Tetrahydro-2,6,6-trimethyl-2-vinyl-4-acetoxypyran	$C_{12}H_{20}O_3$			
Hydrocarbons (see also terpenoids)				
Methane	CH_4	+		
Propene	C_3H_6	+		
Propane	C_3H_8	+		
2-Methylpropene	C_4H_8	+		
Isobutane	C_4H_{10}			+
Isoprene	C_5H_8	+		
2-Methyl-2-butene	C_5H_{10}	+		
Methylcyclobutane	C_5H_{10}		+	
Pentane	C_5H_{12}		+	+
Benzene (IARC, 1982a, 1987a)	C_6H_6		+	+
Methylcyclopentane	C_6H_{12}		+	
Cyclohexane	C_6H_{12}	+	+	
2,2-Dimethylbutane	C_6H_{14}		+	
2,3-Dimethylbutane	C_6H_{14}		+	
2-Methylpentane	C_6H_{14}			+
3-Methylpentane	C_6H_{14}		+	
Hexane	C_6H_{14}		+	+
Toluene	C_7H_8	+		+

Appendix 1 (contd)

Compound	Molecular formula	Identified in		
		Beer	Wine	Spirits
3,4-Dimethyl-2-pentene	C_7H_{14}	+		
Methylcyclohexane	C_7H_{14}		+	+
2,3-Dimethylpentane	C_7H_{16}			+
2,4-Dimethylpentane	C_7H_{16}		+	
2-Methylhexane	C_7H_{16}			+
Heptane	C_7H_{16}		+	+
Styrene (IARC, 1979a, 1987a)	C_8H_8	+	+	+
ortho-Xylene	C_8H_{10}	+		
meta-Xylene	C_8H_{10}		+	
Ethylbenzene	C_8H_{10}	+		
2,2-Dimethylhexane	C_8H_{18}	+		
Indene	C_9H_8		+	
Methylethylbenzene	C_9H_{12}	+		
Isopropyl benzene	C_9H_{12}		+	
Propylbenzene	C_9H_{12}		+	
Naphthalene	$C_{10}H_8$	+	+	+
α-Dimethylstyrene	$C_{10}H_{12}$			+
Isobutylbenzene	$C_{10}H_{14}$	+		
Decane	$C_{10}H_{22}$		+	
Methylnaphthalene	$C_{11}H_{10}$			+
1,3-Dimethylnaphthalene	$C_{12}H_{12}$			+
2,6-Dimethylnaphthalene	$C_{12}H_{12}$			+
Dodecane	$C_{12}H_{26}$		+	
Trimethyldihydronapthalene	$C_{13}H_{16}$		+	
1,1,6-Trimethyl-1,2-dihydronaphthalene	$C_{13}H_{16}$		+	+
1-(2,3,6-Trimethylphenyl)-1,3-butadiene	$C_{13}H_{16}$	+		+
1,1,6-Trimethyltetrahydronaphthalene	$C_{13}H_{18}$		+	+
Anthracene (IARC, 1983c, 1987a)	$C_{14}H_{10}$			+
Phenanthrene (IARC, 1983c, 1987a)	$C_{14}H_{10}$			+
Tetradecane	$C_{14}H_{30}$		+	
Pyrene (IARC, 1983c, 1987a)	$C_{15}H_{10}$			+
Fluoranthene (IARC, 1983c, 1987a)	$C_{16}H_{10}$			+
Hexadecane	$C_{16}H_{34}$		+	
Benzo[*a*]fluorene (IARC, 1983c, 1987a)	$C_{17}H_{12}$			+
Heptadecane	$C_{17}H_{36}$		+	
Benz[*a*]anthracene (IARC, 1983c, 1987a)	$C_{18}H_{12}$			+
Chrysene (IARC, 1983c, 1987a)	$C_{18}H_{12}$			+
Octadecane	$C_{18}H_{38}$		+	
Benzo[*a*]pyrene (IARC, 1983c, 1987a)	$C_{20}H_{12}$			+
Benzo[*e*]pyrene (IARC, 1983c, 1987a)	$C_{20}H_{12}$			+
Benzo[*b*]fluoranthene (IARC, 1983c, 1987a)	$C_{20}H_{12}$			+
Miscellaneous compounds				
Chloroform (IARC, 1979b, 1987a)	$CHCl_3$		+	
Bromoform	$CHBr_3$			+

Appendix 1 (contd)

Compound	Molecular formula	Identified in		
		Beer	Wine	Spirits
Trichloroethylene (IARC, 1979b, 1987a)	C_2HCl_3		+	
1,1,2,3-Tetrachloro-3,3-difluoropropane	$C_3H_2Cl_4F_2$		+	
Ethyl vinyl ether	C_4H_8O			+
Diethyl ether (IARC, 1976c, 1987a)	$C_4H_{10}O$	+	+	+
Diethyl carbonate	$C_5H_{10}O_3$		+	+
Ethyl isopropyl ether	$C_5H_{12}O$		+	
Trichlorotrifluorobenzene	$C_6Cl_3F_3$		+	
2,4,5,6-Tetrachloro-1,3-difluorobenzene	$C_6Cl_4F_2$		+	
Dichlorobenzene (IARC, 1982a, 1987a)	$C_6H_4Cl_2$			+
2,6-Dichlorophenol	$C_6H_4OCl_2$			+
2-Chlorophenol	C_6H_5OCl			+
2,4,6-Trimethyl-1,3,5-trioxane	$C_6H_{12}O_3$			+
Ethyl *tert*-butyl ether	$C_6H_{14}O$		+	
Ethyl *sec*-butyl ether	$C_6H_{14}O$		+	
Dibutyl ether	$C_8H_{18}O$			+
Bis(2-methylbutyl) carbonate	$C_{11}H_{22}O_3$		+	
Diisopentyl carbonate	$C_{11}H_{22}O_3$		+	
1,2,4-Trimethoxy-5-(1-propenyl)benzene, *cis*- (*β*-Asarone)	$C_{12}H_{16}O_3$		+	
Octahydro-4,8a-dimethyl-4a(2*H*)-naphthalenol (Geosmin)	$C_{12}H_{20}O$			+
2,6,6-Trimethyl-10-methylene-1-oxaspiro-[4.5]-8-decene (Vitispirane)	$C_{13}H_{20}O$		+	+
5,7,8,8a-Tetrahydro-2,5,5,8a-tetramethyl-5*H*-1-benzopyran	$C_{13}H_{20}O$			+
1-(2,3,6-Trimethylphenyl)-3-ethoxy-1-butene	$C_{15}H_{22}O$			+
, *trans*-				+
Diphenethyl carbonate	$C_{17}H_{18}O_3$		+	
SOME OTHER COMPOUNDS				
Aflatoxins (IARC, 1976b, 1987a)	$C_{17}H_{12}O_6$	+	+	
Arsenic (IARC, 1980, 1987a)	As		+	
Asbestos (IARC, 1977a, 1987a)	–	+	+	+
Cadmium (IARC, 1976c, 1987a)	Cd		+	
Calcium	Ca	+	+	+
Chromium (IARC, 1980, 1987a)	Cr		+	
Cobalt	Co		+	
Copper	Cu	+	+	
Ethylene thiourea (IARC, 1974, 1987a)	$C_3H_6N_2S$		+	
Fluoride (IARC, 1982b, 1987a)	F		+	
Iron	Fe	+	+	
Lead (IARC, 1980, 1987a)	Pb		+	
Magnesium	Mg		+	+
Manganese	Mn		+	

Appendix 1 (contd)

Compound	Molecular formula	Identified in		
		Beer	Wine	Spirits
Nickel (IARC, 1976c, 1987a)	Ni		+	
Ochratoxin A (IARC, 1983a, 1987a)	$C_{20}H_{18}ClNO_6$	+		
Phosphorus	P	+	+	
Potassium	K	+	+	+
Sodium	Na	+	+	+
Sulphur dioxide	SO_2	+	+	
Sunset Yellow FCF (IARC, 1975, 1987a)	$C_{16}H_{10}N_2Na_2O_7S_2$		+	+
Tannic acid and tannins (IARC, 1976b, 1987)	–		+	+
Trichlorfon (IARC, 1983b, 1987a)	$C_4H_8Cl_3O_4P$		+	
Zearalenone (IARC, 1983a, 1987a)	$C_{18}H_{22}O_5$	+		
Zinc	Zn	+	+	

[a]Based on data from Nykänen & Suomalainen (1983), supplemented by references cited in section 3

Appendix 2
Activity profiles for genetic and related tests

Appendix 2

Activity profiles for genetic and related tests

Methods

The x-axis of the activity profile represents the bioassays in phylogenetic sequence by endpoint, and the values on the y-axis represent the logarithmically transformed lowest effective doses (LED) and highest ineffective doses (HID) tested. The term 'dose', as used in this report, does not take into consideration length of treatment or exposure and may therefore be considered synonymous with concentration. In practice, the concentrations used in all the in-vitro tests were converted to μg/ml, and those for in-vivo tests were expressed as mg/kg bw. Because dose units are plotted on a log scale, differences in molecular weights of compounds do not, in most cases, greatly influence comparisons of their activity profiles. Conventions for dose conversions are given below.

Profile-line height (the magnitude of each bar) is a function of the LED or HID, which is associated with the characteristics of each individual test system — such as population size, cell-cycle kinetics and metabolic competence. Thus, the detection limit of each test system is different, and, across a given activity profile, responses will vary substantially. No attempt is made to adjust or relate responses in one test system to those of another.

Line heights are derived as follows: for negative test results, the highest dose tested without appreciable toxicity is defined as the HID. If there was evidence of extreme toxicity, the next highest dose is used. A single dose tested with a negative result is considered to be equivalent to the HID. Similarly, for positive results, the LED is recorded. If the original data were analysed statistically by the author, the dose recorded is that at which the response was significant ($p < 0.05$). If the available data were not analysed statistically, the dose required to produce an effect is estimated as follows: when a dose-related positive response is observed with two or more doses, the lower of the doses is taken as the LED; a single dose resulting in a positive response is considered to be equivalent to the LED.

In order to accommodate both the wide range of doses encountered and positive and negative responses on a continuous scale, doses are transformed logarithmically, so that effective (LED) and ineffective (HID) doses are represented by positive and negative numbers, respectively. The response, or logarithmic dose unit (LDU_{ij}), for a given test system i and chemical j is represented by the expressions

$$LDU_{ij} = -\log_{10}(\text{dose}), \text{ for HID values; } LDU \leqslant 0$$

and (1)

$$LDU_{ij} = -\log_{10}(\text{dose} \times 10^{-5}), \text{ for LED values; } LDU \geqslant 0.$$

These simple relationships define a dose range of 0 to −5 logarithmic units for ineffective doses (1−100 000 μg/ml or mg/kg bw) and 0 to +8 logarithmic units for effective doses (100 000−0.001 μg/ml or mg/kg bw). A scale illustrating the LDU values is shown in Figure 1. Negative responses at doses less than 1 μg/ml (mg/kg bw) are set equal to 1. Effectively, an LED value ⩾100 000 or an HID value ⩽1 produces an LDU = 0; no quantitative information is gained from such extreme values. The dotted lines at the levels of log dose units 1 and −1 define a 'zone of uncertainty' in which positive results are reported at such high doses (between 10 000 and 100 000 μg/ml or mg/kg bw) or negative results are reported at such low dose levels (1 to 10 μg/ml or mg/kg bw) as to call into question the adequacy of the test.

Fig. 1. Scale of log dose units used on the y-axis of activity profiles

Positive (μg/ml or mg/kg bw)	Negative (μg/ml or mg/kg)	Log dose units
0.001		8
0.01		7
0.1		6
1.0		5
10		4
100		3
1000		2
10 000		1
100 000	1	0
	10	−1
	100	−2
	1000	−3
	10 000	−4
	100 000	−5

LED and HID are expressed as μg/ml or mg/kg bw.

In practice, an activity profile is computer generated. A data entry programme is used to store abstracted data from published reports. A sequential file (in ASCII) is created for each compound, and a record within that file consists of the name and Chemical Abstracts Service number of the compound, a three-letter code for the test system (see below), the qualitative test result (with and without an exogenous metabolic system), dose (LED or HID), citation number and additional source information. An abbreviated citation for each publication is stored in a segment of a record accessing both the test data file and the citation file. During processing of the data file, an average of the logarithmic values of the data subset is calculated, and the length of the profile line represents this average value. All dose values are plotted for each profile line, regardless of whether results are positive or negative. Results obtained in the absence of an exogenous metabolic system are indicated by a bar (–), and results obtained in the presence of an exogenous metabolic system are indicated by an upward-directed arrow (↑). When all results for a given assay are either positive or negative, the mean of the LDU values is plotted as a solid line; when conflicting data are reported for the same assay (i.e., both positive and negative results), the majority data are shown by a solid line and the minority data by a dashed line (drawn to the extreme conflicting response). In the few cases in which the numbers of positive and negative results are equal, the solid line is drawn in the positive direction and the maximal negative response is indicated with a dashed line.

Profile lines are identified by three-letter code words representing the commonly used tests. Code words for most of the test systems in current use in genetic toxicology were defined for the US Environmental Protection Agency's GENE-TOX Program (Waters, 1979; Waters & Auletta, 1981). For this publication, codes were redefined in a manner that should facilitate inclusion of additional tests in the future. If a test system is not defined precisely, a general code is used that best defines the category of the test. Naming conventions are described below.

Dose conversions for activity profiles

Doses are converted to μg/ml for in-vitro tests and to mg/kg bw per day for in-vivo experiments.

1. In-vitro test systems
   (*a*) Weight/volume converts directly to μg/ml.
   (*b*) Molar (M) concentration × molecular weight = mg/ml = 10^3 μg/ml; mM concentration × molecular weight = μg/ml.
   (*c*) Soluble solids expressed as % concentration are assumed to be in units of mass per volume (i.e., 1% = 0.01 g/ml = 10 000 μg/ml; also, 1 ppm = 1 μg/ml).
   (*d*) Liquids and gases expressed as % concentration are assumed to be given in units of volume per volume. Liquids are converted to weight per volume using the density (D) of the solution (D = g/ml). If the bulk of the solution is water, then D = 1.0 g/ml. Gases are converted from volume to mass using the ideal gas law, PV = nRT. For exposure at 20-37°C at standard atmospheric pressure, 1% (v/v) = 0.4 μg/ml × molecular weight of the gas. Also, 1 ppm (v/v) = 4×10^{-5} μg/ml × molecular weight.
   (*e*) For microbial plate tests, concentrations reported as weight/plate are divided by top agar volume (if volume is not given, a 2-ml top agar is assumed). For spot tests, in which concentrations are reported as weight or weight/disc, a 1-ml volume is used as a rough approximation.

(*f*) Conversion of asbestos concentrations given in μg/cm^2 are based on the area (A) of the dish and the volume of medium per dish; i.e., for a 100-mm dish: $A = \pi R^2 = \pi \times (5\ cm)^2 = 78.5\ cm^2$. If the volume of medium is 10 ml, then 78.5 cm^2 = 10 ml and 1 cm^2 = 0.13 ml.

2. In-vitro systems using in-vivo activation

   For the body fluid-urine (BF–) test, the concentration used is the dose (in mg/kg bw) of the compound administered to test animals or patients.

3. In-vivo test systems

   (*a*) Doses are converted to mg/kg bw per day of exposure, assuming 100% absorption. Standard values are used for each sex and species of rodent, including body weight and average intake per day, as reported by Gold *et al.* (1984). For example, in a test using male mice fed 50 ppm of the agent in the diet, the standard food intake per day is 12% of body weight, and the conversion is dose = 50 ppm × 12% = 6 mg/kg bw per day.

   Standard values used for humans are: weight — males, 70 kg; females, 55 kg; surface area, 1.7 m^2; inhalation rate, 20 l/min for light work, 30 l/min for mild exercise.

   (*b*) When reported, the dose at the target site is used. For example, doses given in studies of lymphocytes of humans exposed *in vivo* are the measured blood concentrations in μg/ml.

Codes for test systems

For specific nonmammalian test systems, the first two letters of the three-symbol code word define the test organism (e.g., SA– for *Salmonella typhimurium*, EC– for *Escherichia coli*). In most cases, the first two letters accurately represent the scientific name of the organism. If the species is not known, the convention used is –S–. The third symbol may be used to define the tester strain (e.g., SA8 for *S. typhimurium* TA1538, ECW for *E. coli* WP2*uvrA*). When strain designation is not indicated, the third letter is used to define the specific genetic endpoint under investigation (e.g., ––D for differential toxicity, ––F for forward mutation, ––G for gene conversion or genetic crossing-over, ––N for aneuploidy, ––R for reverse mutation, ––U for unscheduled DNA synthesis). The third letter may also be used to define the general endpoint under investigation when a more complete definition is not possible or relevant (e.g., ––M for mutation, ––C for chromosomal aberration).

For mammalian test systems, the first letter of the three-letter code word defines the genetic endpoint under investigation: A–– for aneuploidy, B–– for binding, C–– for chromosomal aberration, D–– for DNA strand breaks, G–– for gene mutation, I–– for inhibition of intercellular communication, M–– for micronucleus formation, R–– for DNA repair, S–– for sister chromatid exchange, T–– for cell transformation and U–– for unscheduled DNA synthesis.

For animal (i.e., nonhuman) test systems *in vitro*, when the cell type is not specified, the code letters –IA are used. For such assays *in vivo*, when the animal species is not specified, the code letters –VA are used. Commonly used animal species are identified by the third letter (e.g., ––C for Chinese hamster, ––M for mouse, ––R for rat, ––S for Syrian hamster).

For test systems using human cells *in vitro*, when the cell type is not specified, the code letters –IH are used. For assays on humans *in vivo*, when the cell type is not specified, the code letters –VH are used. Otherwise, the second letter specifies the cell type under investigation (e.g., –BH for bone marrow, –LH for lymphocytes).

Some other specific coding conventions used for mammalian systems are as follows: BF– for body fluids, HM– for host-mediated, ––L for leucocytes or lymphocytes *in vitro* (–AL, animals; –HL, humans), –L– for leucocytes *in vivo* (–LA, animals; –LH, humans), ––T for transformed cells.

Note that these are examples of major conventions used to define the assay code words. The alphabetized listing of codes must be examined to confirm a specific code word. As might be expected from the limitation to three symbols, some codes do not fit the naming conventions precisely. In a few cases, test systems are defined by first-letter code words, for example: MST, mouse spot test; SLP, mouse specific locus test, postspermatogonia; SLO, mouse specific locus test, other stages; DLM, dominant lethal test in mice; DLR, dominant lethal test in rats; MHT, mouse heritable translocation test.

References

Garrett, N.E., Stack, H.F., Gross, M.R. & Waters, M.D. (1984) An analysis of the spectra of genetic activity produced by known or suspected human carcinogens. *Mutat. Res.*, *134*, 89-111

Gold, L.S., Sawyer, C.B., Magaw, R., Backman, G.M., de Veciana, M., Levinson, R., Hooper, N.K., Havender, W.R., Bernstein, L., Peto, R., Pike, M.C. & Ames, B.N. (1984) A carcinogenic potency database of the standardized results of animal bioassays. *Environ. Health Perspect.*, *58*, 9-319

Waters, M.D. (1979) *The GENE-TOX program.* In: Hsie, A.W., O'Neill, J.P. & McElheny, V.K., eds, *Mammalian Cell Mutagenesis: The Maturation of Test Systems* (*Banbury Report 2*), Cold Spring Harbor, NY, CHS Press, pp. 449-467

Waters, M.D. & Auletta, A. (1981) The GENE-TOX program: genetic activity evaluation. *J. chem. Inf. comput. Sci.*, *21*, 35-38

TABLE 1. ALPHABETICAL LIST OF TEST SYSTEM CODE WORDS

Endpoint	*Code*	*Definition*
C	ACC	*Allium cepa*, chromosomal aberrations
A	AIA	Aneuploidy, animal cells *in vitro*
A	AIH	Aneuploidy, human cells *in vitro*
G	ANF	*Aspergillus nidulans*, forward mutation
R	ANG	*Aspergillus nidulans*, genetic crossing-over
A	ANN	*Aspergillus nidulans*, aneuploidy
G	ANR	*Aspergillus nidulans*, reverse mutation
G	ASM	*Arabidopsis* species, mutation
A	AVA	Aneuploidy, animal cells *in vivo*
A	AVH	Aneuploidy, human cells *in vivo*
F	BFA	Body fluids from animals, microbial mutagenicity
F	BFH	Body fluids from humans, microbial mutagenicity
D	BHD	Binding (covalent) to DNA, human cells *in vivo*
D	BHP	Binding (covalent) to RNA or protein, human cells *in vivo*
D	BID	Binding (covalent) to DNA *in vitro*
D	BIP	Binding (covalent) to RNA or protein *in vitro*
G	BPF	Bacteriophage, forward mutation
G	BPR	Bacteriophage, reverse mutation
D	BRD	Other DNA repair-deficient bacteria, differential toxicity
D	BSD	*Bacillus subtilis rec* strains, differential toxicity
G	BSM	*Bacillus subtilis*, multigene test
D	BVD	Binding (covalent) to DNA, animal cells *in vivo*
D	BVP	Binding (covalent) to RNA or protein, animal cells *in vivo*
C	CBA	Chromosomal aberrations, animal bone-marrow cells *in vivo*
C	CBH	Chromosomal aberrations, human bone-marrow cells *in vivo*
C	CCC	Chromosomal aberrations, spermatocytes treated *in vivo*, spermatocytes observed
C	CGC	Chromosomal aberrations, spermatogonia treated *in vivo*, spermatocytes observed
C	CGG	Chromosomal aberrations, spermatogonia treated *in vivo*, spermatogonia observed
C	CHF	Chromosomal aberrations, human fibroblasts *in vitro*
C	CHL	Chromosomal aberrations, human lymphocytes *in vitro*
C	CHT	Chromosomal aberrations, transformed human cells *in vitro*
C	CIA	Chromosomal aberrations, other animal cells *in vitro*
C	CIC	Chromosomal aberrations, Chinese hamster cells *in vitro*
C	CIH	Chromosomal aberrations, other human cells *in vitro*
C	CIM	Chromosomal aberrations, mouse cells *in vitro*
C	CIR	Chromosomal aberrations, rat cells *in vitro*
C	CIS	Chromosomal aberrations, Syrian hamster cells *in vitro*
C	CIT	Chromosomal aberrations, transformed animal cells *in vitro*
C	CLA	Chromosomal aberrations, animal leucocytes *in vivo*
C	CLH	Chromosomal aberrations, human lymphocytes *in vivo*
C	COE	Chromosomal aberrations, oocytes or embryos treated *in vivo*
C	CVA	Chromosomal aberrations, other animal cells *in vivo*
C	CVH	Chromosomal aberrations, other human cells *in vivo*
D	DIA	DNA strand breaks, cross-links or related damage, animal cells *in vitro*
D	DIH	DNA strand breaks, cross-links or related damage, human cells *in vitro*
C	DLM	Dominant lethal test, mice
C	DLR	Dominant lethal test, rats
C	DMC	*Drosophila melanogaster*, chromosomal aberrations
R	DMG	*Drosophila melanogaster*, genetic crossing-over or recombination
C	DMH	*Drosophila melanogaster*, heritable translocation test
C	DML	*Drosophila melanogaster*, dominant lethal test
G	DMM	*Drosophila melanogaster*, somatic mutation (and recombination)
A	DMN	*Drosophila melanogaster*, aneuploidy
G	DMX	*Drosophila melanogaster*, sex-linked recessive lethal mutations
D	DVA	DNA strand breaks, cross-links or related damage, animal cells *in vivo*
D	DVH	DNA strand breaks, cross-links or related damage, human cells *in vivo*
G	EC2	*Escherichia coli* WP2, reverse mutation
D	ECB	*Escherichia coli* (or *E. coli* DNA), strand breaks, cross-links or related damage; DNA repair
D	ECD	*Escherichia coli pol* A/W3110-P3478 differential toxicity (spot test)
G	ECF	*Escherichia coli* exclusive of strain K12, forward mutation
G	ECK	*Escherichia coli* K12, forward or reverse mutation
D	ECL	*Escherichia coli pol* A/W3110-P3478, differential toxicity (liquid suspension test)
G	ECR	*Escherichia coli* (other miscellaneous strains), reverse mutation
G	ECW	*Escherichia coli* WP2 *uvrA*, reverse mutation
D	ERD	*Escherichia coli rec* strains, differential toxicity
G	G51	Gene mutation, mouse lymphoma L5178Y cells *in vitro*, all other loci

Table 1 (contd)

Endpoint	Code	Definition
G	G9O	Gene mutation, Chinese hamster lung V79 cells, ouabain resistance
G	GCL	Gene mutation, Chinese hamster lung cells exclusive of V79 *in vitro*
G	GCO	Gene mutation, Chinese hamster ovary cells *in vitro*
G	G9H	Gene mutation, Chinese hamster lung V79 cells, *hprt* locus
G	GIA	Gene mutation, other animal cells *in vitro*
G	GIH	Gene mutation, human cells *in vitro*
G	GML	Gene mutation, mouse lymphoma cells exclusive of L5178Y *in vitro*
G	G5T	Gene mutation, mouse lymphoma L5178Y cells *in vitro*, TK locus
G	GVA	Gene mutation, animal cells *in vivo*
H	HMA	Host-mediated assay, animal cells in animal hosts
H	HMH	Host-mediated assay, human cells in animal hosts
H	HMM	Host-mediated assay, microbial cells in animal hosts
C	HSC	*Hordeum* species, chromosomal aberrations
G	HSM	*Hordeum* species, mutation
I	ICH	Inhibition of intercellular communication, human cells *in vitro*
I	ICR	Inhibition of intercellular communication, animal cells *in vitro*
G	KPF	*Klebsiella pneumonia*, forward mutation
G	MAF	*Micrococcus aureus*, forward mutation
C	MHT	Mouse heritable translocation test
M	MIA	Micronucleus test, animal cells *in vitro*
M	MIH	Micronucleus test, human cells *in vitro*
G	MST	Mouse spot test
M	MVA	Micronucleus test, other animals *in vivo*
M	MVC	Micronucleus test, hamsters *in vivo*
M	MVH	Micronucleus test, human cells *in vivo*
M	MVM	Micronucleus test, mice *in vivo*
M	MVR	Micronucleus test, rats *in vivo*
G	NCF	*Neurospora crassa*, forward mutation
A	NCN	*Neurospora crassa*, aneuploidy
G	NCR	*Neurospora crassa*, reverse mutation
C	PLC	Plants (other), chromosomal aberrations
M	PLI	Plants (other), micronuclei
G	PLM	Plants (other), mutation
S	PLS	Plants (other), sister chromatid exchanges
D	PLU	Plants, unscheduled DNA synthesis
D	PRB	Prophage induction, SOS repair test or DNA strand breaks, cross-links or related damage
C	PSC	*Paramecium* species, chromosomal aberrations
G	PSM	*Paramecium* species, mutation
D	RIA	DNA repair exclusive of unscheduled DNA synthesis, animal cells *in vitro*
D	RIH	DNA repair exclusive of unscheduled DNA synthesis, human cells *in vitro*
D	RVA	DNA repair exclusive of unscheduled DNA synthesis, animal cells *in vivo*
G	SA0	*Salmonella typhimurium* TA100, reverse mutation
G	SA2	*Salmonella typhimurium* TA102, reverse mutation
G	SA3	*Salmonella typhimurium* TA1530, reverse mutation
G	SA4	*Salmonella typhimurium* TA104, reverse mutation
G	SA5	*Salmonella typhimurium* TA1535, reverse mutation
G	SA7	*Salmonella typhimurium* TA1537, reverse mutation
G	SA8	*Salmonella typhimurium* TA1538, reverse mutation
G	SA9	*Salmonella typhimurium* TA98, reverse mutation
D	SAD	*Salmonella typhimurium*, DNA repair-deficient strains, differential toxicity
G	SAF	*Salmonella typhimurium*, forward mutation
G	SAS	*Salmonella typhimurium* (other miscellaneous strains), reverse mutation
G	SCF	*Saccharomyces cerevisiae*, forward mutation
R	SCG	*Saccharomyces cerevisiae*, gene conversion
R	SCH	*Saccharomyces cerevisiae*, homozygosis by mitotic recombination or gene conversion
A	SCN	*Saccharomyces cerevisiae*, aneuploidy
G	SCR	*Saccharomyces cerevisiae*, reverse mutation
G	SGR	*Streptomyces griseoflavus*, reverse mutation
S	SHF	Sister chromatid exchange, human fibroblasts *in vitro*
S	SHL	Sister chromatid exchange, human lymphocytes *in vitro*
S	SHT	Sister chromatid exchange, transformed human cells *in vitro*
S	SIA	Sister chromatid exchange, other animal cells *in vitro*
S	SIC	Sister chromatid exchange, Chinese hamster cells *in vitro*
S	SIH	Sister chromatid exchange, other human cells *in vitro*
S	SIM	Sister chromatid exchange, mouse cells *in vitro*
S	SIR	Sister chromatid exchange, rat cells *in vitro*
S	SIS	Sister chromatid exchange, Syrian hamster cells *in vitro*
S	SIT	Sister chromatid exchange, transformed animal cells *in vitro*
S	SLH	Sister chromatid exchange, human lymphocytes *in vivo*
G	SLO	Mouse specific locus test, other stages
G	SLP	Mouse specific locus test, postspermatogonia
P	SPF	Sperm morphology, F1 mice
P	SPH	Sperm morphology, humans *in vivo*
P	SPM	Sperm morphology, mice
P	SPR	Sperm morphology, rats
D	SSB	*Saccharomyces* species, DNA strand breaks, cross-links or related damage
D	SSD	*Saccharomyces* species, DNA repair-deficient strains, differential toxicity
G	STF	*Streptomyces coelicolor*, forward mutation
G	STR	*Streptomyces coelicolor*, reverse mutation

Table 1 (contd)

Endpoint	*Code*	*Definition*
S	SVA	Sister chromatid exchange, animal cells *in vivo*
S	SVH	Sister chromatid exchange, other human cells *in vivo*
D	SZD	*Schizosaccharomyces pombe*, DNA repair-deficient strains, differential toxicity
G	SZF	*Schizosaccharomyces pombe*, forward mutation
R	SZG	*Schizosaccharomyces pombe*, gene conversion
G	SZR	*Schizosaccharomyces pombe*, reverse mutation
T	TBM	Cell transformation, BALB/c 3T3 mouse cells
T	TCL	Cell transformation, other established cell lines
T	TCM	Cell transformation, C3H 10T1/2 mouse cells
T	TCS	Cell transformation, Syrian hamster embryo cells, clonal assay
T	TEV	Cell transformation, other viral enhancement systems
T	TFS	Cell transformation, Syrian hamster embryo cells, focus assay
T	TIH	Cell transformation, human cells *in vitro*
T	TPM	Cell transformation, mouse prostate cells
T	T7R	Cell transformation, SA7/rat cells
T	TRR	Cell transformation, RLV/Fischer rat embryo cells
T	T7S	Cell transformation, SA7/Syrian hamster embryo cells
C	TSC	*Tradescantia* species, chromosomal aberrations
M	TSI	*Tradescantia* species, micronuclei
G	TSM	*Tradescantia* species, mutation
T	TVI	Cell transformation, treated *in vivo*, scored *in vitro*
D	UBH	Unscheduled DNA synthesis, human bone-marrow cells *in vivo*
D	UHF	Unscheduled DNA synthesis, human fibroblasts *in vitro*
D	UHL	Unscheduled DNA synthesis, human lymphocytes *in vitro*
D	UHT	Unscheduled DNA synthesis, transformed human cells *in vitro*
D	UIA	Unscheduled DNA synthesis, other animal cells *in vitro*
D	UIH	Unscheduled DNA synthesis, other human cells *in vitro*
D	UPR	Unscheduled DNA synthesis, rat hepatocytes *in vivo*
D	URP	Unscheduled DNA synthesis, rat primary hepatocytes
D	UVA	Unscheduled DNA synthesis, other animal cells *in vivo*
D	UVC	Unscheduled DNA synthesis, hamster cells *in vivo*
D	UVH	Unscheduled DNA synthesis, other human cells *in vivo*
D	UVM	Unscheduled DNA synthesis, mouse cells *in vivo*
D	UVR	Unscheduled DNA synthesis, other rat cells *in vivo*
C	VFC	*Vicia faba*, chromosomal aberrations
S	VFS	*Vicia faba*, sister chromatid exchange

ETHANOL[a]

Test code	End point	Test system	Results No act	Act	Dose (LED or HID)	Reference
PRB	D	Prophage induction/SOS repair test/DNA strand breaks, cross-links, etc.	–	0	55000.0000	Kvelland (1983)
ERD	D	Escherichia coli rec strains, differential toxicity	(+)	(+)	25000.0000	De Flora et al. (1984a)
BRD	D	Other DNA repair-deficient bacteria, differential toxicity	–	0	79000.0000	Braun et al. (1982)
SA0	G	Salmonella typhimurium TA100, reverse mutation	–	–	6130.0000	Cotruvo et al. (1977)
SA0	G	Salmonella typhimurium TA100, reverse mutation	–	–	5000.0000	McCann et al. (1975)
SA0	G	Salmonella typhimurium TA100, reverse mutation	–	–	0.0000	Blevins & Shelton (1983)
SA0	G	Salmonella typhimurium TA100, reverse mutation	–	0	0.0000	De Flora et al. (1984a)
SA0	G	Salmonella typhimurium TA100, reverse mutation	(+)	(+)	80000.0000	De Flora et al. (1984b)
SA2	G	Salmonella typhimurium TA102, reverse mutation	–	–	0.0000	Blevins & Shelton (1983)
SA5	G	Salmonella typhimurium TA1535, reverse mutation	–	–	39500.0000	Blevins & Taylor (1982)
SA5	G	Salmonella typhimurium TA1535, reverse mutation	–	–	6130.0000	Cotruvo et al. (1977)
SA5	G	Salmonella typhimurium TA1535, reverse mutation	–	0	0.0000	De Flora et al. (1984a)
SA5	G	Salmonella typhimurium TA1535, reverse mutation	–	–	0.0000	Blevins & Shelton (1983)
SA7	G	Salmonella typhimurium TA1537, reverse mutation	–	–	39500.0000	Blevins & Taylor (1982)
SA7	G	Salmonella typhimurium TA1537, reverse mutation	–	–	6130.0000	Cotruvo et al. (1977)
SA7	G	Salmonella typhimurium TA1537, reverse mutation	–	0	0.0000	De Flora et al. (1984a)
SA7	G	Salmonella typhimurium TA1537, reverse mutation	–	–	0.0000	Blevins & Shelton (1983)
SA8	G	Salmonella typhimurium TA1538, reverse mutation	–	–	39500.0000	Blevins & Taylor (1982)
SA8	G	Salmonella typhimurium TA1538, reverse mutation	–	–	6130.0000	Cotruvo et al. (1977)
SA8	G	Salmonella typhimurium TA1538, reverse mutation	–	0	0.0000	De Flora et al. (1984a)
SA8	G	Salmonella typhimurium TA1538, reverse mutation	–	–	0.0000	Blevins & Shelton (1983)
SA9	G	Salmonella typhimurium TA98, reverse mutation	0	–	29625.0000	Arimoto et al. (1982)
SA9	G	Salmonella typhimurium TA98, reverse mutation	–	–	39500.0000	Blevins & Taylor (1982)
SA9	G	Salmonella typhimurium TA98, reverse mutation	–	–	6130.0000	Cotruvo et al. (1977)
SA9	G	Salmonella typhimurium TA98, reverse mutation	–	0	0.0000	De Flora et al. (1984a)
SA9	G	Salmonella typhimurium TA98, reverse mutation	–	–	6130.0000	Cotruvo et al. (1977)
SAS	G	Salmonella typhimurium (miscellaneous strains), reverse mutation	–	0	39450.0000	Barale et al. (1983)
SCG	R	Saccharomyces cerevisiae, gene mutation	+	0	39500.0000	Harsanyi et al. (1977)
ANG	R	Aspergillus nidulans, genetic crossing-over	+	0	150000.0000	Bandas & Zakharov (1980)
SCF	G	Saccharomyces cerevisiae, forward mutation	+	0	15780.0000	Hamada et al. (1985)
SCF	G	Saccharomyces cerevisiae, forward mutation	(+)	0	39250.0000	Cabeça-Silva et al. (1982)
SCF	G	Saccharomyces cerevisiae, forward mutation	–	0	61320.0000	Gualandi & Bellincampi (1981)
ANF	G	Aspergillus nidulans, forward mutation	+	0	31560.0000	Käfer (1984)
ANN	A	Aspergillus nidulans, aneuploidy	+	0	47000.0000	Morpurgo et al. (1979)
ANN	A	Aspergillus nidulans, aneuploidy	+	0	55230.0000	Gualandi & Bellincampi (1981)
ANN	A	Aspergillus nidulans, aneuploidy	+	0	39500.0000	Harsanyi et al. (1977)
ANN	A	Aspergillus nidulans, aneuploidy	+	0	9200.0000	Schubert et al. (1979)
VFS	S	Vicia faba, sister chromatid exchanges	+	0	782.0000	Cortés et al. (1986)
PLS	S	Plants (other), sister chromatid exchanges	+	0	98625.0000	Ma et al. (1984)
TSI	M	Tradescantia species, micronuclei	–	0	7820.0000	Cortés et al. (1986)
PLI	M	Plants (other), micronuclei	+	0	2300.0000	Rieger & Michaelis (1960)
VFC	C	Vicia faba, chromosomal aberrations	+	0	9200.0000	Schubert et al. (1979)
VFC	C	Vicia faba, chromosomal aberrations	+	0	0.0000	Rieger & Michaelis (1970)

ETHANOL (contd)

Test code	End point	Test system	Results No act	Results Act	Dose (LED or HID)	Reference
VFC	C	*Vicia faba*, chromosomal aberrations	+	0	9200.0000	Rieger et al. (1985)
DMG	R	*Drosophila melanogaster*, genetic crossing-over or recombination	–	0	78900.0000	Graf et al. (1984)
DMM	G	*Drosophila melanogaster*, somatic mutation (and recombination)	–	0	78900.0000	Graf et al. (1984)
DMX	G	*Drosophila melanogaster*, sex-linked recessive lethal mutations	–	0	39450.0000	Vogel & Chandler (1974)
DMX	G	*Drosophila melanogaster*, sex-linked recessive lethal mutations	–	0	237600.0000	Woodruff et al. (1984)
DMX	G	*Drosophila melanogaster*, sex-linked recessive lethal mutations	–	0	30000.0000	Creus et al. (1983)
DMX	G	*Drosophila melanogaster*, sex-linked recessive lethal mutations	–	0	3925.0000	Vogel et al. (1983)
DIA	D	DNA strand breaks, cross-links, etc., animal cells *in vitro*	–	0	7900.0000	Sina et al. (1983)
G5T	G	Gene mutation, mouse lymphoma L5178Y cells *in vitro*, *TK* locus	–	0	31878.0000	Amacher et al. (1980)
SIC	S	Sister chromatid exchange, Chinese hamster cells *in vitro*	+	+	3900.0000	De Raat et al. (1983)
SIC	S	Sister chromatid exchange, Chinese hamster cells *in vitro*	–	+[b]	7360.0000	Darroudi & Natarajan (1987)
SIC	S	Sister chromatid exchange, Chinese hamster cells *in vitro*	–	+	4600.0000	Takehisa & Kanaya (1983)
SIC	S	Sister chromatid exchange, Chinese hamster cells *in vitro*	–	0	790.0000	Obe & Ristow (1977)
SIC	S	Sister chromatid exchange, Chinese hamster cells *in vitro*	–	0	7900.0000	Schwartz et al. (1982)
SIA	S	Sister chromatid exchange, other animal cells *in vitro*	–	0	7900.0000	Garcia Heras et al. (1982)
MIA	M	Micronucleus test, animal cells in vitro	–	0	39450.0000	Lasne et al. (1984)
CIC	C	Chromosomal aberrations, Chinese hamster cells *in vitro*	–	+[b]	7360.0000	Darroudi & Natarajan (1987)
TCM	T	Cell transformation, C3H 10T1/2 mouse cells	(+)	0	0.0000	Abernethy et al. (1982)
TCS	T	Cell transformation, Syrian hamster embryo cells, clonal assay	–	0	3950.0000	Bokkenheuser et al. (1983)
SHL	S	Sister chromatid exchange, human lymphocytes *in vitro*	+	0	395.0000	Alvarez et al. (1980a)
SHL	S	Sister chromatid exchange, human lymphocytes *in vitro*	–	0	15780.0000	Jansson (1982)
SHL	S	Sister chromatid exchange, human lymphocytes *in vitro*	–	0	3950.0000	Obe et al. (1977)
SHL	S	Sister chromatid exchange, human lymphocytes *in vitro*	–	0	3950.0000	Véghelyi & Osztovics (1978)
SHL	S	Sister chromatid exchange, human lymphocytes *in vitro*	–	0	1578.0000	Athanasiou & Bartsocas (1980)
SHL	S	Sister chromatid exchange, human lymphocytes *in vitro*	–	0	3200.0000	Hill & Wolff (1983)
SHL	S	Sister chromatid exchange, human lymphocytes *in vitro*	–	0	7900.0000	Königstein et al. (1984)
SHT	S	Sister chromatid exchange, transformed human cells *in vitro*	–	–	790.0000	Sobti et al. (1982)
SHT	S	Sister chromatid exchange, transformed human cells *in vitro*	–	–	790.0000	Sobti et al. (1983)
CHL	C	Chromosomal aberrations, human lymphocytes *in vitro*	–	0	5000.0000	Cadotte et al. (1973)
CHL	C	Chromosomal aberrations, human lymphocytes *in vitro*	+	0	1160.0000	Badr et al. (1977)
CHL	C	Chromosomal aberrations, human lymphocytes *in vitro*	–	0	3950.0000	Obe et al. (1977)
CHL	C	Chromosomal aberrations, human lymphocytes *in vitro*	–	0	7900.0000	Königstein et al. (1984)
CHL	C	Chromosomal aberrations, human lymphocytes *in vitro*	–	0	7900.0000	Banduhn & Obe (1985)
CHL	C	Chromosomal aberrations, human lymphocytes *in vitro*	–	0	7900.0000	Kuwano & Kajii (1987)
SVA	S	Sister chromatid exchange, animal cells *in vivo*	+	0	6000.0000	Alvarez et al. (1980b)
SVA	S	Sister chromatid exchange, animal cells *in vivo*	–	0	157000.0000	Korte & Obe (1981)
SVA	S	Sister chromatid exchange, animal cells *in vivo*	+	0	3850.0000	Tates et al. (1980)
SVA	S	Sister chromatid exchange, animal cells *in vivo*	+	0	2250.0000	Czajka et al. (1980)
SVA	S	Sister chromatid exchange, animal cells *in vivo*	+	0	13000.0000	Obe et al. (1979)
SVA	S	Sister chromatid exchange, animal cells *in vivo*	–	0	25000.0000	Korte et al. (1981)
SVA	S	Sister chromatid exchange, animal cells *in vivo*	–	0	0.0000	Nayak & Buttar (1986)
MVM	M	Micronucleus test, mice *in vivo*	–	0	53000.0000	Chaubey et al. (1977)
MVM	M	Micronucleus test, mice *in vivo*	–	0	1580.0000	Watanabe et al. (1982)

ETHANOL (contd)

Test code	End point	Test system	Results No act	Act	Dose (LED or HID)	Reference
MVR	M	Micronucleus test, rats in vivo	+	0	1500.0000	Baraona et al. (1981b)
MVR	M	Micronucleus test, rats in vivo	–	0	7700.0000	Tates et al. (1980)
CBA	C	Chromosomal aberrations, animal bone-marrow cells in vivo	–	0	25000.0000	Korte et al. (1981)
CBA	C	Chromosomal aberrations, animal bone-marrow cells in vivo	–	0	13833.0000	Korte et al. (1979)
CBA	C	Chromosomal aberrations, animal bone-marrow cells in vivo	–	0	7700.0000	Tates et al. (1980)
CLA	C	Chromosomal aberrations, animal leucocytes in vivo	–	0	157000.0000	Korte & Obe (1981)
CLA	C	Chromosomal aberrations, animal leucocytes in vivo	–	0	7700.0000	Tates et al. (1980)
CGG	C	Chromosomal aberrations, spermatogonia treated in vivo	–	0	7880.0000	Halkka & Eriksson (1977)
CGG	C	Chromosomal aberrations, spermatogonia treated in vivo	–	0	3906.0000	Kohila et al. (1976)
COE	C	Chromosomal aberrations, oocytes or embryos treated in vivo	+	0	3140.0000	Kozachuk & Barilyak (1982)
COE	C	Chromosomal aberrations, oocytes or embryos treated in vivo	–	0	0.0000	Barilyak & Kozachuk (1983)
DLM	C	Dominant lethal test, mice	?	0	1580.0000	James & Smith (1982)
DLM	C	Dominant lethal test, mice	+	0	1900.0000	Badr & Badr (1975)
DLR	C	Dominant lethal test, rats	+	0	1970.0000	Mankes et al. (1982)
DLR	C	Dominant lethal test, rats	+	0	10000.0000	Klassen & Persaud (1976)
DLR	C	Dominant lethal test, rats	–	0	12835.0000	Chauhan et al. (1980)
AVA	A	Aneuploidy, animal cells in vivo	+	0	2800.0000	Kaufman & Bain (1984a)
AVA	A	Aneuploidy, animal cells in vivo	+	0	2800.0000	Kaufman & Bain (1984b)
AVA	A	Aneuploidy, animal cells in vivo	+	0	3950.0000	Kaufman (1983)
AVA	A	Aneuploidy, animal cells in vivo	+	0	3490.0000	Hunt (1987)
AVA	A	Aneuploidy, animal cells in vivo	–	0	6250.0000	Daniel & Roane (1987)

[a]The genetic activity profile was prepared in collaboration with the Genetic Toxicology Division of the US Environmental Protection Agency, who also determined the doses used. Only results from experimental systems are given.

[b]Plant activation system

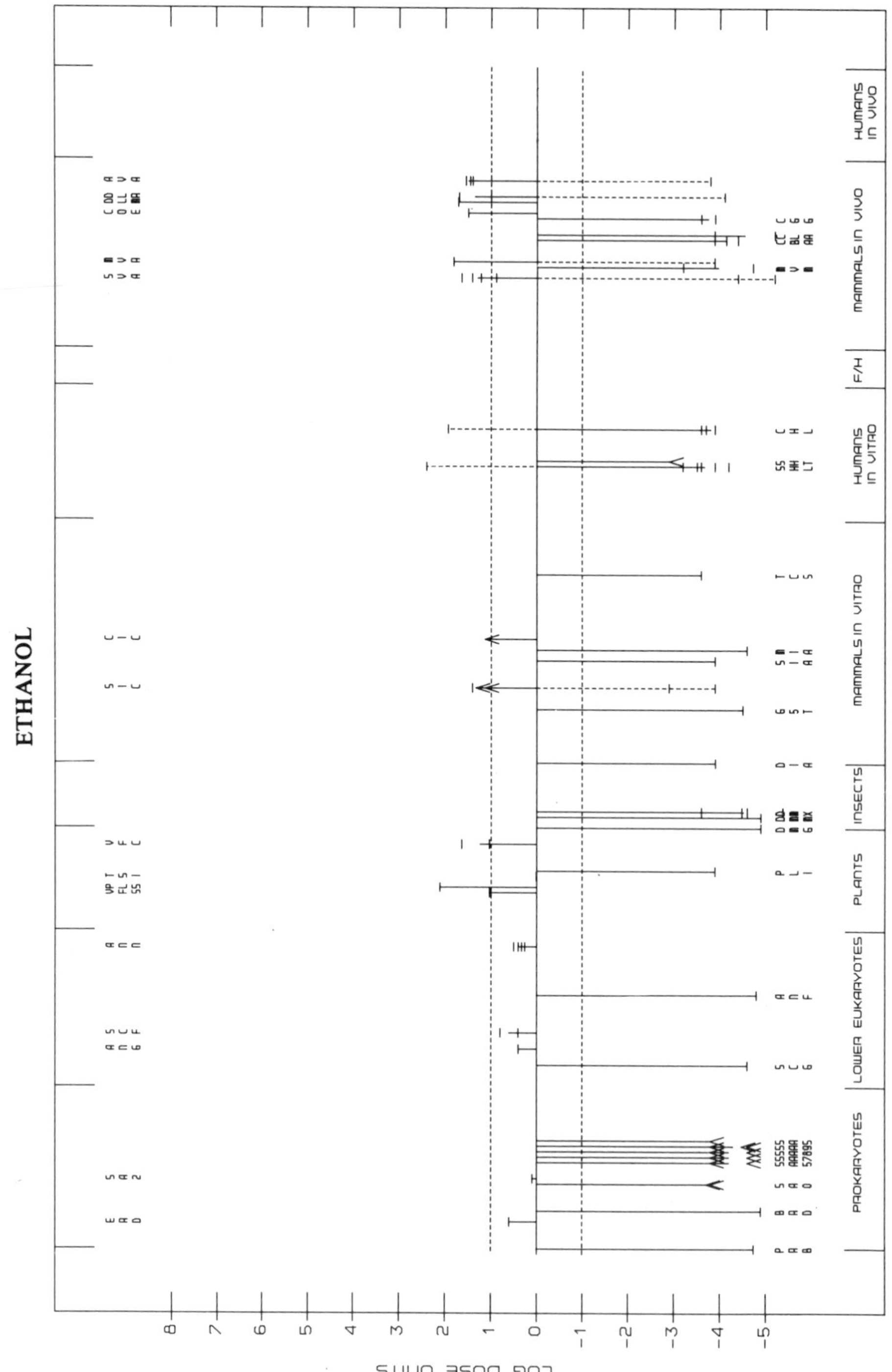
ETHANOL
PROKARYOTES
LOWER EUKARYOTES
PLANTS
INSECTS
MAMMALS IN VITRO
HUMANS IN VITRO
F/H
MAMMALS IN VIVO
HUMANS IN VIVO
LOG DOSE UNITS
8
7
6
5
4
3
2
1
0
-1
-2
-3
-4
-5

ACETALDEHYDE[a]

Test code	End point	Test system	Results No act	Results Act	Dose (LED or HID)	Reference
ERD	D	Escherichia coli rec strains, differential toxicity (spot test)	(+)	0	7800.0000	Rosenkranz (1977)
SA0	G	Salmonella typhimurium TA100, reverse mutation	–	–	5000.0000	Mortelmans et al. (1986)
SA4	G	Salmonella typhimurium TA104, reverse mutation	–	0	2515.0000	Marnett et al. (1985)
SA5	G	Salmonella typhimurium TA1535, reverse mutation	(+)	0	7800.0000	Rosenkranz (1977)
SA5	G	Salmonella typhimurium TA1535, reverse mutation	–	–	5000.0000	Mortelmans et al. (1986)
SA7	G	Salmonella typhimurium TA1537, reverse mutation	–	–	5000.0000	Mortelmans et al. (1986)
SA8	G	Salmonella typhimurium TA1538, reverse mutation	(+)	0	7800.0000	Rosenkranz (1977)
SA9	G	Salmonella typhimurium TA98, reverse mutation	–	–	5000.0000	Mortelmans et al. (1986)
ECW	G	Escherichia coli WP2 uvrA, reverse mutation	+	0	39.0000	Véghelyi et al. (1978)
ECW	G	Escherichia coli WP2 uvrA, reverse mutation	+	0	780.0000	Igali & Gaszo (1980)
SCF	G	Saccharomyces cerevisiae, forward mutation	(+)	0	23400.0000	Bandas (1982)
PLS	S	Plants (other), sister chromatid exchanges	+	0	75.0000	Cortés et al. (1986)
PLI	M	Plants (other), micronuclei	+	0	75.0000	Cortés et al. (1986)
ACC	C	Allium cepa, chromosomal aberrations	+	0	75.0000	Cortés et al. (1986)
VFC	C	Vicia faba, chromosomal aberrations	+	0	220.0000	Rieger & Michaelis (1960)
SIC	S	Sister chromatid exchange, Chinese hamster cells in vitro	+	0	3.9000	Obe & Beek (1979)
SIC	S	Sister chromatid exchange, Chinese hamster cells in vitro	+	0	31.2000	Obe & Ristow (1977)
SIC	S	Sister chromatid exchange, Chinese hamster cells in vitro	+	0	4.0000	Obe et al. (1978)
SIA	S	Sister chromatid exchange, other animal cells in vitro	+	+	7.8000	De Raat et al. (1983)
MIA	M	Micronucleus test, animal cells in vitro	+	0	22.0000	Bird et al. (1982)
CIR	C	Chromosomal aberrations, rat cells in vitro	+	0	4.4000	Bird et al. (1982)
TCM	T	Cell transformation, C3H 10T1/2 mouse cells	–	0	100.0000	Abernethy et al. (1982)
DIH	D	DNA strand breaks, cross-links, etc., human cells in vitro	+	0	0.4400	Lambert et al. (1985)
SHL	S	Sister chromatid exchange, human lymphocytes in vitro	+	0	6.0000	Jansson (1982)
SHL	S	Sister chromatid exchange, human lymphocytes in vitro	+	0	8.0000	Böhlke et al. (1983)
SHL	S	Sister chromatid exchange, human lymphocytes in vitro	+	0	7.8000	Ristow & Obe (1978)
SHL	S	Sister chromatid exchange, human lymphocytes in vitro	+	0	1.8000	Véghelyi et al. (1978)
SHL	S	Sister chromatid exchange, human lymphocytes in vitro	+	0	15.6000	Obe et al. (1978)
SHL	S	Sister chromatid exchange, human lymphocytes in vitro	+	0	4.4000	He & Lambert (1985)
CHL	C	Chromosomal aberrations, human lymphocytes in vitro	+	0	20.0000	Badr & Hussain (1977)
CHL	C	Chromosomal aberrations, human lymphocytes in vitro	+	0	16.0000	Böhlke et al. (1983)
CHL	C	Chromosomal aberrations, human lymphocytes in vitro	+	0	4.0000	Obe et al. (1985)
CHL	C	Chromosomal aberrations, human lymphocytes in vitro	–	0	15.6000	Obe et al. (1979)
CHL	C	Chromosomal aberrations, human lymphocytes in vitro	(+)	0	0.7800	Obe et al. (1978)
CIH	C	Chromosomal aberrations, other human cells in vitro	+	0	7.8000	Obe et al. (1979)
SVA	S	Sister chromatid exchange, animal cells in vivo	+	0	0.4000	Obe et al. (1979)
SVA	S	Sister chromatid exchange, animal cells in vivo	+	0	0.5000	Korte & Obe (1981)
COE	C	Chromosomal aberrations, oocytes or embryos treated in vivo	+	0	7800.0000	Barilyak & Kozachuk (1983)
BID	D	Binding (covalent) to DNA in vitro	+	0	44100.0000	Ristow & Obe (1978)

[a] From IARC (1987b)

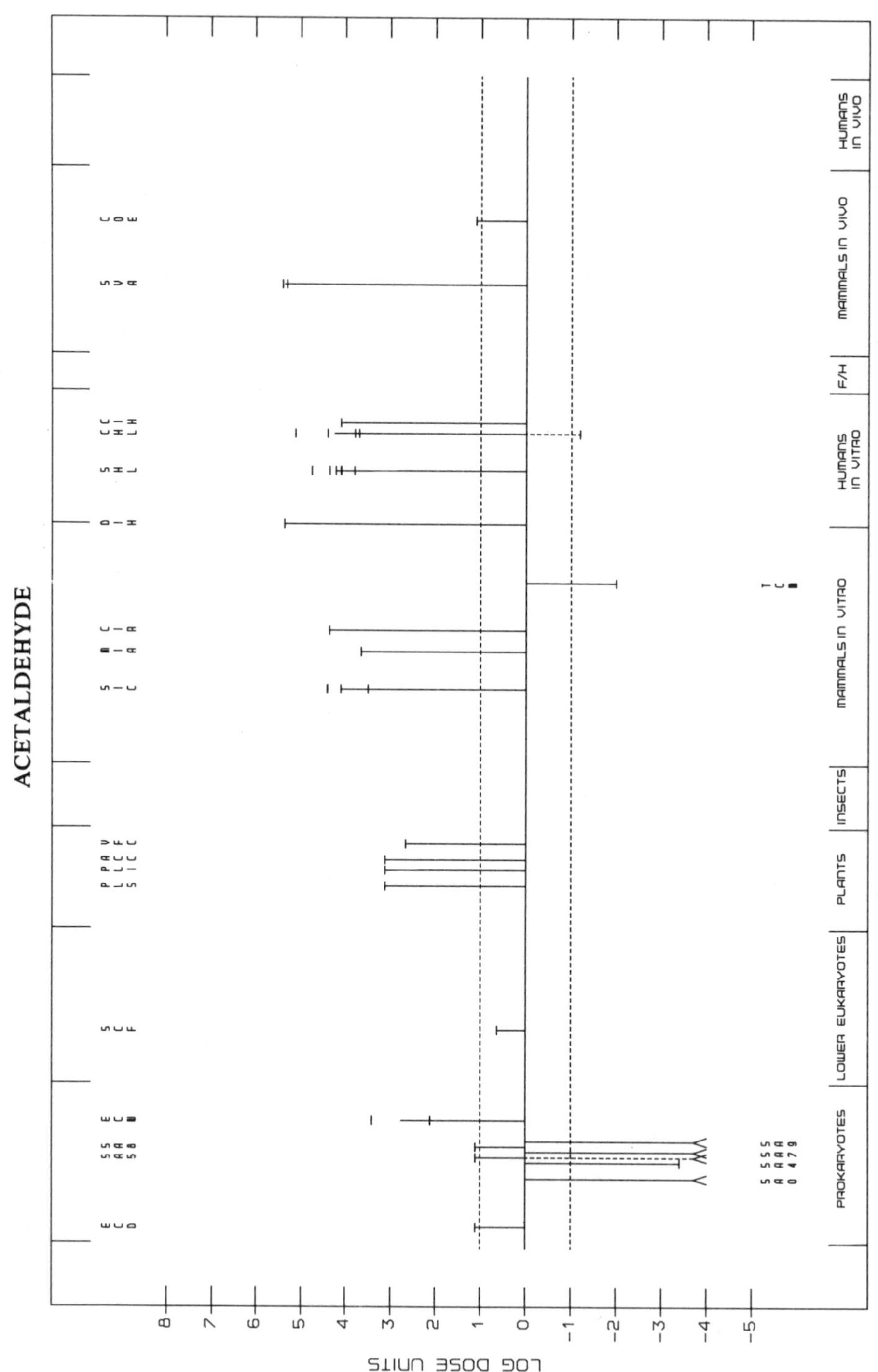
ACETALDEHYDE
LOG DOSE UNITS
8
7
6
5
4
3
2
1
0
-1
-2
-3
-4
-5
PROKARYOTES
LOWER EUKARYOTES
PLANTS
INSECTS
MAMMALS IN VITRO
HUMANS IN VITRO
F/H
MAMMALS IN VIVO
HUMANS IN VIVO

CUMULATIVE CROSS INDEX TO IARC MONOGRAPHS ON THE EVALUATION OF CARCINOGENIC RISKS TO HUMANS

The volume, page and year are given. References to corrigenda are given in parentheses.

B

F

H

I

J

K

L

M

U

Y

Z

PUBLICATIONS OF THE INTERNATIONAL AGENCY FOR RESEARCH ON CANCER

SCIENTIFIC PUBLICATIONS SERIES

(Available from Oxford University Press)
through local bookshops

No. 1 LIVER CANCER
1971; 176 pages; out of print

No. 2 ONCOGENESIS AND HERPESVIRUSES
Edited by P.M. Biggs, G. de-Thé & L.N. Payne
1972; 515 pages; out of print

No. 3 *N*-NITROSO COMPOUNDS: ANALYSIS AND FORMATION
Edited by P. Bogovski, R. Preussmann & E. A. Walker
1972; 140 pages; out of print

No. 4 TRANSPLACENTAL CARCINOGENESIS
Edited by L. Tomatis & U. Mohr
1973; 181 pages; out of print

*No. 5 PATHOLOGY OF TUMOURS IN LABORATORY ANIMALS. VOLUME 1. TUMOURS OF THE RAT. PART 1
Editor-in-Chief V.S. Turusov
1973; 214 pages

*No. 6 PATHOLOGY OF TUMOURS IN LABORATORY ANIMALS. VOLUME 1. TUMOURS OF THE RAT. PART 2
Editor-in-Chief V.S. Turusov
1976; 319 pages
*reprinted in one volume, Price £50.00

No. 7 HOST ENVIRONMENT INTERACTIONS IN THE ETIOLOGY OF CANCER IN MAN
Edited by R. Doll & I. Vodopija
1973; 464 pages; £32.50

No. 8 BIOLOGICAL EFFECTS OF ASBESTOS
Edited by P. Bogovski, J.C. Gilson, V. Timbrell & J.C. Wagner
1973; 346 pages; out of print

No. 9 *N*-NITROSO COMPOUNDS IN THE ENVIRONMENT
Edited by P. Bogovski & E. A. Walker
1974; 243 pages; £16.50

No. 10 CHEMICAL CARCINOGENESIS ESSAYS
Edited by R. Montesano & L. Tomatis
1974; 230 pages; out of print

No. 11 ONCOGENESIS AND HERPESVIRUSES II
Edited by G. de-Thé, M.A. Epstein & H. zur Hausen
1975; Part 1, 511 pages; Part 2, 403 pages; £65.-

No. 12 SCREENING TESTS IN CHEMICAL CARCINOGENESIS
Edited by R. Montesano, H. Bartsch & L. Tomatis
1976; 666 pages; £12.-

No. 13 ENVIRONMENTAL POLLUTION AND CARCINOGENIC RISKS
Edited by C. Rosenfeld & W. Davis
1976; 454 pages; out of print

No. 14 ENVIRONMENTAL *N*-NITROSO COMPOUNDS: ANALYSIS AND FORMATION
Edited by E.A. Walker, P. Bogovski & L. Griciute
1976; 512 pages; £37.50

No. 15 CANCER INCIDENCE IN FIVE CONTINENTS. VOLUME III
Edited by J. Waterhouse, C. Muir, P. Correa & J. Powell
1976; 584 pages; out of print

No. 16 AIR POLLUTION AND CANCER IN MAN
Edited by U. Mohr, D. Schmähl & L. Tomatis
1977; 311 pages; out of print

No. 17 DIRECTORY OF ON-GOING RESEARCH IN CANCER EPIDEMIOLOGY 1977
Edited by C.S. Muir & G. Wagner
1977; 599 pages; out of print

No. 18 ENVIRONMENTAL CARCINOGENS: SELECTED METHODS OF ANALYSIS
Edited-in-Chief H. Egan
VOLUME 1. ANALYSIS OF VOLATILE NITROSAMINES IN FOOD
Edited by R. Preussmann, M. Castegnaro, E.A. Walker & A.E. Wassermann
1978; 212 pages; out of print

No. 19 ENVIRONMENTAL ASPECTS OF *N*-NITROSO COMPOUNDS
Edited by E.A. Walker, M. Castegnaro, L. Griciute & R.E. Lyle
1978; 566 pages; out of print

No. 20 NASOPHARYNGEAL CARCINOMA: ETIOLOGY AND CONTROL
Edited by G. de-Thé & Y. Ito
1978; 610 pages; out of print

No. 21 CANCER REGISTRATION AND ITS TECHNIQUES
Edited by R. MacLennan, C. Muir, R. Steinitz & A. Winkler
1978; 235 pages; £35.-

Prices, valid for October 1988, are subject to change without notice

SCIENTIFIC PUBLICATIONS SERIES

No. 22 ENVIRONMENTAL CARCINOGENS: SELECTED METHODS OF ANALYSIS
Editor-in-Chief H. Egan
VOLUME 2. METHODS FOR THE MEASUREMENT OF VINYL CHLORIDE IN POLY(VINYL CHLORIDE), AIR, WATER AND FOODSTUFFS
Edited by D.C.M. Squirrell & W. Thain
1978; 142 pages; out of print

No. 23 PATHOLOGY OF TUMOURS IN LABORATORY ANIMALS. VOLUME II. TUMOURS OF THE MOUSE
Editor-in-Chief V.S. Turusov
1979; 669 pages; out of print

No. 24 ONCOGENESIS AND HERPESVIRUSES III
Edited by G. de-Thé, W. Henle & F. Rapp
1978; Part 1, 580 pages; Part 2, 522 pages; out of print

No. 25 CARCINOGENIC RISKS: STRATEGIES FOR INTERVENTION
Edited by W. Davis & C. Rosenfeld
1979; 283 pages; out of print

No. 26 DIRECTORY OF ON-GOING RESEARCH IN CANCER EPIDEMIOLOGY 1978
Edited by C.S. Muir & G. Wagner,
1978; 550 pages; out of print

No. 27 MOLECULAR AND CELLULAR ASPECTS OF CARCINOGEN SCREENING TESTS
Edited by R. Montesano, H. Bartsch & L. Tomatis
1980; 371 pages; £22.50

No. 28 DIRECTORY OF ON-GOING RESEARCH IN CANCER EPIDEMIOLOGY 1979
Edited by C.S. Muir & G. Wagner
1979; 672 pages; out of print

No. 29 ENVIRONMENTAL CARCINOGENS: SELECTED METHODS OF ANALYSIS
Editor-in-Chief H. Egan
VOLUME 3. ANALYSIS OF POLYCYCLIC AROMATIC HYDROCARBONS IN ENVIRONMENTAL SAMPLES
Edited by M. Castegnaro, P. Bogovski, H. Kunte & E.A. Walker
1979; 240 pages; out of print

No. 30 BIOLOGICAL EFFECTS OF MINERAL FIBRES
Editor-in-Chief J.C. Wagner
1980; Volume 1, 494 pages; Volume 2, 513 pages; £55.-

No. 31 *N*-NITROSO COMPOUNDS: ANALYSIS, FORMATION AND OCCURRENCE
Edited by E.A. Walker, L. Griciute, M. Castegnaro & M. Börzsönyi
1980; 841 pages; out of print

No. 32 STATISTICAL METHODS IN CANCER RESEARCH. VOLUME 1. THE ANALYSIS OF CASE-CONTROL STUDIES
By N.E. Breslow & N.E. Day
1980; 338 pages; £20.-

No. 33 HANDLING CHEMICAL CARCINOGENS IN THE LABORATORY: PROBLEMS OF SAFETY
Edited by R. Montesano, H. Bartsch, E. Boyland, G. Della Porta, L. Fishbein, R.A. Griesemer, A.B. Swan & L. Tomatis
1979; 32 pages; out of print

No. 34 PATHOLOGY OF TUMOURS IN LABORATORY ANIMALS. VOLUME III. TUMOURS OF THE HAMSTER
Editor-in-Chief V.S. Turusov
1982; 461 pages; £32.50

No. 35 DIRECTORY OF ON-GOING RESEARCH IN CANCER EPIDEMIOLOGY 1980
Edited by C.S. Muir & G. Wagner
1980; 660 pages; out of print

No. 36 CANCER MORTALITY BY OCCUPATION AND SOCIAL CLASS 1851-1971
By W.P.D. Logan
1982; 253 pages; £22.50

No. 37 LABORATORY DECONTAMINATION AND DESTRUCTION OF AFLATOXINS B_1, B_2, G_1, G_2 IN LABORATORY WASTES
Edited by M. Castegnaro, D.C. Hunt, E.B. Sansone, P.L. Schuller, M.G. Siriwardana, G.M. Telling, H.P. Van Egmond & E.A. Walker
1980; 59 pages; £6.50

No. 38 DIRECTORY OF ON-GOING RESEARCH IN CANCER EPIDEMIOLOGY 1981
Edited by C.S. Muir & G. Wagner
1981; 696 pages; out of print

No. 39 HOST FACTORS IN HUMAN CARCINOGENESIS
Edited by H. Bartsch & B. Armstrong
1982; 583 pages; £37.50

No. 40 ENVIRONMENTAL CARCINOGENS: SELECTED METHODS OF ANALYSIS
Edited-in-Chief H. Egan
VOLUME 4. SOME AROMATIC AMINES AND AZO DYES IN THE GENERAL AND INDUSTRIAL ENVIRONMENT
Edited by L. Fishbein, M. Castegnaro, I.K. O'Neill & H. Bartsch
1981; 347 pages; £22.50

No. 41 *N*-NITROSO COMPOUNDS: OCCURRENCE AND BIOLOGICAL EFFECTS
Edited by H. Bartsch, I.K. O'Neill, M. Castegnaro & M. Okada
1982; 755 pages; £37.50

No. 42 CANCER INCIDENCE IN FIVE CONTINENTS. VOLUME IV
Edited by J. Waterhouse, C. Muir, K. Shanmugaratnam & J. Powell
1982; 811 pages; £37.50

SCIENTIFIC PUBLICATIONS SERIES

No. 43 LABORATORY DECONTAMINATION AND DESTRUCTION OF CARCINOGENS IN LABORATORY WASTES: SOME *N*-NITROSAMINES
Edited by M. Castegnaro, G. Eisenbrand, G. Ellen, L. Keefer, D. Klein, E.B. Sansone, D. Spincer, G. Telling & K. Webb
1982; 73 pages; £7.50

No. 44 ENVIRONMENTAL CARCINOGENS:. SELECTED METHODS OF ANALYSIS
Editor-in-Chief H. Egan
VOLUME 5. SOME MYCOTOXINS
Edited by L. Stoloff, M. Castegnaro, P. Scott, I.K. O'Neill & H. Bartsch
1983; 455 pages; £22.50

No. 45 ENVIRONMENTAL CARCINOGENS: SELECTED METHODS OF ANALYSIS
Editor-in-Chief H. Egan
VOLUME 6. *N*-NITROSO COMPOUNDS
Edited by R. Preussmann, I.K. O'Neill, G. Eisenbrand, B. Spiegelhalder & H. Bartsch
1983; 508 pages; £22.50

No. 46 DIRECTORY OF ON-GOING RESEARCH IN CANCER EPIDEMIOLOGY 1982
Edited by C.S. Muir & G. Wagner
1982; 722 pages; out of print

No. 47 CANCER INCIDENCE IN SINGAPORE 1968-1977
Edited by K. Shanmugaratnam, H.P. Lee & N.E. Day
1982; 171 pages; out of print

No. 48 CANCER INCIDENCE IN THE USSR
Second Revised Edition
Edited by N.P. Napalkov, G.F. Tserkovny, V.M. Merabishvili, D.M. Parkin, M. Smans & C.S. Muir,
1983; 75 pages; £12.-

No. 49 LABORATORY DECONTAMINATION AND DESTRUCTION OF CARCINOGENS IN LABORATORY WASTES: SOME POLYCYCLIC AROMATIC HYDROCARBONS
Edited by M. Castegnaro, G. Grimmer, O. Hutzinger, W. Karcher, H. Kunte, M. Lafontaine, E.B. Sansone, G. Telling & S.P. Tucker
1983; 81 pages; £9.-

No. 50 DIRECTORY OF ON-GOING RESEARCH IN CANCER EPIDEMIOLOGY 1983
Edited by C.S. Muir & G. Wagner
1983; 740 pages; out of print

No. 51 MODULATORS OF EXPERIMENTAL CARCINOGENESIS
Edited by V. Turusov & R. Montesano
1983; 307 pages; £22.50

No. 52 SECOND CANCER IN RELATION TO RADIATION TREATMENT FOR CERVICAL CANCER
Edited by N.E. Day & J.D. Boice, Jr
1984; 207 pages; £20.-

No. 53 NICKEL IN THE HUMAN ENVIRONMENT
Editor-in-Chief F.W. Sunderman, Jr
1984: 530 pages; £32.50

No. 54 LABORATORY DECONTAMINATION AND DESTRUCTION OF CARCINOGENS IN LABORATORY WASTES: SOME HYDRAZINES
Edited by M. Castegnaro, G. Ellen, M. Lafontaine, H.C. van der Plas, E.B. Sansone & S.P. Tucker
1983; 87 pages; £9.-

No. 55 LABORATORY DECONTAMINATION AND DESTRUCTION OF CARCINOGENS IN LABORATORY WASTES: SOME *N*-NITROSAMIDES
Edited by M. Castegnaro, M. Benard, L.W. van Broekhoven, D. Fine, R. Massey, E.B. Sansone, P.L.R. Smith, B. Spiegelhalder, A. Stacchini, G. Telling & J.J. Vallon
1984; 65 pages; £7.50

No. 56 MODELS, MECHANISMS AND ETIOLOGY OF TUMOUR PROMOTION
Edited by M. Börszönyi, N.E. Day, K. Lapis & H. Yamasaki
1984; 532 pages; £32.50

No. 57 *N*-NITROSO COMPOUNDS: OCCURRENCE, BIOLOGICAL EFFECTS AND RELEVANCE TO HUMAN CANCER
Edited by I.K. O'Neill, R.C. von Borstel, C.T. Miller, J. Long & H. Bartsch
1984; 1011 pages; £80.-

No. 58 AGE-RELATED FACTORS IN CARCINOGENESIS
Edited by A. Likhachev, V. Anisimov & R. Montesano
1985; 288 pages; £20.-

No. 59 MONITORING HUMAN EXPOSURE TO CARCINOGENIC AND MUTAGENIC AGENTS
Edited by A. Berlin, M. Draper, K. Hemminki & H. Vainio
1984; 457 pages; £27.50

No. 60 BURKITT'S LYMPHOMA: A HUMAN CANCER MODEL
Edited by G. Lenoir, G. O'Conor & C.L.M. Olweny
1985; 484 pages; £22.50

No. 61 LABORATORY DECONTAMINATION AND DESTRUCTION OF CARCINOGENS IN LABORATORY WASTES: SOME HALOETHERS
Edited by M. Castegnaro, M. Alvarez, M. Iovu, E.B. Sansone, G.M. Telling & D.T. Williams
1984; 53 pages; £7.50

No. 62 DIRECTORY OF ON-GOING RESEARCH IN CANCER EPIDEMIOLOGY 1984
Edited by C.S. Muir & G.Wagner
1984; 728 pages; £26.-

No. 63 VIRUS-ASSOCIATED CANCERS IN AFRICA
Edited by A.O. Williams, G.T. O'Conor, G.B. de-Thé & C.A. Johnson
1984; 774 pages; £22.-

SCIENTIFIC PUBLICATIONS SERIES

No. 64 LABORATORY DECONTAMINATION AND DESTRUCTION OF CARCINOGENS IN LABORATORY WASTES: SOME AROMATIC AMINES AND 4-NITROBIPHENYL
Edited by M. Castegnaro, J. Barek, J. Dennis, G. Ellen, M. Klibanov, M. Lafontaine, R. Mitchum, P. Van Roosmalen, E.B. Sansone, L.A. Sternson & M. Vahl
1985; 85 pages; £6.95

No. 65 INTERPRETATION OF NEGATIVE EPIDEMIOLOGICAL EVIDENCE FOR CARCINOGENICITY
Edited by N.J. Wald & R. Doll
1985; 232 pages; £20.-

No. 66 THE ROLE OF THE REGISTRY IN CANCER CONTROL
Edited by D.M. Parkin, G. Wagner & C. Muir
1985; 155 pages; £10.-

No. 67 TRANSFORMATION ASSAY OF ESTABLISHED CELL LINES: MECHANISMS AND APPLICATION
Edited by T. Kakunaga & H. Yamasaki
1985; 225 pages; £20.-

No. 68 ENVIRONMENTAL CARCINOGENS: SELECTED METHODS OF ANALYSIS VOLUME 7. SOME VOLATILE HALOGENATED HYDROCARBONS
Edited by L. Fishbein & I.K. O'Neill
1985; 479 pages; £20.-

No. 69 DIRECTORY OF ON-GOING RESEARCH IN CANCER EPIDEMIOLOGY 1985
Edited by C.S. Muir & G. Wagner
1985; 756 pages; £22.

No. 70 THE ROLE OF CYCLIC NUCLEIC ACID ADDUCTS IN CARCINOGENESIS AND MUTAGENESIS
Edited by B. Singer & H. Bartsch
1986; 467 pages; £40.-

No. 71 ENVIRONMENTAL CARCINOGENS: SELECTED METHODS OF ANALYSIS VOLUME 8. SOME METALS: As, Be, Cd, Cr, Ni, Pb, Se, Zn
Edited by I.K. O'Neill, P. Schuller & L. Fishbein
1986; 485 pages; £20.

No. 72 ATLAS OF CANCER IN SCOTLAND 1975-1980: INCIDENCE AND EPIDEMIOLOGICAL PERSPECTIVE
Edited by I. Kemp, P. Boyle, M. Smans & C. Muir
1985; 282 pages; £35.-

No. 73 LABORATORY DECONTAMINATION AND DESTRUCTION OF CARCINOGENS IN LABORATORY WASTES: SOME ANTINEOPLASTIC AGENTS
Edited by M. Castegnaro, J. Adams, M. Armour, J. Barek, J. Benvenuto, C. Confalonieri, U. Goff, S. Ludeman, D. Reed, E.B. Sansone & G. Telling
1985; 163 pages; £10.-

No. 74 TOBACCO: A MAJOR INTERNATIONAL HEALTH HAZARD
Edited by D. Zaridze & R. Peto
1986; 324 pages; £20.-

No. 75 CANCER OCCURRENCE IN DEVELOPING COUNTRIES
Edited by D.M. Parkin
1986; 339 pages; £20.-

No. 76 SCREENING FOR CANCER OF THE UTERINE CERVIX
Edited by M. Hakama, A.B. Miller & N.E. Day
1986; 315 pages; £25.-

No. 77 HEXACHLOROBENZENE: PROCEEDINGS OF AN INTERNATIONAL SYMPOSIUM
Edited by C.R. Morris & J.R.P. Cabral
1986; 668 pages; £50.-

No. 78 CARCINOGENICITY OF ALKYLATING CYTOSTATIC DRUGS
Edited by D. Schmähl & J. M. Kaldor
1986; 338 pages; £25.-

No. 79 STATISTICAL METHODS IN CANCER RESEARCH. VOLUME III. THE DESIGN AND ANALYSIS OF LONG-TERM ANIMAL EXPERIMENTS
By J.J. Gart, D. Krewski, P.N. Lee, R.E. Tarone & J. Wahrendorf
1986; 219 pages; £20.-

No. 80 DIRECTORY OF ON-GOING RESEARCH IN CANCER EPIDEMIOLOGY 1986
Edited by C.S. Muir & G. Wagner
1986; 805 pages; £22.-

No. 81 ENVIRONMENTAL CARCINOGENS: METHODS OF ANALYSIS AND EXPOSURE MEASUREMENT. VOLUME 9. PASSIVE SMOKING
Edited by I.K. O'Neill, K.D. Brunnemann, B. Dodet & D. Hoffmann
1987; 379 pages; £30.-

No. 82 STATISTICAL METHODS IN CANCER RESEARCH. VOLUME II. THE DESIGN AND ANALYSIS OF COHORT STUDIES
By N.E. Breslow & N.E. Day
1987; 404 pages; £30.-

No. 83 LONG-TERM AND SHORT-TERM ASSAYS FOR CARCINOGENS: A CRITICAL APPRAISAL
Edited by R. Montesano, H. Bartsch, H. Vainio, J. Wilbourn & H. Yamasaki
1986; 575 pages; £32.50

No. 84 THE RELEVANCE OF *N*-NITROSO COMPOUNDS TO HUMAN CANCER: EXPOSURES AND MECHANISMS
Edited by H. Bartsch, I.K. O'Neill & R. Schulte-Hermann
1987; 671 pages; £50.-

SCIENTIFIC PUBLICATIONS SERIES

No. 85 ENVIRONMENTAL CARCINOGENS: METHODS OF ANALYSIS AND EXPOSURE MEASUREMENT. VOLUME 10. BENZENE AND ALKYLATED BENZENES
Edited by L. Fishbein & I.K. O'Neill
1988; 318 pages; £35.-

No. 86 DIRECTORY OF ON-GOING RESEARCH IN CANCER EPIDEMIOLOGY 1987
Edited by D.M. Parkin & J. Wahrendorf
1987; 685 pages; £22.-

No. 87 INTERNATIONAL INCIDENCE OF CHILDHOOD CANCER
Edited by D.M. Parkin, C.A. Stiller, G.J. Draper, C.A. Bieber, B. Terracini & J.L. Young
1988; 402 pages; £35.-

No. 88 CANCER INCIDENCE IN FIVE CONTINENTS. VOLUME V
Edited by C. Muir, J. Waterhouse, T. Mack, J. Powell & S. Whelan
1988; 1004 pages; £50.-

No. 89 METHODS FOR DETECTING DNA DAMAGING AGENTS IN HUMANS: APPLICATIONS IN CANCER EPIDEMIOLOGY AND PREVENTION
Edited by H. Bartsch, K. Hemminki & I.K. O'Neill
1988; 518 pages; £45.-

No. 90 NON-OCCUPATIONAL EXPOSURE TO MINERAL FIBRES
Edited by J. Bignon, J. Peto & R. Saracci
(in press) 1988; approx. 500 pages; £45.-

No. 91 TRENDS IN CANCER INCIDENCE IN SINGAPORE 1968-1982
Edited by H.P. Lee, N.E. Day & K. Shanmugaratnam
1988; 160 pages; £25.-

No. 92 CELL DIFFERENTIATION, GENES AND CANCER
Edited by T. Kakunaga, T. Sugimura, L. Tomatis and H. Yamasaki
1988; 204 pages; £25.-

No. 93 DIRECTORY OF ON-GOING RESEARCH IN CANCER EPIDEMIOLOGY 1988
Edited by M. Coleman & J. Wahrendorf
1988; 662 pages; £26.-

IARC MONOGRAPHS ON THE EVALUATION OF THE CARCINOGENIC RISK OF CHEMICALS TO HUMANS

(English editions only)

(Available from booksellers through the network of WHO Sales Agents*)

Volume 1
Some inorganic substances, chlorinated hydrocarbons, aromatic amines, N-*nitroso compounds, and natural products*
1972; 184 pages; out of print

Volume 2
Some inorganic and organometallic compounds
1973; 181 pages; out of print

Volume 3
Certain polycyclic aromatic hydrocarbons and heterocyclic compounds
1973; 271 pages; out of print

Volume 4
Some aromatic amines, hydrazine and related substances, N-*nitroso compounds and miscellaneous alkylating agents*
1974; 286 pages;
Sw. fr. 18.-

Volume 5
Some organochlorine pesticides
1974; 241 pages; out of print

Volume 6
Sex hormones
1974; 243 pages;
out of print

Volume 7
Some anti-thyroid and related substances, nitrofurans and industrial chemicals
1974; 326 pages; out of print

Volume 8
Some aromatic azo compounds
1975; 357 pages; Sw.fr. 36.-

Volume 9
Some aziridines, N-, S- *and* O-*mustards and selenium*
1975; 268 pages; Sw. fr. 27.-

Volume 10
Some naturally occurring substances
1976; 353 pages; out of print

Volume 11
Cadmium, nickel, some epoxides, miscellaneous industrial chemicals and general considerations on volatile anaesthetics
1976; 306 pages; out of print

Volume 12
Some carbamates, thiocarbamates and carbazides
1976; 282 pages; Sw. fr. 34.-

Volume 13
Some miscellaneous pharmaceutical substances
1977; 255 pages; Sw. fr. 30.-

Volume 14
Asbestos
1977; 106 pages; out of print

Volume 15
Some fumigants, the herbicides 2,4-D and 2,4,5-T, chlorinated dibenzodioxins and miscellaneous industrial chemicals
1977; 354 pages; Sw. fr. 50.-

Volume 16
Some aromatic amines and related nitro compounds — hair dyes, colouring agents and miscellaneous industrial chemicals
1978; 400 pages; Sw. fr. 50.-

Volume 17
Some N-*nitroso compounds*
1978; 365 pages; Sw. fr. 50.

Volume 18
Polychlorinated biphenyls and polybrominated biphenyls
1978; 140 pages; Sw. fr. 20.-

Volume 19
Some monomers, plastics and synthetic elastomers, and acrolein
1979; 513 pages; Sw. fr. 60.-

Volume 20
Some halogenated hydrocarbons
1979; 609 pages; Sw. fr. 60.-

Volume 21
Sex hormones (II)
1979; 583 pages; Sw. fr. 60.-

Volume 22
Some non-nutritive sweetening agents
1980; 208 pages; Sw. fr. 25.-

Volume 23
Some metals and metallic compounds
1980; 438 pages; Sw. fr. 50.-

Volume 24
Some pharmaceutical drugs
1980; 337 pages; Sw. fr. 40.-

Volume 25
Wood, leather and some associated industries
1981; 412 pages; Sw. fr. 60.-

Volume 26
Some antineoplastic and immunosuppressive agents
1981; 411 pages; Sw. fr. 62.-

*A list of these Agents may be obtained by writing to the World Health Organization, Distribution and Sales Service, 1211 Geneva 27, Switzerland

IARC MONOGRAPHS SERIES

Volume 27
Some aromatic amines, anthraquinones and nitroso compounds, and inorganic fluorides used in drinking-water and dental preparations
1982; 341 pages; Sw. fr. 40.-

Volume 28
The rubber industry
1982; 486 pages; Sw. fr. 70.-

Volume 29
Some industrial chemicals and dyestuffs
1982; 416 pages; Sw. fr. 60.-

Volume 30
Miscellaneous pesticides
1983; 424 pages; Sw. fr. 60.-

Volume 31
Some food additives, feed additives and naturally occurring substances
1983; 14 pages; Sw. fr. 60.-

Volume 32
Polynuclear aromatic compounds, Part 1, Chemical, environmental and experimental data
1984; 477 pages; Sw. fr. 60.-

Volume 33
Polynuclear aromatic compounds, Part 2, Carbon blacks, mineral oils and some nitroarenes
1984; 245 pages; Sw. fr. 50.-

Volume 34
Polynuclear aromatic compounds, Part 3, Industrial exposures in aluminium production, coal gasification, coke production, and iron and steel founding
1984; 219 pages; Sw. fr. 48.-

Volume 35
Polynuclear aromatic compounds, Part 4, Bitumens, coal-tars and derived products, shale-oils and soots
1985; 271 pages; Sw. fr.70.-

Volume 36
Allyl compounds, aldehydes, epoxides and peroxides
1985; 369 pages; Sw. fr. 70.-

Volume 37
Tobacco habits other than smoking; betel-quid and areca-nut chewing; and some related nitrosamines
1985; 291 pages; Sw. fr. 70.-

Volume 38
Tobacco smoking
1986; 421 pages; Sw. fr. 75.-

Volume 39
Some chemicals used in plastics and elastomers
1986; 403 pages; Sw. fr. 60.-

Volume 40
Some naturally occurring and synthetic food components, furocoumarins and ultraviolet radiation
1986; 444 pages; Sw. fr. 65.-

Volume 41
Some halogenated hydrocarbons and pesticide exposures
1986; 434 pages; Sw. fr. 65.-

Volume 42
Silica and some silicates
1987; 289 pages; Sw. fr. 65.-

*Volume 43
Man-made mineral fibres and radon
1988; 300 pages; Sw. fr. 65.-

*Volume 44
Alcohol drinking
1988; 416 pages; Sw. fr. 65.-

Supplement No. 1
Chemicals and industrial processes associated with cancer in humans (IARC Monographs, Volumes 1 to 20)
1979; 71 pages; out of print

Supplement No. 2
Long-term and short-term screening assays for carcinogens: a critical appraisal
1980; 426 pages; Sw. fr. 40.-

Supplement No. 3
Cross index of synonyms and trade names in Volumes 1 to 26
1982; 199 pages; Sw. fr. 60.-

Supplement No. 4
Chemicals, industrial processes and industries associated with cancer in humans (IARC Monographs, Volumes 1 to 29)
1982; 292 pages; Sw. fr. 60.-

Supplement No. 5
Cross index of synonyms and trade names in Volumes 1 to 36
1985; 259 pages; Sw. fr. 60.-

*Supplement No. 6
Genetic and related effects: An updating of selected IARC Monographs from Volumes 1-42
1987; 730 pages; Sw. fr. 80.-

*Supplement No. 7
Overall evaluations of carcinogenicity: An updating of IARC Monographs Volumes 1-42
1987; 440 pages; Sw. fr. 65.-

*From Volume 43 onwards, the series title has been changed to IARC MONOGRAPHS ON THE EVALUATION OF CARCINOGENIC RISKS TO HUMANS

INFORMATION BULLETINS ON THE SURVEY OF CHEMICALS BEING TESTED FOR CARCINOGENICITY*

No. 8 (1979)
Edited by M.-J. Ghess, H. Bartsch & L. Tomatis
604 pages; Sw. fr. 40.-

No. 9 (1981)
Edited by M.-J. Ghess, J.D. Wilbourn, H. Bartsch & L. Tomatis
294 pages; Sw. fr. 41.-

No. 10 (1982)
Edited by M.-J. Ghess, J.D. Wilbourn & H. Bartsch
362 pages; Sw. fr. 42.-

No. 11 (1984)
Edited by M.-J. Ghess, J.D. Wilbourn, H. Vainio & H. Bartsch
362 pages; Sw. fr. 50.-

No. 12 (1986)
Edited by M.-J. Ghess, J.D. Wilbourn, A. Tossavainen & H. Vainio
385 pages; Sw. fr. 50.-

No. 13 (1988)
Edited by M.-J. Ghess, J.D. Wilbourn & A. Aitio
404 pages; Sw. fr. 43.-

NON-SERIAL PUBLICATIONS

(Available from IARC)

ALCOOL ET CANCER
By A. Tuyns (in French only)
1978; 42 pages; Fr. fr. 35.-

CANCER MORBIDITY AND CAUSES OF DEATH AMONG DANISH BREWERY WORKERS
By O.M. Jensen
1980; 143 pages; Fr. fr. 75.-

DIRECTORY OF COMPUTER SYSTEMS USED IN CANCER REGISTRIES
By H.R. Menck & D.M. Parkin
1986; 236 pages; Fr. fr. 50.-

*Available from IARC; or the World Health Organization Distribution and Sales Services, 1211 Geneva 27, Switzerland or WHO Sales Agents.

IARC Monographs are distributed by the World Health Organization, Distribution and Sales Service, 1211 Geneva 27, Switzerland and are available from booksellers through the network of WHO Sales Agents.

A list of these Agents may be obtained by writing to the above address.